# ORTHOPEDIC THERAPY of the SHOULDER

# ORTHOPEDIC THERAPY of the SHOULDER

**Martin J. Kelley,** MS, PT
President, University Sports Physical Therapy
University of Pennsylvania Sports Medicine Center
Philadelphia, Pennsylvania

**William A. Clark,** MS, PT, ATC
Senior Physical Therapist
Wyomissing Professional Clinic of Physical Therapy
Wyomissing, Pennsylvania

**with 14 contributors**

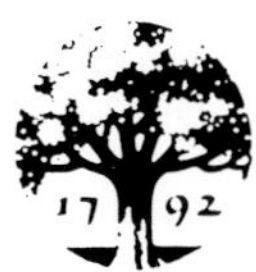


J. B. Lippincott Company
PHILADELPHIA

I dedicate my efforts on this book to my grandfather, Anthony Grennan.
May you rest in peace.

W.A.C.

Acquisitions Editor: Andrew Allen
Sponsoring Editor: Laura Dover
Production Editor: Virginia Barishek
Indexer: Max Weaver
Interior Designer: Nancy Rider
Cover Designer: Larry Pezzato
Production: Textbook Writers Associates
Compositor: Circle Graphics
Printer/Binder: Quebecor/Kingsport



6 5 4 3 2 1

**Library of Congress Cataloging-in-Publication Data**

Orthopedic therapy of the shoulder/edited by Martin J. Kelley, William A. Clark; with 14 contributors

p. cm.

Includes bibliographical references and index.

ISBN 0-307-54830-3 (alk. paper)

1. Shoulder—Wounds and injuries—Treatment. 2. Shoulder—Diseases—Treatment. 3. Shoulder—Wounds and injuries. 4. Shoulder—Diseases. I. Kelley, Martin J. II. Clark, William A. (William Anthony), 1957-

[DNLM: 1. Shoulder—injuries. 2. Shoulder—pathology. 3. Shoulder Joint—pathology. 4. Joint Diseases—rehabilitation. WE 810 077 1995]

RD557.5.068 1995

617.5′72044–dc20

DNLM/DLC

for Library of Congress 94-28214

CIP

Any procedure or practice described in this book should be applied by the health-care practitioner under appropriate supervision in accordance with professional standards of care used with regard to the unique circumstances that apply in each practice situation. Care has been taken to confirm the accuracy of information presented and to describe generally accepted practices. However, the authors, editors, and publisher cannot accept any responsibility for errors or omissions or for any consequences from application of the information in this book and make no warranty, expressed or implied, with respect to the contents of the book.

Every effort has been made to ensure drug selections and dosages are in accordance with current recommendations and practice. Because of ongoing research, changes in government regulations, and the constant flow of information on drug therapy, reactions, and interactions, the reader is cautioned to check the package insert for each drug for indications, dosages, warnings, and precautions, particularly if the drug is new or infrequently used.

∞ This paper meets the requirements of ANSI/NISO Z39.48-1992 (Permanence of Paper).

# Contributors

**Christopher A. Arrigo, M.S., P.T., A.T.C.**
Senior Physical Therapist, HEALTHSOUTH Sports Medicine and Rehabilitation Center, Birmingham, Alabama

**William A. Clark, M.S., P.T., A.T.C.**
Wyomissing Professional Clinic of Physical Therapy, Wyomissing, Pennsylvania; Adjunct Professor, Department of Physical Therapy, Beaver College, Glenside, Pennsylvania; and Adjunct Professor, Philadelphia College of Pharmacy and Science, Philadelphia, Pennsylvania

**David W. Clifton, Jr., B.S., P.T.**
President/CEO, Disability Management Associates, Lester, Pennsylvania; Senior Clinical Instructor, Hahnemann Medical School and University, Program in Physical Therapy, Philadelphia, Pennsylvania; Trustee, Foundation for Physical Therapy Research, Alexandria, Virginia

**G. Kelley Fitzgerald, M.S., P.T., O.C.S.**
Assistant Professor, Department of Orthopaedic Surgery and Rehabilitation, Program in Physical Therapy, Hahnemann University, Philadelphia, Pennsylvania

**Jill L. Frick, P.T.**
Senior Physical Therapist, Sports Medicine, Duke Medical Center, Durham, North Carolina

**Joel A. Henry, P.T., O.C.S., M.T.C.**
Director, Wyomissing Professional Clinic of Physical Therapy, Wyomissing, Pennsylvania

**Joseph P. Iannotti, M.D., Ph.D.**
Associate Professor of Orthopaedic Surgery and Chief of Shoulder Service, Department of Orthopaedic Surgery, Hospital of the University of Pennsylvania, Philadelphia, Pennsylvania

**Martin J. Kelley, M.S., P.T.**
President, University Sports Physical Therapy, University of Pennsylvania Sports Medicine Center, Philadelphia, Pennsylvania; Adjunct Professor, Department of Physical Therapy, Beaver College, Glenside, Pennsylvania

**Terry R. Malone, Ed.D., P.T., A.T.C**
Associate Professor and Director, Division of Physical Therapy, University of Kentucky, Lexington, Kentucky

**Susan L. Michlovitz, P.T., M.S.**
Director of Hand Therapy, Temple University, Philadelphia, Pennsylvania; Adjunct Associate Professor, Department of Orthopaedic Surgery and Rehabilitation, Program in Physical Therapy, Hahnemann University, Philadelphia, Pennsylvania

**Alex J. Petruska, Jr., P.T., A.T.C., S.C.S.**
Senior Physical Therapist, Charles River Sports Therapy West, Inc., Wellesley, Massachusetts

**Gwendolyn Waser Richmond, M.S., P.T.**
Staff Physical Therapist, Tuckahoe Physical Therapy, Richmond, Virginia

**Linda A. Steiner, M.S., P.T., O.C.S.**
Clinic Manager, Women's Physical Therapy Center, Raintree Hospital Rehabilitation Network, Weymouth, Massachusetts; Adjunct Instructor, MGH Institute of Health Professions, Boston, Massachusetts

**Kevin E. Wilk, P.T.**
National Director, Research and Clinical Education and Associate Clinical Director, HEALTHSOUTH Sports Medicine and Rehabilitation Center, Birmingham, Alabama; Director, Rehabilitative Research, American Sports Medicine Institute, Birmingham, Alabama

**Gerald R. Williams, M.D.**
Assistant Professor of Orthopaedic Surgery and Attending Surgeon of Shoulder Service, Department of Orthopaedic Surgery, Hospital of the University of Pennsylvania, Philadelphia, Pennsylvania

**James E. Zachazewski, M.S., P.T., S.C.S., A.T.C.**
Coordinator, Sports Physical Therapy, Physical Therapy Services, Massachusetts General Hospital, Boston, Massachusetts; Assistant Professor, Graduate Program in Physical Therapy, MGH Institute of Health Professions, Boston, Massachusetts; Adjunct Lecturer, Department of Physical Therapy, Sargent College, Boston University, Boston, Massachusetts

# Preface

Interest in the shoulder complex has recently peaked, and justifiably so, since pathology and treatment of this region are clinically consuming and challenging. Therefore, the purpose in writing this book was twofold. First, the editors wanted to provide a comprehensive text on orthopedic rehabilitation of the shoulder. Second, the editors wanted to provide an updated reference on current orthopedic principles as they relate to clinical management of shoulder dysfunction.

The first three chapters—anatomy, biomechanics, and pathology—concentrate on the basic sciences relative to the shoulder region. A thorough appreciation of these subjects provides the sound foundation necessary for successful management of shoulder disorders. Chapters 4 and 5 complement one another in an effort to clarify the decision-making process involved in proper physician diagnosis of the surgical and nonsurgical client as well as the necessary, although all too often overlooked, evaluation conducted by the rehabilitation specialist. It remains the hope of the editors that Chapter 4 helps to clarify diagnostic testing, surgical technique, and physicians' expectations of progression in rehabilitation. Likewise, Chapter 5 attempts to outline the key elements of a thorough clinical examination combined with contemporary clinical thinking.

The remaining chapters are devoted to the mechanics of rehabilitation, with Chapters 6, 7, and 8 covering the broad topics of modalities, manual therapy, and exercises. As in the preceding chapters, the editors and contributing authors strove to support clinical concepts with the most recent valid research. Two specific client profiles—the athlete and the injured worker—are given additional attention in Chapters 9 and 10. These two patient profiles often present additional challenges to the rehabilitation specialist. Chapter 11 presents four case studies in an attempt to demonstrate direct clinical application of the aforementioned concepts and principles.

The editors and contributing authors are optimistic that this text will benefit graduate students in physical therapy, occupational therapy, and sports medicine, as well as provide a comprehensive shoulder rehabilitation text for the clinical specialist treating patients with orthopedic and sports medicine–related shoulder dysfunction. Likewise, the editors and contributing authors welcome constructive feedback on this, the first edition of *Orthopedic Therapy of the Shoulder.*

*Martin J. Kelley, MS, PT*
*William A. Clark, MS, PT, ATC*

# Acknowledgments

To all those who contributed to my education, encouraging both critical and creative thinking. To my secretary, Barbara O'Connor, whose assistance was unending and always available. To my co-editor, Will Clark, for his special friendship, both personal and professional. To my wife, Ann, for patience and love beyond the imaginable. To my children, Meaghan and Madeline, who put life in perspective. Lastly, to God, for being step by step along the path.

*M.J.K.*

After 4 years of effort, there are many who deserve special recognition and heartfelt thanks. To my wife, Andrea, who sacrificed and persevered. To my co-editor, Marty Kelley, without your fortitude, knowledge, and persistence, this project would never have been completed. Being able to call you my friend and colleague is a true privilege. To the team at J.B. Lippincott Company, for your support and assistance throughout. To all the contributing authors and the illustrator for your fine work and cooperation. To Humbert (Buddy) A. Fontana, P.T., you were so instrumental in shaping and refining my clinical mind and hands, and in doing so inspired me to want to share with others what you so graciously taught me. To all those who contributed to my academic pursuits, especially Micheal Bome, P.T., and Cheryll Reigger-Krug, P.T., your teaching excellence has inspired me to reach for higher goals throughout my professional career. To my parents and family, especially my mom, who believed in my abilities and instilled in me the desire and confidence to succeed. And finally, to God, the One ultimately responsible for giving me the opportunity to be enriched by all those people mentioned above, as well as all the patients I have had the privilege of learning from.

*W.A.C.*

# Contents

# ORTHOPEDIC THERAPY
# of the
# SHOULDER

# Chapter 1

William A. Clark

# Anatomy



Martin J. Kelley and William A. Clark: ORTHOPEDIC THERAPY OF THE SHOULDER.

*Anatomy*: the dissecting of an animal or plant in order to study its structure; the science of the structure of animals or plants; the structure of an organism or body; a detailed analysis.[30] With respect to the shoulder, structure, by definition, implies an anatomic region as opposed to a single joint. Thus a discussion of shoulder anatomy requires considerable time and attention.

This chapter is divided into three sections: comparative, developmental, and descriptive anatomy. In all three sections an emphasis is placed on those points which are most pertinent to the treatment of orthopedic disorders of the shoulder region.

# Comparative Anatomy

*Comparative anatomy*, as defined by *Taber's Medical Dictionary*, is a comparison of homologous structures of different animals.[4] A study in comparative anatomy assists one in understanding and explaining the differences between animals in response to changes in the organism's environment, functional demands, and posture. In studying comparative anatomy, one traces the topographic and morphologic changes that have occurred between different forms of animal life. *Topographic changes* refer to changes in the presence of, location of, or relationship of structures. *Morphologic changes* refer to changes in the shape and size of individual structures.

Controversy exists among scholars as to the validity of individual theories regarding evolutionary changes. The lateral-fin theory and the gill-arch theory are the two most often debated theories concerned with the origin of the upper and lower extremities. The lateral-fin theory is more widely accepted and appears to be the most plausible explanation for the origin of the extremities in humans.[5]

## Lateral-Fin Theory

This theory states that the extremities began as longitudinal folds of epidermis located on the lateral aspect of the main torso of the most primitive form of sea life.[5] This pair of folds began just behind the gills and extended to the anus (Fig. 1-1a). By accentuation of the anterior and posterior portions and suppression of the intermediate portions, the pectoral and pelvic fins were differentiated (see Fig. 1-1b).

The next step in evolution marked migration of muscle tissue into the primitive folds. This development provided the folds with purposeful movement and power for locomotion. The muscle buds were arranged in a radial manner and derived innervation from the ventral roots of the adjoining spinal nerves (Fig. 1-2). At the base of the pectoral fin the peripheral nerves demonstrated a series of divisions, giving rise to a nerve plexus.[5,23] A direct relationship existed between the number of spinal nerves that contributed to the plexus and the number of myotomies present in the fin.[5]

The next significant topographic change marked the appearance of cartilaginous rays that

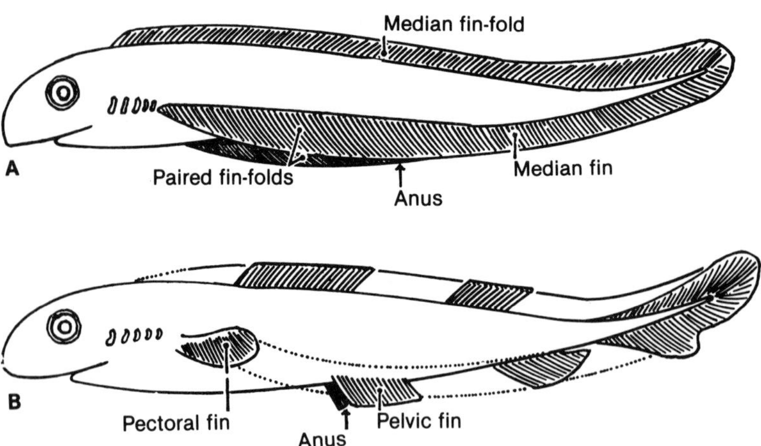


**Figure 1-1.** The lateral-fin theory states that the extremities began as (a) a pair of longitudinal folds on the lateral aspect of the main torso of the most primitive form of sea life, and then (b) by accentuation of the anterior and posterior portions and suppression of the intermediate portions, the pectoral and pelvic fins were differentiated. (After Weidersheim, in Neal HV, Rand HW. Chordate anatomy. New York: Blakiston, Div. McGraw-Hill, 1936.)

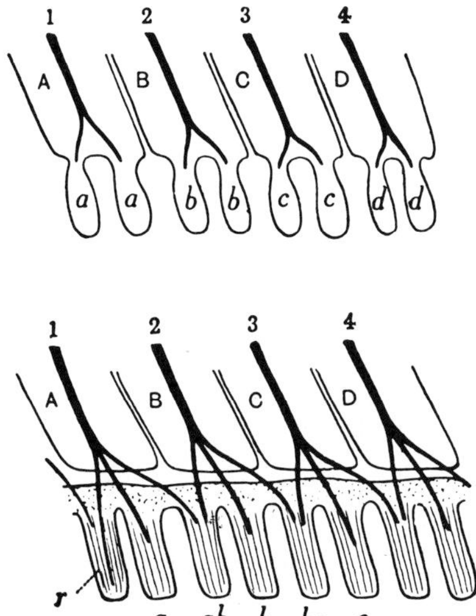


**Figure 1-2.** Formation of adult radial muscles from embryonic muscle buds, and their motor nerve supply. (*Above*) Embryonic stage with a pair of buds to each segment. (*Below*) Adult stage with radial muscles compounded of material from adjacent buds. 1–4, Four spinal nerves; A–D, four myomeres; *a–d*, muscle buds; *r*, radial muscle. (From Goodrich ES. Studies on the structure and development of vertebrates. London: Macmillan, 1930: 134.)

developed between the radial muscles. Soon after their appearance, the proximal ends of the rays concentrated and fused, forming basal cartilages, or basilia. Together these skeletal elements provided additional strength and support to the fins.

# Evolution of the Pectoral Girdle

## SEA DWELLERS

In sea-dwelling creatures, the most primitive pectoral girdle resembled an inverted arch that crossed the anterior surface of the body and extended in a posterior direction on either side of the body just above the articulation in the basilia. The girdle consisted of a ventral segment, or coracoid, and a dorsal segment, or scapula (Fig. 1-3). The point where these two joined each other formed a primitive glenoid fossa, which in turn articulated with the basal cartilages of the primitive limb.[5] The dorsal segment demonstrated an additional change through development of a suprascapula.

Prior to primitive forms of life adapting to land, a girdle of membranous bones emerged. Each half of this girdle consisted of four membranous bones: post-temporal, supracleithrum, cleithrum, and clavicle[5] (Figs. 1-4 and 1-5). Both halves of this girdle united with each other by way of a single skeletal element, the interclavicle. Prior to the presence of amphibia, the membranous girdle and the basal girdle united[5] (see Fig. 1-4).

## AMPHIBIA

When the earliest forms of life ventured from the sea to terrestrial habitat, several significant topographic and morphologic changes took place.

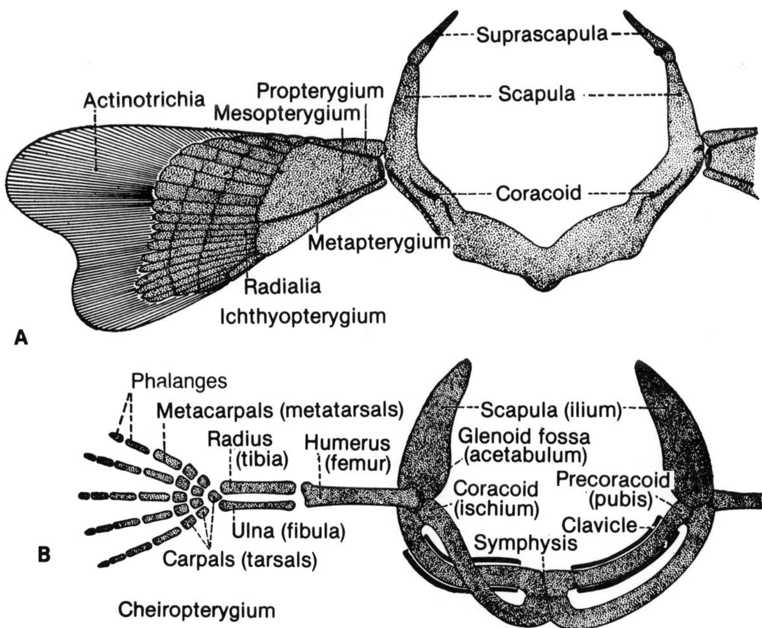


**Figure 1-3.** The functional demand for a freely movable fin necessitated the presence of an articulation. This topographic change appeared in the basilia and formed the precursor of the glenohumeral joint. (From Neal HV, Rand HW. Chordate anatomy. New York: Blakiston, Div. McGraw-Hill, 1936.)

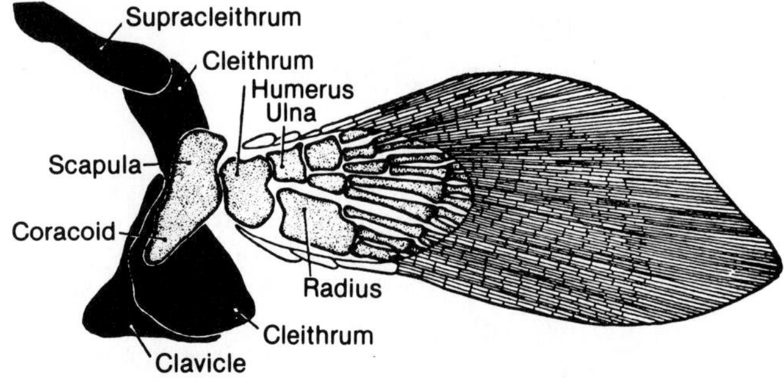


**Figure 1-4.** Prior to primitive forms adapting to land, a girdle of membranous bones emerged. Each half of this girdle consisted of four bones: posttemporal, supracleithrum, cleithrum, and clavicle. (Redrawn from Brown, in Neal HW, Rand HV. Chordate anatomy. New York: Blakiston, Div. McGraw-Hill, 1936.)

The membranous girdle decreased in size and eventually disappeared; along with this change, the skull was completely freed from all attachments to the girdle (see Fig. 1-5b–e). The cartilaginous girdle became more defined and assumed a more significant role in meeting the new functional and environmental demands.[5] In becoming more defined, the pectoral girdle of the amphibia demonstrated for the first time a tripartite structure; the coracoid, represented by the ventral bar, segmented into two structures: the anterior procoracoid, represented by the clavicle, and the posterior coracoid. The suprascapula and scapula remained essentially unaltered.[5,16]

In amphibians, the scapula was positioned close to the cervical spinal elements but freed from any attachment to the skull. The size of the scapula was massive, and the glenoid cavity was directed laterally. The articular surface, as described by Howell,[8] was screw-shaped and indicative of awkward limb movement. The limbs were positioned in a coronal plane and held horizontal to the ground.[5,8,16] This arrangement suited these forms of life for excellent locomotion in water and just barely adequate locomotion on land (consider the forelimb movements of an alligator on land compared with in water). The humerus was a massive skeletal element that appeared flattened and was considerably

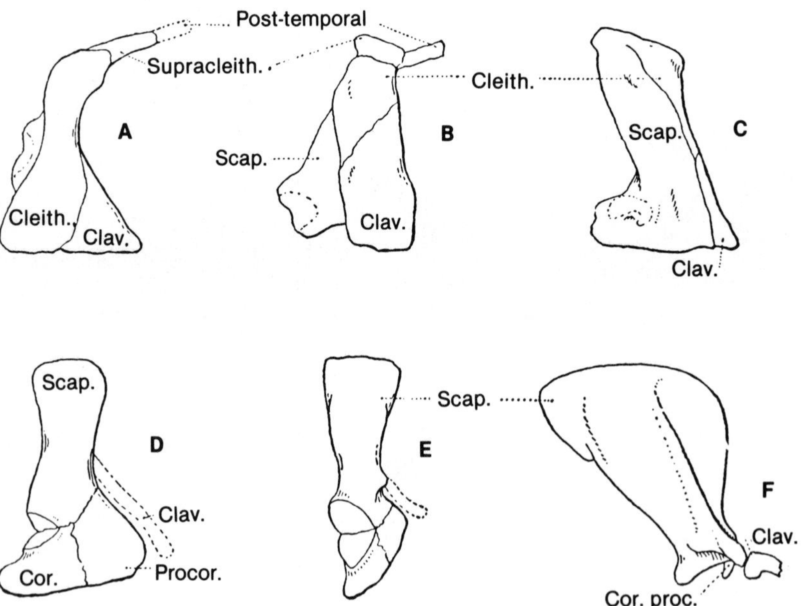


**Figure 1-5.** Phylogenesis of the pectoral girdle. (a) Sauropterus (Devonian crossopterygian lung fish). (b) Eogyrinus (Carboniferous embolomerous amphibian). (c) Eryops (Permian rhachitomous amphibian). (d) Moschops (Permian dinocephalian reptile). (e) Cynognathus (Triassic theriodont reptile). (f) Macaca (an Old-World Recent monkey). (From Howell AB. Speed in animals. Chicago: University of Chicago Press, 1944:138.)

larger at its distal end.[3,5] The increase in size of its distal end provided for the attachment of the large, powerful muscles in the forearm necessary for locomotion.

The amphibians were the first to demonstrate the basic pattern of the pentadactyl limb.[5,16] The pentadactyl limb consisted of a proximal segment linked to two middle segments, which in turn articulated with several distal elements (see Fig. 1-4). The proximal element is considered the precursor to the humerus; the two middle elements, precursors to the ulna and radius; and the distal elements, precursors to the carpals, metacarpals, and phalanges. Eventually, the principal distal skeletal element on the radial side evolved into the thumb, and the remaining four distal elements on the ulnar side evolved into the four digits. In all remaining steps in evolution up to and including human beings, this basic pattern is maintained.[5,16]

## REPTILES

During the reptilian stage, the cleithrum, a membranous bone that previously had attached the pectoral girdle to the skull, disappeared entirely[5,23] (see Fig. 1-5d–e). With this topographic change, the entire pectoral girdle migrated a considerable distance from the skull. The pectoral girdle became further defined, consisting of a scapula, a procoracoid, and a coracoid. The clavicle eventually replaced the procoracoid by a gradual reduction in the size and presence of this skeletal element (see Fig. 1-5d–e). In some reptiles, the clavicle is absent and the pectoral girdles are greatly reduced or have disappeared altogether.[5,16] In early reptilian forms, the scapula remained relatively massive in size. With later forms the scapula gradually reduced in size and the glenoid shifted from its lateral position to face in an inferior and posterior direction. With this change in the direction of the glenoid came a significant alteration in the direction of the forelimb from lateral to forward. With these changes the humerus was brought into a more forward relationship to the trunk and now was positioned beneath the body. Along with this change in position, the size of the humerus diminished, and two nodules appeared in the proximal end of the bone. These nodules developed into anterior and posterior tuberosities and formed the precursors to the greater and lesser tuberosities found in humans.[5] These adaptations assisted reptiles with weight bearing and locomotion on land.

## MAMMALS

In mammals, four main variations of the pectoral girdle are noted. Mammals adapted for running have lost their clavicle, and their scapula is relatively narrow so as to provide greater mobility. Mammals adapted for swimming also have lost their clavicle, but their scapula is wider to provide for more versatility. Mammals that fly demonstrate a large, long, well-developed clavicle with a small, narrow, curved scapula. Mammals noted for climbing or brachiating, including humans, have strong clavicles, a large coracoid, and a broad, strong scapula.[5,23] In the lowest order of mammals, the coracoid remains a large and significant skeletal structure situated between the sternum and the glenoid fossa. In higher forms, the coracoid size is significantly reduced to the point of just being a small bony projection on the anterior surface of the scapula (see Fig. 1-5f). Along with the reduction in size of the coracoid came development of the coracoid ligament. Occasionally, small masses of isolated cartilage can be found in this structure, leaving one to wonder if this original design was bone rather than ligament.[5,23] These changes in skeletal structure freed the scapula from all attachments to the axial skeleton.

When mammals assumed an upright posture, the anteroposterior dimension of the thorax diminished as a relative flattening of the thoracic cavity took place (Fig. 1-6). This adaptation placed the scapula at approximately a 45-degree

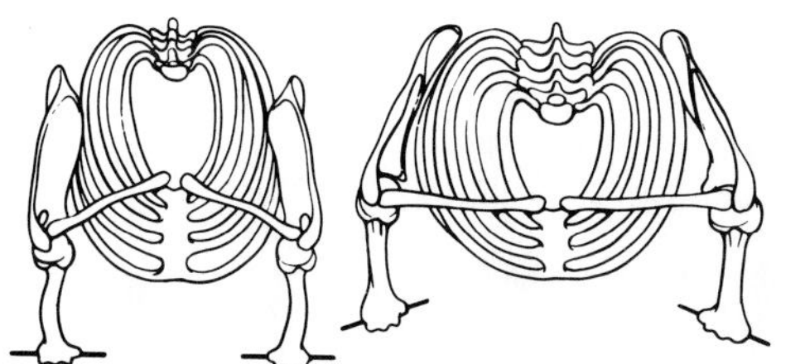

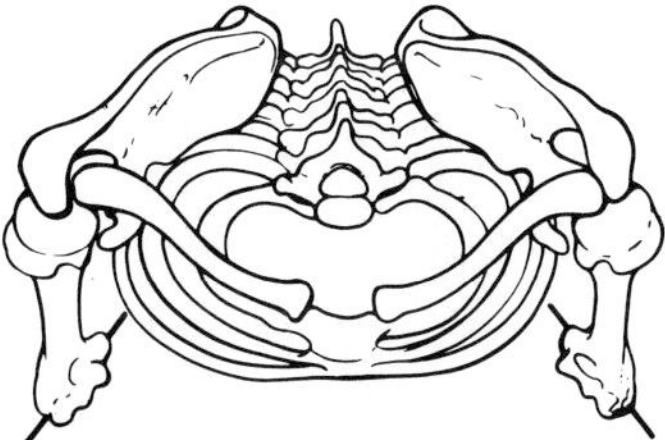

**Figure 1-6.** The anteroposterior dimension of the thoracic cage has decreased over time, with the scapula approximately 45 degrees to the midline. The scapula and the old fossa also assumed a more dorsal position in the thoracic cage. This led to the glenoid fossa being directed laterally. Consequently, a relative external rotation of humeral head and an internal rotation of the shaft occurred. (From Rockwood C, Matsen F. The shoulder, Vol. 1. Philadelphia: WB Saunders, 1990.)

angle to the midline of the torso.[5,23] This led to the glenoid fossa being directed laterally, a significant alteration in anatomy and biomechanics.

In mammals, the scapular spine appeared, the procoracoid disappeared, and the coracoid diminished in size to resemble the coracoid process found in humans. Additional morphologic changes took place in the size of the scapula in response to functional requirements and changes in posture. In pronogrades (quadripeds), where the primary function is to support a heavy frame, the body of the scapula is broad and massive. In other mammals, where the forelimb is designed for prehensile activity and the change in posture is from pronograde to orthograde (bipeds), the scapula more closely resembles that which is found in humans.

Comparisons of shape of the scapula can be drawn between different species by using a scapular index (Fig. 1-7). This index is the ratio of the breadth, measured along the scapular spine, and the length, measured from superior angle to inferior angle, of the scapula.[5,9] As life forms approach human beings, the overall size of the scapula is reduced, and the ratio of breadth to length diminishes as a result of a relative increase in breadth and decrease in length. Along with the increase in the breadth of the scapula, the dimensions of the infraspinous and supraspinous regions changed. Comparisons again can be drawn between species by using an infraspinous index, which is the ratio between the size of area above the spine and the size of area below the spine. As life forms approach human beings and the breadth of the scapula increases, both the infraspinous and supraspinous regions grow. However, the size of the infraspinous region grew to a greater extent than the size of the supraspinous region. Along with this morphologic change, the infraspinatus, teres minor, and subscapularis increased in size and power, and the direction of their force moments changed. These morphologic changes in the body of the scapula and associated musculature significantly altered the biomechanics of the shoulder and more specifically the glenohumeral joint and rotator cuff musculature. In summary, as life forms approach human beings, the scapular index progressively decreases, but the infraspinous index and the supraspinous index progressively increase.

In addition to the changes in the body of the

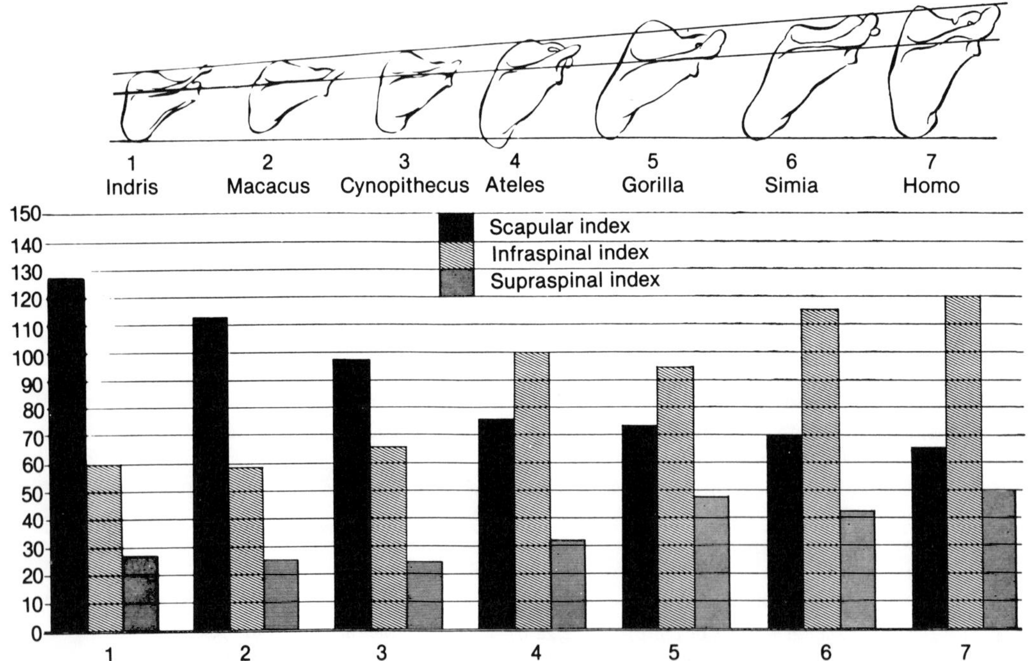


**Figure 1-7.** Progressive decrease in scapular index in successive stages from pronograde to orthgrade. (Redrawn from Inman VT, Saunders JB de C, and Abbott LC: Observations of the function of the shoulder joint. J Bone Joint Surg 1944;26:2.)

scapula, the acromion process progressively increased in size from a nearly insignificant process in a pronograde to a much larger and significant structure in an orthograde[5] (Fig. 1-8). This morphologic alteration has had profound influences on the overall power and leverage of the deltoid musculature.

Other significant changes in the humerus occurred when mammals assumed an upright posture. In mammals, whose forelimb is used primarily for weight bearing and running, the torsion angle of the humerus is approximately 90 degrees[5] (Fig. 1-9). In primates, where the posture changes to orthograde, the functional demands required the upper extremity to be capable of performing movements anterior to the body and the elbow to be maintained in a parasagittal plane. To satisfy these demands, the humeral shaft developed an increase in internal torsion.[5] In association with a change in the torsion angle of the humerus, rotation of the articular surfaces took place. The proximal end rotated internally, and the distal end rotated externally. This created a medial displacement of the tuberosities and the bicipital groove. In pronogrades, the biceps tendon passes over the center of the humeral head and is capable of performing as a primary elevator of the humerus. In contrast, in orthogrades, the biceps tendon is displaced medially, and its ability to act as a powerful elevator of the humerus is compromised.[3,5,9]

In addition to medial displacement of the tuberosities, changes were noted in their size. In pronogrades, the tuberosities are of nearly equal size. In orthogrades, there is a marked reduction in the size of the lesser tuberosity and an increase in the size of the greater tuberosity.[5,31] Once again, the relative importance of the mus-

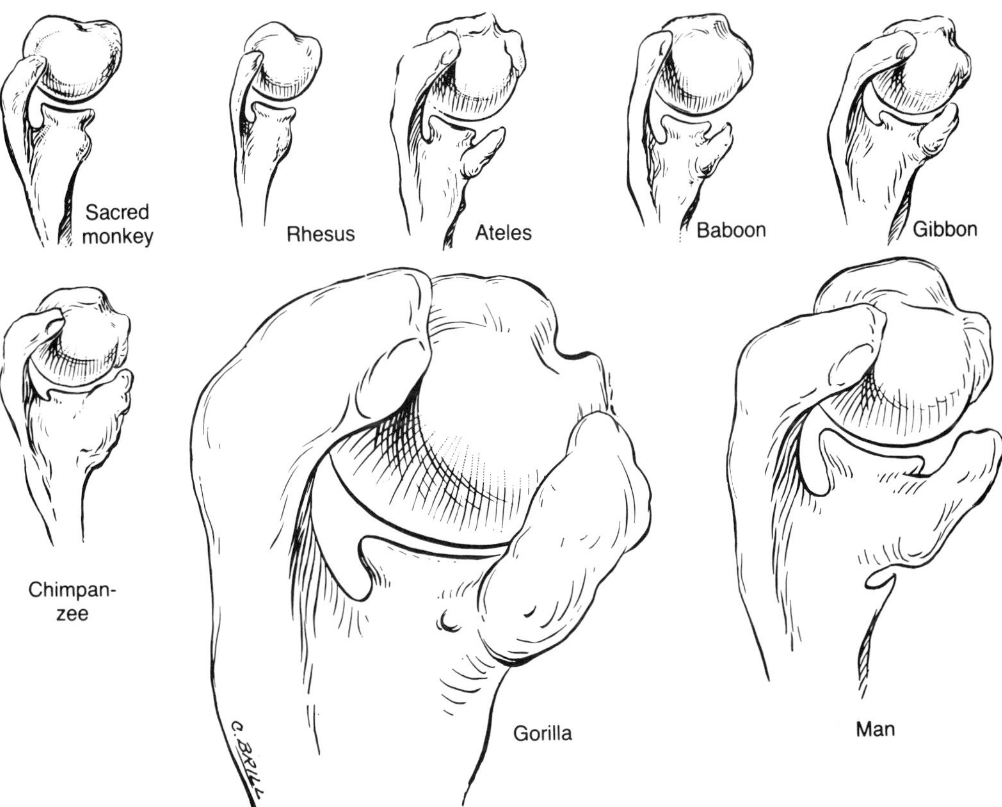


**Figure 1-8.** Gradual increase in spine of the scapula and the acromion process during development from the pronograde to the orthograde. This change reflects the increasing importance of the deltoid muscle. Also note the increase in size of the coracoid process, the inequality of the two tuberosities of the head of the humerus, and the inner displacement of the intertubercular sulcus in successive stages of development. (From Depalma AF. Surgery of the shoulder. 3rd ed. Philadelphia: JB Lippincott, 1983.)

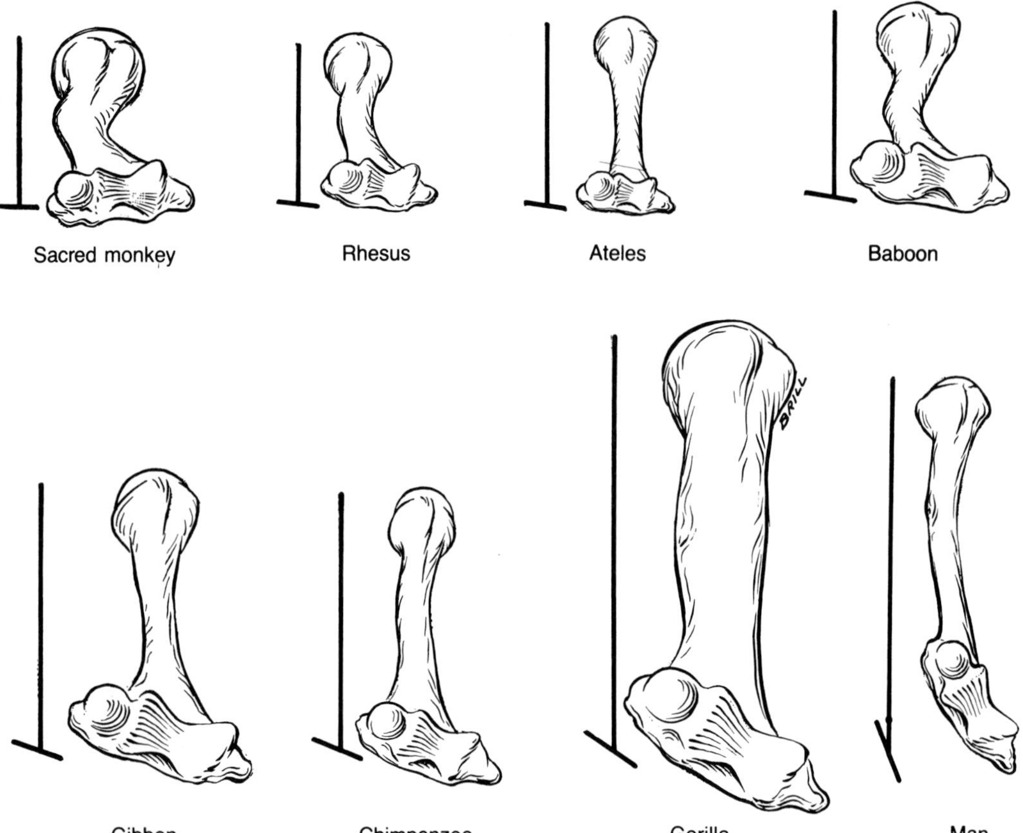


**Figure 1-9.** Progressive increase in torsion in shaft of the humerus, resulting in inward rotation of the bicipital groove. The articular surfaces at either end of the humerus rotate in opposite directions. (From Depalma AF. Surgery of the shoulder. 3rd ed. Philadelphia: JB Lippincott, 1983.)

cles of the rotator cuff is evident. With evolution, the deltoid tubercle demonstrates a progressive shift to a more distal position on the humeral shaft (Fig. 1-10). This distal migration, coupled with the significant increase in the size of the acromion process, provided this powerful muscular unit with additional leverage. All these morphologic and topographic changes demonstrate the significance of structure dictating function. Mammals who rely on their forelimbs for reaching, climbing, and prehension require powerful, well-coordinated, and synchronized neuromuscular mechanisms and force couples.

## Evolution of Upper Extremity Muscles

The muscles of the shoulder region have demonstrated significant changes in response to changes in posture and new functional demands. Preamphibian forms demonstrated primitive muscular elements that began as single sheets of tissue. Their action was limited to simple movement of the pectoral limb (fin) for locomotion in water. With the shift to amphibian forms, these single sheets of muscle tissue defined themselves more clearly into separate elements.

Inman et al.,[9] in their classical work on the shoulder, have provided the most comprehensive and detailed review of the changing role of the shoulder musculature. Their description divides the musculature into three topographic units: scapulohumeral, axiohumeral, and axioscapular.

### SCAPULOHUMERAL

As the name suggests, these are muscular units that connect the scapula to the humerus. Included in this group are the deltoid, supraspinatus, infraspinatus, teres minor, and subscapularis muscles.

The supraspinatus, infraspinatus, and subscapularis muscles developed from the same

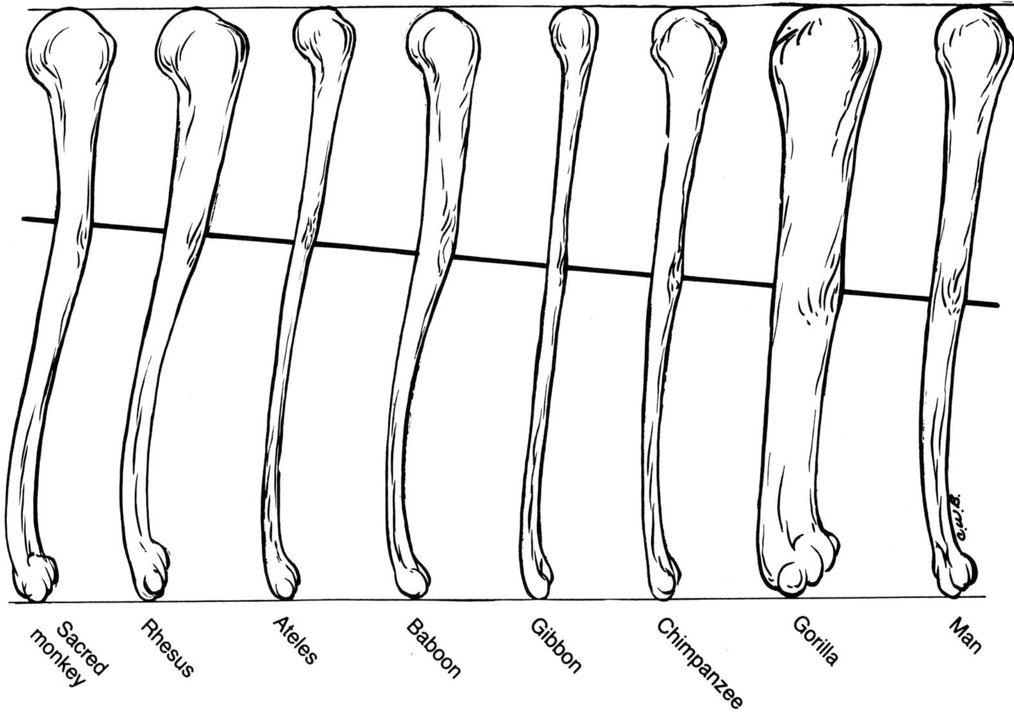


**Figure 1-10.** Deltoid insertion migrates progressively to a lower level on the shaft of the humerus, indicating the significant role played by the deltoid in higher primates. (From Depalma AF. Surgery of the shoulder. 3rd ed. Philadelphia: JB Lippincott, 1983.)

muscle sheet as the pectoral muscles. The deltoid and teres minor muscles developed from a single muscle sheet, and as the deltoid further detailed itself, the supraspinatus, infraspinatus, and subscapularis muscles began to separate themselves from the pectoral muscle group.

In later forms of terrestrial (land) existence, the forelimb freed itself from the axial skeleton, and the deltoid muscle mass increased considerably. At the same time, the relative mass of the supraspinatus decreased. In humans, the deltoid comprises 41 percent of the total mass of this group, while the supraspinatus comprises 18 percent.[5,9] The infraspinatus initially was not a distinct element. As the scapula increased in size, this muscle emerged. With the progressive increase in the infraspinous region, the size of this muscle increased. In humans it constitutes approximately 16 percent of the total mass of this group.[5,9] The subscapularis began as single muscle sheet on the anterior surface of the scapula. As the scapula elongated, the overall area of attachment and the number of fasciculi at its origin increased. In humans it comprises 20 percent of the total mass of this group.[5,9] The teres minor was the last of this group to emerge. In early mammals it cannot be distinguished separately from the deltoid. With later forms of mammalian life, the teres minor emerges as a single entity. With the progressive increase in the infraspinous region, the relative size of this muscle increased. In humans the teres minor comprises 5 percent of the total mass of this group.[5,9]

## AXIOSCAPULAR

As the name suggests, these are the muscular units that connect the scapula to the axial skeleton. Included in this group are the serratus anterior, rhomboid, levator scapula, trapezius, and sternocleidomastoid muscles.[5,9]

The serratus anterior, rhomboid, and levator scapula muscles in primitive forms functioned as a single unit to control movements of the scapula. The muscle fibers originated on the first eight or ten ribs and corresponding transverse processes of the same vertebrae and inserted into the vertebral border of the scapula. Alterations in posture and function created the separation of this primitive structure into individual elements.[5] The individual elements emerged as a result of concentration of their proximal and distal fibers and progressive reduction of their intermediate fibers. Those fibers concerned with dorsal displacement of the scapula emerged as the rhomboid muscles, those with cranial displacement became the levator scapula, and those with ventral displacement became the serratus anterior.[5,9] With change from pronograde to orthograde, the scapula displaced in a dorsal direction and the thoracic cage flattened. These alterations, along with the force of gravity, likely prompted the serratus anterior to secure the vertebral border of the scapula to the thorax.

The trapezius and sternocleidomastoid muscles emerged from a single muscle sheet connected to the membranous girdle and the primitive pectoral girdle in preamphibian forms. In amphibian forms, this muscle sheet extends from the occipital region to the torso. In later forms of terrestrial life, this muscle sheet extends from the occiput, midcervical, and thoracic regions to the spine, acromion process, and body of the scapula.[5,9] The only noteworthy changes to have occurred in this region during the evolution of primates included concentration of the proximal and distal fibers, a gradual decrease in the middle fibers, greater distinction between the two muscles, and advancement of the trapezius to the distal third of the clavicle in humans.

### AXIOHUMERAL

Although the name suggests that these units connect the humerus to the torso, subtle characteristics of the individual muscles in humans do not strictly follow what is implied. Included in this group are the pectoralis major and minor, latissimus dorsi, and teres major muscles.

The pectoral muscles emerged from a single sheet which in preamphibian forms connected the primitive coracoid to the humerus.[5,9] In later forms of reptiles and early forms of mammals, the changes in posture and the functional demands placed on the forelimb prompted displacement of part of this muscle sheet dorsally. This dorsal division gained attachment to the scapula and in later forms of mammals led to the emergence of the supraspinatus, infraspinatus, and subscapularis muscles. The remaining portion of this muscle sheet migrated from the procoracoid and the coracoid to the sternum, and the pectoralis major emerged as a distinct muscular element. The pectoralis major later demonstrated additional changes by dividing into a deep and a superficial layer. From the deep layer emerged the pectoralis minor, and in higher primates the attachment of this muscle shifted from the humerus to the coracoid process.[5,9] A division of the superficial layer migrated from the sternum to the clavicle, giving rise to a clavicular head and a sternal head.

The latissimus dorsi and teres major muscles evolved from a single sheet that extended from the main torso to the humerus. In primates, the two components became separate elements, with the teres major connecting the scapula to the humerus and the latissimus dorsi maintaining its relationship with the main torso. In humans, the latissimus dorsi often demonstrates an attachment to the inferior angle of the scapula. In higher primates, particularly those specialized in climbing, these two muscular units are unusually well developed, and their individual and total masses are significantly increased.[5,9]

### BICEPS AND TRICEPS

Both these muscles emerged from two distinct brachial sheets. From a ventral sheet emerged the biceps, and from a dorsal sheet emerged the triceps. By proximal migration along a fascial plane, these elements gained attachment to the scapula.[5,9]

In earlier forms of life, including the earliest forms of mammals, the biceps is a single muscular element that acts with the supraspinatus to position the forelimb ahead of the body.[3,5,9] In changing to an upright posture, alterations in the torsion angle of the humerus significantly reduced the ability of the biceps to perform elevation of the humerus. In primates, the biceps demonstrates two heads of origin.

The triceps, in comparison with the biceps, has demonstrated very minor changes. With evolution, the dorsal sheet further defined itself into three distinct muscle units: long head, lateral head, and medial head.[5] As one might suspect, this muscle group is more developed in primates specialized in climbing.

## Developmental Anatomy

*Developmental anatomy* is defined as embryology of the organism from the time of egg fertilization until skeletal maturity.[4] In 1901, Bardeen and Lewis[1] provided the medical community with an in-depth study of the developmental processes involved in formation of the extremities in human beings. In 1953, Gardner and Gray[6] provided additional insight into the developmental processes involved in the formation of synovial joints. These studies provide most of what is known about developmental anatomy of the shoulder.

The human embryo begins life as a mass of undifferentiated tissue. This mass of tissue divides into three germ cell layers: ectoderm, endoderm, and mesoderm. During prenatal development, the individual cells of these germ layers divide, migrate, aggregate, and differentiate in precise patterns to form the highly specialized tissues and organs of the body.

Prenatal development is divided into two periods. The *embryonic period* begins at fertilization and ends in the eighth week. The *fetal period* begins during week 8 and ends at full term. *Skeletal maturation* is defined as the point in time when the growth centers for the bones unite. This discussion of developmental anatomy of the shoulder region is outlined in a chronologic sequence beginning with the fourth week in the embryonic period and ending with skeletal maturation. Because of the numerous changes that occur during the embryonic period, the skeletal and muscular developments will be reviewed separately.

## Week 4

During the fourth week of intrauterine development, four minute swellings or buds appear on the anterolateral aspect of the embryo[1,5] (Fig. 1-11). The upper limb bud is a sac of ectoderm filled with mesoderm and constructed in such a manner that a sulcus is present on its dorsal surface and a pit on its ventral surface.[23] The base of the bud is positioned opposite to and extending from the fourth cervical to the first thoracic spinal segments. The upper limb buds appear slightly earlier than the lower ones, and they extend toward the embryo's head. The head and neck develop more rapidly than the rest of the embryo, so the four limb buds are positioned disproportionately low on the embryo's torso. The entire embryo measures approximately 4 to 5 mm in length.[5]

During week 4, the upper limb buds rapidly increase in size so that by the end week 4 the limb bud itself measures approximately 3 mm in length.[23] It is comprised of loosely organized embryonic connective tissue whose cells posses the ability to differentiate into fibroblasts, chondroblasts, and osteoblasts.

During week 4, the nerves of the brachial plexus enter the base of the limb at right angles (Fig. 1-12). The development of muscle tissue in the shoulder region first begins at 4½ weeks. At this time, premuscle masses are noted extending from the main torso toward the base of the limb bud (Fig. 1-13). At the end of week 4, there is no evidence of nerve, muscle, or skeletal elements in the limb bud, but the raw materials for these specialized structures exist within the mesenchymal cells of the limb bud.[5]

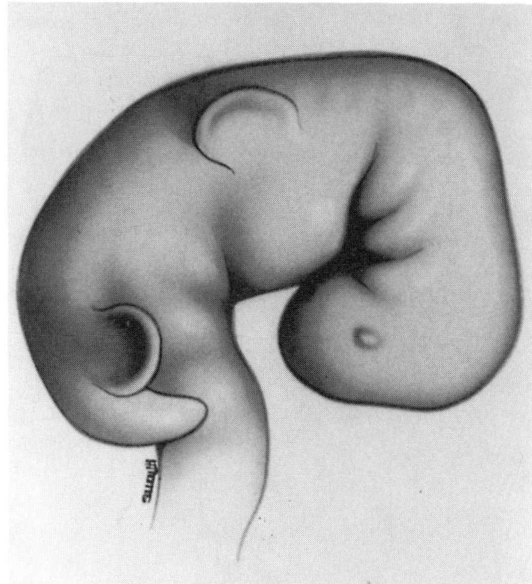

**Figure 1-11.** During the fourth week of intrauterine development, four minute swellings or buds appear on the anterolateral aspect of the embryo. The upper limb bud is a sac of ectoderm filled with mesoderm and constructed in such a manner that a sulcus is present on its dorsal surface and a pit on its ventral surface. Development of the head and neck occurs in advance of the rest of the embryo, resulting in disproportionately low positions of the upper and lower limb buds on the embryo's trunk. (From Rockwood C, Matsen F. The shoulder. Vol. 1. Philadelphia: WB Saunders, 1990.)

## Week 5

The first evidence of skeletal elements appears early in week 5.[5,23] The scapula appears at the level of the fourth and fifth cervical segments, and the clavicle appears for the first time. Some of the mesenchymal cells located centrally in the limb bud condense in a longitudinal central core referred to as the *blastema*.[5,23,31] The blastema demonstrates chondrification in its central core that rapidly expands from its caudal end to its base.[5] The blastema then differentiates into individual cartilaginous elements. Although an articulation or shoulder joint does not yet exist, a clearly discernible area can be noted between the scapula and blastema where chondrification does not occur (Fig. 1-14). This area, referred to as the *interzone*, is the first step in the formation of the glenohumeral joint. The interzone consists of three discernible layers of cells: two cartilaginous layers placed on either side of a layer of

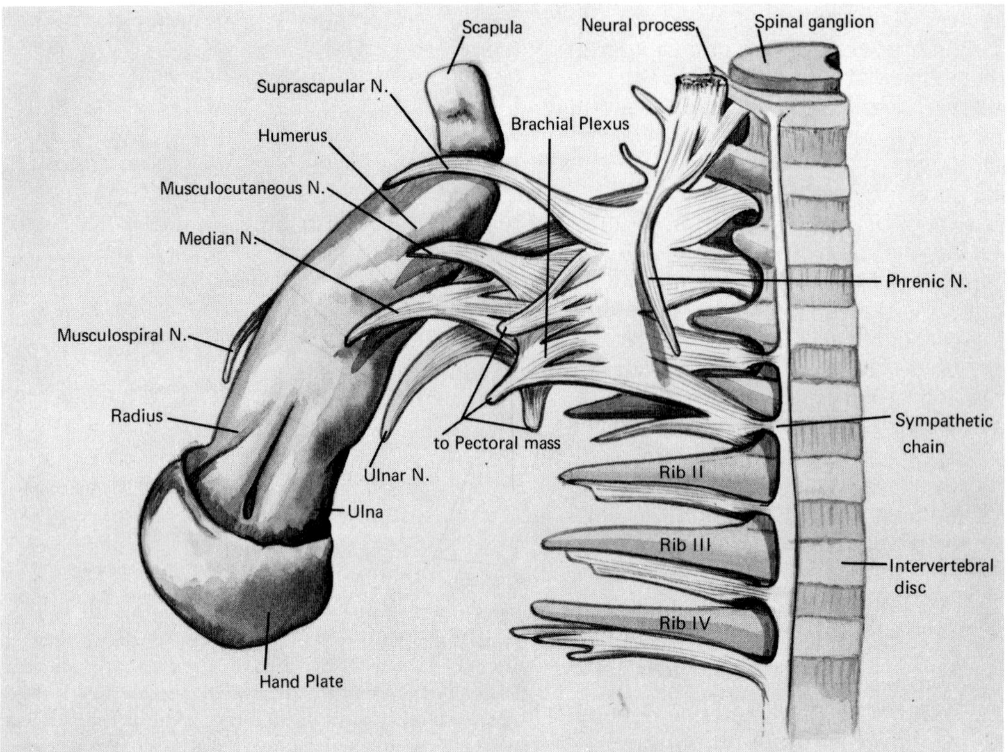


**Figure 1-12.** At 4½ weeks (embryo 9 mm). The nerves of the brachial plexus enter the base of the arm at right angles without any downward inclination. (Redrawn from Lewis WH. The development of the arm in man. Am J Anat 1901–1902;1:156.)

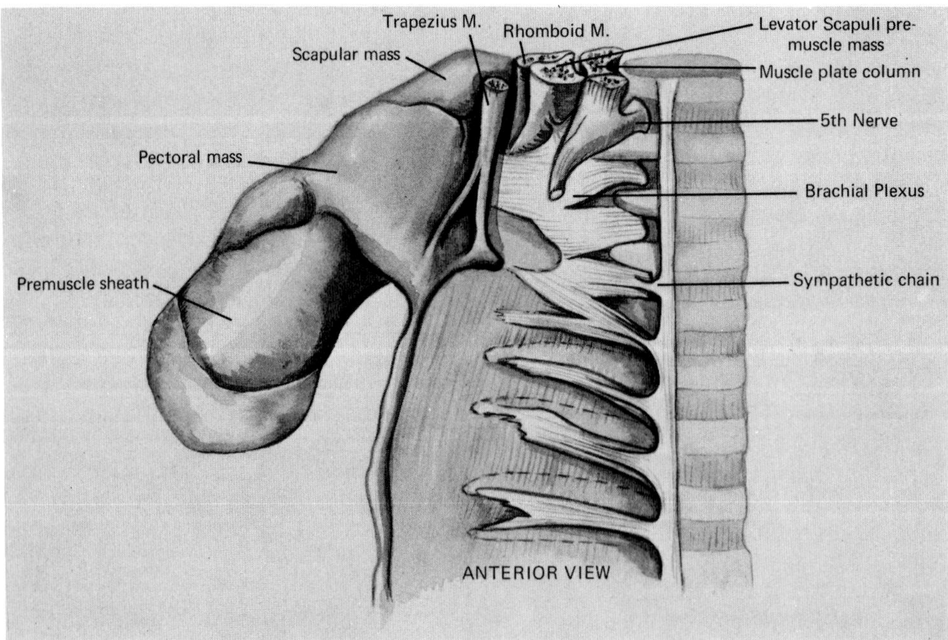


**Figure 1-13.** Same embryo as shown in Figure 1-12, ventral view. At 4½ weeks, premuscle masses are noted extending from the main torso toward the base of the limb bud. (Redrawn from Lewis WH. The development of the arm in man. Am J Anat 1901–1902;1:156.)

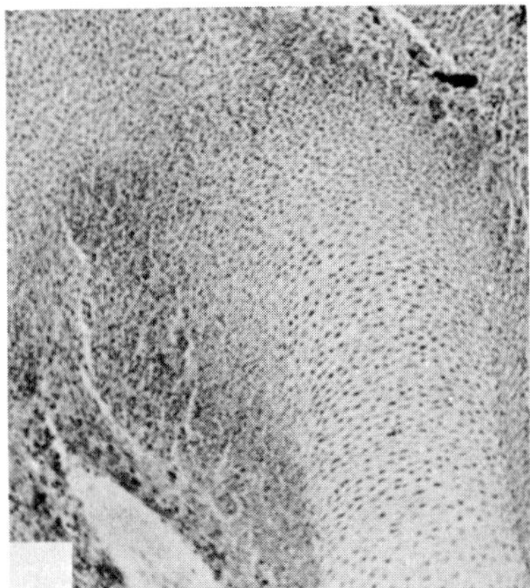

**Figure 1-14.** At approximately 5 weeks (12 mm). The central core of the humerus begins to chondrify but a homogeneous interzone remains between the scapula and the humerus. (From Gardner E, Gray DJ. Prenatal development of the human shoulder and acromioclavicular joints. Am J Anat 1953;92:219.)

loose cells. This three-layered structure is surrounded by mesenchymal tissue that later in the fetal period differentiates into the joint capsule, synovial membrane, menisci/labrum, ligaments, and bursa. The second step, the creation of a joint cavity, occurs during week 7 and will be reviewed then.[5,6] This two-step process is the same for all the joints of the shoulder region.

During week 5, numerous developments occur simultaneously in the rapidly growing limb. The outer portion of the central core differentiates into recognizable muscle masses, and nerves invade the base of the limb. This invasion of nervous tissue into the limb bud stimulates the development of limb musculature. By the end of week 5, the nervous elements have delineated themselves as individual branches of the brachial plexus. The individual peripheral nerves extend into the premuscle sheaths, which are now encircling the blastema. The development of the individual muscles occurs rapidly during week 5, and by cellular condensation, tendons are formed.[5]

## Week 6

Early in week 6, the blastema differentiates into separate skeletal elements. The humerus, ulna, and radius are clearly distinguishable and demonstrate advanced chondrification. The clavicle appears during week 6 as a condensation of tissue projecting from the acromion toward the first rib and only spanning approximately a third of this distance.[5] Soon after the emergence of the clavicle, the coracoclavicular ligaments emerge as a poorly defined mass of tissue extending from the clavicle to the coracoid process. By week 6, the scapula has enlarged and shifted to occupy a position that spans from the fourth cervical segment to the first thoracic segment. By the end of week 6, initial bone formation develops in the limb as a periosteal collar forms around the shaft of the humerus, and all the individual skeletal elements of the shoulder region are clearly delineated.[5-7] During week 6, a condensation of cells occurs around the glenoid fossa of the scapula, forming the glenoid lip (Fig. 1-15). The individual skeletal elements continue to develop unique structural characteristics (Fig. 1-16). The mesodermal cells of the limb bud rearrange themselves to form deep, intermediate, and superficial layers. This arrangement is created by a difference in the rate of growth of these tissues.[23,31] The difference in growth rates also stimulates bending of the upper limb at the elbow. In association with bending of the limb bud, the muscles, by virtue of their position, divide into dorsal extensors and ventral flexors.

## Week 7

Early in week 7 the limbs extend in a ventral direction and the limb buds rotate in opposite directions. The upper limbs rotate laterally along their longitudinal axes approximately 90 degrees such that the elbow faces posteriorly and the extensor muscles face posteriorly and laterally.[23]

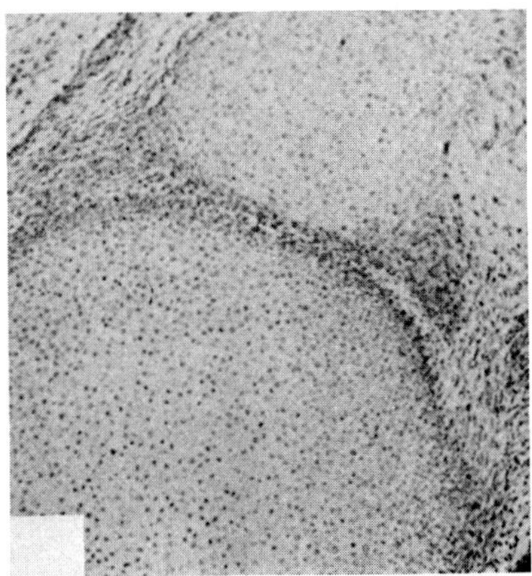

**Figure 1-15.** Three layered interzone at 21 mm (approximately 6 weeks). Note the condensation around the glenoid to form the glenoid lip; the interzone assumes a three-layered configuration. (From Gardner E, Gray DJ. Prenatal development of the human shoulder and acromioclavicular joints. Am J Anat 1953;92:219.)

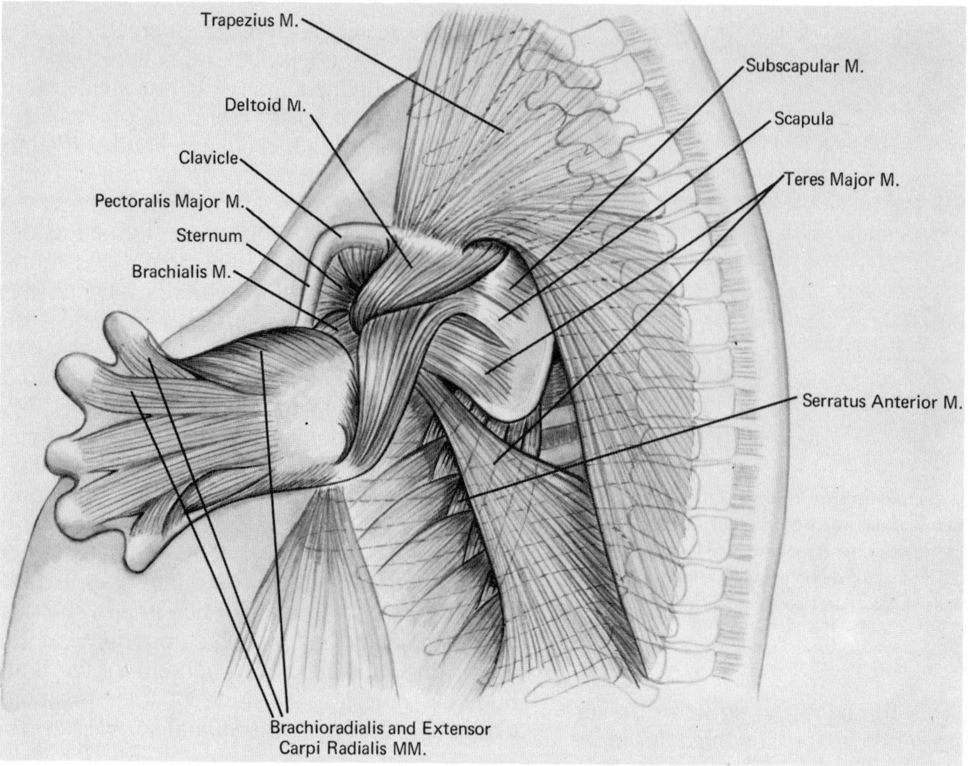


**Figure 1-16.** At 6½ to 7 weeks (embryo 14 mm). The trapezius has descended and gained attachment to the clavicle and the scapula; it extends from the occiput to the fifth rib. (Redrawn from Lewis WH. The development of the arm in man. Am J Anat 1901–1902;1:184.)

During week 7, chondrification of the humerus and scapula occurs at a rapid pace, and the humeral head appears[5] (Fig. 1-17). The head becomes more defined and rapidly increases in size. By the end of week 7, the humeral head demonstrates a characteristic rounded shape, bony prominences are noticeable, indicating development of the greater and lesser tubercles, and the outline of the humeral head is clearly delineating itself from the shaft of the humerus by formation of the anatomic and surgical neck. The scapula rapidly increases in size, and the acromion, spine, and coracoid process define themselves. The clavicle now extends its full length, and its medial end blends with the first rib and sternum.

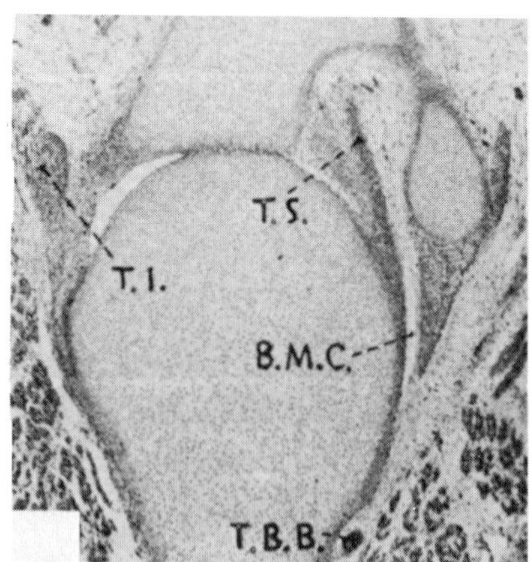


**Figure 1-17.** At approximately 7 weeks (27 mm). The joint is well formed; the humeral head is spherical and is delineated from the shaft of the humerus. The scapula shows advanced chondrification. The tendons of the infraspinatus (T.I.), subscapularis (T.S.), and the biceps (T.B.B.) are clearly seen, as is the bursa of the coracobrachialis muscle (B.M.C.). (From Gardner E, Gray DJ. Prenatal development of the human shoulder and acromioclavicular joints. Am J Anat 1953;92:219.)

During week 7, the second step in the formation of the glenohumeral joint takes place. There is an invasion of vascular tissue into the surrounding mesenchymal tissue and the middle layer of cells in the interzone. Enzymes leaking from the blood vessels are specific to destruction of the loose layer of cells, creating, in essence, a cavity.[5,6] By being highly specific, these enzymes do not damage the two layers of cartilaginous cells or the surrounding mesenchymal tissue and its supportive elements. With proliferation and condensation, the mesenchymal cells outline the fibrous capsule and most of the ligaments, including the three glenohumeral ligaments. The middle layer of the interzone continues to lose its cellular density by enzyme activity. A cavity or true joint space is formed and is lined by a synovial membrane.[5,6]

At this point in time the scapula has descended to a position where it lies between the first and fifth intercostal spaces. With descent of the scapula, the muscles attached to it elongate and the brachial plexus demonstrates a definite downward inclination (Fig. 1-18).

## Week 8

By week 8, the scapula has descended further such that only a small portion of it lies above the first intercostal space, and the inferior angle is positioned over the fifth intercostal space. Now the brachial plexus demonstrates a pronounced downward inclination and is stretched over the first rib. At this point in time, the ribs are on the same plane as the vertebrae from which they originate. At a later point in time, the rib cage descends obliquely downward, and with this the scapula demonstrates a final few degrees of descent.[5]

By the end of the embryonic period, the entire shoulder region is formed. The human embryo measures approximately 23 mm in length, and the upper limbs extend so that the hands are stretched and the forearms are pronated (Fig. 1-19). The musculoskeletal and neuromuscular structures resemble in all characteristics the adult shoulder.

## Embryologic Development of Muscle

The embryologic development of the muscles of the shoulder region is outlined separately because their progression is more easily understood as an evolution from premuscle sheets to well-defined structures. Muscles most closely associated with the trunk develop first, followed by those which connect the arm to the trunk, and finally those of the forearm and hand. The invasion of nerve tissue into these masses stimulates and directs the development of the individual muscles.

By the fifth week, five premuscle masses are discernible: the trapezius and sternocleidomas-

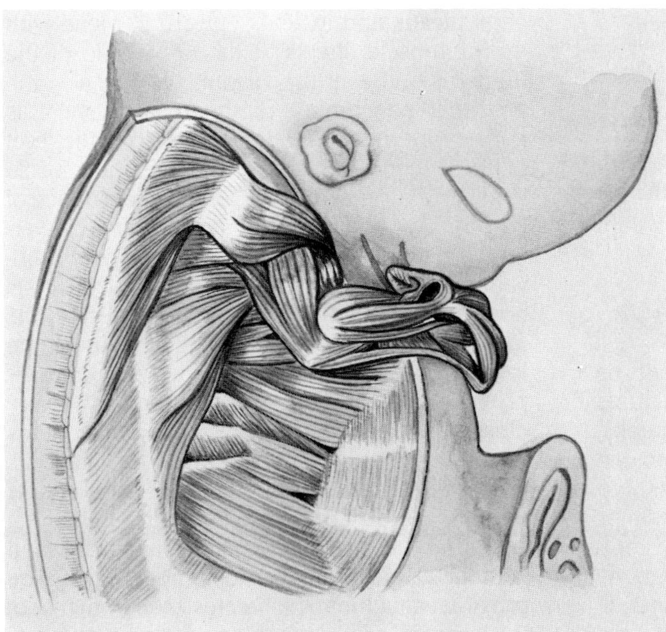

**Figure 1-18.** At the end of the 7th week (embryo 20 mm). The greater part of the scapula lies below the level of the first rib and the arm assumes a downward inclination, pulling the brachial plexus downward. (Redrawn from Bardeen CR, Lewis WH. Am J Anat 1901;1:1.)

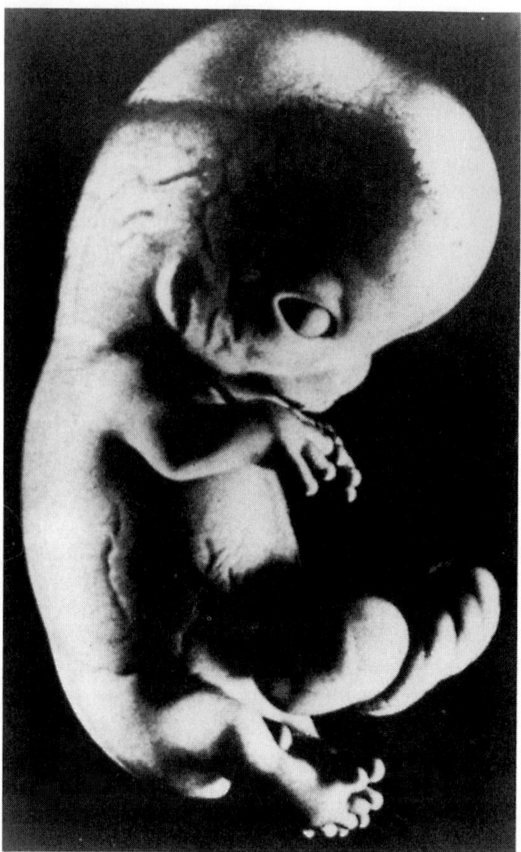

**Figure 1-19.** At the eighth week of gestation the embryo is about 23 mm long. Through growth of the upper limb, the hands are stretched with the arms pronated. The firm musculature is now clearly defined. (From Rockwood C, Matsen F. The shoulder. Vol. 1. Philadelphia: WB Saunders, 1990.)

toid, the levator scapula and serratus anterior, the latissimus dorsi and teres major, the pectoralis major and minor, and the rhomboid major and minor.

## TRAPEZIUS AND STERNOCLEIDOMASTOID

The premuscle sheet of this group presents as a single sheet arising from a position high up near the cranium and cervical region. At 5½ weeks, it is positioned directly opposite the first four cervical segments.[5] The sheet quickly divides into a dorsal and ventral portion. From the dorsal portion evolves the trapezius, and from the ventral portion evolves the sternocleidomastoid. At 6 weeks, the spinal accessory nerve invades this structure. The dorsal sheet then migrates distally and extends caudally. By week 7, the distal end of the trapezius is level with the fifth thoracic vertebrae and has attached itself to the scapula and clavicle. The ventral portion also migrates caudally and extends ventrally so that at 7 weeks the sternocleidomastoid has attached itself to the sternum and the clavicle. As these muscle sheets extend in a caudal direction, the accessory nerve is pulled in a downward direction. By week 8, the distal end of the trapezius is level with the sixth thoracic vertebrae.

## LEVATOR SCAPULAE AND SERRATUS ANTERIOR

The premuscle sheet of this group, discernible at 5½ weeks, arises in the upper cervical region, and by week 6 it extends from the first cervical vertebrae to the ninth rib. The mass is invaded by nerves from the second through seventh cervical vertebrae. The mass demonstrates advanced differentiation, but as yet it does not demonstrate any attachment to the scapula. During week 7, the serratus anterior distinguishes itself as a thin sheet extending from the dorsal border of the scapula to the first nine ribs. By week 8, the muscle mass separates into two individual muscles in all areas of attachment, with the exception of the superior angle of the scapula, where it remains a united structure.[5]

## LATISSIMUS DORSI AND TERES MAJOR

These two muscles evolve from a single sheet discernible at 5 weeks. It lies dorsal to the brachial plexus and extends upward to blend with the premuscle sheets at the upper end of the humerus and over the scapula. At 6 weeks, the proximal attachment of the muscle sheet is joined with the sternocleidomastoid at the level of the second cervical vertebrae. The muscle sheet extends distally along the lateral surface of the embryo as far as the second thoracic vertebrae. During week 6, the muscle sheet is invaded by nerve tissue. By week 7, the latissimus dorsi presents as a broad, thin sheet that has migrated distally and gained attachment to the lower thoracic and upper lumbar vertebrae. Its proximal attachment is to the humerus in very close connection with the teres major. The teres major occupies a position that is identical to its position in the adult shoulder.[5] By the end of week 8, the distal fibers of the latissimus dorsi extend to the ninth intercostal space and blend with the fascia of the thoracolumbar region. The proximal attachment separates itself from that of the teres major and twists on itself prior to insertion on the humerus. As these muscles migrate distally and laterally, they pull their individual nerve branches with them.

## PECTORALIS MAJOR AND MINOR

The pectoral premuscle mass is discernible by week 5. This sheet is positioned directly opposite the premuscle sheet of the latissimus dorsi. It lies anterior to the brachial plexus and blends with the sheet of the upper end of the humerus.[5] By week 6, the pectoral mass extends from the second intercostal region and the clavicle to the upper end of the humerus. At this time the bulk of the pectoral mass lies above the level of the first rib. The portion of this mass destined to become the pectoralis minor projects toward the coracoid process. Before the end of week 6, nerve tissue invades this muscle sheet from the fifth, sixth, and seventh cervical nerves. During week 7, the premuscle sheet divides into two individual muscles. The pectoralis minor, now a distinct structure, lies deep to the pectoralis major and extends from the second through the fourth ribs to the coracoid process. The pectoralis major is well defined, and its sternal and clavicular portions are clearly distinguishable from each other. The fibers of these two heads blend with one another to extend toward the humerus, where they attach by a single tendon (Fig. 1-20).

## RHOMBOID MAJOR AND MINOR

The muscle mass of the rhomboids presents at 5½ weeks. At this point in time, the premuscle sheet is level with the fifth cervical vertebrae and is subsequently invaded by nerve tissue from this level.[5] With distal migration of the scapula, this sheet extends downward so that by week 7 it lies opposite the sixth cervical vertebrae. By week 8, it extends from the seventh to the fourth thoracic vertebrae. This sheet then separates into major and minor masses. By the end of week 8, the muscles demonstrate firm attachment to the scapula.

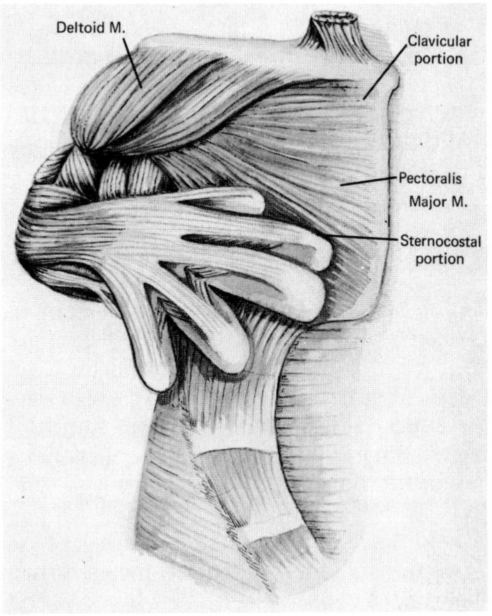


**Figure 1-20.** At 7 weeks (embryo 20 mm). The pectoral mass has divided into its clavicular and sternocostal portions. (Redrawn from Bardeen CR, Lewis WH. Am J Anat 1901;1:1.)

## DELTOID AND ROTATOR CUFF

At approximately 5½ weeks, the proximal aspect of the limb bud differentiates itself from a bulging mass of mesenchymal tissue to a more clearly defined mass of premuscle tissue. This premuscle sheet clearly distinguishes itself from the aforementioned muscles of the shoulder region, but the ability to discern between the individual muscles of this group is not possible.[5] Initially, the deltoid presents as a large mass of tissue extending from the acromion process and clavicle to the humerus. It lies over and intimately blends with the premuscle sheet of the rotator cuff. At this point in time, the premuscle tissue lying distal to the acromion cannot be separated, whereas the premuscle tissue lying proximal to the acromion are easily distinguishable. The deltoid clearly arises from the acromion; the supraspinatus, from the upper medial surface of the scapula; the infraspinatus, from the dorsal and lateral surfaces of the scapula; and the subscapularis, from the ventral and medial surfaces of the scapula. The insertion of the subscapularis onto the humerus lies very close to the insertion of the teres major, and it is difficult to separate them. A clear distinction between the deltoid and teres minor is not possible either.[5]

By week 6, the axillary nerve invades the deltoid muscle sheet and sends a separate branch to its lower portion. This branch passes between the subscapularis and teres major and pierces the premuscle tissue at a point that will later distinguish itself as the teres minor. The suprascapular nerve invades the supraspinatus and infraspinatus muscles, and the upper and lower subscapular nerves invade the subscapularis muscle.[5]

By week 7, the shape and physical characteristics of the deltoid, supraspinatus, infraspinatus, and subscapularis muscles are identical to those of the adult (Fig. 1-21). Although the deltoid and teres minor muscles still share a very close relationship, they have clearly separated themselves from one another.[5] In a similar way, the insertions of the subscapularis and teres major muscles are clearly separated. By the end of week 8, all the muscles of this group have evolved to the point

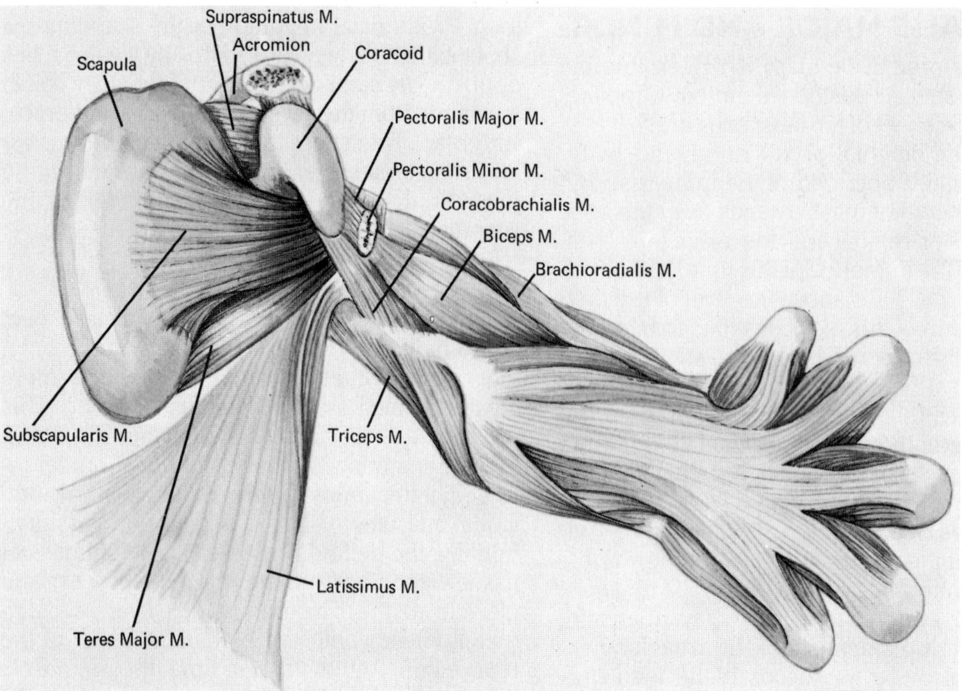


**Figure 1-21.** At 7 weeks (embryo 20 mm). The triceps has elongated and its heads are distinguishable. The biceps has also elongated, and its two heads are separating; the short head is closely associated with the coracobrachialis. (Redrawn from Lewis WH. The development of the arm in man. Am J Anat 1901–1902;1:145.)

where they are nearly identical in physical characteristics to those of the adult shoulder.

## BICEPS, CORACOBRACHIALIS, AND TRICEPS

At approximately 5½ weeks, the undifferentiated tissue that surrounds the blastema of the upper limb is invaded by terminal branches of the brachial plexus and blood vessels.[5] By the beginning of week 6, the biceps and coracobrachialis are recognizable and are noted to extend from the coracoid process to the humerus and radius. At this point, the two heads of the biceps remain very closely united. During week 6, the base of the coracoid process and the long head of the biceps migrate from each other. The long head, at its point of origin, forms the supraglenoid tubercle. The short head remains attached to the tip of the coracoid process in close association with the coracobrachialis. By week 7, the biceps clearly demonstrates two heads of origin, and they are distancing themselves from one another. At the end of the embryonic period, the long head of the biceps arises from the supraglenoid tubercle, passes through the glenohumeral joint space, lies in the intertubercular groove, and is covered by the transverse humeral ligament.

During week 6, the triceps begins to appear on the posterolateral surface of the humerus, extending from the scapula to the ulna. The muscle is invaded by the radial nerve, and all three heads are recognizable, although they are not clearly separated from one another. By week 7, the triceps elongates, and its three heads begin to separate into a lateral, medial, and long head. By the end of the embryonic period, all three heads are now well developed, and they converge distally with the anconeus muscle to form a common tendon of insertion on the ulna.

# Fetal Period

At the end of the embryonic period, the components of the shoulder region are adult in configuration but miniature in size.[5] During the fetal period, these structures continue to grow in size. With respect to the shoulder region, the most significant changes occur in the collagenous tissues of the bones, ligaments, cartilage, and tendons.

Early in the fetal period, the epiphyses of the bones of the shoulder region are invaded by a fine network of blood vessels.[5] The tendons and ligaments also demonstrate an increase in vascularization. This increase in vascularity is the primary stimulus for additional growth and provides the nutrients necessary for skeletal maturation. As the length of the bones increases, the overall size of the fetus increases, and the soft tissues, namely, tendons, muscles, nerves, and ligaments, are forced to lengthen. In addition to changes in length, movements of the fetus provide an additional stimulus for increases in the size and strength of the musculoskeletal structures. During the transition from embryo to fetus, migration of the numerous muscle masses takes place. With this lengthening process, several important soft-tissue structures in the shoulder region mature. These include the articular synovial capsule, the three glenohumeral ligaments, the glenoid labrum, and the bursa.

## ARTICULAR SYNOVIAL JOINT CAPSULE

The synovial joints of the shoulder region demonstrate significant development and growth during the fetal period. The cavities that have already formed increase in size, and associated growth occurs in the synovial capsule. The superior part of the capsule is anchored along the articular hyaline cartilage of the humeral head, while the inferior part is attached to the neck of the humerus. The inferior part is attached so low down on the neck of the humerus that a part of the metaphysis of the humerus is intracapsular. On the internal surface, the synovial lining demonstrates active proliferation. On its external surface, the fibrous elements proliferate as well, and within the substance of the anterior capsule, the glenohumeral ligaments develop.

## GLENOHUMERAL LIGAMENTS

During the fetal period, the glenohumeral ligaments develop as fibrous thickenings within the collagenous structure of the anterior capsule. The relationship of the ligaments to the capsule and the subscapularis bursa is established during the fetal period (Fig. 1-22). However, like the adult, the size, shape, number, and location of the ligaments demonstrate considerable variation.[5] By the end of the fetal period, the glenohumeral ligaments as well as all the other ligaments of the shoulder region resemble those of the adult shoulder in form and sites of attachment.

## GLENOID LABRUM

Early in the fetal period, the lip of the glenoid fossa assumes a triangular appearance, and fibrous elements increase in number and thickness.[5] Soon after the glenoid lip matures, a transitional zone of fibrocartilage appears between the lip of the glenoid and the hyaline cartilage of the fossa (Fig. 1-23). This area continues to mature so that at full term a dense area of fibrocartilage and elastic cartilage is present on the entire surface of the glenoid lip.

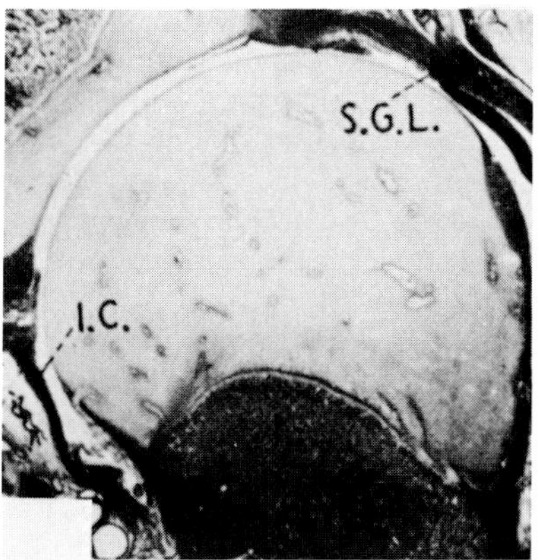


**Figure 1-22.** A fetus 348 mm (at term). The superior glenohumeral ligament (S.G.L.) and the inferior capsule (I.C.) are clearly seen. (From Gardner E, Gray DJ. Prenatal development of the human shoulder and acromioclavicular joints. Am J Anat 1953;92:219.)

## BURSAE

The bursae of the shoulder region are either present prior to or begin developing at the start of the fetal period.[5] The subdeltoid bursa begins as a small space between the undersurface of the deltoid and the outermost surface of the rotator cuff. By full term, this structure is well defined and has markedly increased in size such that it extends throughout the subacromial region, cov-

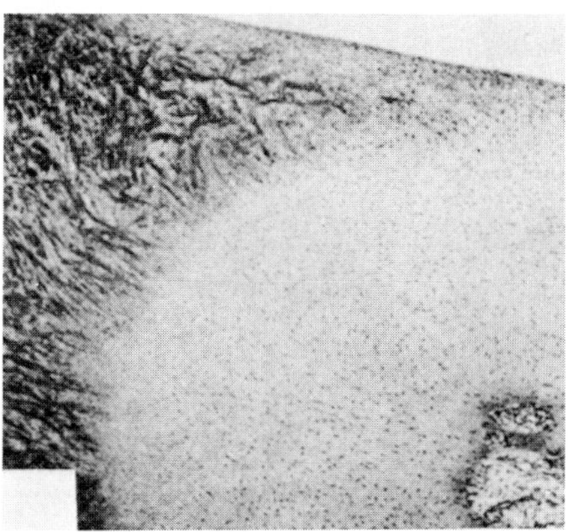

**Figure 1-23.** A fetus 366 mm (at term). The labrum, a dense fibrous structure, is clearly delineated from the hyaline cartilage. The area next to the scapula consists of cellular elements suggesting fibrocartilage. (From Gardner E, Gray DJ. Prenatal development of the human shoulder and acromioclavicular joints. Am J Anat 1953;92:219.)

ering the entire external surface of the rotator cuff and the entire undersurface of the deltoid.[5] The subcoracoid bursa, an extension of the subdeltoid, usually develops later during the fetal period. By full term, this bursa is always fully developed and often demonstrates an open communication with the glenohumeral joint through an opening in the synovial capsule.

The subscapular bursa develops during the fetal period and, like the subcoracoid bursa, usually demonstrates an open communication with the synovial capsule of the glenohumeral joint. The area where the subscapular bursa and the anterior capsule communicate is referred to as the *subscapular recess*. In the adult shoulder, the location and presence of the subscapular recess, the subscapular bursa, and its relationship with the glenohumeral ligaments demonstrate considerable variation.[5] By full term, these structures and their relationships are clearly defined.

# Postnatal Development

After birth, the soft-tissue structures of the shoulder region do not reveal any significant changes other than an increase in size and strength and ultimately achieving their respective adult proportions.[5] Postnatal development of the shoulder region is earmarked by significant changes in the skeletal elements. These changes include, first, the appearance of ossification centers and, then later, fusion of these centers.

## HUMERUS

The humerus develops from seven and occasionally eight centers of ossification: one center for the shaft, one for the humeral head, one for each tuberosity, one for the head of the radius, one for the trochlear portion of the articular surface of the elbow, and one for each condyle.[7] The nucleus for the shaft appears near the center of the shaft during week 8 and extends toward the extremities. At full term, the shaft demonstrates nearly full ossification through its entire length. Ossification of the humeral head is accomplished by three centers, one for the humeral head and one for each tuberosity (Fig. 1-24). In some rare instances, an isolated, ovoid-shaped nucleus of ossification for the humeral head is noted at birth. More often this nucleus appears between 4 and 6 months of age.[5] On occasion, a single center appears for both tuberosities, but more often than not,[7] a separate center for the greater tuberosity appears during the third year, and a smaller center for the lesser tuberosity appears during the fifth year. The two ossification centers for the tuberosities usually fuse with one another during the fifth or sixth year, and they

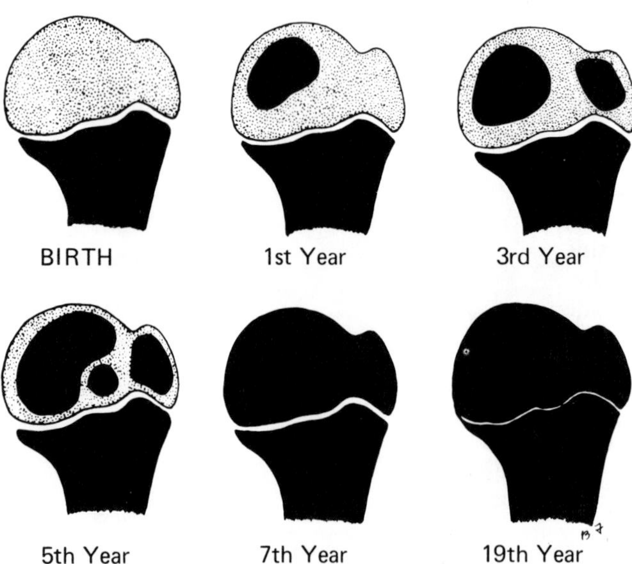


**Figure 1-24.** Ossification of the upper epiphysis is accomplished by three centers: one for the head, which appears between the fourth and sixth months; one for the greater tuberosity, appearing usually during the third year; and one for the lesser tuberosity, appearing about the fifth year. The epiphyses of the tuberosities fuse into one mass at about the fifth year, and this, in turn, unites with the epiphysis of the head about the seventh year. The head and the shaft of the humerus unite at about the nineteenth year. (From Depalma AF. Surgery of the shoulder. 3rd ed. Philadelphia: JB Lippincott, 1983.)

usually unite with the center for the humeral head by the beginning of the seventh year.[5] However, the union of the tuberosities with the humeral head may not take place until 14 years of age. The union of the humeral head with the shaft of the humerus usually occurs during the nineteenth year. Because of this timetable, radiographic diagnosis of injuries to the upper end of the humerus at birth, during childhood, and in early adolescence can be difficult.

## SCAPULA

The scapula develops from seven or more centers, one for the body, two for the coracoid process, two or three for the acromion process, one for the vertebral border, and one for the inferior angle[7] (Fig. 1-25). Ossification of the body of the scapula occurs during the second month of fetal life. Initially, it presents as an irregular quadrilateral plate lying immediately behind the glenoid cavity. This plate extends to form the chief part of the scapula. The spine emerges from its posterior surface during the third month of fetal life.

At birth, a large part of the scapula is osseous; however, the coracoid process, inferior angle, acromion process, glenoid cavity, and posterior border are cartilaginous[7] (see Fig. 1-25a). The vertebral border and inferior angle each have a single center of ossification that usually appears at the time of puberty and fuses by the twenty-second year (see Fig. 1-25b). The two processes and the glenoid fossa are outlined further.

The formation of the acromion process occurs in at least two ways. First, the base of the acromion is formed in part by an extension of the center of ossification for the spine. Second, two or three centers in the body of the process appear during puberty and usually fuse by 22 years of age. These then unite with one another, and then all three or more centers unite with the base.[5] Occasionally, the centers fail to unite and may be mistaken on x-ray for a fracture (see Fig. 1-25c). Recently, nonfusion of the extremity of the acromion has been implicated as a possible source of painful impingement.[15,23]

The coracoid process has three centers of ossification, one in the center, one at the base, and one at the tip. The one in the center of the process appears during the first year. The one at the base appears during the tenth year and contributes to the formation of the upper portion of the glenoid fossa (see Fig. 1-25b). The one at the tip usually appears during puberty. This center is initially wafer-like in shape, and occasionally it fails to fuse with the rest of the process.[5] At 15 years of age, the centers of the process fuse with the body of the scapula.

The glenoid cavity forms from two separate centers of ossification, one for the upper one-third and one for the lower two-thirds (see Fig. 1-25b). The first center appears during the tenth

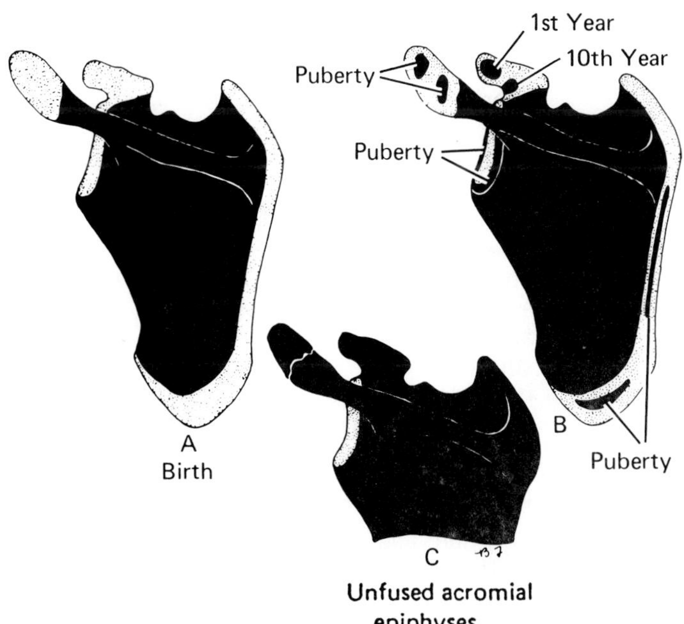


**Figure 1-25.** Date of appearance of the ossification centers of scapula, coracoid, acromion, and glenoid fossa. (From Depalma AF. Surgery of the shoulder. 3rd ed. Philadelphia: JB Lippincott, 1983.)

year and contributes to formation of the superior margin of the glenoid fossa and base of the coracoid process.[5] Fusion between this center and the scapula usually occurs during the fifteenth year. The second center appears during puberty and contributes to formation of the inferior margins of the glenoid fossa. This second center contributes to formation of the glenoid fossa to a greater degree than the first.[5] These two centers usually fuse at 15 years of age.

### CLAVICLE

The clavicle first appears as a dense bar of mesenchymal tissue. Chondrification of this skeletal element begins early in the embryonic period.[2,5] Initially, the clavicle has two centers of ossification that lie very close to one another, situated at the junction of the outer two-thirds and the inner one-third. When chondrification is completed, the two centers unite, and ossification proceeds laterally toward the acromion and medially toward the sternum (Fig. 1-26a). The shaft of the clavicle is one of the first bones in the human body to ossify.[5] The clavicle also demonstrates a thin ossification center at its sternal end and a scale-like center at its acromial end (see Fig. 1-26b). The sternal end and the acromial end begin to ossify at about 18 years of age, and they fuse with the main shaft at approximately 22 years of age. By 23 years of age, all skeletal elements of the shoulder region have matured, their epiphyseal centers have closed, and their surface markings are firmly developed.

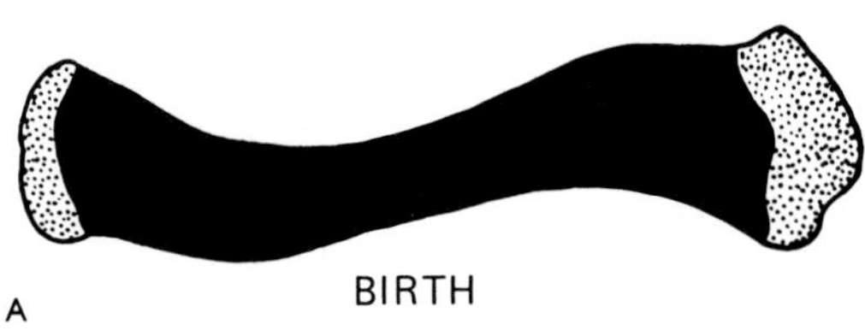


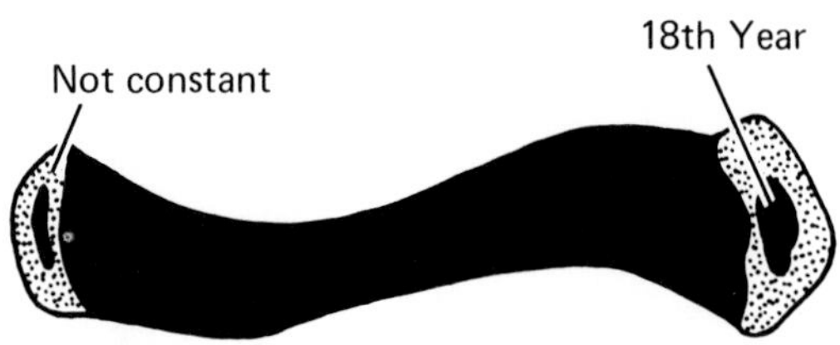


**Figure 1-26.** Date of appearance of ossification centers of the clavicle. (From Depalma AF. Surgery of the shoulder. 3rd ed. Philadelphia: JB Lippincott, 1983.)

# Descriptive Anatomy

# Osteology

*Osteology* is the division of human anatomy concerned with the study of bones. The bones of the human body are classified by their shape: long, flat, short, and irregular. The shape of any bone relates directly to its function within the skeletal system.

There are three bones responsible for the skeletal framework of the shoulder region: the clavicle, scapula, and humerus. Each bone displays individual features and physical characteristics.

### CLAVICLE

The clavicle derives its anatomic name from the latin word *clavius*, which means "key."[7] Anatomists have speculated that this bone received its name because its curved shape resembles a key. The clavicle, considered a long bone, consists of a shaft and two extremities (Fig. 1-27). The shaft extends from the midline of the body to the acromion process of the scapula and presents with a double curvature. The right clavicle is generally longer, thicker, and rougher than the left, and in females this bone is generally shorter, thinner, and smoother than in males.[7]

The length of the clavicle is divided into thirds, with the coracoid process the dividing point between the proximal two-thirds and the distal one-third. The proximal two-thirds has a convexity directed forward, and the distal one-third has a convexity directed backward. The proximal two-thirds is prismatic in shape, and the distal one-third is relatively flat. The surface markings of these two sections are quite different.

#### SURFACE MARKINGS

##### The Distal One-Third

The distal one-third presents with two surfaces, an upper and lower, and two borders, an anterior and posterior. The upper surface is flat but not smooth. It presents with a roughened texture created by impressions located near the anterior and posterior borders that serve as points of attachments for the anterior deltoid and trapezius muscles (see Fig. 1-27a). A small area located between these two rough areas is smooth in texture and can be palpated subcutaneously.

The lower surface is relatively flat but also presents with roughened areas. On the posterior border near the junction of the proximal two-thirds and the distal one-third, a rough eminence projects downward toward the coracoid process

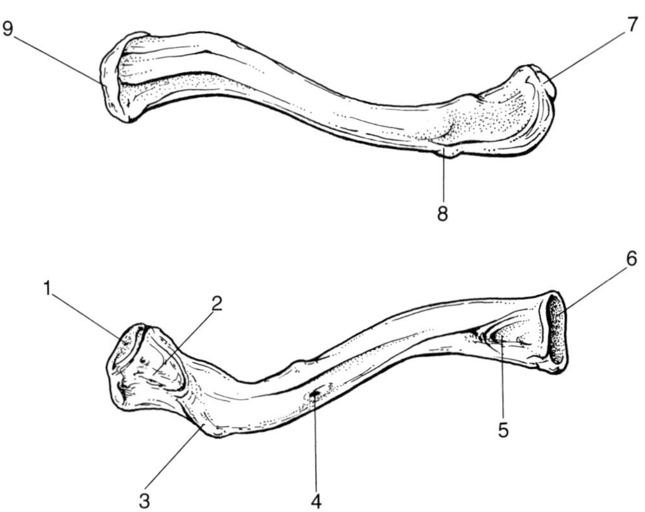


**Figure 1-27.** Right clavicle. (a) Superior surface. (b) Inferior surface. 1, articular surface for acromioclavicular joint; 2, trapezoid line; 3, conoid tubercle; 4, vascular foramen; 5, attachment site for costoclavicular ligament; 6, articular surface for sternoclavicular joint; 7, articular surface for acromioclavicular joint; 8, conoid tubercle; 9, articular surface for sternoclavicular joint.

of the scapula. This conoid tubercle serves as the site of attachment for the conoid portion of the coracoclavicular ligament (see Fig. 1-27b). From where this tubercle begins, there is an oblique line that extends in a lateral direction toward the acromion process. This ridge, referred to as the *trapezoid line*, serves as the site of attachment for the trapezoid portion of the coracoclavicular ligament.

On the anterior border there is a rough area that occasionally begins as a prominence near the midline of the clavicle and tapers to a thin impression laterally. This tubercle is the site of attachment for the anterior deltoid. The posterior border is broader than the anterior border, convex in shape, and presents with a roughened texture to provide for firm attachment of the upper trapezius.[7]

### The Proximal Two-Thirds

The proximal two-thirds of the clavicle presents with three borders, anterior, posterior, and superior, and three surfaces, anterior, posterior, and inferior.[7] These surfaces and borders create a prismatic shape that is quite different from the thin, flattened shape of the distal one-third. The curvature of the proximal two-thirds is such that the convexity is directed forward and the concavity is directed backward (see Fig. 1-27).

***Borders.*** The anterior border is smooth and remains continuous with the anterior border at the distal end. At its distal extent, it defines an interval between the attachment of the anterior deltoid and the pectoralis major muscles. At its proximal end, it provides for attachment of the clavicular portion of the pectoralis major (see Fig. 1-27a).

The posterior border extends from the conoid tubercle of the distal end to the rhomboid impression of the proximal end (see Fig. 1-27b). This border defines the posterior and inferior surfaces by effectively separating them, and it provides an attachment site for the subclavius and the fascia that envelops the omohyoid muscle.[7]

The superior border is continuous with the posterior border of the distal end. It is smooth and round at its distal end but rough at its proximal end for attachment of the sternocleidomastoid muscle.

***Surfaces.*** The anterior surface is defined by the anterior and superior borders. Its external surface is covered only by the attachment of the platysma, thus giving it a smooth and easily palpable texture. A prominent line on the anterior surface divides this surface into an upper and lower half.[7] The upper half provides attachment for the sternocleidomastoid, and the lower half provides attachment for the pectoralis major. The anterior surface faces forward and slightly upward at its sternal end but gradually shifts to face outward and upward at its acromial end. This change in direction is a result of twisting that takes place in the shaft of the clavicle.

The posterior surface is defined by the superior and posterior borders. This surface is smooth and flat and faces backward toward the neck region. At its proximal end it provides for attachment of the sternohyoid muscle. In its midline there is a nutrient foramen that permits the primary nutrient artery to enter the clavicle (see Fig. 1-27b). At approximately the junction of the first two-thirds and the distal one-third, the posterior surface lies very close to the nerves of the brachial plexus and the subclavian vessels. The entire posterior surface of the proximal end is concave. This allows for unrestricted passage of and added protection to the great vessels and nerves located between the clavicle and the first rib.

The inferior surface is defined by the anterior and posterior borders. At its proximal end it is continuous with the articular surface of the sternoclavicular joint and often presents with a small facet for articulation with the first rib. Just lateral to the proximal end there is a roughened area where the rhomboid ligament (costoclavicular ligament) attaches (see Fig. 1-27b). The remaining length of the inferior surface presents as a longitudinal groove that provides for attachment of the subclavius muscle. Occasionally, the groove is divided by a thin line that anchors the subclavius muscle by way of an intermuscular septum.[7]

***Articular surfaces.*** The two extremities of the clavicle present with articular surfaces that are surrounded by a synovial membrane, joint capsule, supportive ligaments, and more often than not separated by a meniscus. The presence of a meniscus, the extent of ligamentous structures, and the size and shape of the articular surfaces are discussed further in the section on arthrology.

## SCAPULA

On initial observation, the scapula is relatively flat, has a triangular shape, and presents with three borders and three angles. Closer inspection reveals a concavity on its ventral surface and a convexity on its dorsal surface (Fig. 1-28). Additional observation reveals three sharp angles and several prominences and depressions.

### SURFACE MARKINGS

#### Anterior Surface

The ventral surface is concave in contour so as to lie comfortably over the convexity of the thoracic wall (see Fig. 1-28a). This matching of surfaces

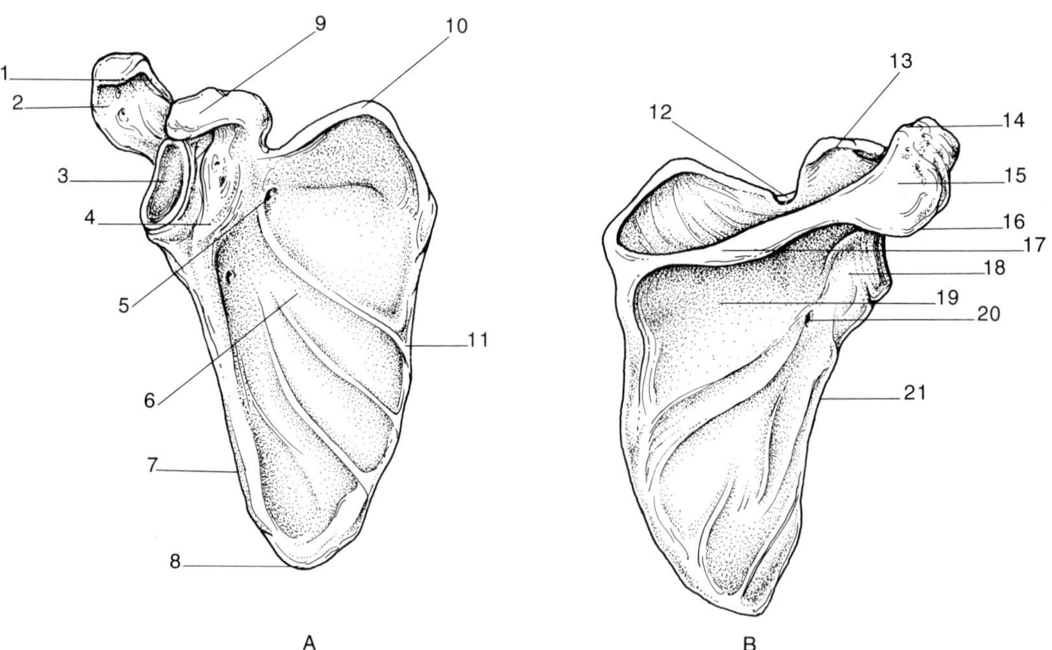


**Figure 1-28.** Right scapula. (a) Costal surface. (b) Dorsal surface. 1, articular surface for acromioclavicular joint; 2, acromion; 3, glenoid fossa; 4, neck; 5, vascular foramen; 6, subscapular fossa; 7, lateral (axillary) border; 8, inferior angle; 9, coracoid process; 10, superior angle; 11, medial (vertebral) border; 12, scapular notch; 13, coracoid process; 14, articular surface for acromioclavicular joint; 15, acromion; 16, spine acromion; 17, spine; 18, neck; 19, infraspinous fossa; 20, vascular foramen; 21, lateral (axillary) border.

allows for free gliding movements of the scapula. For the most part, the ventral surface, referred to as the *subscapular fossa*, is covered by the attachment of the subscapularis muscle. If one removes the subscapularis from the anterior surface, close inspection reveals that the surface is divided into thirds. The medial two-thirds provides a roughened area for attachment of the subscapularis muscle. The roughened surface is created by several ridges that arise from the medial border and project in a superior and lateral direction. These oblique ridges provide points of attachment for the tendinous portions of the subscapularis, and the areas in between provide deeper and broader surfaces for anchoring of the fleshy fibers of the subscapularis.[7] At its most medial margin, the anterior surface presents a narrow edge that extends from the superior to the inferior angle. This surface feature effectively separates the anterior surface from the vertebral border and provides for attachment of the serratus anterior muscle. The superior margin presents with a curved appearance that extends in a transverse direction, giving the impression that the bone is bending on itself. This region, referred to as the *subscapular angle*, effectively increases the strength of the scapula and provides a base of support for the spine and acromion process. It is in this region that the scapula exposes its deepest depression and the thickest portion of the subscapularis. This portion of the subscapularis has a direct line of pull that is perpendicular to the plane of the glenoid cavity (plane of the scapula).[7] The significance of this relationship to glenohumeral joint biomechanics and other facts related to the plane of the scapula will be discussed further in Chapter 2. The lateral one-third of the anterior surface is relatively smooth and free of any attachment to the subscapularis.

#### Posterior Surface

The posterior surface of the scapula presents with a convex contour from top to bottom and a mixture of convexity and concavity from medial to lateral (see Fig. 1-28b). The surface is unevenly divided by the spine of the scapula into a superior region, or supraspinous fossa, and an inferior region, or infraspinous fossa.

***Supraspinous fossa.*** The supraspinous fossa is the smallest of the two. It presents as a smooth concavity deepened further by the superior arch of the spine of the scapula. The width of the fossa is broad medially and tapers laterally to form the supraspinatus outlet. The supraspinatus muscle fills the entire fossa but only attaches itself to the medial two-thirds.[7] The remaining one-third is covered by the musculotendinous portion of the supraspinatus muscle as it extends through the outlet to form the superior part of the rotator cuff.[11]

***Infraspinous fossa.*** The infraspinous fossa is much larger than the supraspinous fossa, and through most of its extent it provides for attachment of the infraspinatus muscle. This surface is convex centrally but concave along the arch of the spine and over the superior aspect of the medial border. The lateral border presents with a deep groove defined by a ridge medially that extends in a downward and backward direction from the lower part of the glenoid cavity to just above the inferior angle. This ridge separates the fossa from the lateral border and provides for attachment of a strong aponeurosis that separates the infraspinatus from the teres major and minor muscles. The surface between the ridge and the border is narrow in its upper two-thirds, where it provides for attachment of the teres minor. At the center of the lateral border exists a small groove that permits passage of and protection to the dorsal scapular vessels (circumflex scapular artery). The lower one-third of the lateral (axillary) border presents as a triangular surface that provides for attachment of the teres major muscle. The upper two-thirds and lower one-third are separated by an oblique line that extends in a transverse direction from the lateral border to the ridge. Attached to this line is an aponeurosis that separates the teres minor from the teres major.

#### Spine

The spine of the scapula, a prominent plate of bone, extends in an oblique direction from the vertebral border to the acromion process (see Fig. 1-28b). It begins as a smooth triangular surface and then proceeds in a lateral and upward direction, moving away from the body of the scapula and eventually terminating as the acromion process.[7] The spine is roughly triangular in shape with its apex near the vertebral border and its base near the neck of the scapula.

The spine presents with two surfaces. The concave superior surface forms the wall of the supraspinous fossa and provides a firm area of attachment for the supraspinatus muscle. The concave inferior surface forms the roof of the infraspinous fossa and provides for attachment of the infraspinatus muscle. Near the center of the inferior surface of the spine there is a small nutrient foramen that permits the passage of nutrient vessels into the body of the scapula (see Fig. 1-28b).

The spine presents with three borders. The anterior border is where the spine meets the body of the scapula. The posterior border, also called the *crest*, lies directly opposite the anterior border. The crest presents as a broad surface defined by a superior and inferior ridge. The superior ridge affords attachment to the upper trapezius, and the inferior ridge affords attachment to the posterior deltoid. The roughened area between the two ridges provides for the attachment of tendinous fibers from both muscles. The external border, which is slightly concave, extends from the external surface at the neck of the scapula to the undersurface of the acromion process. A narrow portion of bone, referred to as the *greater scapular notch* (*spinoglenoid notch*), exists between the root of the external border and the glenoid fossa (see Fig. 1-28b). This notch connects the infraspinous and supraspinous fossae.

### Acromion Process

The acromion process presents as a large, oblong, triangular process that appears to be flat when viewed from behind. At first this process is directed a little outward but quickly changes its direction, curving forward and upward to form a roof over the glenoid cavity[7] (see Fig. 1-28). The external surface is convex and rough so as to provide for attachment of the deltoid muscle. The outer-most border is thick and presents as an irregular surface with three or more tubercles for the tendinous insertions of the deltoid.[7] The concave inner margin provides for attachment of the trapezius muscle. At the center of the inner margin is a small oval articular facet that articulates with the acromial end of the clavicle, effectively forming the acromioclavicular joint (see Fig. 1-28). The apex of the acromion is located at the front, where the outer and inner margins meet. This area is relatively thin and provides for attachment of the coracoacromial ligament. Occasionally, the coracoacromial ligament demonstrates partial ossification prior to its attachment. The shape and contour of the undersurface and the apex of the acromion have been studied by several researchers. Bigliani and coworkers[23] have identified three types of acromions based on shape (see Fig. 1-29). Type I acromions are relatively flat, type II acromions are rounded, and type III acromions are hooked. The hooked acromion has been implicated as a source of painful impingement.

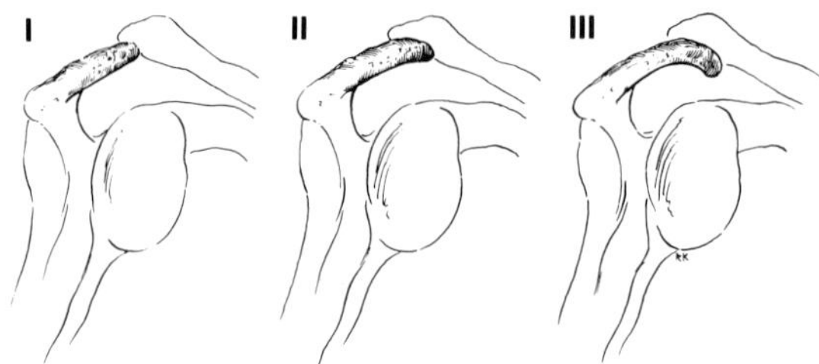


**Figure 1-29.** The three types of acromion morphology defined by Bigliani and Morrison. Type I, with its flat surface, provided the least compromise of the supraspinatus outlet, whereas Type III's sudden discontinuity or hook was associated with the highest rate of rotator cuff pathology in a series of cadaver dissections. (From Rockwood C, Matsen F. The shoulder. Vol. 1. Philadelphia: WB Saunders, 1990:45.)

## BORDERS

Of the three scapular borders, the superior is the shortest and thinnest.[7] This concave border extends from the superior angle to the coracoid process. At its outer margin it presents with a deep semicircular notch that is transformed into a hole by being covered by the transverse ligament (see Fig. 1-28b). This opening provides for protected passage of the suprascapular nerve from the supraspinous fossa to the infraspinous fossa. Occasionally, the suprascapular notch is a site of painful nerve entrapment or blunt trauma causing supraspinatus and infraspinatus weakness and atrophy.

The external border, which is the thickest of the three borders, commences at the lower margin of the glenoid cavity and extends obliquely downward and backward to terminate at the inferior angle (Fig. 1-30a). It commences as a rough impression, the infraglenoid tubercle. This tubercle is the site of attachment for the long head of the triceps. The anterior margin of this border presents with a longitudinal groove extending as far distally as the lower one-third. This groove

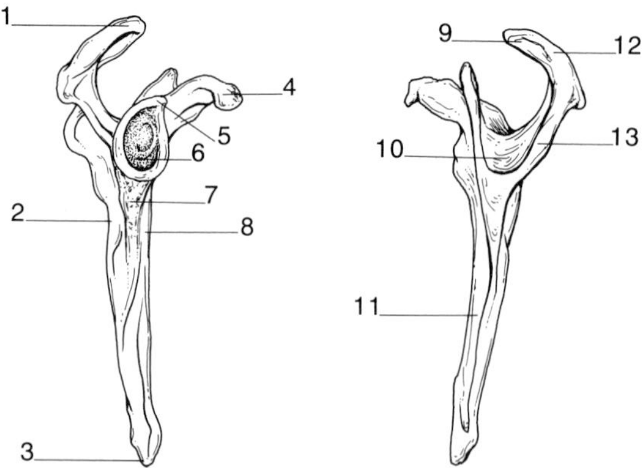


**Figure 1-30.** Right scapula. (a) Lateral aspect. (b) Medial aspect. 1, acromion; 2, infraspinous fossa; 3, inferior angle; 4, coracoid process; 5, supraglenoid tubercle; 6, glenoid fossa; 7, infraglenoid tubercle; 8, subscapular fossa; 9, articular surface for acromioclavicular joint; 10, supraspinous fossa; 11, medial border; 12, acromion; 13, spine.

provides for attachment of lower part of the subscapularis muscle. The posterior and anterior surfaces of the lower one-third are thin in comparison with the upper two-thirds, and this affords attachment to the teres major and subscapularis, respectively.

The medial or vertebral border, also called the *base* of the scapula, is the longest of the three borders, extending from superior to inferior angle (see Fig. 1-30b). This border is not as thick as the external border and not as thin as the superior border. It presents as an arched or curved surface, and the portion above the level of the spine is bent outward to form an obtuse angle with the lower portion.[7] This border presents with an anterior lip, a posterior lip, and an intermediate space. The anterior lip provides for attachment of the serratus anterior muscle. The posterior lip provides for attachment of the supraspinatus muscle above the spine and the infraspinatus muscle below the spine. The intermediate space provides for attachment of levator scapulae and rhomboid major and minor muscles.[7] The intermediate space above the spine presents as a broad triangular surface defined by the superior angle where the levator scapulae attaches. The edge of the superior angle and triangular surface is where the rhomboid minor attaches. The edge of the superior angle and triangular surface is where the rhomboid minor attaches. The rhomboid major attaches to the vertebral border by way of a fibrous arch to the triangular surface and the area directly below the spine.[7]

The scapula presents with three angles: superior, inferior, and anterior. The superior angle is formed by the meeting of the superior and vertebral borders. It presents as a thin, smooth, rounded surface that is inclined slightly outward to afford attachment for the levator scapulae. The inferior angle, thicker than the superior, is formed by the meeting of the vertebral (medial) and axillary (lateral) borders. Its external surface provides for attachment of the teres major muscle and occasionally a few fibers from latissimus dorsi muscle. The anterior angle is the thickest portion of the scapula and is more commonly referred to as the *head* of the scapula[7] (see Fig. 1-28b). This area presents as an extension of the body of the scapula and gives rise to the glenoid cavity. The neck of the scapula is a slightly depressed area that encircles the anterior angle or head of the scapula. The neck is more distinct on the posterior surface than on the anterior surface and more distinct on the inferior margin than on the superior margin.

The glenoid cavity presents as a shallow articular surface that resembles an inverted comma, with its inferior margin wider than its superior margin. At the most superior extent of the glenoid cavity, referred to as the *apex*, lies the supraglenoid tubercle, which provides for attachment of the long head of the biceps (see Fig. 1-30a). The most peripheral margin of the glenoid cavity is slightly raised and provides for attachment of the glenoid labrum.

### CORACOID PROCESS

The coracoid process, so called because it resembles a crow's beak, arises from the neck of the scapula by way of a broad base (see Fig. 1-28a). This structure extends upward and inward as a thick, curved process. Becoming more tapered, it projects in a forward and outward direction. The ascending portion of this process presents as a smooth concave surface over which passes the tendon of the subscapularis. The horizontal portion is flattened from above downward, its upper surface is convex and irregular, and its undersurface is smooth. Its inner and outer borders are rough and provide for attachment of several tendons and ligaments. At the base of the coracoid process, a rough impression on the inner side provides for attachment of the conoid portion of the coracoclavicular ligament. Extending from this roughened impression is a ridge that runs in an oblique direction forward and outward along the upper surface of the horizontal portion. This ridge provides for attachment of the trapezoid portion of the coracoclavicular ligament. The outer border of the horizontal portion presents with a roughened area for attachment of the coracoacromial ligament. The very tip of the coracoid process provides for attachment of the conjoined tendon formed by the union of the coracobrachialis and the short head of the biceps muscle. The apex also provides for attachment of the costocoracoid ligament.

### STRUCTURE

The thickened portions of the scapula are formed of cancellous bone, whereas the rest is comprised of a thin layer of dense, compact bone. The center of the supraspinous fossa and occasionally the upper part of the infraspinous fossa present as semitransparent. In rare instances, bone tissue is missing, and the adjacent muscles come in contact with one another.[7]

## HUMERUS

The humerus is the longest bone of the upper extremity, presenting with a shaft and two extremities (Fig. 1-31). The shaft, constructed of a cylinder of hard, compact bone, is thickest at its

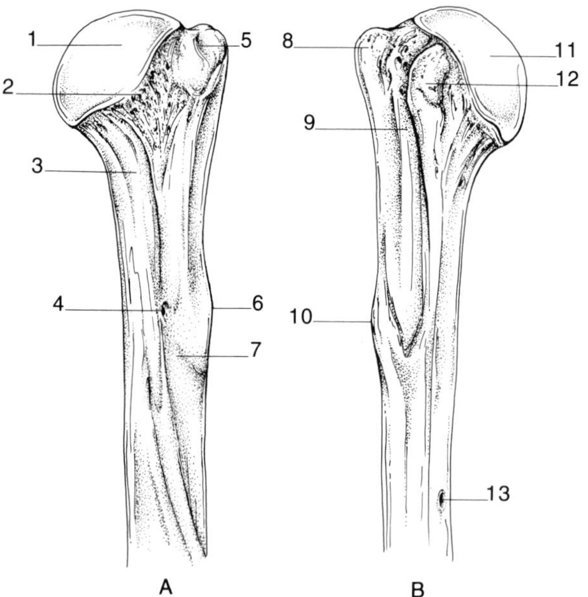


**Figure 1-31.** Right humerus. (a) Posterior aspect. (b) Anterior aspect. 1, head and articular surface; 2, anatomic neck; 3, surgical neck; 4, vascular foramen; 5, greater tubercle; 6, deltoid tuberosity; 7, groove for radial nerve; 8, greater tubercle; 9, bicipital (intertubecular) groove; 10, deltoid tuberosity; 11, head; 12, lesser tubercle; 13, vascular foramen.

center and thinnest at the extremities. The two extremities are constructed of cancellous bone covered with a thin layer of compact bone. The proximal extremity, referred to as the *head* of the humerus, forms the articular surface of the glenohumeral joint.

## HUMERAL HEAD

The humeral head presents as a large, rounded surface connected to the shaft by a constricted portion of bone referred to as the *surgical neck*. The head, not nearly a perfect sphere, is directed in an upward, inward, and backward direction.[7] The rounded appearance of the humeral head is disturbed by two bony eminences, the greater and lesser tuberosities (see Fig. 1-31). The most proximal extent of the humeral head articulates with the glenoid fossa of the scapula to form the glenohumeral joint. The articular surface is smooth and coated with hyaline cartilage. The circumference of the articular surface is slightly constricted and is referred to as the *anatomic neck*. This is a clearly demarcated area separate from the surgical neck that is located near the shaft of the humerus (see Fig. 1-31a). The anatomic neck forms an obtuse angle with the shaft of the humerus as it faces in an oblique direction. This region is more clearly demarcated in the lower half of the circumference than in the upper half. In the upper half, it presents as a narrow groove effectively separating the articular surface from the tuberosities. The anatomic neck affords attachment to the glenohumeral joint capsule and ligaments. This area is also perforated in numerous places by vascular foramina that provide nutrition to the head of the humerus.[7]

### Greater Tuberosity

The greater tuberosity is located on the outer margin of the humeral head. Its upper surface is rounded and defined by three flattened areas referred to as *facets*. The upper most facet provides for attachment of the supraspinatus muscle, the middle facet provides for attachment of the infraspinatus muscle, and the lower-most facet and adjacent area on the shaft provide for attachment of the teres minor muscle. The outer surface of the tuberosity, which is convex and rough, is continuous with the shaft of the humerus.

### Lesser Tuberosity

The lesser tuberosity, located on the front of the humeral head, faces in an inward and forward direction. The summit or peak of this tuberosity presents with a facet that provides for attachment of the subscapularis muscle.

### Bicipital Groove

The tuberosities are separated from one another by a deep groove that contains the tendon of the long head of the biceps muscle and a branch of the anterior humeral circumflex artery. This depression, referred to as the *bicipital groove*, begins at the top of the humeral head, courses obliquely downward and slightly inward, terminating at the junction of the proximal one-third and distal two-thirds of the shaft of the humerus[7] (see Fig. 1-31b). Where the groove begins, it is deep and narrow; as it descends, it becomes shallow and broader. The floor of the groove is lined with hyaline cartilage and provides for attachment of the latissimus dorsi muscle. The medial lip, a prolongation of the lesser tuberosity, provides for attachment of the teres major muscle. The lateral lip, a prolongation of the greater tuberosity, provides for attachment of the pectoralis major muscle.

## SHAFT

The shaft of the humerus is almost cylindrical in its upper half, but gradually it becomes prismatic and flattened in its lower half, where it broadens to form the epicondylar characteristics of the elbow joint. The shaft presents with three borders, anterior, external, and internal, and three surfaces, external internal and posterior.

### Borders

The anterior border extends from the anterior margin of the greater tuberosity to the conoid depression at the elbow, and it effectively separates the internal and external surfaces (see Fig. 1-31b). The proximal extent of the anterior border is very prominent and rough is its appearance, being synonymous with the lateral lip of the bicipital groove. At approximately its center it forms the medial margin of the deltoid tubercle. At its distal extent it is smooth and more rounded in appearance, providing for attachment of the brachialis anticus muscle.

The external border begins on the posterior margin of the greater tuberosity and terminates on the lateral epicondyle of the elbow. This border effectively separates the external and posterior surfaces of the shaft. The border is rounded and clearly demarcated in its upper half, where it provides for attachment of the teres minor muscle and the long head of triceps. The center is traversed by a broad but shallow groove that courses in an oblique direction from medial to lateral. This groove provides direction and protection to the radial nerve and the superior profundus artery. The distal extent, prominent and rough in appearance, terminates as the lateral supracondylar ridge of the humerus.[7]

The internal border extends from the lesser tuberosity to the medial epicondyle. The proximal one-third is synonymous with the medial lip of the bicipital groove and provides for attachment of the tendon of the teres major muscle. At about its center it provides for attachment of the coracobrachialis, and just distal to this there presents a foramen for entrance to the nutrient canal of the humeral shaft[7] (see Fig. 1-31b). The distal third is synonymous with the medial supracondylar ridge of the elbow. The anterior margin provides for attachment of the brachialis anticus, and the posterior margin provides for the attachment of the medial head of triceps muscle.

### Surfaces

The external surface is defined by the anterior border medially and the external border laterally. This surface initially faces outward and is covered by the deltoid muscle. It presents as a smooth, rounded surface but gradually shifts to a concave surface from above to below, directing itself in an outward but slightly forward direction. At about the middle of its extent it presents a roughened triangular groove that courses in an oblique direction from behind, forward, and downward.[7] This is the start of the radial groove. At about the same location is found the deltoid tubercle, which affords attachment to the deltoid tendon.

The internal surface formed by the anterior border laterally and the internal border medially is less extensive than the external surface. Initially, this surface faces inward, and then, as it descends, it faces in both an inward and forward direction.[7] This surface, initially very narrow, commences as the floor of the bicipital groove. As it descends, it broadens and becomes rougher in its appearance to provide for attachment of the coracobrachialis tendon. As it terminates, it presents once again a smooth concave surface that provides for attachment of the brachialis anticus muscle.

The posterior surface appears somewhat twisted such that its proximal extent faces a little inward and its distal extent faces backward and slightly outward.[7] Nearly the whole surface is covered by the lateral and medial heads of the triceps muscles. These two muscles are separated by the radial groove.

## SURGICAL ANATOMY

There are several points of interest with regard to surgical anatomy of the proximal humerus. First, one should recall that the proximal epiphysis is the first to demonstrate ossification but the last to unite with the shaft. It is responsible for the ultimate length of the humerus more so than any other part of this bone. Amputations of the upper limb in young children must consider these facts because the proximal end of the humerus will continue to grow, and lengthening of the stump will progress over time.

Fractures in children and adolescents of the

upper end of the humerus mandate particular and specific considerations associated with maintaining normal development. Separation of the proximal epiphysis sometimes occurs in young children and is readily determined by a characteristic deformity created by the lower fragment. The shoulder presents with an abrupt projection of bone at the front of the joint just inferior to the coracoid process. Fractures in children may be due to direct or indirect trauma. A frequent cause of fracture in the humerus is muscular action, and the region most susceptible to this type of fracture is the shaft just below the deltoid tubercle.

Fractures can and often do occur in the region of the anatomic neck, surgical neck, and/or separation of the greater tuberosity. Fractures of the anatomic neck rarely occur, and in fact, many authorities doubt if fractures ever occur here. These types of fractures are classified as intracapsular but are more than likely part intracapsular and part extracapsular, since the lower part of the capsule inserts below the anatomic neck and the upper part inserts directly into the anatomic neck.[7] Fractures of the humeral head are classified as either impacted or nonimpacted. In most cases, the fragments are not displaced on account of the capsule either in whole or in part remaining attached to the lower fragment. Occasionally, a very remarkable alteration in position takes place such that the upper fragment turns on its own axis. When this occurs, the cartilaginous surface of the head of the humerus rests against the upper end of the lower fragment. When the fractured end is entirely separated from all its surroundings and its vascular supply is fully compromised, one can expect it to undergo necrosis, but this occurs rarely. In fractures of the shaft of the humerus, the lesion can occur anywhere along the length of the humerus but appears more often in the lower half than in the upper half. Several points of interest in connection to fractures of the shaft need mentioning. First, the radial nerve lies in a precarious position in the groove on the posterior surface of the humerus, leaving this nerve very susceptible to trauma. Second, nonunion fractures appear to be more common in the humerus than in any other bone of the body.[7] Several facts may offer an explanation for this. The ability to fixate fractures in the shoulder and the elbow joint is often difficult if not impossible. Often movement occurs not in the joint but rather between the fracture fragments. On rare occasions, muscle tissue effectively separates the bony fragments. The want of support of the distal end of the humerus can create a drag on the proximal humerus and effectively separate the proximal fragments.

Tumors of the humerus also occur with some frequency. A common place for a chondroma to develop is the shaft of the humerus in the neighborhood of the deltoid tubercle. Sarcomata also frequently develop in the shaft of the humerus.[24] Refer to Chapters 3 and 4 for additional information on these points.

# Arthrology: Articulations of the Shoulder Region

The bones of the human body are connected to one another by way of an articulation or joint. The study of these anatomic structures is referred to as *arthrology*. The term *arthrology* is derived form the Greek word *arthron* and has been widely adopted into standard clinical terminology as in arthroscopic, arthritis, and arthrodesis.[24] The articulations of the body vary considerably in structure. The structure of any articulation in the body is an expression of the function it performs.

The articulations of the body have been divided into three distinct classes: fibrous, cartilaginous, and synovial. By definition, a *synovial joint* consists of two articular surfaces covered with articular cartilage and separated by a potential space filled with synovial fluid and enclosed by an articular capsule that connects the two bones to one another.[24] The shoulder region consists of three synovial joints: the sternoclavicular, acromioclavicular, and glenohumeral.

## STERNOCLAVICULAR JOINT

The sternoclavicular joint is regarded by most anatomists as a synovial joint. The parts entering into its formation are the sternal end of the clavicle, the upper and lateral surface of the first part of the sternum, and the cartilage of the first rib (see Fig. 1-32). The articular surface of the clavicle is much larger than the sternum, and the layer of cartilage on the clavicle is considerably thicker.[7] The sternal end of the clavicle is triangular in shape and presents with a convex surface in the coronal plane and a concave surface in the transverse plane. The joint angles in a posterior and medial direction. The two articular surfaces are relatively flat and are separated by a fibrocartilaginous meniscus. The meniscus attaches to the superior margin of the articular surface of the clavicle, and the inferior margin is continuous with the undersurface of the clavicle. The posterior margin projects backward, effectively increasing the articular surface area and the stability of this articulation. The aforementioned structures are secured to one another by a series of ligaments and a joint capsule.

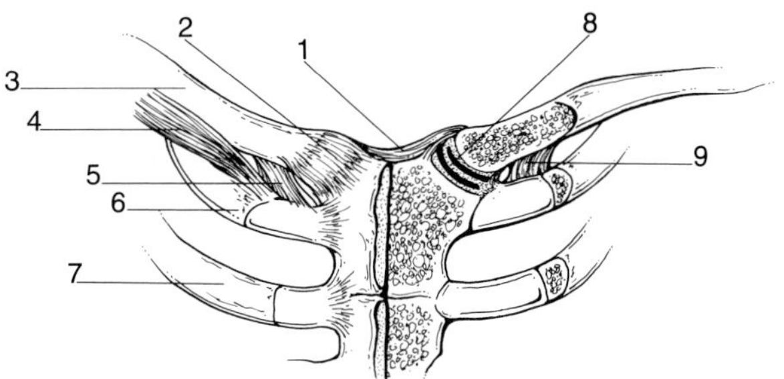


**Figure 1-32.** The sternoclavicular joint. 1, interclavicular ligament; 2, anterior sternoclavicular ligament; 3, clavicle; 4, subclavius muscle; 5, costoclavicular (rhomboid) ligament; 6, first rib; 7, second rib; 8, interarticular meniscus; 9, costoclavicular (rhomboid) ligament.

## SYNOVIAL CAPSULE

The joint capsule completely surrounds the articulating structures. It consists of fibrous tissue that varies in thickness and strength. The fibers extending across the front and back of the capsule are considerably thicker, and the thickest bands form the anterior and posterior sternoclavicular ligaments. Those fibers extending across the top and bottom of the capsule are relatively thin and scant in appearance and resemble more closely thin connective tissue than firm fibrous tissue.[7]

## LIGAMENTS

The anterior ligament forms a broad band of fibrous tissue that covers the anterior surface of the joint. The fibers attach to the front portion of the upper-most part and inner-most edge of the clavicle. They then pass obliquely downward and inward toward their attachment to the upper anterior part of the first section of the sternum. The ligament is covered in front by the sternocleidomastoid tendon and its related connective tissue and behind blends with the interarticular meniscus and the two synovial membranes.

The posterior ligament forms a broad band of fibrous tissue that covers the posterior surface of the joint. This ligament blends in front with the synovial membrane and the interarticular meniscus and behind binds to the tendons of the sternothyroid and sternohyoid muscles.

The interclavicular ligament is a flattened band of tissue that varies in thickness from one individual to another. The ligament, whether it is well formed or barely noticeable, extends from the upper inner edge of one clavicle to the upper inner edge of the other. The ligament passes in a curved direction and on its path from one clavicle to the other binds to the upper margin of the sternum.

The costoclavicular ligament is a short, flat, rhomboid-shaped structure that passes from the first rib to the clavicle. The fibrous bands begin on the upper and inner portion of the cartilage of the first rib. They ascend in an oblique direction backward and outward and attach to the undersurface of the clavicle on a roughened area referred to as the *rhomboid impression*. The ligament lies in close relationship with the subclavius muscle in front and the subclavian vein behind.

## MENISCUS

The interarticular meniscus is a flat, nearly circular disc of fibrocartilage that lies between the articular surfaces of the clavicle and the sternum. The meniscus attaches above to the upper and posterior border of the articular surface of the clavicle and below to the cartilage of the first rib and its articulation with the sternum (Fig. 1-32). The peripheral margin of the meniscus is attached to the anterior, posterior, and interclavicular ligaments. The meniscus is thicker at its periphery, especially at its upper and posterior margins, and thinner at its center and near its lower margins. The meniscus effectively divides the joint into two cavities, each of which is provided with a separate synovial membrane. One of the synovial membranes extends from the sternal end of the clavicle to the adjacent surface of the meniscus and to the cartilage of the first rib. The second membrane, which is the larger of the two, extends between the articular surface of the sternum and the adjacent surface of the meniscus.

## SURGICAL ANATOMY

Dislocation of the sternoclavicular joint occurs rarely; more often the clavicle is fractured. The reasons for this are twofold. First, the forces are more often transmitted along the long axis of the clavicle, and second, the strength of the ligamentous structures leads more often to a fracture than to displacement. When dislocation does occur, the direction of the displacement depends more on the direction in which the force is applied than on the anatomic construction of the joint. A force that causes the clavicular end to displace in a posterior direction is the most serious. It can cause a life-threatening situation by compromising vital neurovascular structures that lie directly behind this joint. Once a dislocation of this joint has occurred, the likelihood of recurrence is extremely high. This is due in large part to the anatomic construction of the articulation. The articulating surfaces are not congruent, and the stability of the joint is dependent on the ligaments. Once the ligaments have been traumatized, their ability to provide dynamic and static stability is challenged. To maintain proper alignment of the joint often requires internal fixation. The mechanism for providing internal fixation offers a challenge to orthopedic surgeons. Pin fixation can lead to postoperative complications of pin migration. Discussion of surgical options is explored further in Chapter 4.

## ACROMIOCLAVICULAR JOINT

The acromioclavicular joint is considered a synovial articulation and is stated to be the only articulation between the scapula and the clavicle, although others have noted from cadaver dissection that in some rare instances a coracoclavicular bar or joint connecting the coracoid process and clavicle exists.[23] The acromioclavicular joint is formed by the distal end of the clavicle and the inner margin of the acromion process (Fig. 1-33a). The distal end of the clavicle is positioned higher than the acromion, and the acromion is angled or slanted downward. The clavicle presents with a small, flat, oval articulating surface. The shape of the distal end directs the extremity outward and forward, and the articular surface faces in a downward direction. The two articulating surfaces are far from being considered congruent. More often than not they are separated by a fibrocartilaginous meniscus. Unlike the sternoclavicular joint, this joint is usually formed by a single joint cavity surrounded by a single synovial capsule. In some rare instances, cadaver dissection has revealed a construction similar to the sternoclavicular joint. In either case, the acromioclavicular joint capsule is strengthened by the presence of the interarticular cartilage and by a superior and inferior acromioclavicular ligament. Further support is provided by the coracoclavicular ligaments, which extend across the coracoid process of the scapula to the undersurface of the distal end of the clavicle.

### LIGAMENTS

The superior ligament is a quadrilateral band that effectively covers the superior surface of this articulation. The ligament extends from the upper portion of the outer end of the clavicle to the superior surface of the acromion process. This structure intimately blends with the connective tissue or aponeuroses of the deltoid and upper trapezius muscles. The undersurface of the ligament intimately blends with the synovial membrane and interarticular meniscus. Proper tension of this ligament and associated structures assists in maintaining the position of the superior capsule and meniscus at rest and during movement.

The inferior ligament is considerably thinner than the superior ligament, but the two ligaments are continuous with each other by way of connective tissue. This ligament extends from the undersurface of the clavicle to the adjoining undersurface of the acromion. The superior surface blends with the synovial membrane and in some instances with the meniscus. The inferior surface often blends with the connective tissue of the supraspinatus tendon.

#### Coracoacromial Ligament

The coracoacromial ligament extends from the base of the coracoid process to the undersurface of the acromion. At its point of origin it is somewhat broader; as it extends toward the acromion, it tapers but still maintains a rather broad insertion into the undersurface of the acromion, extending out to and investing the tip of the acromion. In arthritic changes of the undersurface of the acromion, osteophytic changes often involve this ligament, and surgical intervention often sacrifices this structure in an attempt to increase subacromial space.

#### Coracoclavicular Ligaments

The coracoclavicular ligaments extend from the coracoid process of the scapula to the undersurface of the clavicle and are not actually part of the acromioclavicular joint. However, their primary function is to maintain the normal position of this joint, and they are discussed with this articulation. The ligament consists of two distinct bands that are named according to their respective shapes.

***Conoid.*** The conoid ligament is composed of a dense band of fibers that are conical in shape with its summit directed downward and its base directed upward[7] (see Fig. 1-33a). The ligament extends from a rough impression at the base of the coracoid process to the conoid tubercle and a line extending from the tubercle half an inch on the undersurface of the clavicle. This ligament lies more medial and more posterior than the trapezoid.

***Trapezoid.*** The trapezoid ligament, quadrilateral in shape, is a broad, thin band extending from the upper surface of the coracoid process in an

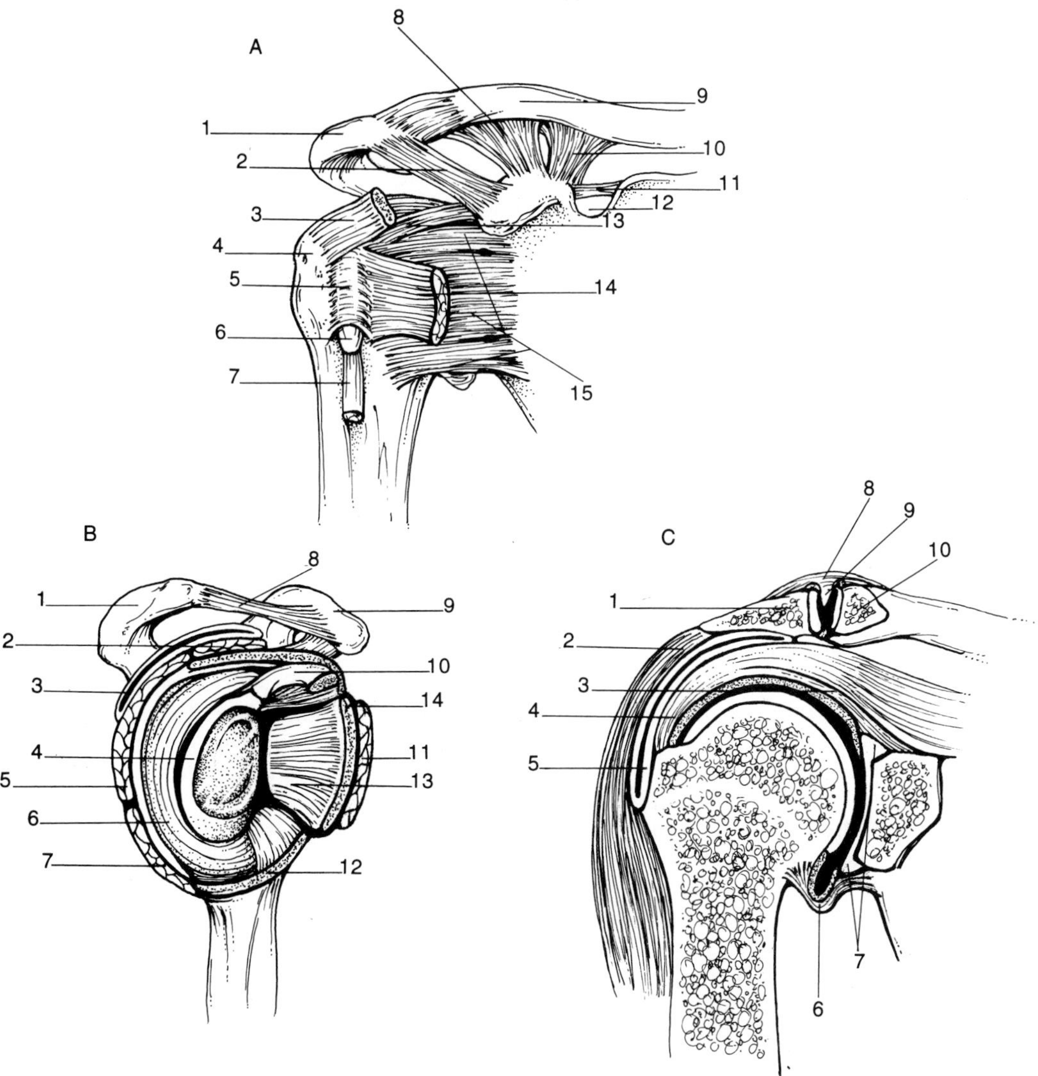


**Figure 1-33.** The acromioclavicular and glenohumeral joints. (a) Anterior view. 1, acromion; 2, coracoacromial ligament; 3, supraspinatus tendon (cut); 4, greater tubercle; 5, transverse ligament of intertubecular groove; 6, extension of synovial sheath covering the bicipital tendon; 7, long head of the biceps tendon; 8, trapezoid portion of the coracoclavicular ligaments; 9, clavicle; 10, conoid portion of the coracoclavicular ligaments; 11, superior transverse ligament; 12, scapular notch; 13, coracohumeral ligament; 14, subscapularis tendon (cut); 15, superior, middle, and inferior glenohumeral ligaments. (b) Opened lateral view. 1, acromion; 2, supraspinatus tendon; 3, subdeltoid bursa; 4, labrum; 5, infraspinatus tendon; 6, inner lining of the synovial membrane; 7, teres minor tendon; 8, coraocoacromial ligament; 9, coracoid process; 10, biceps tendon; 11, subscapularis tendon; 12, inferior glenohumeral ligament; 13, middle glenohumeral ligament; 14, superior glenohumeral ligament. (c) Coronal section. 1, acromion; 2, deltoid muscle; 3, capsular ligament; 4, supraspinatus tendon; 5, subdeltoid bursa; 6, inferior capsular fold; 7, labrum; 8, superior acromioclavicular ligament; 9, interarticular meniscus; 10, clavicle.

oblique direction to the oblique line on the undersurface of the clavicle[7] (see Fig. 1-33a). The conoid and trapezoid ligaments join together as they meet on the undersurface of the clavicle. The two ligaments lie posterior to the anterior deltoid and subclavius and anterior to upper trapezius. Their primary function is to maintain the distal end of the clavicle in proper alignment with the acromion process.

## MENISCUS

In most situations, the meniscus partially separates the two articulating surfaces and occupies the upper part of the joint cavity, being well connected to the superior ligament and synovial membrane.[7] On occasion, it is completely absent, and very rarely it divides the joint into separate cavities. The meniscus consists of fibrocartilage, and it serves to distribute forces evenly within the joint, providing additional stability.

### SURGICAL ANATOMY

The acromioclavicular joint is often the site of arthritic changes, anatomic variants and osteophyte formation. The shape of the acromion varies considerably from one individual to the next, and it is believed by many that the shape of the acromion determines to a considerable extent one's likelihood of rotator cuff injuries. On occasion, the acromion remains unfused and has been implicated as a possible source of impingement.[15,23] Liberson[13] classified the different types as the preacromion, mesacromion, metacromion, and basiacromion center. In his study, an unfused acromion was noted in 1.4 percent of the roentgenograms, and when noted, the abnormality was bilateral in 62 percent of subjects. The most common defects were of the mesacromion and metacromion types. Neer,[17,18] in his reporting of acromioplasties, found no increased incidence of unfused epiphyses. Orthopedic procedures are often used to effect changes in the undersurface of the acromion and the distal end of the clavicle in what is commonly referred to as an *acromioplasty*. A Mumford procedure consists of removal of the distal end of the clavicle.

Subluxation and dislocation of this joint most often occur in a downward direction such that the acromion process of the scapula is displaced under the distal end of the clavicle. Dislocations in the opposite direction have been described but are much less common. Dislocation of the acromioclavicular joint is referred to as a *shoulder separation*. Often the displacement is incomplete on account of the coracoclavicular ligaments remaining intact or being only partially torn.[7] With acromioclavicular separation, a cosmetic complaint alone is often managed without surgical correction. When the trauma is violent enough to cause complete disruption of these ligaments, then the joint is truly dislocated. Like the sternoclavicular joint, the acromioclavicular joint dislocation presents with a likelihood of recurrence and often requires internal fixation. Very often this is managed by reestablishing the coracoclavicular distance through the use of a screw, wire, or sutures. For further information on surgical management, refer to Chapter 4.

## GLENOHUMERAL JOINT

The glenohumeral articulation is considered a spheroidal or ball-and-socket joint. The articulating surfaces are formed by the head of the humerus and the glenoid cavity of the scapula. The head of the humerus is two to three times larger than the glenoid, and the glenoid fossa is very shallow (see Fig. 1-33c). Although it is provided with additional depth by the presence of the labrum, the additional concavity does not provide adequate stability to this articulation. The relationship shared by the two articular surfaces has been likened to that of a golf ball and a golf tee.[26] This articulation relies on an intact capsuloligamentous-labral complex along with a strong rotator cuff for stability (see Fig. 1-33b).

### ARTICULAR SURFACES

In a study of 20 shoulders Saha,[27,28] described the humeral articular surface as highly irregular and not a perfect sphere. He classified the articular surfaces as one of three types. Type A presents with a humeral surface with a radius of curvature smaller than that of the glenoid and more curved than the glenoid, with a small circular contact area. Type B presents with a humeral head and glenoid surface that have similar curvatures. In this type, there is better fit, with a larger circular contact area. Type C presents with a humeral surface that has a radius of curvature larger than that of the glenoid, which is then more curved. The contact surface is ring-shaped and limited to the peripheral margins of the articular surfaces. In addition to the imbalance in the size of the two articular surfaces, there also exist differences in the angles formed between the articular surfaces and their respective bones. The head of the humerus is directed in a posterior, medial, and superior direction. The glenoid cavity is directed in a anterior, lateral, and superior direction. Despite these differences in size and angulations, the two surfaces complement each other in such a manner as to permit the greatest freedom of motion of any articulation within the body.

The articular surface of the humeral head is covered by articular cartilage that is thicker at its center and thinner at its peripheral margin. The articular surface represents approximately one-third of an irregular sphere with a radius of curvature of about 2.25 cm. The average vertical dimension of the surface is 48 mm, with a 25-mm radius of curvature; the average transverse dimension is 45 mm, with a 22-mm radius of curvature.[29] The head is inclined and retroverted relative to the shaft. According to Testut,[32] the angle of inclination is between 130 and 150 degrees, and the angle of retroversion is estimated to be 20 to 30 degrees.[10,27–29] In addition to these incongruencies, the head of the humerus is not a perfect sphere but presents with a changing curvature and diameter throughout its surface.

The glenoid is teardrop-shaped, with its superior margin being narrower than its inferior margin, and its shape has been described as resembling an inverted comma (see Fig. 1-33b). The oval concave glenoid surface has an average vertical dimension of 35 mm and a transverse diameter of only 25 mm.[29] The articular surface of the glenoid is thicker at its peripheral margins and thinner at its center.[7] The most peripheral margin of the glenoid is slightly raised to form a rim. Attached to this rim is a fibrocartilaginous labrum. The inner surface of the labrum is covered with synovium and is continuous with the articular surface of the glenoid. The outer surface attaches to the capsule and is continuous with the periosteum of the scapular neck. The shape of the labrum changes with rotation of the humeral head, and for this reason there exists debate over the presence of the labrum and its function. Moseley and Overgaard[14] consider the labrum a redundant fold of capsular tissue. They state that the labrum is composed of dense fibrous connective tissue that is devoid of any fibrocartilage except in a small transitional zone at its site of attachment on the glenoid rim.

The superior portion of the labrum and the long head of the biceps blend together at their attachment to the supraglenoid tubercle. This labrum-tendon complex has been recognized recently as a site of pathology in shoulder instability and impingement. In a similar fashion, the long head of the triceps blends with the labrum as it attaches to the infraglenoid tubercle; however, this does not appear to be a site of mechanical stress. On the anterior aspect of the glenoid rim, the labrum passes over the glenoid notch and forms a osteofibrous tunnel through which an extension of the synovial capsule may communicate with the subscapularis bursa.[7]

## CAPSULE

The capsule of the glenohumeral joint completely encircles the articulation. It is attached to the entire circumference of the glenoid cavity just medial to the glenoid rim and extends across the entire articulation to anchor firmly onto the anatomic neck of the humerus. In general, the capsule is a loose and redundant structure, stated to be twice the surface area of the humeral head.[23] The capsule is thickest in its superior and inferior extents. At its superior attachment on the humeral head it encroaches on the articular cartilage much more closely than at any other point. The capsule also extends down the length of the intertubercular groove. The inferior capsule extends for a considerable distance onto the shaft of the humerus and presents with a redundant fold (see Fig. 1-33c). Obliteration of this fold in the capsule has been implicated as a cause of adhesive capsulitis.[19]

## SYNOVIAL MEMBRANE

The capsule is lined throughout by a synovial membrane that is reflected inferiorly along the anatomic neck of the humerus, blending with hyaline cartilage of the humeral head. Proximally, the capsule extends for varying distances over the glenoid labrum, blending with its superficial fibers but not reaching the articular surface of the glenoid. In the anterior region, the synovial membrane is loose, redundant, and extends along the anterior surface of the neck of the scapula as far as the root of the coracoid process. The synovial membrane is also prolonged distally to line the bicipital groove, where it is reflected over the biceps tendon.

## SYNOVIAL RECESSES

Synovial recesses are often present in the anterior portion of the capsule (81.8 percent).[5] The most frequent opening is located between the superior and middle ligaments. When this opening is present, the anterior capsule communicates with the subscapularis and subcoracoid bursae. The number and location of recesses in the shoulder can vary considerably. Moseley and Overgaard[14] identified four variations in the anterior capsule, and DePalma[5] classified six (Fig. 1-34). DePalma observed that the number and size of the recesses depended to a certain extent on where the synovial capsule began. When the capsule begins close to the labrum and glenoid rim, the number and size of the recesses are less. When the capsule originates more medially on the neck of the glenoid, the recesses are generally more numerous and larger. He speculates that shoulders with a larger capsule and more numerous recesses are predisposed to instability.

## LIGAMENTS

The anterior aspect of the capsule is reinforced by three thickenings referred to as the *glenohumeral ligaments*. The ligaments are named in relation to their location on the anterior capsule: superior, middle, and inferior.

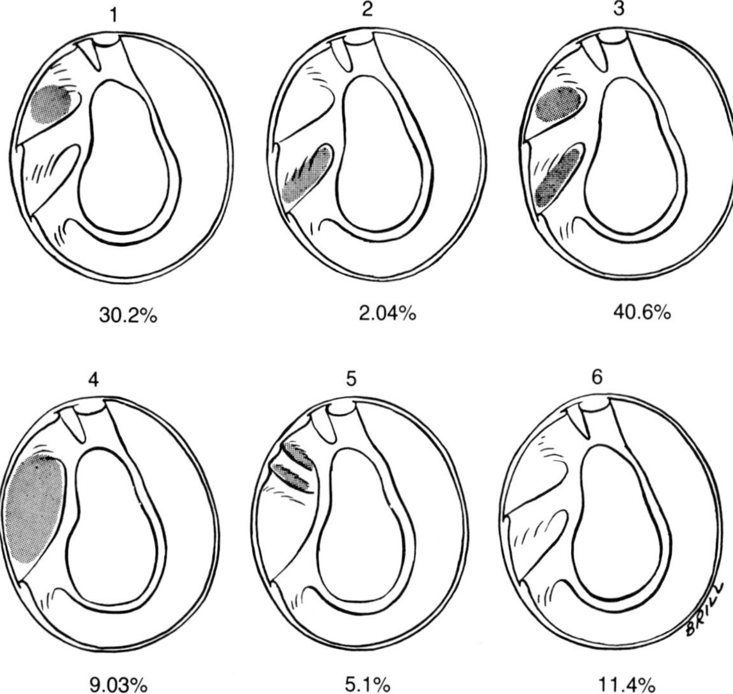


**Figure 1-34.** Six types of arrangement of the synovial recesses, and their incidence: (1) Characterized by one synovial recess above the middle glenohumeral ligament. (2) One synovial recess below the glenohumeral ligament. (3) Two synovial recesses: a superior subscapular recess above the glenohumeral ligament, and an inferior subscapular recess below the glenohumeral ligament. (4) One large synovial recess above the inferior glenohumeral ligament; the middle glenohumeral ligament is absent. (5) The middle ligament exists as two small synovial folds. (6) Complete absence of synovial recesses. (From Depalma AF. Surgery of the shoulder. 3rd ed. Philadelphia: JB Lippincott, 1983.)

**Superior Glenohumeral Ligament**

The superior ligament blends with the labrum and biceps tendon on the superior rim of the glenoid near the upper pole of the glenoid fossa and the base of the coracoid process. The ligament extends to the fovea capitis of the humerus adjacent and just superior to the lesser tuberosity in conjunction with the coracohumeral ligament. Testut[32] states that the ligament is directed transversely and lies slightly anterior to and underneath the coracohumeral ligament, inserting into the anatomic neck between the upper segment of the lesser tuberosity and the articular surface. O'Brien and coworkers[21] have described three common variations in the origin of the superior glenohumeral ligament (Fig. 1-35). DePalma[5] noted in 73 of 96 specimens that the superior glenohumeral ligament is attached to the biceps tendon, labrum, and middle glenohumeral ligament. In 20 of the specimens the ligament attached to the biceps tendon and labrum, and in one the ligament attached to the biceps tendon alone. Other investigators have noted the presence of the superior ligament as well. Schlemm considered it to be a deeper portion of the coracohumeral ligament, and Welcher and others compared it with the ligamentum teres and round ligament of the hip joint, occasionally referring to it as "Flood's ligament."[7] According to DePalma,[5] of the three ligaments, the superior is the most constant, being present in 94 of 96 specimens studied. In a more recent investiga-

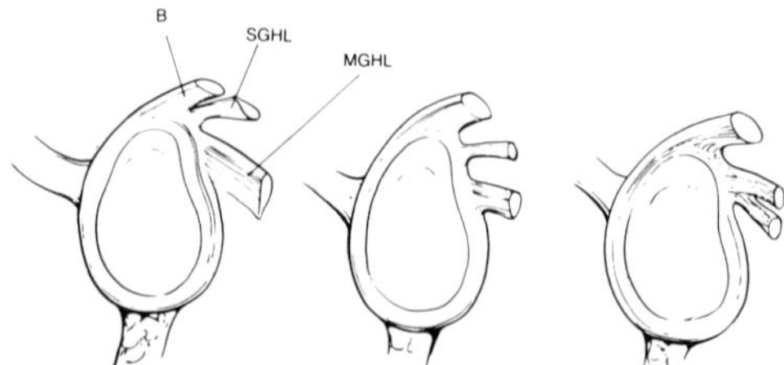


**Figure 1-35.** Three common variations of the origin of the superior glenohumeral ligament (SGHL). B, biceps tendon; MGHL, middle glenohumeral ligament. (From Rockwood C, Matsen F. The shoulder. Vol. 1. Philadelphia: WB Saunders, 1990:18.)

tion, O'Brien et al.[21] noted its presence to be approximately 90 percent.

The most important feature of this structure's anatomy is its relationship to the biceps tendon and superior labrum. The region where these structures are united to one another represents an area of mechanical stress. DePalma[5] noted that the labrum in this area demonstrated a tendency to be pulled away from the glenoid rim in specimens as young as 20 years of age. Furthermore, he noted that the frequency and severity of this abnormality increase with age. He speculated that the reason for this may be due in part to the superior ligament and biceps tendon exerting a distracting force on the labrum, pulling it away from the glenoid rim. Recently, this pathologic entity has gained attention, possibly in conjunction with advanced technology in arthroscopic surgery. Refer to Chapters 3 and 4 for further information on these lesions.

### Middle Glenohumeral Ligament

The middle glenohumeral ligament, when present, usually arises from the labrum just inferior to the attachment of the superior ligament. Turkel et al.[33] described the origin as extending from the superior aspect of the glenoid rim to the region between the middle and inferior thirds of the rim. The ligament then courses in an oblique direction downwardly and laterally and gradually enlarges to insert just medial to the lesser tuberosity. Near its point of insertion, the ligament lies either beneath or adherent to the subscapularis tendon. DePalma[5] noted a considerable degree of variation in the specimens he studied. The ligament was easily identifiable in 68 percent, poorly defined in 16 percent, and absent in 12 percent. O'Brien and coworkers[21] reported that the ligament was absent in 27 percent of the specimens they studied. Both these groups state that the ligament demonstrates a considerable degree of variation in size. Occasionally, the ligament presents as a double thickening on the anterior capsule with no attachment to the labrum. In other specimens, the size of the ligament varied from a thin wisp to a well-defined, thick structure resembling the long head of the biceps.[23] When the ligament is well defined, it does provide a significant restraint to anterior translation of the humeral head, especially when the anterior portion of the inferior glenohumeral ligament is damaged.[21]

### Inferior Glenohumeral Ligament

The inferior glenohumeral ligament is receiving greater attention lately, and its significance in instability is gaining further appreciation. DePalma[5] described this ligament as a triangular structure arising from the glenoid labrum and blending with the anterior capsule in the region between the subscapularis and the triceps tendons. He characterized this ligament as an indistinct diffuse thickening of the capsule well noted in 54 specimens, poorly defined in 18, and absent in 24. Turkel et al.[33] described this ligament as having a superior band consisting of a thickened anterosuperior edge, an anterior axillary pouch, and a posterior axillary pouch. Others have described the inferior glenohumeral ligament as having an anterior band, a posterior band, and an axillary pouch. They describe the origin of the bands from the glenoid rim in terms of the face of a clock, the anterior band originating from various positions between 2 and 4 o'clock and the posterior band originating between 7 and 9 o'clock. These investigators note that the method of attachment to the humeral head was one of two types. In some it was collar-like, varying in thickness and located just inferior to the articular edge (Fig. 1-36). In others the ligament demonstrated a V-shaped fashion, with the anterior and posterior bands attaching close to the articular surface and the axillary pouch attaching to the humerus at the apex of the V, further from the articular edge. If one can imagine the axillary pouch as a hammock with the anterior and posterior bands being the strong, thick, tight borders of the hammock, then one can better appreciate that this complex acts as a sling to support the head of the humerus. The anterior and posterior bands of this complex

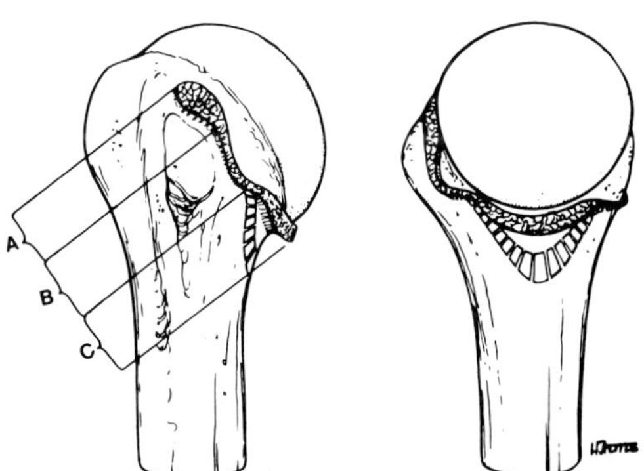


**Figure 1-36.** The attachment sites of the glenohumeral ligaments. *Left*, the superior glenohumeral ligament inserts into the fovea capitis line just superior to the lesser tuberosity (a). The middle glenohumeral ligament inserts into the humerus just medial to the lesser tuberosity (b). The inferior glenohumeral ligament complex has two common attachment mechanisms (c). It may attach in a collar-like fashion, or it may have a V-shaped attachment to the articular edge (*right*). (From Rockwood C, Matsen F. The shoulder. Vol. 1. Philadelphia: WB Saunders, 1990:16.)

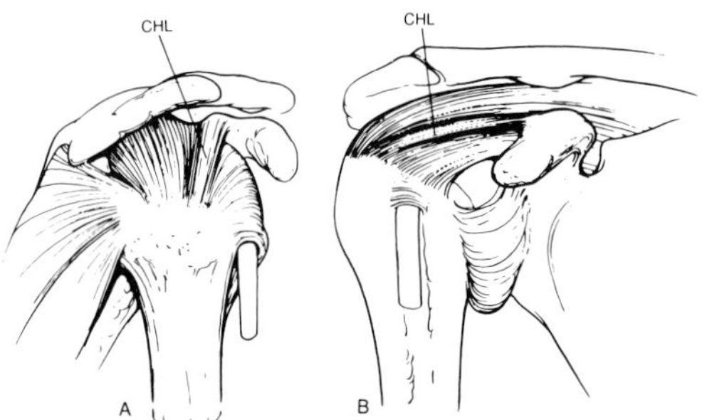


**Figure 1-37.** (a,b) The coracohumeral ligament (CHL) is a strong band originating from the base of the lateral border of the coracoid process, just below the coracoacromial ligament and merging with the capsule laterally to insert on the greater tuberosity. This ligament may have importance as a suspensory structure for the adducted arm. (From Rockwood C, Matsen F. The shoulder. Vol. 1. Philadelphia: WB Saunders, 1990:16.)

show great variation in thickness, but these investigators have been able to identify them in all specimens. When noted to be a distinct structure, this capsuloligamentous complex is the largest and strongest of the three glenohumeral ligaments.

The stability of the glenohumeral joint is dependent on all the capsuloligamentous structures. Failure in part or in whole of any one of these structures adversely affects shoulder function. Chapters 2 through 4 discuss this in greater detail.

### Coracohumeral Ligament

The coracohumeral ligament is described as a strong band extending from base and lateral border of the coracoid process, just below the coracoacromial ligament, to the greater tuberosity of the humeral head (Fig. 1-37). The anterior surface of the ligament is rather distinct, but as one moves laterally, the ligament blends with the capsule. The posterior surface of the ligament is virtually indistinguishable from the capsule. Resection of this ligament is often performed for decompression of the subcoracoacromial space. For more details on the significance of this ligament, refer to Chapters 2 and 4.

### Transverse Humeral Ligament

The transverse humeral ligament crosses the intertubercular groove and effectively controls the position of the long head of biceps. The fibers of this ligament cross from the lesser to the greater tuberosity in a transverse fashion, and the thickness and width of the ligament vary from one individual to the next.

## ROTATOR INTERVAL

Nobuhara and Ikeeda[20] in 1980 described the anterior capsule as having an interval between the tendons of the supraspinatus and subscapularis. In this region lies the superior glenohumeral ligament, coracohumeral ligament, biceps tendon, and middle glenohumeral ligament. Some surgeons consider this an area of structural weakness and advocate obliterating it during surgical reconstruction for anterior instability.[20,26]

## BURSAE

There are said to be approximately 50 named bursae in the body, and several important ones exist in the shoulder region. Codman[3] names 13 within the shoulder region (Fig. 1-38). He states that the bursae should not be regarded as simply "sacs filled with fluid found in various places where friction occurs between different layers or structures." Rather, he describes them as "spaceless spaces, not filled with fluid, but supplied with a most wonderful self-oiling mechanism, such that their walls glide on one another with their surfaces no farther apart than the thickness of the thinnest sheet of paper."[3] The ana-

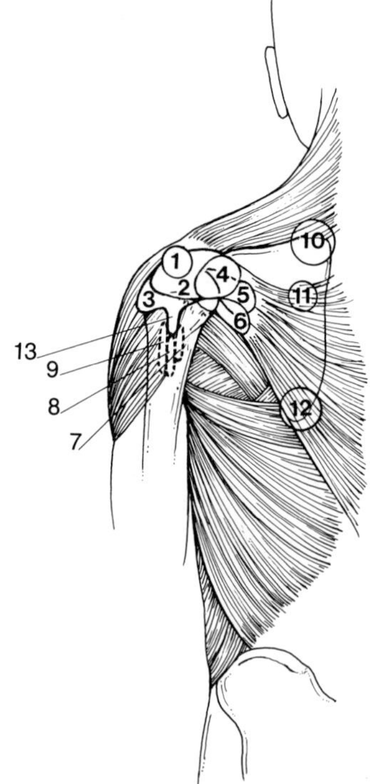


**Figure 1-38.** Normal bursae about the shoulder. 1, subcutaneous acromial bursa; 2, subacromial bursa; 3, subdeltoid bursa; 4, bursa of the coracobrachialis muscle; 5, bursa of the infraspinatus muscle; 6, subscapular bursa; 7, bursa of the latissimus dorsi; 8, bursa of the teres major. Codman states that the bursae numbered 2, 3, and 4 are essentially one bursa, although they are often separated by thin films of tissue. Numbers 5, and 6 are actually extensions of the joint, as is 13, which is a synovial lining of the bicipital groove. The bursae numbered 9, 10, 11, and 12 are inconstant and have no official anatomic names. (Adapted from Codman EA. The shoulder. Boston: Thomas Todd, 1934.)

tomic dissection he describes is outstanding and lends convincing proof to his understanding of shoulder anatomy.

### SUBDELTOID BURSA

Codman considered the subdeltoid bursa to be the largest in the human body and quite complex. He refers to it as a secondary scapulohumeral joint and notes that the subdeltoid, subacromial, and subcoracoid bursae are one and the same. He states that on occasion a thin membrane of synovium may seem to separate the three portions. He states that the size of the bursa is better appreciated by observing its different components during passive movement. He points out that filling the bursa with any material causes the periphery of the bursa to contract, effectively reducing the expansiveness of its natural state. The bursa consists of a roof and a base.

> Its base is firmly attached to the upper and outer three-fourths inch of the greater tuberosity, as well as to about three-fourths of an inch of the rotator cuff tendons where they attach to the tuberosities. Part of its base covers the bicipital groove. The roof firmly attaches to the undersurface of the acromion, the undersurface of the coracoacromial ligament, and to the fibers of origin of the deltoid from the edge of the acromion. The periphery extends loosely downward under the deltoid, backward and outward under the acromion, inward under the coracoid, between it and the subscapularis, and under the common origin of the short head of the biceps and the coracobrachialis.[3]

The roof and base are in intimate contact with one another, and they are lined by a thin, nearly transparent synovial membrane that secretes enough synovial fluid to permit near frictionless movement. Codman[3] noted that beneath this membrane existed a very fine network of blood vessels that permit the synovial membrane to increase or decrease its secretions as needed. He speculated further that this arrangement also permits the bursa to become congested rather quickly when irritated. The subacromial bursa is an essential component of the glenohumeral joint, and when this structure is inflamed, it can lead to a significant loss of motion.

### SUBSCAPULARIS BURSA

The subscapularis bursa lies between the subscapularis tendon and the neck of the scapula. It is important to distinguish this bursa from the subcoracoid bursa. The subcoracoid bursa lies under the coracoid process and on top of the subscapularis tendon, whereas this bursa lies underneath the subscapularis tendon and may communicate freely with the glenohumeral joint through the openings between the superior and middle glenohumeral ligaments. The bursa's primary function is to protect the subscapularis tendon as it passes under the base of the coracoid process and over the neck of the scapula. On occasion, loose bodies are noted in this structure, and it is often involved in synovitis of the shoulder.

### INFRASPINATUS BURSA

On occasion, a bursa exists between the tendon of the infraspinatus and the joint capsule; however, in this situation, there does not appear to be open communication between the bursa and the capsule. Codman[3] considered both the infraspinatus and subscapularis bursae to be extensions and reinforcements of the joint capsule noticeable at rest but obliterated with movements of internal and external rotation. Similar forms of bursae are also noted near the insertion sites of the teres major, latissimus dorsi, and pectoralis major muscles.

### SCAPULAR BURSAE

The scapula has a varying number of bursae associated with it: a subtrapezoid bursa located beneath the upper trapezius at its insertion on the superior angle, an infraserratus bursa located between the inferior angle of the scapula and the chest wall, and a subscapular bursa between the anterior surface of the scapula and the posterior surface of the first three ribs. Surgeons have attributed subscapular crepitus to involvement in one or more of these bursae. Codman openly challenged the surgeons of his time who sought to attribute painful crepitus to disorders of these bursae and questioned treating these patients surgically. Other bursae have been noted between the coracoid process and the pectoralis minor, between the subcutaneous tissue of the skin and the acromion, and between the latissimus dorsi and the inferior angle of the scapula.[3,7]

# Myology: Anatomy of Shoulder Musculature

## MUSCLES OF THE TRUNK

Muscles of the trunk that are considered muscles of the shoulder region include the trapezius, latissimus dorsi, levator scapulae, rhomboid minor, and rhomboid major muscles (Fig. 1-39).

### TRAPEZIUS

The trapezius is a broad, flat, triangular muscle located immediately beneath the skin and superficial fascia of the upper and posterior aspects of the cervical spine, thoracic spine, and shoulders. This paired muscle arises from the external oc-

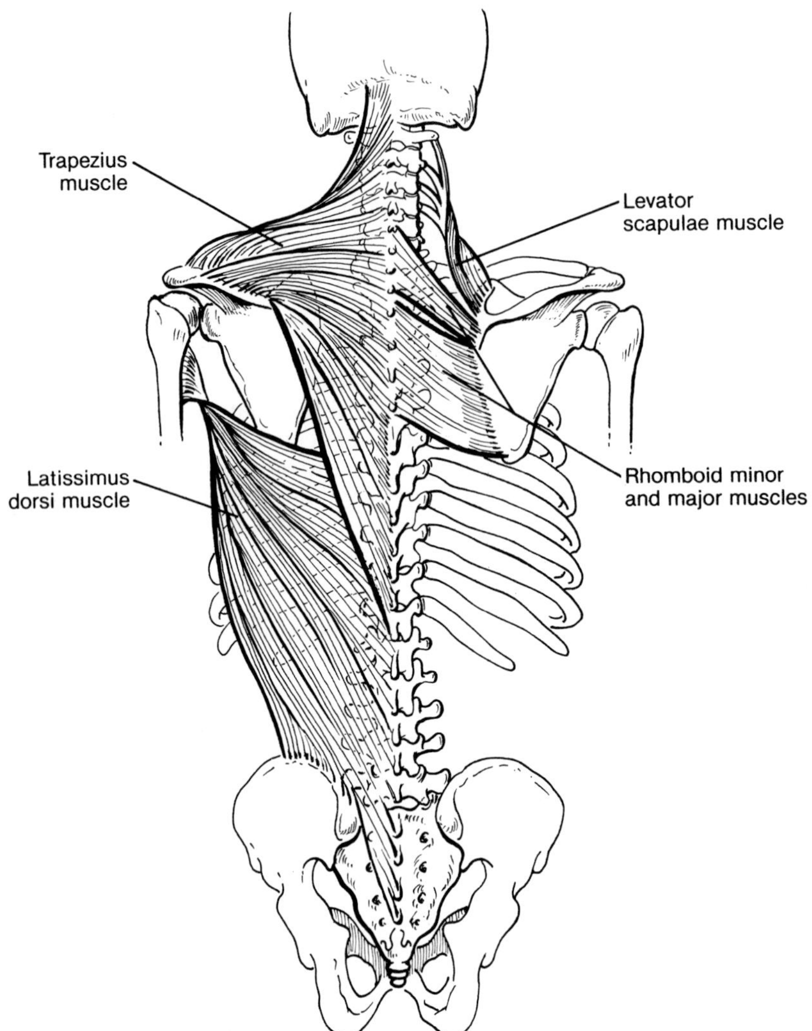


**Figure 1-39.** Muscles of the trunk. (From Pratt NE. Clinical musculoskeletal anatomy. Philadelphia: JB Lippincott, 1991.)

cipital protuberance and inner third of the superior nuchal line of the occipital bone, ligamentum nuchae, and spinous processes of the seventh cervical and all thoracic vertebrae. The muscle is divided into the upper, middle, and lower fibers. The upper fibers proceed in an outward and downward direction to insert on the posterior border of the distal third of the clavicle. The middle fibers proceed in a horizontal direction to insert on the inner margin of the acromion process and superior aspect of the spine of the scapula. The lower fibers proceed in upward and outward direction and merge with one another to form a triangular aponeurosis that inserts into a tubercle on the external surface of the scapula near the meeting of the spine and superior angle. If the trapezius is dissected out on both sides, the two muscles together resemble a diamond-shaped quadrangle, two angles corresponding to the shoulders, a third to the occipital protuberance, and the fourth to the last thoracic vertebra. For the most part, the muscle consists of fleshy tissue, with tendinous tissue noted only at its sites of attachment.[7] The undersurface of the muscle is innervated by the spinal accessory nerve and branches from the third and fourth cervical nerves. This is also the location of its blood supply, from the superior cervical artery.

## LATISSIMUS DORSI

The latissimus dorsi is a broad, flat tissue that arises by a series of tendinous fibers from the spinous processes of the last six thoracic vertebrae and through an aponeurotic attachment to the thoracolumbar fascia. By way of the fascial attachment, it is connected to the spinous processes of all lumbar and sacral vertebrae, as well as from the external lip of the iliac crest and the last three or four ribs. From this extensive origin, the fibers course in different directions. The upper fibers run in a horizontal direction, the middle fibers run in an oblique upward direction, and the lower fibers run in an upward and vertical direction. All the fibers converge to form a thick fasciculus that either attaches to or crosses over the inferior angle of the scapula. After passing the inferior angle, the tendon courses around the lower border of the teres major muscle, and on crossing the inferior capsule of the glenohumeral joint, the tendon twists on itself so that the superior fibers change their position from posterior to inferior and the vertical fibers from anterior to superior.[7] The distal end of the tendon terminates as a quadrilateral structure about 3 inches in length that passes in front of the tendon of the teres major and inserts onto the floor of the bicipital groove at a slightly higher position on the humerus than the tendon of the pectoralis major. The lower border of the tendon unites with the teres major tendon, and the two are often separated by a bursa. An additional bursa often exists between the muscle and the inferior angle of the scapula. The tendon also gives off an expansion to the deep fascia of the arm near its point of insertion. Often a muscular slip arises from the upper edge of the tendon near the posterior fold of the axilla and crosses the axilla in front of the axillary vessels and nerves to join with the undersurface of the pectoralis major tendon, the coracobrachialis tendon, or the fascia over the biceps. This muscular slip is approximately 3 to 4 inches in length and 1/4 to 3/4 inches in thickness.[7] All these expansions of the tendon suggest that the latissimus has a significant influence on the static and dynamic forces acting on the glenohumeral joint. The latissimus dorsi is innervated by the thoracodorsal nerve.

### LEVATOR SCAPULAE

The levator scapulae, located on the posterior and lateral aspect of the cervical spine, originates as a series of tendinous slips extending from the transverse processes of atlas as well as the posterior tubercles of the transverse processes of the second, third, and fourth cervical vertebrae. The tendinous slips quickly merge with the substance of the muscle to form a flat muscle that courses in a downward and backward direction. The muscle terminates on the posterior border of the scapula in a flattened area between the superior angle and the root of the scapular spine. This muscle is innervated by small nerve branches from the anterior divisions of the third and fourth cervical nerve roots as well as a branch of the dorsal scapular nerve.

### RHOMBOID MAJOR AND MINOR

The rhomboid minor, located slightly higher than the rhomboid major, arises from the ligamentum nuchae and spinous processes of the seventh cervical and first thoracic vertebrae. The tendinous portions quickly develop into fleshy fibers that course in an outward and downward direction and unite with the fibers of the rhomboid major. The rhomboid minor inserts into the smooth triangular surface of the scapula at the root of the scapular spine.

The rhomboid major, located immediately below the rhomboid minor, arises by tendinous slips from the spinous processes of the first four or five thoracic vertebrae. The tendons quickly merge into fleshy fibers of muscle tissue that course in an outward and upward direction to insert into a narrow tendinous arch that extends from the root of the spine to the superior angle. The musculotendinous fibers often extend onto the body of the scapula itself. Both the minor and major are innervated by the dorsal scapular nerve.

## MUSCLES OF THE UPPER EXTREMITY

The muscles of the upper extremity that function at the shoulder are divided into the following groups: anterior thoracic region, lateral thoracic region, acromial region, anterior and posterior scapular regions, and anterior and posterior humeral regions.

### ANTERIOR THORACIC REGION

#### Pectoralis Major

The pectoralis major is a broad, thick, triangular muscle that originates from the anterior surface of the sternum, the anterior surface of the sternal half of the clavicle, and the cartilages of the first six or seven ribs, and by way of aponeurotic expansions, the muscle blends with the fibers of the opposite pectoralis major and the external oblique of the same side (Fig. 1-40). The clavicular fibers pass in an oblique downward and outward direction. The fibers from the lower ribs and lower half of the sternum pass upward and outward, and those from the middle of the sternum pass in a horizontal direction. All the fibers converge to form a large, flattened tendon that is approximately 2 inches in width.[7] This tendon attaches by way of a broad insertion into the lateral lip of the bicipital groove.

The construction of this muscle's tendon of

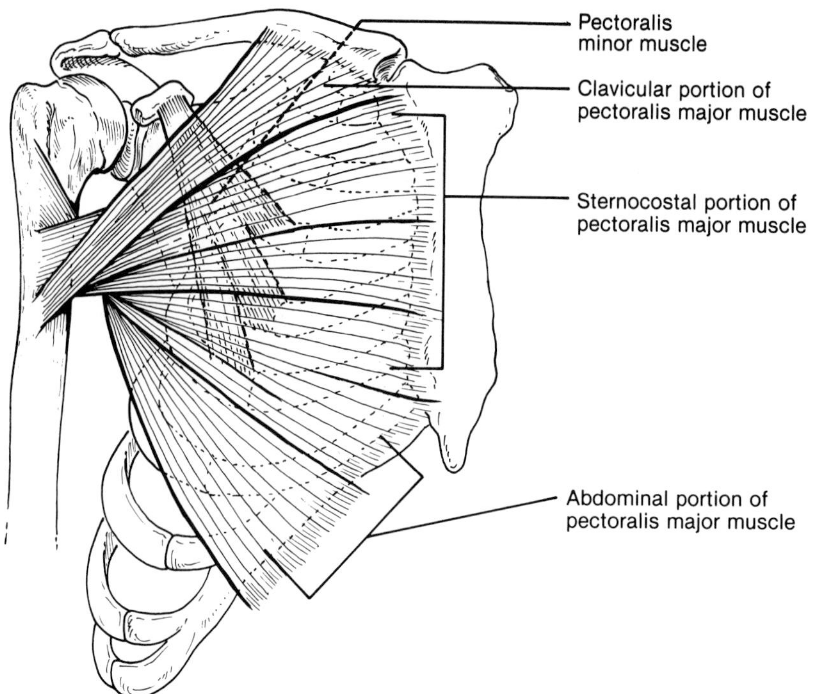


**Figure 1-40.** The pectoralis major and minor. (From Pratt NE. Clinical musculoskeletal anatomy. Philadelphia: JB Lippincott, 1991.)

insertion is unique. The tendon consists of two laminae, one placed in front of the other and blended together at its lowest portion.[7] The anterior lamina, which is the thickest of the two, receives the fibers from the clavicle and the upper half of the sternum and ribs. The posterior lamina receives the fibers from the lower half of the sternum and the deeper fibers from the costal cartilages. These two sets of fibers blend with the posterior lamina in such a way as to twist so that the deeper fibers and those from the lower costal cartilages turn backward successively behind the superficial ones. The posterior lamina inserts higher up on the humerus than the anterior lamina, and in addition to inserting into the bicipital lip, it also gives off an expansion that effectively covers the bicipital groove and blends with the glenohumeral joint capsule.

The pectoralis major helps to define the axilla by forming the anterior wall of the axillary space and providing cover for the axillary vessels and nerves, as well as the coracobrachialis and biceps muscles. The upper-most border of this muscle lies nearly parallel to the deltoid, being separated by only a slight interspace in which lies deeply the cephalic vein and the humeral branch of the acromial thoracic artery.[7] The lower border of this muscle forms the anterior margin of the axilla, and at first, this border is clearly separated from the latissimus dorsi by a considerable distance, but as these two tendons approach their respective sites of insertion, they converge towards one another.

#### Pectoralis Minor

The pectoralis minor is a thin, flat, triangular muscle located in the upper part of the thorax that lies deep to the pectoralis major and is separated from it by the costocoracoid membrane. This muscle arises by way of three tendinous digitations from the third, fourth, and fifth ribs near their costal cartilages and from a strong aponeurosis covering the intercostal muscles. The fibers run in an oblique direction sharply upward and slightly outward. They merge with one another to form a flattened tendon that inserts on the inner border and upper surface of the coracoid process. The axillary artery and vein as well as the cords of the brachial plexus lie directly beneath the tendon of the pectoralis minor. This region can present with neurovascular compromise due to tightness of the pectoralis minor and related connective tissue.

The pectoralis major and minor muscles are innervated by the medial and lateral pectoral nerves, which receive nerve branches from all the spinal nerves that contribute to the brachial plexus.[7] The pectoralis minor receives its innervation from the medial pectoral branch, and the pectoralis major receives its innervation from both the medial and lateral pectoral branches.

### Subclavius

The subclavius is a small, triangular muscle situated in the space between the undersurface of the clavicle and the uppermost surface of the first rib. It arises by a short, thick tendon from the first rib and its cartilaginous attachment to the sternum. Lying in front of the rhomboid ligament, the fibers proceed in an oblique direction upward and outward to insert in a deep groove on the undersurface of the clavicle. The subclavius is separated from the external surface of the first rib by the subclavian artery and vein and the nerves of the brachial plexus. This muscle is innervated by a specific branch from the fifth cervical spinal nerve.

## LATERAL THORACIC REGION

### Serratus Anterior

The serratus anterior is a thin, irregularly shaped quadrilateral muscle placed between the ribs and the scapula that arises by nine tendinous slips or digitations from the first eight ribs, giving the impression of a serrated edge (Fig. 1-41). These tendinous slips originate on the external surface and upper border of the first eight ribs and by an expansion to the aponeurosis covering the intercostal muscles that correspond to these ribs. From this extensive origin, the tendons give way to fibers that pass in a backward direction, lying closely adherent to the chest wall. Ultimately these fibers insert on the vertebral border of the scapula in the following manner: The first two digitations insert into a triangular area on the anterior surface of the superior angle. The next two digitations spread to form a thin, triangular sheet that inserts into nearly the whole length of the anterior surface of the vertebral border. The last five digitations form a fan-shaped structure that inserts into a triangular impression on the anterior surface of the inferior angle.[7] The serratus is innervated by the long thoracic nerve, which is formed by branches from the fifth, sixth, and seventh cervical spinal nerves.

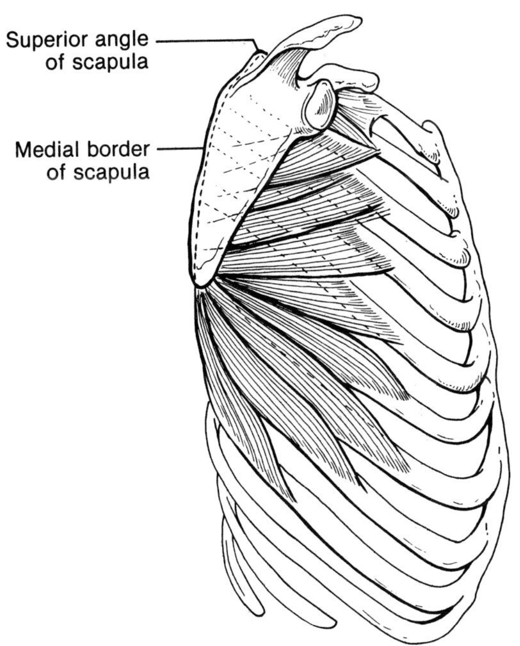


**Figure 1-41.** The serratus anterior. (From Pratt NE. Clinical musculoskeletal anatomy. Philadelphia: JB Lippincott, 1991.)

## ACROMIAL REGION

### Deltoid

The deltoid is a large, thick, triangular muscle that arises from the outer third of the anterior border and superior surface of the clavicle, from the outer margin and superior surface of the acromion process, and from the lower lip of the posterior border of the spine of the scapula. From this extensive origin, the fibers converge in the following manner: Fibers of the middle deltoid pass vertically, those of the anterior deltoid pass obliquely backward, and those of the posterior deltoid pass obliquely forward (Fig. 1-42). All the fibers unite to form a thick tendon that anchors itself strongly to the deltoid tubercle, which lies on the external surface of the humeral shaft approximately halfway down its length. Tendinous expansions also unite with the deep fascia of the arm.[7] The muscle is rather coarse in its texture, and the arrangement of the fibers is unique.

The middle fibers, especially the central portion, arise in a bipenniform manner from four tendinous intersections that arise from the acromion and pass downward parallel to each other within the substance of the muscle. The oblique fibers then insert into three tendinous intersections that pass upward from the deltoid insertion. The tendinous portions of the middle deltoid alternate with one another by way of intramuscular septa within the substance of the muscle belly. The fibers of the anterior and posterior deltoid, not arranged in such an elaborate manner, pass directly from their points of origin to their point of insertion.[7] The deltoid is innervated by the axillary nerve.

## ANTERIOR SCAPULAR REGION

### Subscapularis

The subscapularis a large, triangular muscle that arises from the anterior surface of the scapula (Fig. 1-43). The tendon of origin begins on the

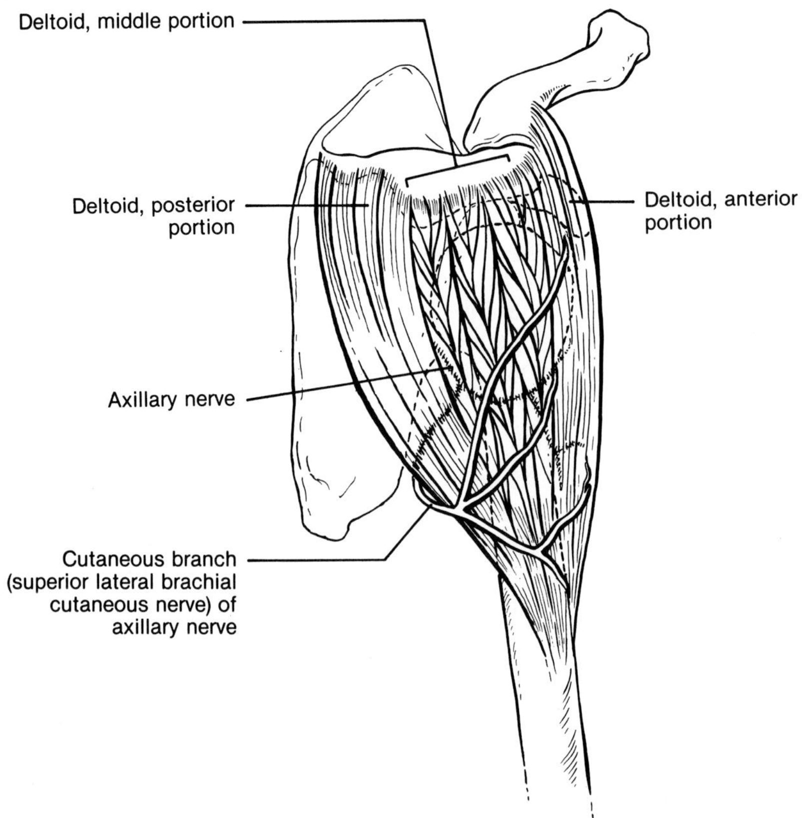


**Figure 1-42.** The deltoid. (From Pratt NE. Clinical musculoskeletal anatomy. Philadelphia: JB Lippincott, 1991.)

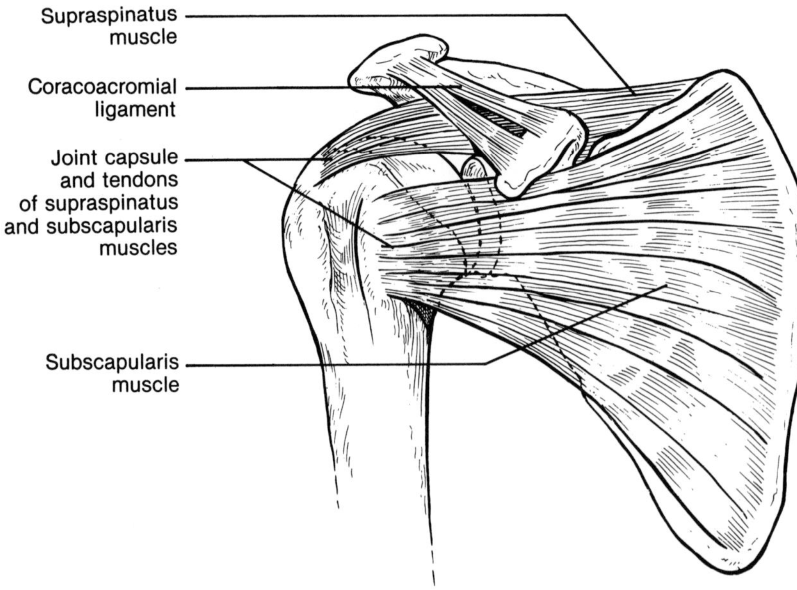


**Figure 1-43.** The subscapularis. (From Pratt NE. Clinical musculoskeletal anatomy. Philadelphia: JB Lippincott, 1991.)

medial two-thirds of the anterior surface as well as the anterior surfaces of the inferior and superior angles and the lower two-thirds of the axillary border. Some of the fibers arise from tendinous laminae that intersect the muscle and attach to ridges on the surface of the scapula. Other fibers arise from an aponeurosis that separates the subscapularis from the teres major and the long head of the triceps.[7] Before becoming a tendon, the anterior surface of the subscapularis forms a considerable part of the posterior wall of the axilla. In doing so, it effectively provides a floor for the tendons of the coracobrachialis, biceps, and serratus anterior, as well as the axillary vessels and nerves of the brachial plexus. The lower border of the subscapularis is continuous with the teres major and latissimus dorsi muscles. All the fibers pass in an outward direction and eventually merge to terminate in a single tendon of insertion. The tendon of the subscapularis passes over the anterior capsule of the glenohumeral joint, is firmly anchored to the lesser tuberosity of the humerus, and effectively forms the anterior component of the rotator cuff. This muscle is supplied by the upper and lower subscapular nerves, which receive their nerve bundles from the fifth and sixth cervical nerves.

## POSTERIOR SCAPULAR REGION

### Supraspinatus

The supraspinatus muscle located within the supraspinous fossa is encased in a dense, thick fascial sleeve. The supraspinous fascia, together with the fossa, forms a fibro-osseous tunnel. The fibers of the supraspinatus arise from the medial two-thirds of the floor of the fossa and the internal surface of the fascia. The muscular fibers converge to a tendon that passes through the supraspinatus outlet formed by the coracoacromial arch and the superior aspect of the glenohumeral joint. The tendon passes over and is intimately adherent to the superior portion of the capsule. It effectively forms the superior portion of the rotator cuff and then extends to firmly anchor itself to the highest facet on the greater tuberosity of the humerus (Fig. 1-44). The tendon is flattened but of considerable thickness in a healthy state. Its attachment to the greater tuberosity is strengthened by having a broad site of insertion. In addition to this, the point of insertion is further strengthened by having a transitional zone that transforms itself from fibrous tissue to fibrocartilaginous to cartilaginous and ultimately to osseous tissue.[3] The supraspinatus

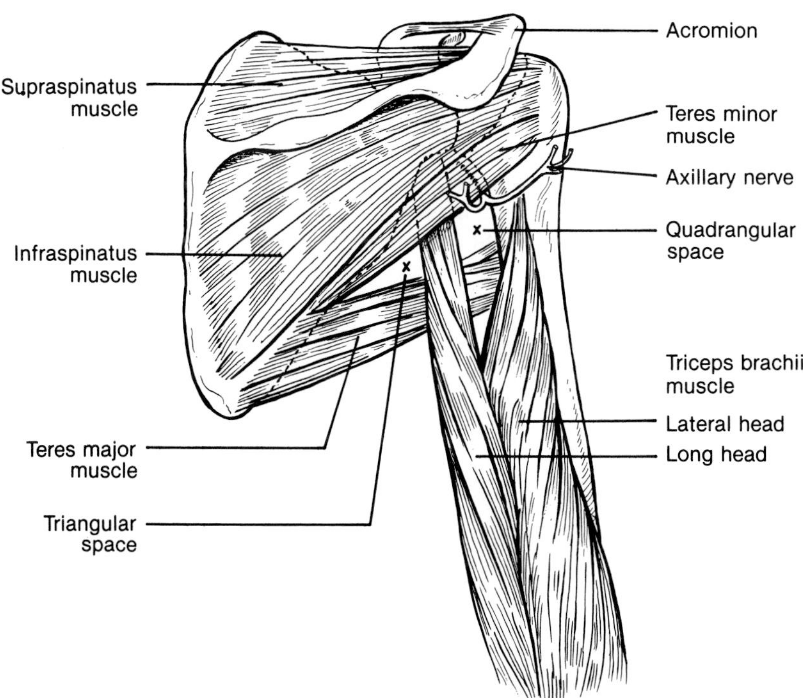


**Figure 1-44.** The supraspinatus, infraspinatus, and teres minor muscles. (From Pratt NE. Clinical musculoskeletal anatomy. Philadelphia: JB Lippincott, 1991.)

receives its innervation from the suprascapular nerve and its blood supply from the suprascapular artery.

**Infraspinatus**

The infraspinatus is a thick, triangular muscle that arises by way of fleshy fibers from the internal two-thirds of the posterior surface of the scapula and by way of tendinous fibers from the ridges on the posterior surface. The infraspinatus, like the supraspinatus, is covered by a dense fibrous membrane, and some of the muscle fibers adhere to the undersurface of this fascia. This fascia separates the infraspinatus from the teres minor and major muscles. Where the infraspinatus is covered by the posterior deltoid, the fascia divides into two layers, one that passes over the deltoid and blends with the deltoid fascia and another that passes beneath the deltoid and lies over the glenohumeral joint.[7] The fibers of the infraspinatus converge to a single tendon that glides over the external border of the spine of the scapula, passes over the posterior part of the glenohumeral joint capsule, and inserts into the middle facet of the greater tuberosity of the humerus. On occasion, the tendon is separated from the spine of the scapula by a bursa that may or may not communicate with the synovial cavity of the glenohumeral joint. After the suprascapular nerve courses along the undersurface of the supraspinatus, it passes through the spinoglenoid notch to innervate the infraspinatus.

**Teres Minor**

The teres minor is a narrow, elongated muscle that arises from the dorsal surface of the axillary border of the scapula and from two laminae, each of which separates the teres minor from the teres major and the infraspinatus. The fibers pass obliquely upward and outward to terminate as a broad, flattened tendon that inserts on the lower facet of the greater tuberosity as well as the shaft of the humerus immediately below the tuberosity. The tendon passes directly over and is intimately adherent to the posterior capsule of the glenohumeral joint. The teres minor is innervated by the posterior division of the axillary nerve after the nerve passes through the quadrangular space.

**Teres Major**

The teres major is a thick but relatively flattened muscle that arises from an oval-shaped surface on the dorsal aspect of the inferior angle of the scapula as well as from a fibrous septum that lies between it and the teres minor and the infraspinatus. The fibers are directed in a upward and outward direction and terminate in a flat tendon that passes inferior to the glenohumeral joint lying behind the tendon of the latissimus dorsi muscle. On occasion, the tendons of the teres major and latissimus dorsi are separated by a bursa; however, for a considerable extent, the two tendons are united to one another. The tendon of the teres major is roughly 2 in in length and is inserted into the medial lip of the bicipital groove of the humerus. The teres major is innervated by the lower subscapular nerve.

## ANTERIOR HUMERAL REGION

**Coracobrachialis**

The coracobrachialis is located at the upper and medial part of the arm and arises by fleshy fibers from the apex of the coracoid process in common with the short head of the biceps and from the intermuscular septum located between these two muscles. The fibers pass in a downward, backward, and outward direction to terminate in a flat tendon that inserts onto an impression on the medial surface of the shaft of the humerus between the origins of the triceps and the brachialis anticus (Fig. 1-45). The coracobrachialis is innervated by the musculocutaneous nerve, which receives its supply primarily from the seventh cervical nerve.

**Biceps Brachii**

The biceps brachii is a long, fusiform muscle that consists of two heads. The short head arises by a thick, flattened tendon from the apex of the coracoid process in conjunction with the coracobrachialis. The long head arises from the upper-most margin of the glenoid fossa on a prominence known as the *supraglenoid tubercle*. The tendon of the long head shares a point of origin with the superior glenohumeral ligament and glenoid labrum. From its point of origin, the long head arcs over the head of the humerus in a self-contained synovial sheath that is an extension of the synovial membrane of the glenohumeral joint. The posterior surface of the long tendon lies against the superior and superomedial aspects of the humeral head as well as the anteromedial aspect of the humeral head and neck. The tendon passes through an opening in the capsule of the glenohumeral joint and descends the shaft of the humerus in a groove created by elongations of the greater and lesser tuberosities. The tendon is retained within the groove by the transverse humeral ligament, a fibrous band from the tendon of the pectoralis major. Each tendon then proceeds to an elongated muscle belly. Each muscle belly remains a separate entity until just above the elbow joint, where the two unite to form a single entity prior to the formation of a single tendon. The proximal portion of the biceps is overlapped by the pec-

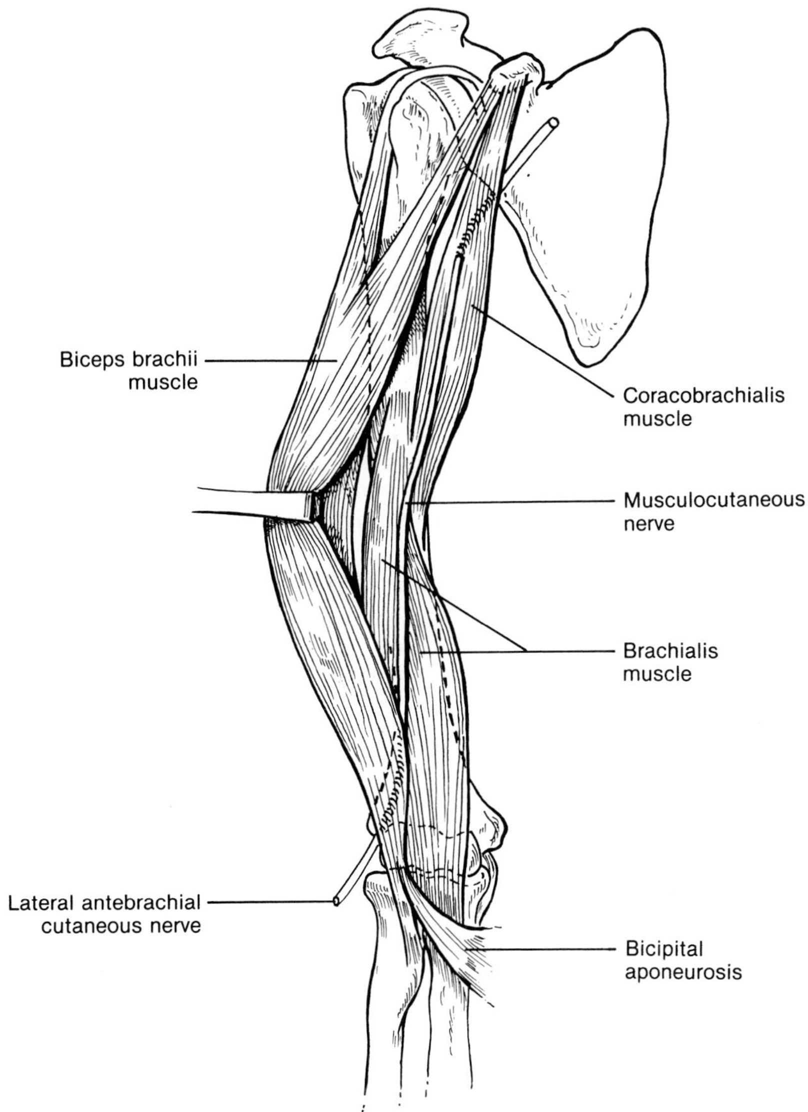


**Figure 1-45.** The biceps and coracobrachialis muscles. (From Pratt NE. Clinical musculoskeletal anatomy. Philadelphia: JB Lippincott, 1991.)

toralis major and deltoid muscles, while the rest of the muscle is covered only by superficial and deep fascia. The biceps is innervated by the musculocutaneous nerve with primary supply from the fifth and sixth cervical nerve roots.

## POSTERIOR HUMERAL REGION

### Triceps

The triceps is located on the posterior surface of the humerus, extending the entire length of the humerus. The muscle is rather large and consists of three heads referred to as long, medial, and lateral. The long head arises from the inferior surface of the glenoid cavity by way of a flat tendon that is attached to a rough triangular impression referred to as the *infraglenoid tubercle*. The long head descends between the teres minor and teres major, effectively dividing the triangular space between these two muscles and the humerus into two smaller spaces, one triangular in shape and the other quadrangular. The triangular space formed by the teres minor above, the teres major below, and the long head of the triceps laterally permits safe passage of the dorsal scapular vessels. The quadrangular space is formed by the teres minor above, the teres major below, the long head of the triceps medially, and the humerus laterally. This anatomic landmark permits passage of the posterior humeral circumflex artery and vein as well as the posterior branch of the axillary nerve. This neurovascular bundle is often tender to palpation and often can be mistaken for posterior cuff tendinitis. The medial and lateral heads arise from the posterior surface of the humerus and thus do not cross the shoulder joint. All three heads pass downward and merge with one another to form a common tendon of insertion that is firmly anchored to the olecranon process of the ulna. The triceps, primarily a powerful extensor of the elbow, also contributes to extension and horizontal abduction of the shoulder. The triceps is innervated by the radial nerve, which receives its nerve bundles from the seventh and eighth cervical nerve roots.

## Neuroanatomy: Nerves and Nerve Plexuses of the Shoulder Region

The peripheral nerves that provide innervation to the skin, fascia, muscles, bones, and joints of the shoulder region begin as either a cranial nerve, as in the case of the spinal accessory nerve, or as spinal nerves, as in the case of the cervical and brachial plexuses.

### CRANIAL NERVE XI: SPINAL ACCESSORY NERVE

Of the 12 cranial nerves, the eleventh cranial nerve, or spinal accessory nerve, is the only one to have a direct influence on the shoulder region. This nerve has two parts: the accessory and the spinal divisions. The spinal portion is the larger division and the one of concern in neuroanatomy of the shoulder.

The spinal division originates as a superficial and deep portion. The superficial portion begins as several filaments from the lateral tract of the spinal cord as low down as the sixth cervical nerve rootlets. The deep portion originates from the anteromedial-lateral tract of the spinal cord. The two portions ascend together, coursing between the ligamentum denticulatum and the posterior roots of the spinal cord. Together they enter the foramen magnum and direct themselves outward to the jugular foramen. The spinal and accessory portions pass through the jugular foramen, lying in a common sheath but separated from one another by a fold of arachnoid. While in the foramen, the spinal portion receives one or two filaments from the accessory portion. Upon exiting the foramen, the two portions separate, and the spinal portion courses in a backward direction, lying either in front of or behind the internal jugular vein. The nerve bundle descends in an oblique direction behind the digastric and stylohyoid muscles to enter the substance of the sternocleidomastoid muscle near its origin.[7] After piercing and innervating the sternocleidomastoid muscle, the nerve bundle continues in an oblique direction across the posterior triangle and terminates in the undersurface of the trapezius. The nerve yields several branches to the sternocleidomastoid, and some of these terminal branches mingle with branches from the second and third cervical nerves in the substance of this muscle. In the posterior triangle, the nerve also mingles with branches from the second and third cervical nerves, and on the undersurface of the trapezius, the branches mingle with the third and fourth cervical nerves to form a plexus that innervates the entire trapezius.[7]

### SPINAL NERVES

The spinal nerves take origin from the spinal cord and are transmitted through the intervertebral foramina on either side of the spinal column. Each spinal nerve begins as two separate rows of rootlets. The rootlets unite in groups to form a dorsal and a ventral nerve root. Within the spinal canal these two roots unite to form a mixed spinal nerve. Each spinal nerve then exits through the intervertebral foramen, and once having exited the foramen, the nerve divides again into a dorsal and a ventral nerve root. These divisions, referred to as the *anterior* and *posterior primary rami*, supply motor and sensory innervation to the anterior and posterior portions of the human body.

The posterior primary rami, generally smaller than the anterior, pass directly posterior and quickly divide into internal and external branches. Both branches innervate the musculoskeletal structures and integument of the spine.

The anterior primary rami are responsible for innervating the parts of the body in front of the spine, including the limbs. In the thoracic region, the anterior primary rami remain distinctly separate from one another and uniform in their distribution. In the cervical, lumbar, and sacral regions, however, the anterior primary rami form intricate plexuses prior to their distribution.

### CERVICAL PLEXUS

The cervical plexus is formed by the anterior divisions of the first four cervical nerves (Fig. 1-46). The plexus is situated opposite the first four cervical vertebrae, lying on the external surface of the levator scapula and scalenus medius

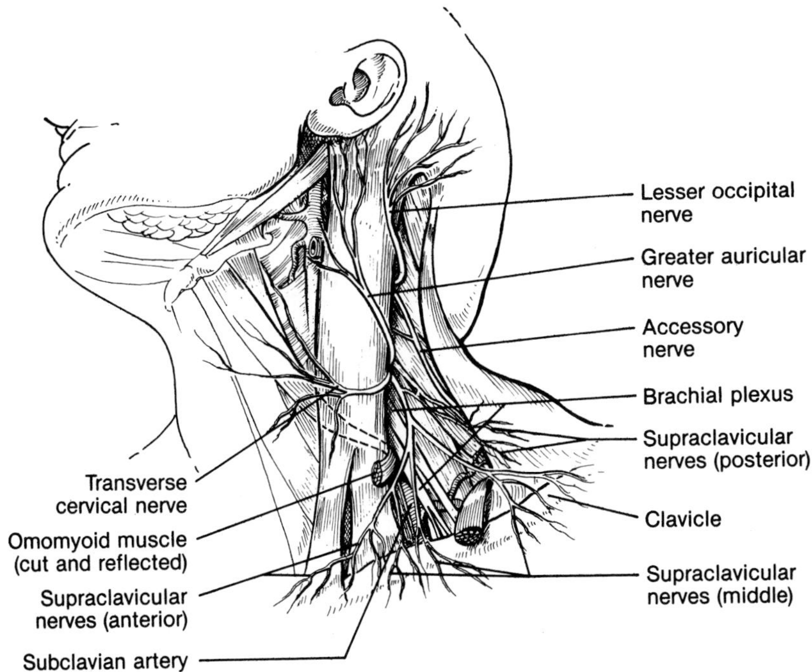


**Figure 1-46.** The cervical plexus and the supraclavicular nerves. (From Pratt NE. Clinical musculoskeletal anatomy. Philadelphia: JB Lippincott, 1991.)

muscles and protectively covered by the sternocleidomastoid muscle.[7] The branches of the plexus can be divided into superficial and deep branches. The superficial branches are further divided into the ascending and descending branches. There are three ascending branches, the occipitalis minor, auricularis magnus, and superficialis colli, and one descending branch, the supraclavicular. Only the supraclavicular branch has a direct influence on the shoulder region.

## SUPRACLAVICULAR NERVE

The supraclavicular branch arises from the third and fourth cervical nerves. It emerges from beneath the posterior border of the sternocleidomastoid muscle and then descends in the posterior triangle beneath the platysma and the deep cervical fascia. Near the clavicle it perforates the fascia and platysma to become cutaneous (see Fig. 1-46). At this point, the branch divides into three groups: suprasternal (medial), supraclavicular (intermediate), and supraacromial (lateral). The suprasternal branches cross obliquely over the external jugular vein and the insertion of the sternocleidomastoid on the clavicle and sternum. These branches innervate the sternoclavicular joint. The supraclavicular branches cross the clavicle and supply the integument over the deltoid and pectoral muscles. The supraacromial branches pass obliquely across the external surface of the trapezius and the acromion and innervate the integument over the superior and posterior part of the shoulder.[7]

The deep branches of the cervical plexus can be divided into the internal and external branches. The internal branches consist of the communicating branches, muscular branches, a communicating branch to the hypoglossal nerve, and a communicating branch to the phrenic nerve. The external branches include communicating branches and muscular branches. The external branches have a direct influence on the shoulder region and are reviewed in greater detail.

The communicating branches lie within the substance of the sternocleidomastoid, in the posterior triangle, and underneath the trapezius. These nerves communicate with the spinal accessory nerve. The muscular branches are distributed to the sternocleidomastoid, trapezius, levator scapulae, and scalenus medius muscles. The sternocleidomastoid is innervated principally by the second cervical nerve, the trapezius and levator scapulae are innervated principally by the third and fourth cervical nerves, and the scalenus medius is innervated by the third or fourth cervical nerves and on occasion by both levels.[7]

## BRACHIAL PLEXUS

The brachial plexus is formed by the union of the anterior divisions of the lower four cervical nerves and the greater part of the first thoracic nerve. In most situations, there is also a small fasciculus from the fourth cervical nerve and on occasion a small contribution from the second thoracic nerve. The plexus extends from the lower part of the cervical spine to the axilla. Where it begins, it is quite broad and does not resemble a plexus but rather a series of nerve roots (Fig. 1-47). It is narrower where it lies opposite the clavicle. Then, as it travels within the axilla, it is once again quite broad and presents with a dense interlacing arrangement, resembling more closely a complicated plexus. As the plexus reaches a point opposite the coracoid process, it divides into numerous branches that remain rather distinct peripheral nerves destined to innervate the musculature and integument of the upper limb.[7]

### ROOTS

The cervical nerves from the fifth to the eighth are rather small in size, and the method in which they communicate shows considerable variation. As the mixed spinal nerves exit their respective foramina, they divide into an anterior and a posterior primary rami. The nerves lie on the external surface of the scalenus medius and are in relation to the outer border of the scalenus anticus.[7]

Prior to formation of the trunks, the fifth cervical nerve communicates with the cervical plexus by a branch extending from the fourth cervical nerve and often contributes to the phrenic nerve. The anterior rami of the fifth and sixth cervical nerves, as well as the eighth cervical and first thoracic nerves, merge with one another soon after their point of exit (see Figs. 1-47 and 1-48). Once having merged, these roots are referred to as *trunks*.

### TRUNKS

The fifth and sixth cervical nerves unite with one another just after their exit from the intervertebral foramen to form the upper trunk (superior). The seventh cervical nerve exits the intervertebral foramen and remains isolated as the middle trunk. The eighth cervical nerve and the first thoracic

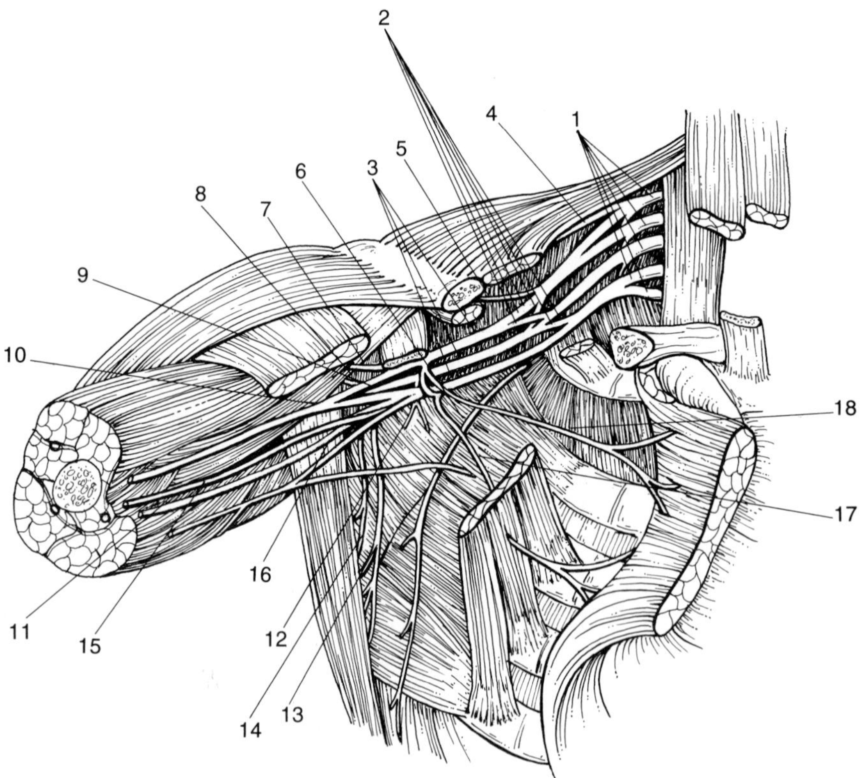


**Figure 1-47.** Neuroanatomy of the shoulder region. 1, nerve roots C5 to C8 and T1; 2, divisions anterior/posterior; 3, cords lateral/posterior/medial; 4, dorsal scapular nerve; 5, suprascapular nerve; 6, long thoracic nerve; 7, musculocutaneous nerve; 8, axillary nerve; 9, radial nerve; 10, median nerve; 11, ulnar nerve; 12, upper subscapular nerve; 13, thoracodorsal nerve; 14, lower subscapular nerve; 15, medial antebrachial cutaneous nerve; 16, medial brachial cutaneous nerve; 17, medial pectoral nerve; 18, lateral pectoral nerve.

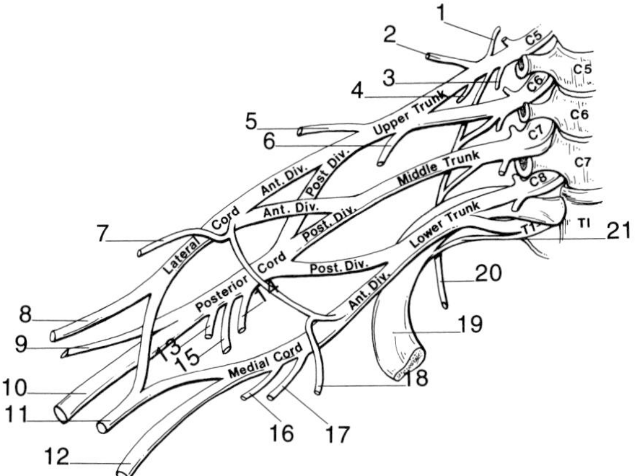


**Figure 1-48.** The brachial plexus common arrangement. 1, contribution from C4 nerve root; 2, dorsal scapular nerve; 3, branch to anterior cervical muscles; 4, branch to phrenic nerve; 5, suprascapular nerve C5, 6; 6, subclavian nerve C5, 6; 7, lateral pectoral nerve C5, 6, 7; 8, musculocutaneous nerve C5, 6, 7; 9, axillary nerve C5, 6; 10, radial nerve C6, 7, 8, T1; 11, median nerve C5, 6, 7, 8, T1; 12, ulnar nerve C8, T1; 13, lower subscapular nerve C5, 6; 14, upper subscapular nerve C5, 6; 15, thoracodorsal nerve C6, 7, 8; 16, medial antebrachial cutaneous C8, T1; 17, medial brachial cutaneous T1; 18, medial pectoral nerve C8, T1; 19, first rib; 20, long thoracic nerve C5, 6, 7; 21, first intercostal nerve T1.

nerve unite with one another just after exiting their respective foramina to form the lower trunk (inferior).

## DIVISIONS

As the trunks pass beneath the clavicle, each one divides into an anterior (ventral) and a posterior (dorsal) division. The posterior divisions of all three trunks merge with one another, while the anterior division of the middle trunk merges with the anterior division of the upper trunk. The anterior division of the lower trunk remains isolated.

## CORDS

The anterior divisions of the upper and middle trunks unite to form a single cord that lies on the lateral surface of the middle part of the axillary artery. The anterior division of the lower trunk forms a cord that lies on the medial surface of the middle part of the axillary artery. The posterior divisions of all three trunks unite to form a single cord that lies underneath the middle part of the axillary artery. These cords are intimately bound by fascial tissue to the external surface of the axillary artery and are named lateral, medial, and posterior according to their relationship with the artery.

## RELATIONSHIPS

In the cervical region the brachial plexus lies within the posterior triangle protected by the skin, platysma muscle, and deep cervical fascia[7] (see Fig. 1-47). The posterior belly of the omohyoid and the transversalis colli artery cross the roots and trunks of the plexus. The posterior scapular artery usually passes between the roots of the plexus. Most often the plexus lies between the anterior and middle scaleni muscles as well as above and to the outer border of the subclavian artery. Once having crossed the subclavian artery, the trunks dive under the clavicle and lie posterior to the subclavius muscle. The posterior aspect of the trunks lies against the first digitation of the serratus anterior and the upper-most slips of the subscapularis muscle.[7] At this point the trunks divide into the divisions. Once reaching the axilla, the divisions lie lateral to the first part of the axillary artery. The divisions quickly form the cords and envelope the second part of the axillary artery, lying lateral, medial, and posterior to it. At the lower part of the axillary space, the cords divide further into the terminal branches that form the peripheral nerves of the upper extremity.

## BRANCHES—PERIPHERAL NERVES

The branches of the plexus are numerous, and they are more easily appreciated by dividing those which arise above from those which arise below the clavicle. Branches above the clavicle consist of communicating branches and muscular branches, as well as the dorsal scapular nerve, subclavian nerve, long thoracic nerve, and suprascapular nerve.

### Branches Above the Clavicle

***Communicating branches.*** Communicating branches from the fifth and sixth cervical nerves join with the phrenic nerve on the surface of the scalenus anticus muscle, and others join with the nerves of the autonomic ganglion.[7]

***Muscular branches.*** Small muscular branches from the lower cervical nerves arise just as these nerves exit their respective foramina and innervate the scaleni and longus colli muscles.

***Dorsal scapular nerve.*** The dorsal scapular nerve arises from the fifth cervical nerve just prior to the formation of the upper trunk (see Figs. 1-47 and 1-48). This nerve pierces the substance of the scalenus medius and passes in a posterior direction under cover from the levator scapula to innervate this muscle, as well as descending further to innervate the rhomboid major and minor.

***Subclavian nerve.*** The subclavian nerve arises from the fifth cervical nerve at the formation of the upper trunk (see Figs. 1-47 and 1-48). This small filament descends in front of the third part of the subclavian artery and innervates the subclavius muscle.

***Long thoracic nerve.*** The long thoracic nerve, considered quite unique because of its remarkably long course, arises by two or three filaments from the fifth, sixth, and sometimes the seventh cervical nerves immediately after they exit their foramina[7] (see Figs. 1-47 and 1-48). These two or three filaments unite in the substance of the scalenus medius, and then a single nerve emerges and descends posterior to the plexus and the axillary vessels. This nerve lies against the anterior surface of the serratus and extends down the length of the thoracic wall to the lower border of the serratus, innervating each digitation by way of a slender filament.

***Suprascapular nerve.*** The suprascapular nerve arises from the upper trunk and passes obliquely outward beneath the trapezius and the omohyoid muscles (see Figs. 1-48 and 1-49). This nerve then enters the supraspinous fossa through the suprascapular notch and lies on the floor of the fossa beneath the supraspinatus muscle (see Fig. 1-49a). In the fossa the nerve gives off two branches to the supraspinatus muscle and an articular filament to the glenohumeral joint. The nerve curves around the external border of the spine of the scapula and enters the infraspinous fossa through the spinoglenoid notch (see Fig. 1-49b). In the infraspinous fossa, the nerve gives off two branches to the infraspinatus muscle and several filaments to the scapula and the glenohumeral joint.

### Branches Below the Clavicle

The branches below the clavicle arise from the three cords of the brachial plexus. The lateral cord gives rise to the lateral pectoral nerve, the musculocutaneous nerve, and the lateral contribution to the median nerve. The medial cord gives rise to the medial pectoral nerve, the medial brachial cutaneous nerve, the medial antebrachial cutaneous nerve, the nerve of Wrisberg, the ulnar nerve, and the medial contribution to

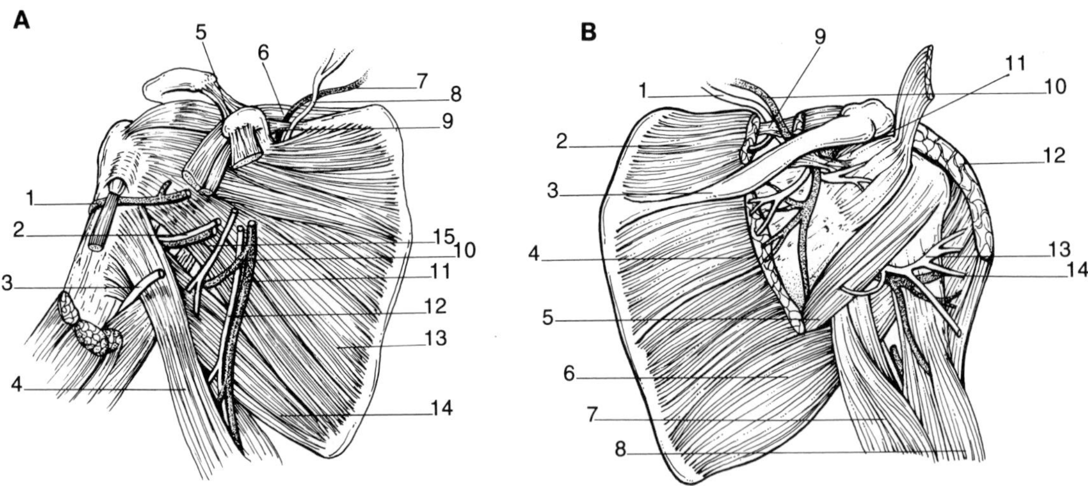


**Figure 1-49.** (a) Anterior view. 1, anterior humeral circumflex artery; 2, axillary nerve and posterior humeral circumflex artery; 3, radial nerve; 4, latissimus dorsi muscle; 5, coracoacromial ligament; 6, supraspinatus muscle; 7, suprascapular artery; 8, suprascapular nerve; 9, transverse scapular ligament and notch; 10, circumflex scapular artery; 11, thoracodorsal artery; 12, thoracodorsal nerve; 13, subscapularis muscle; 14, teres major; 15, lower subscapular nerve. (b) Posterior view. 1, suprascapular nerve; 2, supraspinatus muscle (cut); 3, spine; 4, infraspinatus muscle (cut); 5, teres minor muscle; 6, teres major muscle; 7, triceps long head; 8, triceps lateral head; 9, superior transverse scapular ligament; 10, suprascapular artery; 11, inferior transverse scapular ligament; 12, deltoid muscle (cut); 13, axillary nerve; 14, posterior humeral circumflex artery.

the median nerve. The posterior cord gives rise to the upper and lower subscapular nerves. The middle subscapular nerve, also known as the *thoracodorsal nerve*, arises from the posterior division of the upper trunk just prior to where it joins with the other posterior divisions in formation of the posterior cord. The posterior cord divides into the radial and axillary nerves.

***Lateral and medial pectoral nerves.*** The lateral pectoral nerve arises from the lateral cord, passes inward across the axillary artery and vein, pierces the costocoracoid membrane, and innervates the undersurface of the pectoralis major[7] (see Fig. 1-47). It also sends down a branch that loops under the axillary artery and joins with the medial pectoral nerve. The medial pectoral nerve arises from the medial cord, passes behind the first part of the axillary artery, and then curves forward between the axillary artery and vein, where it joins with the looping branch from the lateral pectoral nerve. The medial pectoral nerve then passes deep to the pectoralis minor, where it divides into numerous filaments that perforate and innervate the pectoralis minor and then pass on to innervate the undersurface of the pectoralis major.[7] The lateral pectoral nerve is supplied by the fifth, sixth, and seventh cervical nerves, and the medial pectoral nerve is supplied by the eighth cervical and first thoracic nerves.

***Subscapular nerves.*** The subscapular nerves are three in number. They innervate the subscapularis, teres major, and latissimus dorsi muscles. All three nerves are supplied by the fifth, sixth, seventh, and eighth cervical nerves (see Figs. 1-47 and 1-50).

***Upper subscapular.*** The upper subscapular nerve is the smallest of the three. It arises from the posterior cord and quickly enters the upper part of the subscapularis. On occasion, this nerve is represented by two branches.

***Middle subscapular (thoracodorsal).*** The middle subscapular nerve, referred to as the *thoracodorsal nerve*, is the largest of the three. This nerve more often than not arises from the posterior division of the upper trunk as it is blending with the other two posterior divisions to form the posterior cord. This nerve then follows the course of the subscapular artery along the posterior wall of the axilla, lying against latissimus dorsi. The thoracodorsal nerve extends to the lower border of latissimus dorsi, innervating the substance of this large, powerful muscle.

***Lower subscapular.*** The lower subscapular nerve arises from the posterior cord distal to the origin of the upper and middle subscapular nerves. It courses outward and enters the axillary border of the subscapularis muscle, which it innervates. It then courses further distally to innervate the teres major.

***Axillary nerve.*** The axillary nerve arises from the posterior cord of the brachial plexus in common with the radial nerve. At its origin it lies posterior to the axillary artery situated between the artery and the subscapularis muscle (see Figs. 1-47 and

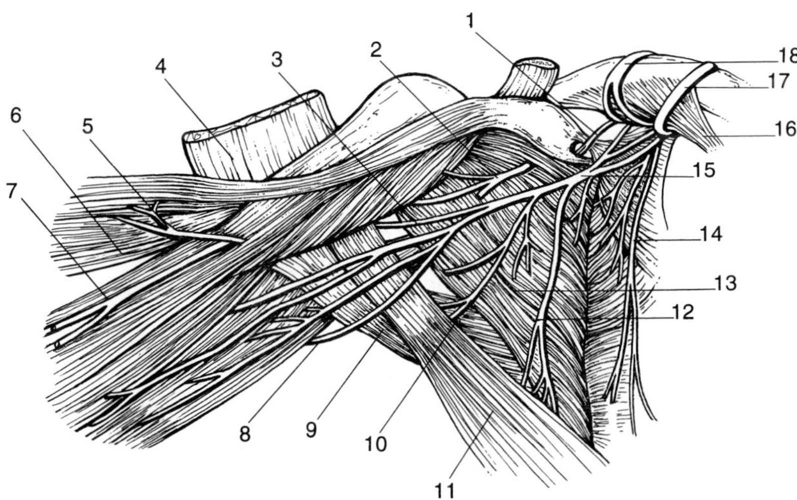


**Figure 1-50.** Posterior cord and peripheral branches. 1, suprascapular nerve; 2, musculocutaneous nerve; 3, axillary nerve; 4, pectoralis major tendon (cut); 5, musculocutaneous nerve; 6, biceps muscle; 7, musculocutaneous nerve; 8, posterior cutaneous nerve of the upper arm; 9, teres major; 10, lower subscapular nerve innervating the teres major; 11, latissimus dorsi; 12, thoracodorsal nerve innervating latissimus dorsi; 13, subscapularis muscle; 14, long thoracic nerve innervating serratus anterior; 15, posterior cord; 16, subclavius muscle; 17, medial cord; 18, lateral cord.

1-50). The axillary nerve then passes in a downward and outward direction to the lateral border of the subscapularis muscle. In this location the axillary nerve gives off a filament that enters the glenohumeral joint capsule just under the tendon of the subscapularis (see Figs. 1-47, 1-50, and 1-51). The axillary nerve then courses backward with the posterior circumflex artery and perforates the quadrilateral space posterior to the glenohumeral joint (Fig. 1-52). This neurovascular bundle lies very close to the glenohumeral joint and the posterior portion of the rotator cuff. Once having exited the quadrilateral space, the nerve divides into an upper and a lower branch. The upper branch winds around the surgical neck of the humerus, beneath the deltoid, in intimate association with the posterior humeral circumflex artery. This branch extends as far as the anterior border of the deltoid, which it innervates. The numerous filaments that innervate the deltoid from below also pierce the substance of the deltoid and innervate the integument of the shoulder and upper arm. At the point of origin,

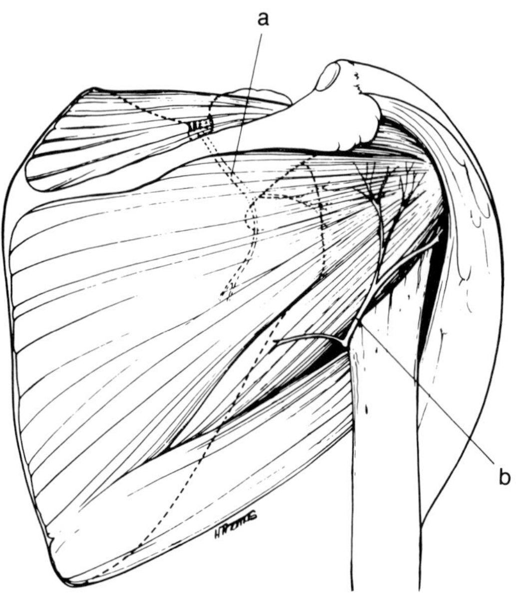


**Figure 1-52.** The posterior innervation of the shoulder joint. The primary nerves are the suprascapular (a) and the axillary (b). (From Rockwood C, Matsen F. The shoulder. Vol. 1. Philadelphia: WB Saunders, 1990:31.)

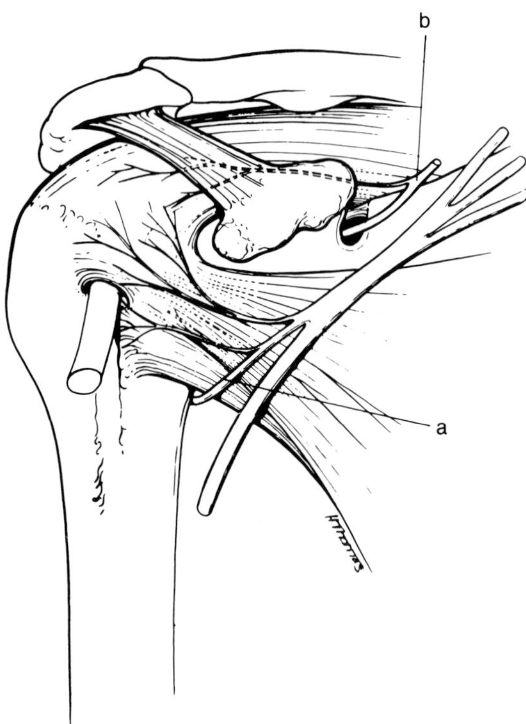


**Figure 1-51.** The innervation of the anterior portion of the shoulder the ancillary (a) and suprascapular (b) nerves form most of the nerve supply to the capsule and the glenohumeral joint. In some instances the musculocutaneous nerve may send some twigs to the anterosuperior portion of the joint. (From Rockwood C, Matsen F. The shoulder. Vol. 1. Philadelphia: WB Saunders, 1990:30.)

the lower branch, by way of some filaments, innervates the teres minor and the posterior portion of the deltoid. The nerve then pierces the deep fascia from underneath and supplies the integument over the lower two-thirds of the posterior surface of the deltoid as well as that covering the long head of the triceps. The terminal branches also provide innervation to the glenohumeral joint capsule and the head of the humerus through articular stems. The axillary nerve receives filaments from the fifth and sixth cervical nerve roots.[7]

***Musculocutaneous nerve.*** The musculocutaneous nerve arises from the lateral cord just opposite to the lower border of the pectoralis minor (see Fig. 1-50). This nerve pierces the coracobrachialis, innervating this muscle very close to where the nerve first originates. Once having passed through the substance of the coracobrachialis, it travels in an oblique direction, lying between the biceps and brachialis and sending several filaments to innervate both these muscles. The nerve then continues its descent down the arm, where it winds around the lateral border of the biceps tendon just above the cubital fossa of the elbow. From underneath the deep fascia of the arm the nerve pierces this fascial sheath and becomes cutaneous in its final distribution. The musculocutaneous nerve receives filaments from the fifth, sixth, and seventh cervical nerves.[7]

***Medial brachial cutaneous nerve.*** The medial brachial cutaneous nerve is one of the smallest branches of the plexus. It arises from the medial cord in conjunction with the ulnar nerve and the medial contribution to the median nerve. It is situated on the inner-most surface of the axillary artery. It courses down the medial aspect of the arm, providing numerous filaments to the integument of the upper arm in the area occupied by the biceps. It derives its supply from the eighth cervical and first thoracic nerves.[7]

***Medial antebrachial cutaneous nerve.*** The medial antebrachial cutaneous nerve is the smallest branch of the entire brachial plexus. This nerve arises from the medial cord in close association with the medial brachial cutaneous and ulnar nerves. It passes through the axillary space, first lying behind the axillary artery and then on the inner side of the axillary vein. This nerve descends along the inner side of the brachial artery to the middle of the arm. At this point it pierces the deep fascia of the arm and supplies the integument on the back part of the lower third of the arm, extending as far distally as the elbow. This nerve receives a filament from the first thoracic nerve.

***Median nerve.*** The median nerve is named for its course down the midline of the arm and forearm to the hand. This nerve arises by way of two contributions, one from the lateral cord and one from the medial cord. These two unite near the lower part of the axillary artery and embrace this vessel over its anterior or lateral surface. The nerve descends the arm, at first lying very close to the lateral surface of the brachial artery. It then crosses the anterior surface of the brachial artery and continues down the arm on the medial aspect of the artery. When it reaches the elbow, it lies deep to the bicipital fascia. The median nerve passes between the two heads of the pronator teres and lies between the undersurface of the flexor digitorum superficialis and the outer surface of the flexor digitorum profundus. The median nerve receives its supply from the sixth, seventh, and eighth cervical nerves and the first thoracic nerve.[7] This nerve does not provide any innervation to the shoulder region.

***Ulnar nerve.*** The ulnar nerve, smaller than the median nerve, arises from the medial cord alone. At its origin it lies on the inner surface of the axillary artery and continues to occupy a similar relationship with the brachial artery in the arm. Two-thirds of the way down the arm the nerve courses obliquely over the short head of the triceps, pierces the internal intermuscular septum, and descends downward to enter the bony groove formed behind the medial epicondyle of the humerus and the olecranon process of the ulna. This nerve receives its supply from the eighth cervical nerve and first thoracic nerve.[7] It provides articular branches to the elbow and wrist, muscular branches to the forearm and hand, and cutaneous branches to the forearm and hand. It does not innervate any structures in the shoulder region.

***Radial nerve.*** The radial nerve is the largest branch of the brachial plexus. This nerve arises from the posterior cord in common with the axillary nerve (see Figs. 1-47 and 1-50). It courses behind the axillary artery and remains posterior to the upper part of the brachial artery. It descends in front of the tendons of the latissimus dorsi and teres major. Once having passed by these tendons, the nerve winds posteriorally around the shaft of the humerus and lies in the radial groove. The nerve travels in this groove with the superior profunda brachial artery. These two structures pass from the inner to the outer side of the humerus, lying between and beneath the medial and lateral heads of the triceps. The radial nerve then pierces the external intermuscular septum and descends between the brachialis and the supinator muscles. Near the lateral epicondyle of the humerus the nerve divides into the posterior interosseous nerve and the radial nerve of the forearm. The radial nerve contains numerous muscular and cutaneous branches. This nerve receives filaments from the sixth, seventh, and eighth cervical nerves and in some instances from the fifth cervical nerve.[7] Other than its relationship with the triceps, this nerve does not have any influence on the shoulder region.

# Vascular Anatomy

The main artery that supplies the upper extremity begins as a single vessel and continues as such from its origin at the sternum to the forearm (Fig. 1-53). Different portions of the main vessel have different names according to the region in which the vessel is located.

## SUBCLAVIAN ARTERY

### FIRST PART

The arteries in their first part differ significantly in length, direction, and relationship with neighboring structures.

#### Right Subclavian Artery

The first part of the right subclavian artery arises from the innominate artery opposite the right sternoclavicular joint. It passes upward and outward to the inner margin of the scalenus anticus

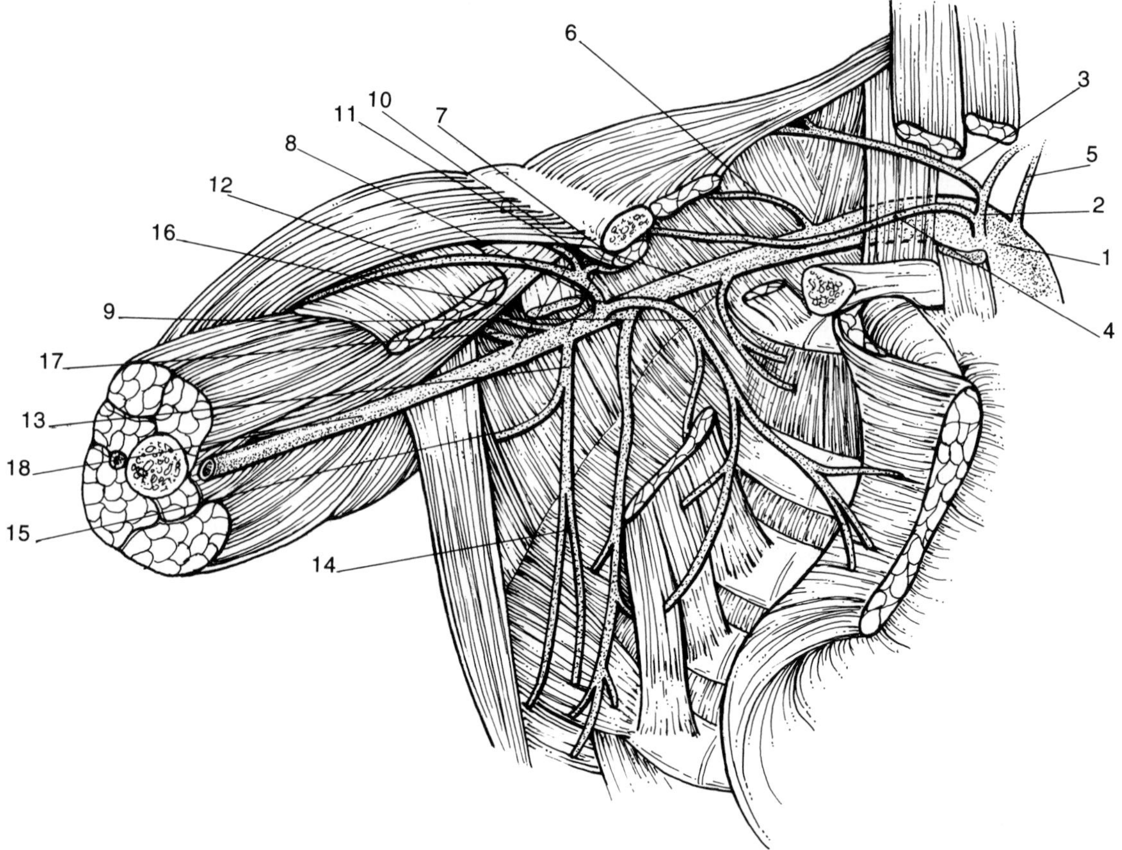


**Figure 1-53.** Vascular anatomy of the shoulder region. 1, subclavian artery parts 1, 2, and 3; 2, thyrocervical artery; 3, transverse cervical artery; 4, suprascapular artery; 5, vertebral artery; 6, dorsal scapular artery; 7, axillary artery parts 1, 2, and 3; 8, thoracoacromial artery; 9, pectoral branch; 10, clavicular branch; 11, acromial branch; 12, deltoid branch; 13, subscapular artery; 14, thoracodorsal artery; 15, circumflex scapular artery; 16, anterior circumflex humeral artery; 17, posterior circumflex humeral artery; 18, brachial artery.

muscle. In this portion the artery ascends slightly above the clavicle, varying in height from one individual to the next.[7]

**Left Subclavian Artery**

The first part of the left subclavian artery arises from the end of the arch of the aorta opposite the fourth thoracic vertebra. The vessel ascends nearly vertical to the inner margin of the scalenus anticus muscle. The first part of the left subclavian artery is considerably longer than the right. It is located deep within the chest cavity, and it is directed nearly straight upward, as opposed to the right, which arches outward.[7]

## SECOND PART

The second part of the subclavian artery is relatively the same for right and left. This portion lies directly underneath the scalenus anticus muscle, is very short, and forms the peak of the arch of the artery (see Fig. 1-53). It is covered in front by the scalenus anticus, sternocleidomastoid, deep cervical fascia, platysma, superficial fascia, and skin. Lying behind this artery one finds the scalenus medius and the pleural membrane.[7] Situated just above the artery are the nerves of the brachial plexus and just below it the pleura.

## THIRD PART

The third part of the subclavian artery passes downward and outward from the lateral border of the scalenus anticus to the outer border of the first rib. The artery lies partly within the posterior triangle of the neck and partly behind the clavicle in the subclavian triangle. It is covered in front by the nerve to the subclavius, the transverse cervical vein, the suprascapular artery and vein, the subclavius, clavicle, deep cervical fascia, descending clavicular branches of the cervical plexus, platysma, superficial fascia, and skin.[7] Behind the artery lies the scalenus medius and the lower trunk of the brachial plexus. Lying above and to the outer side of the artery one finds the middle and upper trunk of the brachial plexus. At its lowest extent it lies against the upper surface of the first rib.

## BRANCHES FROM THE SUBCLAVIAN ARTERY

Four branches arise from the subclavian artery: the vertebral artery, the thyrocervical trunk, the internal mammary artery, and the superior intercostal artery (see Fig. 1-53). On the left side, all four branches arise from the first part of the subclavian, whereas on the right side, the superior intercostal artery arises from the second part.[7] On both the left and right sides, the first three branches arise close to one another near the inner margin of the scalenus anticus muscle. In most cases, the interval between the origin of the subclavian artery and the origin of the first branch is between 1/2 and 1 in.[7]

### Vertebral Artery

The vertebral artery arises from the upper and posterior surface of the subclavian artery and courses in an upward direction, traveling within the transverse foramen of the first six cervical vertebrae. Once having ascended to the first cervical level, the artery twists behind the articulations between the base of the occiput and atlas and enters the foramen magnum, where it anastomoses with the circle of Willis. This artery is responsible for supplying circulation to the proximal portion of the brachial plexus.[23]

### Thyrocervical Trunk

The thyrocervical trunk arises as a short, thick artery off the anterior surface of the subclavian artery very close to the inner border of the scalenus anticus (see Fig. 1-53). The artery quickly divides into the inferior thyroid, suprascapular, and transverse cervical arteries.

***Inferior thyroid.*** This artery passes in an upward direction anterior to the vertebral artery and the longus colli muscle, which lies against the anterior surface of the cervical vertebrae. The artery turns inward under cover from the sheath over the carotid artery and internal jugular vein. It extends to the thyroid gland, where it divides into several smaller branches which then supply the thyroid gland, trachea, larynx, and esophagus, as well as the bones, nerves, and muscles of the cervical spine.[7]

***Suprascapular artery.*** The suprascapular artery arises from the first part of the subclavian artery and passes obliquely outward across the root of the neck. The artery passes obliquely outward across the scalenus anticus muscle and phrenic nerve under cover from the sternocleidomastoid muscle and crosses over the subclavian artery and the cords of the brachial plexus (see Fig. 1-53). The artery then courses outward, again lying parallel to the clavicle and subclavius muscle. Once this artery reaches the superior border of the scapula, it passes over the transverse ligament, effectively separated from the suprascapular nerve (see Fig. 1-49). As the artery passes over the ligament, it sends a branch toward the subscapular fossa, which anastomoses with subscapular arteries located beneath the subscapularis muscle. The artery also sends a branch to the acromioclavicular joint and the glenohumeral joint and a nutrient artery to the clavicle.[7] The artery then enters the supraspinous fossa and lies close the floor of the fossa, supplying nutrition to both the scapula and the supraspinatus muscles. The artery continues laterally until it reaches the neck of the scapula, where it passes downward behind the neck to reach the infraspinous fossa. Within the infraspinous fossa, the artery anastomoses with the dorsal scapular artery and the posterior scapular arteries. Along its long course this artery supplies the sternocleidomastoid and subclavius muscles, the sternal end of the clavicle, and the skin over the upper part of the chest. Also, by way of a supraacromial branch, it supplies the skin over the acromion (Fig. 1-54). This artery is important in providing adequate circulation to many vital structures within the shoulder region.

***Transversalis colli.*** The transversalis colli artery arises from the first part of the subclavian artery. The artery takes a transverse course across the upper part of the subclavian triangle to the anterior margin of the upper trapezius. The artery then passes under the trapezius and divides into two arteries, the superficial cervical and the posterior scapular arteries. The superficial cervical artery ascends under the trapezius and distributes smaller branches to the structures in the cervical region. The posterior scapular artery passes under the levator scapulae near its insertion on the superior angle of the scapula and then descends along the posterior border of the scapula as far distally as the inferior angle. As it courses along the scapula, it supplies the rhomboid, trapezius, and latissimus dorsi muscles. It also anastomoses with the suprascapular and subscapular arteries.[7] This artery provides important nutrition to the shoulder region by direct and collateral circulation.

### Internal Mammary Artery

The internal mammary artery arises from the undersurface of the first part of the subclavian artery just opposite the thyrocervical trunk.[7] This

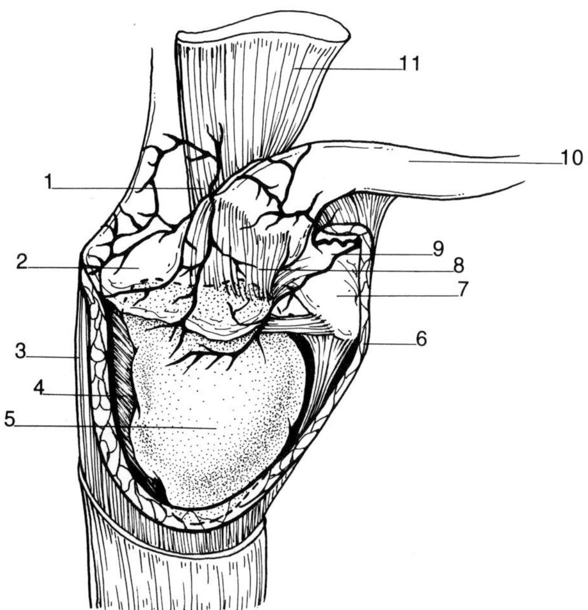


**Figure 1-54.** Branches of the suprascapular artery and others. 1, acromial branches of the suprascapular artery; 2, acromion; 3, posterior deltoid (cut); 4, posterior rotator cuff; 5, subdeltoid bursa; 6, anterior deltoid (cut); 7, coracoid process; 8, superior acromioclavicular ligament; 9, acromial branches of the thoracoacromial artery; 10, clavicle; 11, supraspinatus muscle.

artery passes downward and inward behind the costal cartilage of the first rib and travels a long way, lying on the inner surface of the anterior chest wall. Ultimately, the artery divides into the musculophrenic and superior epigastric arteries.

#### Superior Intercostal Artery

The superior intercostal artery arises from the second part of the subclavian artery off its upper and posterior surface. The artery courses backward and gives off a deep cervical branch. Upon descending behind the pleura, it lies in front of the first two ribs, where it anastomoses with the first aortic intercostal artery.[7]

## AXILLARY ARTERY

The axillary artery is a continuation of the subclavian artery that begins at the outer border of the first rib and terminates at the lower border of the teres major muscle, where the same vessel continues as the brachial artery (see Fig. 1-53). Where the artery begins, it is situated very deep and is surrounded by the cords of the brachial plexus. In contrast, where the artery ends in the axilla, it is very superficial, being covered only by fascia and skin.[7] Like the subclavian artery, dividing the axillary artery into three parts facilitates a description of the artery and an appreciation of its relationship to other key anatomic structures.

### FIRST PART

The first part of the axillary artery lies above the pectoralis minor muscle. Lying in front of the artery one finds the clavicular portion of the pectoralis major, the costocoracoid membrane, the external anterior thoracic nerve, and the acromiothoracic and cephalic veins. Lying behind the artery one finds the first intercostal space, the corresponding intercostal musculature, the second and third digitations of the serratus anterior muscle, and the posterior thoracic and internal anterior thoracic nerves. On its most external surface one will notice the brachial plexus, which is separated from the first portion of the artery by a cellular interval. On the inner surface of the artery is situated the axillary vein.[7]

### SECOND PART

The second part of the axillary artery lies directly behind the pectoralis minor. Lying in front of the artery is the lower portion of the pectoralis major and the width of the pectoralis minor as it tapers toward its insertion on the coracoid process. Lying behind the artery is a cellular interval that effectively separates the artery from the subscapularis muscle. On the inner side of the artery lies the medial cord of the brachial plexus and the axillary vein. On the outer side lies the lateral cord, and on the posterior or undersurface lies the posterior cord.

## THIRD PART

The third part of the axillary artery lies below the pectoralis minor. Initially, the artery is covered in front by the lower border of the pectoralis major. As the artery descends into the axilla, it is only under cover from the fascia and integument. The median nerve transects this section of artery, and lying behind the artery one finds the lower border of the subscapularis tendon and the tendons of latissimus dorsi and teres major muscles. Lying across the outer surface of the artery one finds the coracobrachialis tendon and muscle, and on the inner surface lies the axillary vein.[7] The peripheral nerves of the brachial plexus lie in close proximity to the artery. The median nerve lies external to the artery, the musculocutaneous nerve lies behind the artery for a very short distance, while the ulnar nerve lies between the artery and vein. The lesser internal cutaneous nerve lies just to the inside of the axillary vein. The terminal branches of the posterior cord lie behind the axillary artery, just as they did previously. The axillary nerve follows the course of the axillary artery to the lower border of the subscapularis, where the nerve then passes in a posterior direction to enter the quadrangular space. The radial nerve continues to follow the artery to the point where the artery crosses the lower border of the teres major.

## BRANCHES OF THE AXILLARY ARTERY

The first part of the artery gives rise to the superior thoracic and acromial thoracic arteries. The second part gives rise to the long thoracic and alar thoracic arteries. The third part gives rise to the subscapular, posterior humeral circumflex, and anterior humeral circumflex arteries.

### Superior Thoracic Artery

The superior thoracic artery arises from the axillary artery as a single trunk or in common with the acromial thoracic artery. The artery runs in a forward and inward direction along the upper border of the pectoralis minor muscle. The artery passes between the pectoralis minor and major muscles to the lateral aspect of the chest, where it anastomoses with the internal mammary and intercostal arteries.[7]

### Acromial Thoracic Artery

The acromial thoracic arises as a short trunk from the anterior surface of the axillary artery under cover from the upper border of the pectoralis minor muscle. The trunk projects forward to the upper border of the pectoralis minor, where it divides into three sets of branches: thoracic, acromial, and descending. The thoracic consists of two or three branches that distribute themselves to the serratus anterior and pectoral muscles, and ultimately, they anastomose with the internal mammary and intercostal arteries. The acromial branches are directed outward toward the acromion, supplying the deltoid muscle and anastomosing on the surface of the acromion with the suprascapular and posterior humeral circumflex arteries (see Fig. 1-53). The descending branch passes in the potential space that exists between the pectoralis major and the deltoid in association with the cephalic vein. This artery supplies the deltoid and the pectoral muscles as well as giving rise to a small branch, referred to as the *clavicular artery*, that passes upward to supply the subclavius muscle.

### Long Thoracic Artery

The long thoracic artery arises from the second part of the axillary artery and courses in a downward and inward direction along the border of the pectoralis minor muscle to the side of the chest, where it supplies the serratus anterior and pectoral muscles, the mammary gland, and by way of branches extending across the axilla the axillary glands and the subscapularis muscle. The artery ultimately anastomoses with the internal mammary and intercostal arteries.[7]

### Alar Thoracic Artery

This artery is a rather small branch that supplies the glands and areolar tissue of the axilla. Often it receives collateral circulation from the other thoracic arteries.

### Subscapular Artery

The subscapular artery is the largest branch of the axillary artery. This large vessel arises from the lower border of the subscapularis muscle and courses in a downward and backward direction to reach to the inferior angle of the scapula, where it then anastomoses with the long thoracic and intercostal arteries as well as the posterior scapular artery, which is a branch of the transversalis colli artery. About 1½ in from its origin, the subscapular trunk gives off a large branch, the dorsal scapular artery, that terminates by supplying several branches to the muscles in the interscapular region.[7]

### Dorsal Scapular Artery

The dorsal scapular artery arises from the trunk of the subscapular artery near its point of origin, and in general, this is a larger vessel than the remaining portion of the subscapular artery. The dorsal scapular artery curves around the axillary border of the scapulae, leaving the axilla through the triangular space. The artery enters the infraspinous fossa under cover from the teres minor.

While under the teres minor, the artery anastomoses with the posterior scapular and subscapular arteries. During its course, the artery gives off two sets of branches: one that enters the subscapular fossa underneath the subscapularis and another that continues along the axillary border of the scapula between the teres major and minor. The set of arteries that enters the subscapular fossa anastomoses with the posterior scapular and suprascapular arteries. The second set of arteries reaches to the inferior angle of the scapula and anastomoses with the posterior scapular artery. A small set of arterial branches also distributes blood flow to the posterior deltoid and the long head of the triceps and then anastomoses with the ascending branch of the superior profunda artery, a branch of the brachial artery.

#### Posterior Humeral Circumflex Artery

The posterior humeral circumflex artery arises from the posterior surface of the axillary artery just opposite the lower border of the subscapularis. The artery courses backward through the quadrangular space in association with the axillary veins and nerve. After exiting this space, the artery winds around the surgical neck of the humerus and distributes blood flow to the deltoid muscle and glenohumeral joint (Fig. 1-55a). The artery anastomoses with the anterior humeral circumflex artery and the acromial thoracic arteries, as well as with the superior profunda branch of the brachial artery.

#### Anterior Humeral Circumflex Artery

The anterior humeral circumflex artery arises from the anterior surface of the axillary artery nearly opposite the origin of the posterior humeral circumflex (see Fig. 1-55b). The artery passes horizontally outward beneath the coracobrachialis and the short head of the biceps and lies against the forepart of the surgical neck of the humerus. Upon reaching the bicipital groove, it gives off an ascending branch, the arcuate artery. This branch ascends the bicipital groove to reach the head of the humerus, where it supplies the glenohumeral joint. The anterior humeral circumflex then continues outward beneath the deltoid, supplying it and ultimately anastomosing with the posterior humeral circumflex artery.

## BRACHIAL ARTERY

The brachial artery commences at the lower margin of the teres major and then passes downward along the anterior and medial aspect of the humerus. The brachial artery extends as far distally as 1/2 in below the bend of the elbow, where it then divides into the radial and ulnar arteries.[7]

## VASCULAR ANATOMY OF THE ROTATOR CUFF

Numerous studies have investigated the vascular anatomy of the rotator cuff.[12,14,22,25] The findings suggest that six arteries regularly contribute to the arterial supply of the rotator cuff: the suprascapular, the anterior humeral circumflex by way of the arcuate artery, the posterior humeral circumflex, the thoracoacromial, the suprahumeral, and the subscapular[23] (see Fig. 1-55). Moseley and Overgaard[14] noted that the blood supply to the rotator cuff is derived from one of three sets of vessels: osseous, muscular, and tendinous.

Osseous arteries supply the humeral head and in doing so provide nutrients to the tendons of the rotator cuff. An example of this is the arcuate artery, an ascending branch of the anterior humeral circumflex. Small arterioles run from the arcuate artery toward the articular cartilage and to the zone of the tendinous insertions of the rotator cuff. The arcuate artery gives rise to a branch just before entering the bicipital groove that courses in an upward direction to the rotator cuff. This is a superficial branch that anastomoses with the vessels of the subdeltoid bursa and with the vascular network of the tendinous portion of the supraspinatus muscle.

The muscular vessels are derived from the suprascapular and subscapular arteries. The muscles receive two or three main arteries that ultimately split into smaller vessels which anastomose quite frequently with each other and carry this anastomotic network through the musculotendinous junction into the substance of the tendon. These vessels run a longitudinal course, and with age, they tend to become coiled and tortuous and the number of vessels in the tendinous portion have a tendency to diminish.

The tendinous vessels arise from a network of muscular and osseous arteries that anastomose with each other over the tendons. With age, these vessels also become more tortuous and less viable. There are no main vessels that provide direct supply to the tendons of the rotator cuff. Therefore, these tendons must rely on the muscular and osseous arteries and their forms of collateral circulation. Some investigators speculate that the relative lack of blood flow to the tendons, coupled with direct forces of pressure from the humeral head and subacromial structures, may contribute in whole or in part to failure within the rotator cuff tendons.[22]

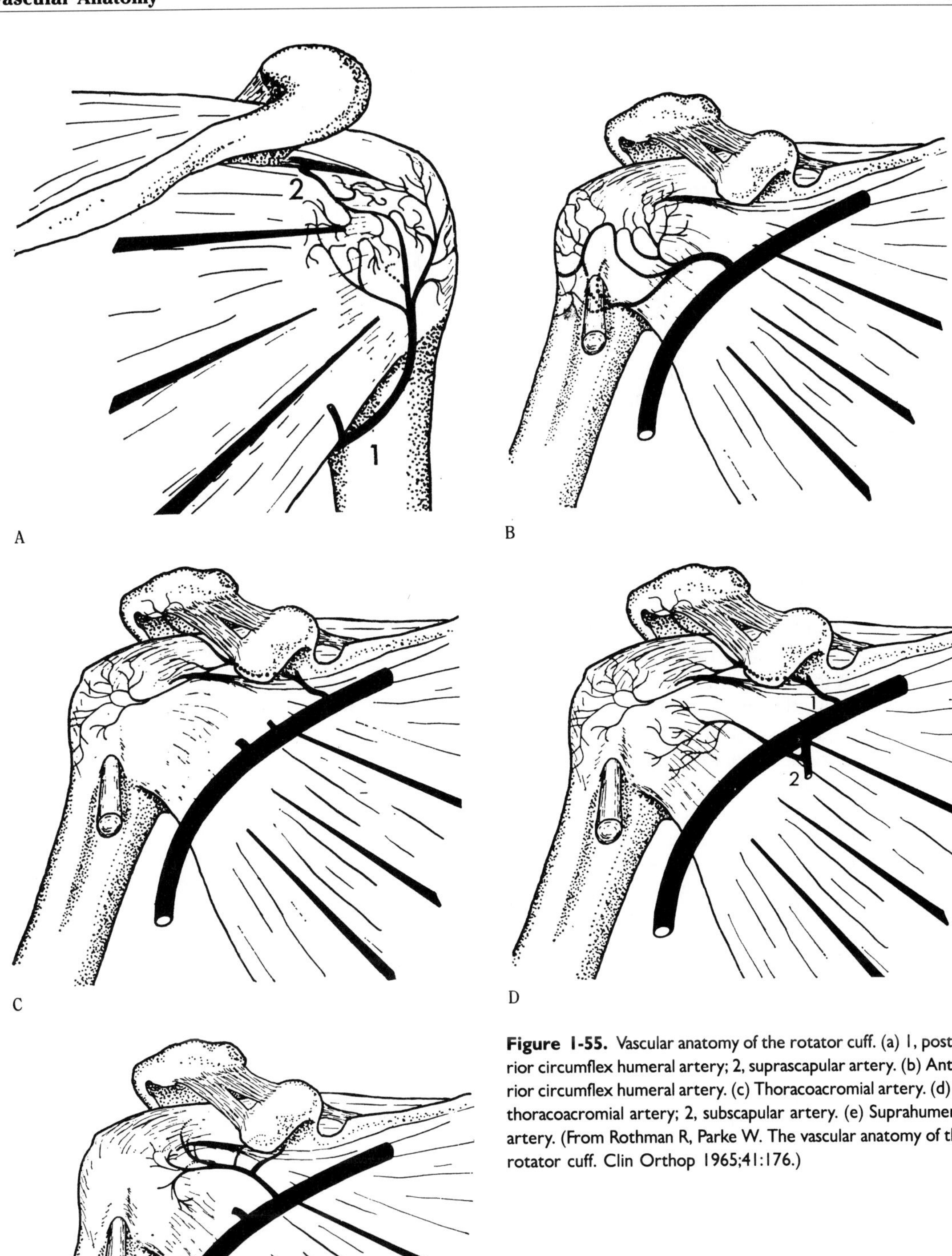


**Figure 1-55.** Vascular anatomy of the rotator cuff. (a) 1, posterior circumflex humeral artery; 2, suprascapular artery. (b) Anterior circumflex humeral artery. (c) Thoracoacromial artery. (d) 1, thoracoacromial artery; 2, subscapular artery. (e) Suprahumeral artery. (From Rothman R, Parke W. The vascular anatomy of the rotator cuff. Clin Orthop 1965;41:176.)

# Summary

Tracing evolution of the shoulder is, as Bateman[2] stated, a study in purposeful evolution. Numerous remarkable changes had to take place for human beings to acquire the degree of accuracy and dexterity noted in movement of the arm and hand. From a primitive fold of epidermis in a sea-dwelling creature, to the awkward movement of a reptile, to the overhead freedom of movement in humans, numerous topographic and morphologic changes took place. The most significant alterations noted were a decrease in the scapular index, an increase in the infraspinous index, the changing torsion angle of the humerus, an increase in the size of the greater tuberosity, an increase in the size of the acromion, distal migration of the deltoid tubercle, and the increasingly important role of the rotator cuff musculature in stabilizing and producing motion at the glenohumeral joint.

As remarkable as the study of comparative anatomy is, one can only marvel at the study of developmental anatomy. Here, one witnesses the miracle of human development. It is astounding to realize that the blueprint for the upper limb is contained within the union of sperm and ovum and that this process, from a hidden blueprint locked within genetic material to full construction of the arm, including such fine and delicate structures as the glenoid labrum, occurs in a mere 8 weeks. Even more astounding is the fact that the extremities do not make their primitive appearance until the fourth week of intrauterine development, thus allowing only 4 weeks for the progression from a minute swelling of undifferentiated tissue to a miniature replica of the adult arm. By the end of the eighth week, the embryo has been transformed into a fetus with four perfectly developed and functioning limbs. Not only is the upper limb functional, but the entire fetus also has developed to the point where this tiny human being is capable of performing such delicate and self-nurturing movements as placing one's thumb in one's mouth.

The third section of this chapter reviewed descriptive anatomy in considerable detail. The intention was to provide a detailed look at shoulder anatomy with an emphasis on clinical orthopedics. In striving to be clinically effective in the management of orthopedic disorders of the shoulder, one soon realizes how instrumental it is to develop a sound working knowledge of anatomy. With advancements in technology such as arthroscopy and magnetic resonance imaging, we can study human anatomy, both normal and pathologic, better than ever before, and it is highly likely that we have barely scratched the surface of our understanding. To remain effective, even the most seasoned veteran of clinical practice finds himself or herself frequently picking up and thumbing through textbooks and articles of anatomy. Hopefully, this chapter has rekindled the readers' flame of enthusiasm for reading further on human anatomy.

# References


1. Bardeen CR, Lewis WH. Development of limbs of body wall and back. Am J Anat 1901;1:1.
2. Bateman JE. The shoulder and neck. Philadelphia: WB Saunders, 1972.
3. Codman EA. The shoulder. Boston: Thomas Todd, 1934.
4. Davis FA: Taber's medical dictionary. Thomas CL, ed. Philadelphia: 1981.
5. DePalma AF. Surgery of the shoulder. 3rd ed. Philadelphia: JB Lippincott, 1983.
6. Gardner E, Gray DJ. Prenatal development of the human shoulder and acromioclavicular joints. Am J Anat 1953;92:219.
7. Gray H, Pick TP, Howden R, eds. Anatomy, descriptive and surgical. American rev ed From 15th English ed. New York: Bounty Books, 1977.
8. Howell AB. Speed in animals. Chicago: University of Chicago Press, 1944.
9. Inman VT, Saunders JB de CM, Abbott LC. Observations on the function of the shoulder joint. J Bone Joint Surg 1944;26A:1.
10. Johnston TB. The movements of the shoulder joint: a plea for the use of the "plane of the scapula" as the plane of reference for movements occurring at the humero-scapular joint. Br J Surg 1937–38;25:252.
11. Kapandji IA. The physiology of the joints. Vol. 1. Edinburgh: Churchill Livingstone, 1970.
12. Laing PG. Arterial supply of the adult humerus. J Bone Joint Surg 1956;38A:1105.
13. Liberson F. Os acromiale—a contested anomaly. J Bone Joint Surg 1937;19:683.
14. Moseley HF, Overgaard B. The anterior capsular mechanism in recurrent anterior dislocation of the shoulder. J Bone joint Surg 1962;44B:913.
15. Mudge MK, Wood VE, Frykman GK. Rotator cuff tears associated with os acromiale. J Bone Joint Surg. 1984;66A:427.
16. Neal HV, Rand HW. Chordate anatomy. Philadelphia: Blakiston, 1936.
17. Neer CS II. Impingement lesions. Clin Orthop 1983;173:70.
18. Neer CS II, Welsh RP. The shoulder in sports. Orthop Clin North Am 1977;8:583.
19. Nevaiser JS. Arthrography of the shoulder joint: a study of the findings in adhesive capsulitis of the shoulder. J Bone Joint Surg 1962;44A:1321.
20. Nobuhara K, Ikeeda H. Rotator interval lesion. Clin Orthop 1987;223:44.
21. O'Brien SJ, Warren RF, Schwartz E. Anterior shoulder instability. Orthop Clin North Am 1987;18:395.
22. Rathbun JB, McNab T. The microvascular pattern of the rotator cuff. J Bone Joint Surg 1970;52B:540.
23. Rockwood CA, Matsen FA III, eds. The shoulder. Philadelphia: WB Saunders, 1990.
24. Romanes GJ. Cunningham's textbook of anatomy. 12th ed. Oxford: Oxford University Press, 1981.
25. Rothman RH, Parke WW. The vascular anatomy of the rotator cuff. Clin Orthop 1965;41:176.
26. Rowe CR. The shoulder. New York: Churchill Livingstone, 1988.
27. Saha AK. Theory of shoulder mechanism: descriptive and applied. Springfield, Ill.: Charles C Thomas, 1961.
28. Saha AK. Mechanism of shoulder movements and a plea for the recognition of "zero position" of the glenohumeral joint. Clin Orthop 1983;173:3.
29. Sarrafian SK. Gross and functional anatomy of the shoulder. Clin Orthop 1983;173:11.
30. Simon and Schuster, Webster's New World Dictionary. Newfeldt V, ed. 3rd collegiate ed. New York: 1988.
31. Streeter W. Developmental horizons in human embryology. Carnegie Series on Embryology 1949;33:151.

32. Testut L. Traite' d'Anatomie Humaine. 7th ed., Vol. I: Osteologie, Arthologie, Myologie. Paris: Doin, 1921:503.
33. Turkel SJ, Panio MW, Marshall JL, Girgis FG. Stabilizing mechanisms preventing anterior dislocation of the glenohumeral joint. J Bone Joint Surg 1981;63A:1208.

# Bibliography

Anderson JE. Grant's atlas of anatomy. 8th ed. Baltimore: Williams & Wilkins, 1983.

Bardeen CR, Lewis WH. Development of limbs of body wall and back. Am J Anat 1901;1:1.

Bateman JE. The shoulder and neck. Philadelphia: WB Saunders, 1972.

Bateman JE. The diagnosis and treatment of ruptures of the rotator cuff. Surg Clin North Am 1963;43:1523.

Bassett RW, Cofield RH. Acute tears of the rotator cuff: the timing of surgical repair. Clin Orthop 1983;175:18.

Bigliani LU, Norris TR, Fischer J, et al. The relationship between the unfused acromial epiphysis and subacromial impingement lesions. Orthop Trans 1983;7:138.

Bigliani LU, Morrisson D, April EW. The morphology of the acromion and its relationship to rotator cuff tears. Orthop Trans 1986;10:228.

Brewer BJ. Aging of the rotator cuf. Am J Sports Med 1979;7:102.

Codman EA. The shoulder. Boston: Thomas Todd, 1934.

Cofield RH. Current concepts review rotator cuff disease of the shoulder. J Bone Joint Surg 1985;67A:974.

Davis FA, Taber's Medical Dictionary. Thomas CL, ed. Philadelphia: FA Davis, 1981.

Depalma AF. Surgery of the shoulder. 3rd ed. Philadelphia: JB Lippincott, 1983.

Fukada H. Rotator cuff tears. Geka Chiryo (Osaka) 1980;43:28.

Gardner E, Gray DJ, O'Rahilly R. Anatomy. 4th ed. Philadelphia: WB Saunders, 1975.

Gardner E, Gray DJ. Prenatal development of the human shoulder and acromioclavicular joints. Am J Anat 1953;92:219.

Goodrich ES. Studies on the structure and development of vertebrates. London: Macmillian, 1930.

Gray H, Pick TP, Howden R, eds. Anatomy, descriptive and surgical. American rev ed From 15th English ed. New York: Bounty Books, 1977.

Harryman DT II, Wang KA, Mack LA, et al. Functional results of rotator cuff repair: correlation with tear size and cuff integrity. Presented at the American Academy of Orthopaedic Surgeons, New Orleans, February 1990.

Hawkins RJ, Kennedy JC. Impingement syndrome in athletes. Am J Sports Med 1980;8:151.

Howell AB. Speed in animals. Chicago: University of Chicago Press, 1944.

Inman VT, Saunders JB de CM, Abbott LC. Observations on the function of the shoulder joint. J Bone Joint Surg 1944;26A:1.

Jackson D. Shoulder surgery in the athlete. Rockville, Md.: Aspen Publishers, 1985.

Jobe FW, Moynes DR. Delineation of diagnostic criteria and a rehabilitation program for rotator cuff injuries. Am J Sports Med 1982;10:336.

Jobe FW, Jobe CM. Painful athletic injuries of the shoulder. Clin Orthop 1983;173:117.

Johnston TB. The movements of the shoulder joint: a plea for the use of the "plane of the scapula" as the plane of reference for movements occurring at the humero-scapular joint. Br J Surg 1937–38;25:252.

Kapandji IA. The physiology of the joints. Vol. 1. Edinburgh: Churchill Livingstone, 1970.

Kent BE. Functional anatomy of the shoulder complex. Phys Ther 1971;51:867.

Laing PG. Arterial supply of the adult humerus. J Bone Joint Surg 1956;38A:1105.

Lewis WH. The development of the arm in man. Am J Anat 1902;145: 184.

Liberson F. Os acromiale—a contested anomaly. J Bone Joint Surg 1937;19:683.

MacNab I. Rotator cuff tendinitis. Ann R Surg Engl 1973;53:4.

Martin CP. The movements of the shoulder joint, with special reference to rupture of the supraspinatus tendon. Am J Anat 1940;66:213.

Mayer L. Rupture of the supraspinatus tendon. J Bone Joint Surg 1937;19A:640.

McLaughlin HL. Lesions of the musculotendinous cuff of the shoulder: the exposure and treatment of tears with retraction. J Bone Joint Surg 1944;26:31.

McLaughlin HL. Rupture of the rotator cuff. J Bone Joint Surg 1962; 44A:979.

McLaughlin HL. Repair of major cuff ruptures. Surg Clin North Am 1963;43:1535.

McMasters PE. Tendon and muscle ruptures: clinical and experimental studies on the causes and location of subcutaneous ruptures. J Bone Joint Surg 1933;15A:705.

Moseley HF, Goldie I. The arterial pattern of the rotator cuff of the shoulder. J Bone Joint Surg 1963;45B:780.

Moseley HF, Overgaard B. The anterior capsular mechanism in recurrent anterior dislocation of the shoulder. J Bone Joint Surg 1962; 44B:913.

Mudge MK, Wood VE, Frykman GK. Rotator cuff tears associated with os acromiale. J Bone Joint Surg 1984;66A:427.

Neal HV, Rand HW. Chordate anatomy. Philadelphia: Blakiston, 1936.

Neer CS II. Impingement lesions. Clin Orthop 1983;173:70.

Neer CS II, Welsh RP. The shoulder in sports. Orthop Clin North Am 1977;8:583.

Nevaiser JS. Ruptures of the rotator cuff. Clin Orthop 1954;3:92.

Nevaiser JS. Arthrography of the shoulder joint: a study of the findings in adhesive capsulitis of the shoulder. J Bone Joint Surg 1962;44A: 1321.

Nevaiser JS. Tears of the rotator cuff. Orthop Clin North Am 1980; 11:295.

Nixon JE, DiStefano V. Ruptures of the rotator cuff. Orthop Clin North Am 1975;6:423.

Nobuhara K, Ikeeda H. Rotator interval lesion. Clin Orthop 1987; 223:44.

O'Brien SJ, Warren RF, Schwartz E. Anterior shoulder instability. Orthop Clin North Am 1987;18:395.

Pratt NE. Clinical musculoskeletal anatomy. Philadelphia: JB Lippincott, 1991.

Rathbun JB, McNab T. The microvascular pattern of the rotator cuff. J Bone Joint Surg 1970;52B:540.

Rockwood CA, Matsen FA III, eds. The shoulder. Philadelphia: WB Saunders, 1990.

Romanes GJ. Cunningham's textbook of anatomy. 12th ed. Oxford: Oxford University Press, 1981.

Rothman RH, Parke WW. The vascular anatomy of the rotator cuff. Clin Orthop 1965;41:176.

Rowe CR. The shoulder. New York: Churchill Livingstone, 1988.

Saha AK. Theory of shoulder mechanism: descriptive and applied. Springfield, Ill.: Charles C Thomas, 1961.

Saha AK. Mechanism of shoulder movements and a plea for the recognition of "zero position" of the glenohumerla joint. Clin Orthop 1983;173:3.

Sarrafian SK. Gross and functional anatomy of the shoulder. Clin Orthop 1983;173:11.

Schwartz RE, O'Brien SJ, Warren RF, et al. Capsular restraints to anterior-posterior motion of the abducted shoulder: a biomechanical study. Orthop Trans 1988;12(3):727.

Simon and Schuster, Webster's New World Dictionary. NewFeldt V, ed. 3rd collegiate ed. New York: 1988.

Steindler A. Kinesiology of the human body under normal and pathologic conditions. Springfield, Ill.: Charles C Thomas, 1955.

Streeter W. Developmental horizons in human embryology. Carnegie Series on Embryology 1949;33:151.

Testut L. Traite' d'Anatomie Humaine. 7th ed., Vol. I: Osteologie, Arthologie, Myologie. Paris: Doin, 1921:503.

Turkel SJ, Panio MW, Marshall JL, Girgis FG. Stabilizing mechanisms preventing anterior dislocation of the glenohumeral joint. J Bone Joint Surg 1981;63A:1208.

WB Saunders Company, Dorland's medical dictionary. Fried J, ed. 26th ed. Philadelphia: 1974.

Chapter 2

*Martin J. Kelley*

# Biomechanics of the Shoulder



Martin J. Kelley and William A. Clark: ORTHOPEDIC THERAPY OF THE SHOULDER.

The shoulder complex has been studied and admired for centuries. This complex ensemble of bone, joint, and soft tissue functions in complete harmony thousands of times per day. Everything from complex sporting activities to simply reaching forward depends on synchronized, rhythmic motion of the multiple components. The glenohumeral joint is the center of activity, having a dual function of mobility and stability. The scapulothoracic joint and muscles provide a movable yet stable base for the humerus. The acromioclavicular and sternoclavicular joints further enhance motion of the shoulder girdle through their common link, the clavicle. Although the shoulder complex is intricate, its predominate function is quite basic, to mobilize the hand in space.

## Resting Position

Ideally, the shoulder girdle musculature should be well balanced with respect to strength and length to allow proper osseous orientation that results in optimal upper extremity function. Spinal alignment significantly influences shoulder girdle resting position due to the direct effect thoracic position has on the scapulothoracic joint and considering the muscular linkages from the thoracic and cervical spine to the shoulder's bony components.[14]

Resting position is highly variable, depending on postural habits, hand dominance, occupation, muscle tone, and age. For example, the professional baseball pitcher's dominant shoulder girdle tends to fall forward and down. This is the result of the repetitive throwing cycle that stretches the posterior scapular muscles while shortening the anterior musculature. In contrast, prolonged static posture, as seen in the 50-year-old "desk jockey," can result in significantly forward shoulders and an increased kyphosis. Evaluation of resting posture can disclose vital information about muscle and joint dysfunction and is integral to all shoulder examinations.

Suspension of the shoulder girdle is attributed to the sternoclavicular ligaments,[8] upper trapezius,[6,102] levator scapulae,[6,102] sternocleidomastoid,[8] fascia,[82] and atmospheric pressure.[102] Alignment can be easily modified through muscular contraction, relaxation, and particularly the body's position with respect to gravity.

## Scapula

The scapula is a premier product of evolution. Man's fall from the trees to upright, ground-dwelling beings has actually resulted in scapular regression.[9] As a consequence of this evolutionary transformation, the scapula condensed and the thorax flattened, altering scapular orientation. The scapula has a slightly concave ventral surface that floats on the convex posterior thoracic wall. This compatible relationship places the scapula in an orientation directing the glenoid fossa 30 to 45 degrees anterior to the coronal plane. Therefore, this is referred to as the *plane of the scapula*[19,54,94] (Fig. 2-1).

The superior angle of the scapula is level with the spinous process of T2, while the inferior

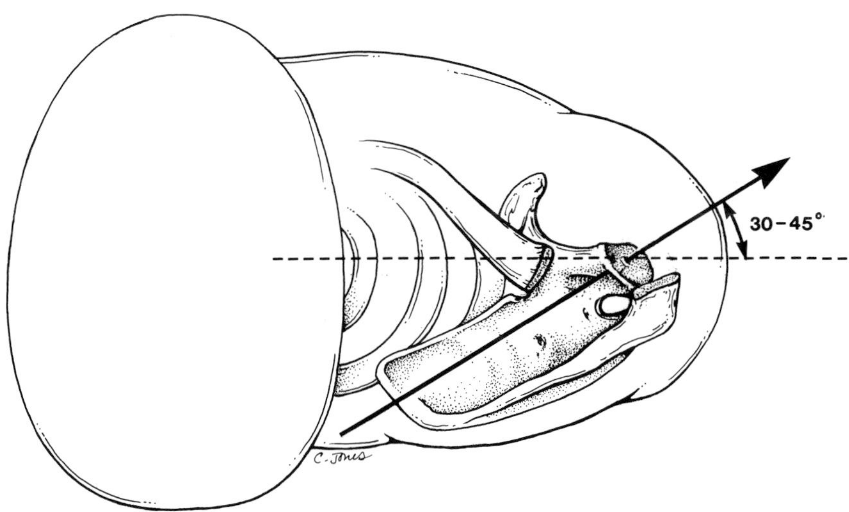


**Figure 2-1.** Scapular orientation in the plane of the scapula.

angle corresponds to the T7 spinous process. The average distance from the spinous processes to the scapular medial border is 5 to 6 cm,[57] although Laumann[64] found 8 to 9 cm to be the normal distance in 40 healthy male subjects (Fig. 2-2a). Rotational orientation has been investigated, but results demonstrate some disparity. Roentgenographic studies revealed the scapulothoracic angle to be −4.5 degrees (varying from −1 to 10 degrees[84]), −5.3 degrees,[36] and 3 degrees.[64] The first two studies indicated an actual resting position of medial rotation, while the third study indicated lateral rotation (see Fig. 2-2a). Variation of initial alignment may affect the setting phase of scapulohumeral rhythm during elevation.

When viewing the scapula from the side, ideal alignment places the acromion in a vertical line extending just anterior to the lateral malleolus to the mastoid process.[58] A 20-degree sagittal plane anterior scapular tilt was found between the lateral scapular border and the vertical[64] (see Fig. 2-2b).

The glenoid fossa is considered to be 7 degrees retroverted[96] with respect to the scapular neck and inclined approximately 5 degrees.[3] The

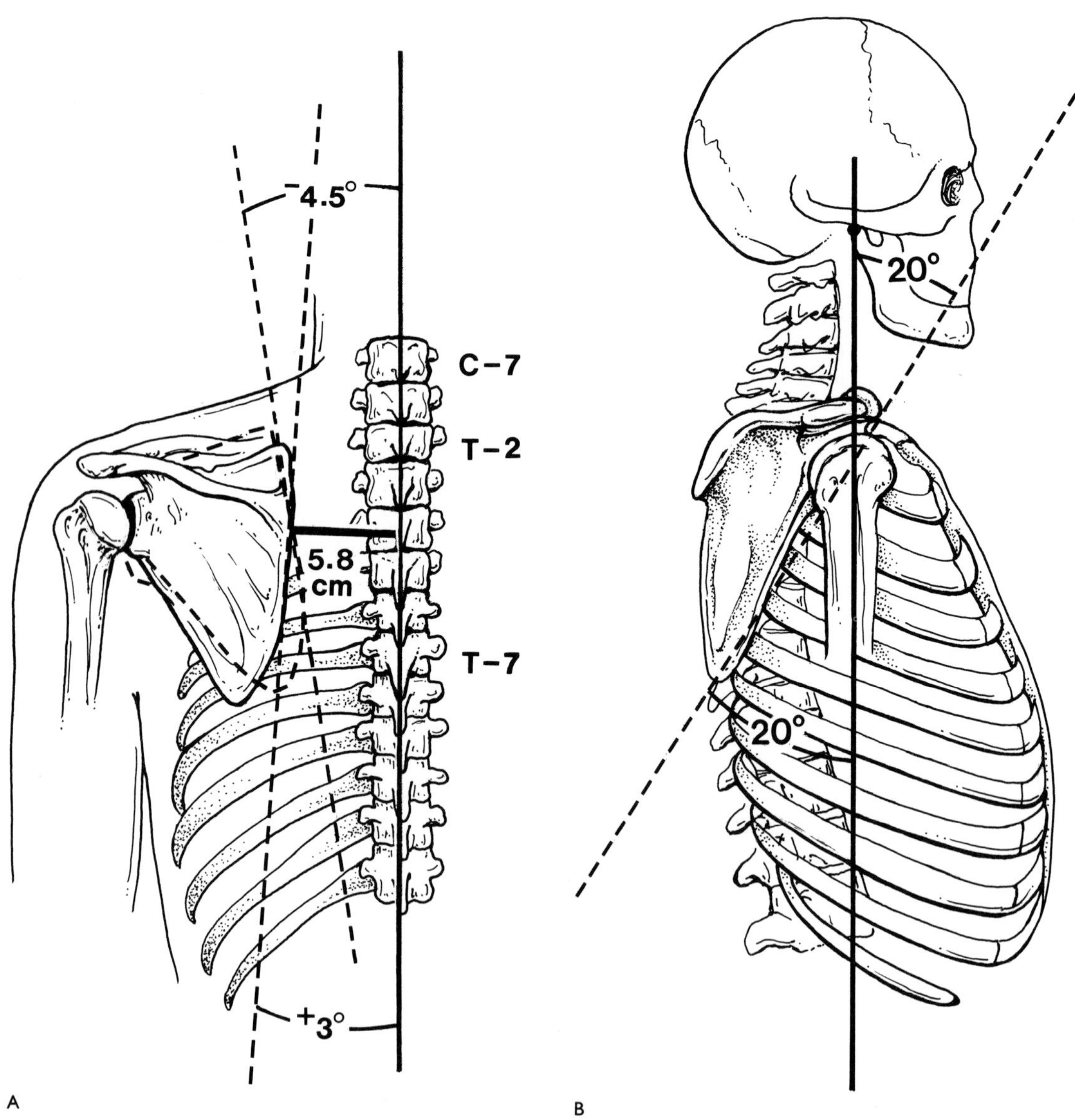


**Figure 2-2.** The resting position of the scapula relative to the head and spine. (a) Posterior view, resting position; scapular distance from the spinous processes and rotational orientation. (b) Normal scapular tilt.

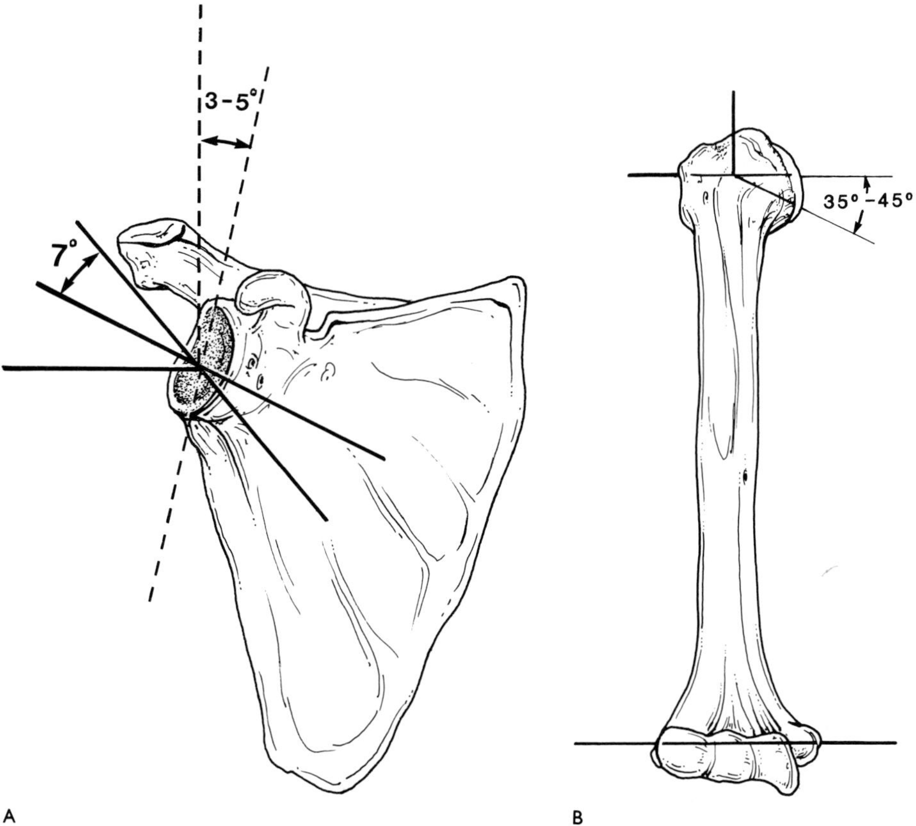


**Figure 2-3.** (a) Normal retroversion and vertical inclination of the glenoid fossa. (b) Normal retroversion of the humeral head with respect to the epicondyles.

humeral head is retroverted approximately 30 degrees from the humeral long axis, corresponding to the 30-degree anterior orientation of the glenoid fossa (Fig. 2-3). A resting position of slight glenohumeral adduction between 0.5 and 4.5 degrees was found.[31,36]

## Planes of Motion

The shoulder complex motion is described in relation to cardinal planes: sagittal, coronal, and horizontal. Flexion and extension occur in the sagittal plane, abduction and adduction in the coronal plane, and horizontal abduction (extension) and adduction (flexion) in the horizontal plane (Fig. 2-4a). Rotation takes place through the long axis of the humerus and can occur in an infinite number of planes. It is typically assessed at 90 degrees of coronal plane abduction or with the arm at the side (see Fig. 2-4b, c).

## Plane of the Scapula

The Academy of Orthopaedic Surgeons (AAOS) no longer differentiates the plane of motion in which the arm is brought overhead; instead, the AAOS has adopted the term *elevation*. Part of the reason for this change came from previous arguments from Codman,[19] Johnston,[54] McGreggor,[71] and Saha.[93,94] These individuals were strong advocates of elevation in the scapular plane (30 to 45 degrees in front of the coronal plane). They realized that regardless of the plane in which the arm was elevated or the direction of rotation, the end position was always the same, the medial epicondyle facing forward[19,54,93] (Fig. 2-5). This, in fact, is the concept of *Codman's paradox*.[19] Elevation in the scapular plane was herald to be true abduction.[38,54] *Gray's Anatomy*[38] actually refers to flexion and extension at right angles to the scapular plane. The articulating bones maintain optimal alignment through this plane of motion compared with abduction in the coronal plane, which incorporates a certain amount of horizontal abduction.[34,54] Motion in the scapular plane is

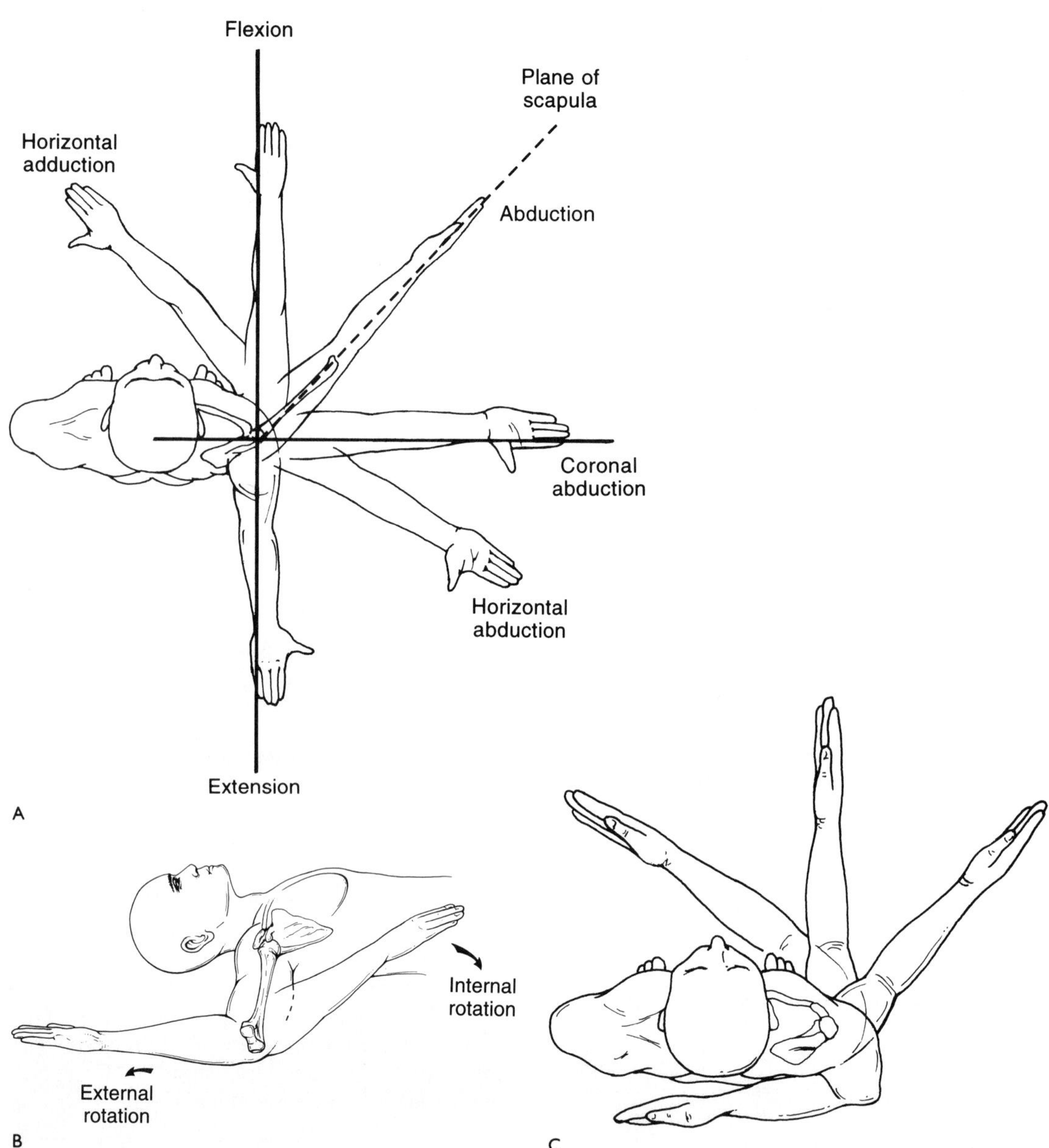


**Figure 2-4.** (a) Superior view showing planes of motion. (b) Humeral external and internal rotation at 90 degrees of coronal plane abduction. (c) Pure glenohumeral rotation at neutral and functional internal rotation.

actually arm movement relative to the scapula as opposed to the trunk. This suggests that the plane of the scapula is not truly fixed, since the scapula translates forward during elevation.[102]

There are several biomechanical and anatomic features of scapular plane elevation that are unique:

1. The joint surfaces have greater conformity.[34,54]
2. During elevation, the inferior capsuloligamentous complex remains untwisted and the associated rotator cuff remains relatively relaxed. This results because humeral rotation is not required[54] (Fig. 2-6).
3. The supraspinatus and deltoid are optimally aligned for elevation.[54]
4. Most functional activities are performed in this plane.[71]

These characteristics, specific to the scapular plane, can greatly enhance shoulder rehabilitation. For example, if treating a patient with rotator

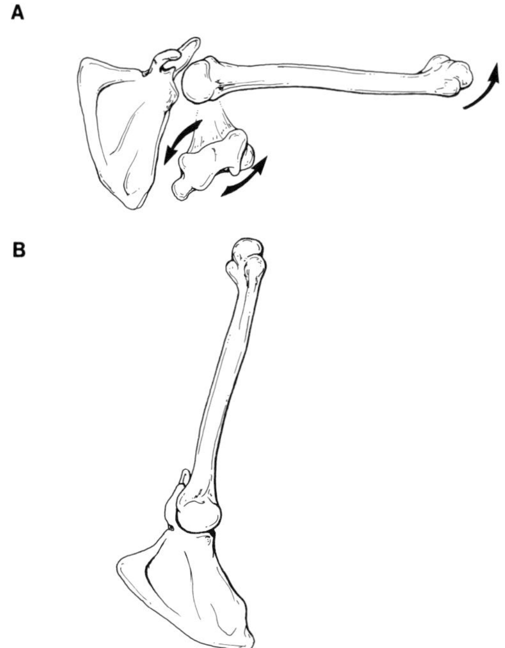


**Figure 2-5.** Whether elevation occurs in the sagittal plane, requiring internal rotation, or the coronal plane, requiring external rotation, the medial epicondyle is oriented anteriorly at end range.

cuff compromise or glenohumeral instability, exercising in the scapular plane can optimize rotator cuff muscle strength yet minimize unwanted passive tension on the rotator cuff tendons and the capsuloligamentous structures.

# Scapulohumeral Rhythm

Scapulohumeral rhythm is an essential concept of shoulder function. It is the synchronous culmination of shoulder girdle joint harmony. Although each joint will be discussed later in detail, we will briefly describe this phenomenon.

As the humerus actively elevates up to 30 degrees of coronal plane or scapular plane abduction and 60 degrees of flexion, the scapula seeks a position of stability. This is called the *setting phase* and is quite individual.[49] Following this phase, the humerus and scapula maintain a certain relationship, described as a *ratio of movement*, as the arm is elevated. This ratio has been investigated both radiographically and goniometrically.

Inman et al.[49] found a 2:1 ratio during both flexion and abduction in the coronal plane between 30 and 170 degrees. Other studies have examined elevation in the scapular plane. Saha[94] found a ratio of 2.3:1, which is very similar to that of Inman et al. Freedman and Munro[36] observed a 3:2 ratio from 0 to 135 degrees in adult males between 17 and 24 years of age. Scapulothoracic contribution decreased from 135 degrees to maximum elevation. Doody and coworkers[31] goniometrically determined a 1.74:1 ratio from 0 to 180 degrees in females between 17 and 21 years of age. They found varied input from the scapulothoracic and glenohumeral joints at different stages, with the former contributing more during the middle phases of abduction (90 to 140 degrees). Adding resistance caused increased scapular rotation in the early phases. Poppen and Walker[84] discovered a 4.3:1 ratio from 0 to 30 degrees and a 1.25:1 or 5:4 ratio from 30 to 180 degrees in subjects 22 to 63 years of age.

The results vary somewhat due to the measurement technique used. However, the rapport between glenohumeral and scapulothoracic motion is critical and generally considered to be 2:1, culminating in 120 and 60 degrees, respectively. Caution is required when comparing passive and active glenohumeral to scapulothoracic ratios and their phases of contribution. During passive motion, the muscles that drive the scapula are inactive; thus initiation of scapular movement

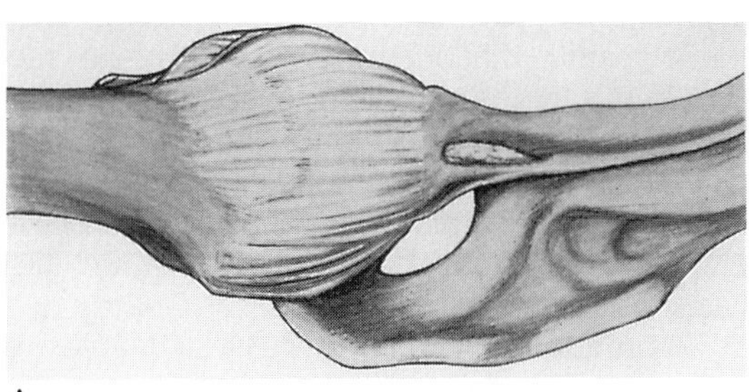


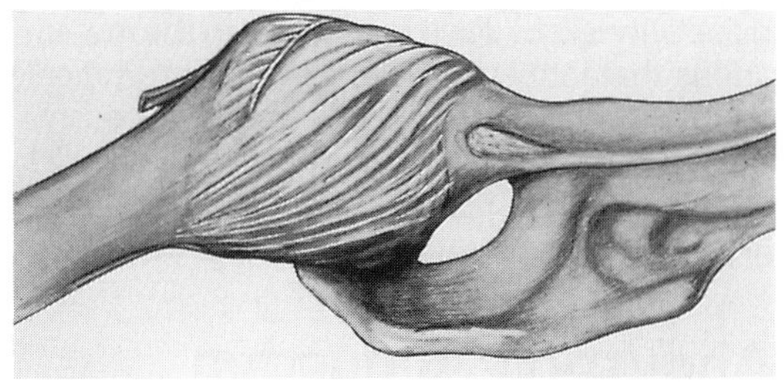


**Figure 2-6.** An inferior view of the glenohumeral joint and capsuloligamentous complex in (a) scapular plane abduction and (b) coronal plane abduction. (From Johnston TB. The movements of the shoulder joint: a plea for the use of the "plane of the scapula" as the plane of reference in movements occurring at the humeroscapular joint. Br J Surg 1937;25:252. By permission of the publishers Butterworth-Heinemann Ltd.)

will lag compared with active motion, being dependent on the glenohumeral capsuloligamentous structure's elasticity and expansion. This is why scapular motion may not be detected until 70 to 90 degrees of elevation when the arm is moved passively. If adhesions exist in the capsuloligamentous complex, early movement is noted of the scapula. For this reason, passive rather than active assessment of scapulohumeral rhythm tends to be more sensitive in determining restrictions of the capsuloligamentous complex.

Evaluation of active shoulder movement is necessary to determine dysfunctional scapulohumeral rhythm. A scapular lag may be noted on arm elevation, many times indicating functional weakness of the serratus anterior muscle. Weakness of the rotator cuff muscles typically results in compensation by the patient shrugging or elevating the scapula. Certainly pain or contracture of the glenohumeral capsuloligamentous complex will cause increased scapular elevation and lateral rotation during active arm trunk motion.

## Range of Motion

When assessing "shoulder" motion, the joints of the shoulder complex primarily are being evaluated. An area often omitted from range-of-motion studies and certainly clinical assessment is the contribution of the spine and thorax to arm-trunk total elevation. Contribution occurs in two ways: (1) the thoracic and mostly lumbar spine extension and side bending and (2) rib expansion. Rib expansion is dictated by available motion at both the costovertebral and transversocostal joints, the intercostal muscles, fascia extensibility, and the pliability of the costal cartilage. It is generally accepted that aging and poor posture significantly reduce their contribution.

Investigations of normal shoulder range of motion conclude dependence on age,[12] gender,[75] and activity level.[37] Factors inherent to the investigations that influence results are measurement technique, stabilization, active versus passive movement, and examiner expertise. Table 2-1 summaries range-of-motion studies. Note the differences in range among the various studies.

### Abduction/Adduction

Scapular plane abduction occurs in a plane 30 to 45 degrees in front of the coronal (see Fig. 2-4a). This plane requires no true rotation of the humerus about its long axis.[54]

Coronal plane *abduction* refers to the humerus moving relative to the body opposed to the scapula (see Fig. 2-4a). This requires the humerus to be horizontally abducted with respect to the glenoid. To achieve full motion, obligatory humeral external rotation occurs to prevent the greater tuberosity from contacting the coracoacromial arch.[19,28,38,54,102] The need for humeral external rotation and horizontal abduction when elevating in the coronal plane places excessive tension across the anterior/inferior glenohumeral capsuloligamentous structures. This explains why individuals who have capsuloligamentous adhesions are much more restricted in coronal plane abduction than scapular plane abduction.

Coronal plane range of motion is generally accepted as 180 degrees.[1,6,28,57,102,105] Murray et al.[75] investigated active coronal plane abduction in males and females in two separate age groups. Interestingly, they found no significant difference between age groups or sexes.

*Adduction* is defined as return from abduction in either the coronal or scapular plane, thus being equal to abduction range of motion.

### Flexion

*Flexion* occurs in the sagittal plane and is accompanied by humeral internal rotation[11,33,67] (Fig. 2-4a). Without rotation, the lesser tubercle impinges against the coracoacromial arch.[71] This mechanism is under less voluntary control than external rotation in abduction, being dependent on the glenohumeral capsuloligamentous complex (CLC), primarily the posterior portion. Tightness of the posterior capsule can lead to restricted flexion but is also suspected to contribute to superior humeral head migration and subacromial impingement.[40] Motion is commonly considered to be 180 degrees[1,6,28,57,102]

### Extension

*Extension* is movement posterior from the anatomic position that occurs in a sagittal plane (see Fig. 2-4a) In the strictest sense, this motion should be considered purely glenohumeral. Once the capsuloligamentous complex and associated muscle pliability is exhausted, the clavicle begins to rotate down, and the scapula elevates while tilting anteriorly.[6]

The AAOS[1] found an average of 60 degrees of extension. This correlates well with other investigations, which found 58 degrees[75] and 62 degrees.[12] A significant difference of 10 degrees was reported for subjects over and under 19 years of age.[12]

**Table 2-1**

**Studies of Normal Range of Motion**

| Motion | Investigator | Technique | *n* | Gender | Age (years) | Range of Motion (degrees) |
|---|---|---|---|---|---|---|
| Abduction (coronal) | Murray | Goniometric | 20 | M/F | 25–36 | 179 |
| | | | | | 55–66 | 178 |
| | AAOS | Goniometric | | | | 180 |
| Abduction (POS) | Boone | Goniometric | 109 | M | 1–19 | 185 |
| | | | | | 20–44 | 182 |
| | Doody | Goniometric | 25 | F | 17–21 | 176 |
| | Freedman | Radiographic | 61 | M | 17–24 | 167 |
| | AAOS | * | | | | 180 |
| Flexion | Boone | * | * | * | 1–19 | 164 |
| | | | | | 20–44 | 165 |
| | Germain | Goniometric | 88 | M/F | 20–70 | 174 |
| | Murray | * | * | * | 25–36 | 171 |
| | | | | | 55–66 | 165 |
| | AAOS | * | | | | 180 |
| Hyperextension | Boone | * | * | * | 1–19 | 67 |
| | | | | | 20–44 | 57 |
| | Murray | * | * | * | 25–36 | 57 |
| | | | | | 55–66 | 58 |
| | AAOS | * | | | | 60 |
| External rotation 90° (coronal plane) | Boone | * | * | * | 1–19 | 108 |
| | | | | | 20–44 | 100 |
| | Murray | * | * | * | 25–36 | 97 |
| | | | | | 55–66 | 88 |
| | AAOS | * | | | | 90 |
| External rotation 0° | Clarke | Goniometric | 10 | M | 20–28 | 67 |
| | AAOS | * | | | | 60 |
| Internal rotation 90° (coronal plane) | Boone | * | * | * | 1–19 | 70 |
| | | | | | 20–44 | 67 |
| | Murray | * | * | * | 25–36 | 51 |
| | | | | | 55–66 | 57 |
| | AAOS | * | | | | 70 |
| Horizontal adduction | Boone | * | * | * | 1–19 | 140 |
| | | | | | 20–44 | 141 |
| | AAOS | * | | | | 135 |
| Horizontal abduction | Boone | * | * | * | 1–19 | 47 |
| | | * | * | * | 20–44 | 44 |

* Indicates study methods and materials are the same as previously described.

## External Rotation

External rotation can occur in any position except full elevation.[19,28,93] Assessment is typically performed in 90 degrees of coronal plane abduction (see Fig. 2-4b) or from a neutral position (see Fig. 2-4c). A significant difference up to 30 degrees can be found between the two measurements. This is directly related to the constraining effect of the subscapularis and the glenohumeral CLC in the neutral position. Turkel et al.[108] demonstrated the correlation between restricting effects and position of these structures related to external rotation from 0 to 90 degrees of abduction (see Capsuloligamentous Complex, p. 81).

Normal range-of-motion studies investigating values of external rotation performed at neutral are few. Clark et al.[17] found an average of 67 degrees. Normal external rotation (at 90 degrees of abduction) is accepted to be 90 degrees.[1,6,94,105] Murray et al.[75] found a significant difference between men and women between 55 and 65 years of age, while significant differences also were found between those over and under 19 years of age.[12] External rotation is considered purely glenohumeral; overestimation of this motion commonly results from allowing scapular substitution. If scapular substitution is allowed when assessing at 90 degrees of coronal plane abduction, the scapula tilts posteriorly (defined by the superior angle direction) and depresses. The scapula will adduct and compress into the thoracic wall when allowed to substitute during external rotation range assessment at zero abduction.

## Internal Rotation

Internal rotation is also considered entirely glenohumeral motion. Internal rotation measured at 90 degrees of abduction is the accepted position for evaluation (see Fig. 2-4b). Internal rotation is difficult to assess at neutral because the forearm contacts the trunk; motion can be measured in this position and is considered to be 90 degrees (see Fig. 2-4c). Typically, internal rotation is less than external rotation when measured at 90 degrees.[1,12,74] Scapular stabilization is necessary to prevent scapular substitution and determine true internal rotation end range at the 90-degree abducted position. Normal range is recognized as 70 degrees.[1,12]

Many clinicians assess internal rotation by reaching behind the back and touching the thumb to the highest spinous process (see Fig. 2-4c). Although this motion is composed largely of internal rotation, concomitant shoulder extension and adduction, as well as elbow and wrist motion, must occur. This can be considered a functional test and is certainly useful in the evaluation process.

## Horizontal Abduction/ Adduction

Horizontal abduction (extension) and adduction (flexion) occur in the horizontal plane (see Fig. 2-4a). Horizontal adduction is measured from the coronal plane passing through the sagittal plane. Normal motion is accepted as 135 degrees.[1,6] Horizontal abduction, measured from the coronal plane posteriorly, is 45 degrees.[6]

In summary, to standardize the measurement of human motion, arm movement has been described relative to the trunk or scapula. In reality, a combination of motion and planes is necessary for the upper extremity to perform the multitude of tasks that are required each day. Restriction by pain, adhesions, or weakness limits full rhythmic motion in one or all planes.

# Osteokinematics and Arthrokinematics

## Sternoclavicular Joint

The sternoclavicular joint serves as the only articular link the shoulder girdle has to the trunk. This is a monumental responsibility, particularly since the amount of articular contact is the least of all the major joints in the body.[27] The small percentage of dislocations is somewhat surprising, since stability is predominantly mediated by the capsule and ligaments.

The sternoclavicular joint is a saddle-type joint separated by an intraarticular disc. The sternal articular surface is concave in the midportion or in the coronal plane and convex in its anteroposterior aspect.[97,102] The medial articular surface of the clavicle has a corresponding concave/convex surface.[73] There is also an inferior articulation with the costal cartilage of the first rib.

Three degrees of freedom are available at the sternoclavicular joint. Elevation and depression occur through an axis in the sagittal plane. Elevation occurs up to 45 degrees, while 5 degrees of depression is allowed.[73] Motion is possible by gliding between the medial clavicle and intraarticular meniscus.[27] Elevation is limited by tension of the costoclavicular ligament[8,15,27,102] (Fig. 2-7b).

Although only 5 degrees of active depression is available, greater excursion results particularly when the clavicular suspensory muscles are lacking. The posterosuperior capsule is the

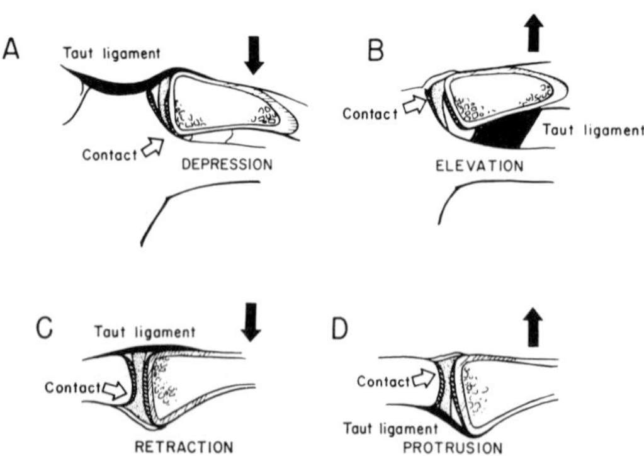


**Figure 2-7.** Sternoclavicular motion through two axes. (a, b) Depression and elevation through the sagittal axis. (c, d) Retraction and protraction through the superomedial to inferolateral oblique axes corresponding restraints. (From Dempster WT. Mechanisms of shoulder movement. Arch Phys Med Rehabil 1965;46:49.)

major ligamentous constraint against unwanted lateral clavicle settling. This assists in maintaining proper resting orientation when the arm is dependent.[8] Although the interclavicular ligament tightened, clavicular position was not altered upon loading the distal clavicle with up to 20 lb.[8] Bony contact between the clavicular inferomedial surface and sternum also adds to stability[27] (see Fig. 2-7a).

Clavicular protraction and retraction occur through an oblique axis oriented superomedially to inferolaterally.[102] Approximately 15 degrees of motion is present in each direction.[73] Because the axis is oblique, retraction is accompanied by elevation, while protraction combines with depression.[8,73,102] Gliding between the meniscus and sternum mediates motion in this plane.[27] Protraction is limited by the posterior fibers of the costoclavicular ligament, posterior sternoclavicular capsule, and posterior fibers of the interclavicular ligament[8,27] (See Fig. 2-7d). Retraction is restricted by the anterior costoclavicular fibers and anterior sternoclavicular capsule[8] (see Fig. 2-7c).

Rotation occurs through the longitudinal axis of the clavicle. Inman et al.[49] demonstrated approximately 40 degrees of upward rotation, defined by the direction of the anterior edge, during flexion and abduction. This motion begins at approximately 90 degrees of elevation and continues, becoming somewhat greater at end range.[49] Upward rotation is dependent on mounting tension of the coracoclavicular ligaments. As scapular rotation advances, the base of the coracoid process, which is the insertion of the coracoclavicular ligaments, begins to move distally. This produces a downward pull on the posterior clavicle, thus causing upward clavicular rotation (Fig. 2-8). Normal laxity of the sternoclavicular capsuloligamentous complex permits the clavicle to rotate about its medial end until tension develops in the complex as they "screw up."[8] Approximately 10 degrees of downward rotation is available.[73]

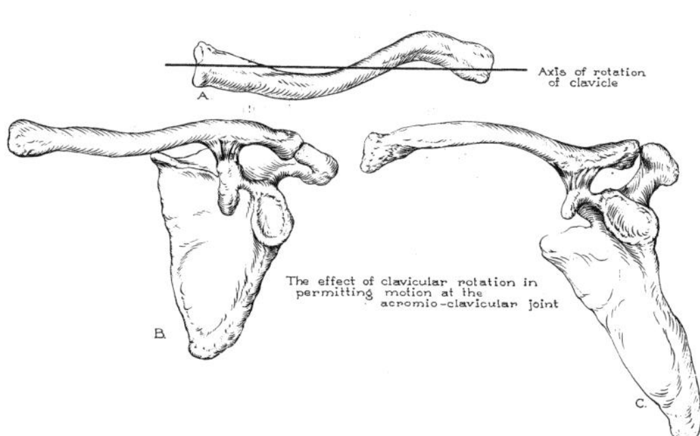


**Figure 2-8.** Scapular rotation causing coracoclavicular tautening and upward clavicular rotation. Corresponding motion also occurs at the sternoclavicular and acromioclavicular joints. (From Inman VT, Saunders JB, Abbott LC. Observations on the function of the shoulder joint. J. Bone Joint Surg 1944;26:1.)

# Acromioclavicular Joint

The acromioclavicular joint is the articulation between the acromial end of the distal clavicle and scapula. This linkage is further aided by the coracoclavicular ligaments, the conoid, and the trapezoid. These ligaments serve not only as a second junction between the scapula and the clavicle but also as an acromioclavicular joint stabilizing structure. The total system is known as the *claviscapular joint*.[27]

The acromioclavicular joint is a plane-type joint having an intraarticular meniscus. The articular surface design varies, but the distal clavicle is usually convex or flattened, while the acromial surface is concave.[102] A dense fibrous capsule encases the joint and is reinforced by the superior, inferior, anterior, and posterior acromioclavicular ligaments. The superior aspect is augmented by the upper trapezius tendinous attachment.

Three degrees of freedom are available at the acromioclavicular joint; however, they rarely occur individually.[73] First, motion occurs through a vertical axis, allowing the scapular vertebral border to"wing" and the glenoid fossa to face anteriorly[27,73] (Fig. 2-9a). The acromion glides forward and backward as the scapula's medial border swings away from and into the thorax. Motion is checked by tension in the conoid and trapezoid.[27]

An axis projects through the sagittal plane and allows scapular abduction and adduction, as described by Mosley[73] (see Fig. 2-9b). Abduction may be more accurately termed *lateral rotation of the scapula*.[27] This motion is checked by the coracoclavicular ligaments and inferior acromioclavicular ligament. Adduction, or *medial rotation*, is limited by impingement of the coracoid on the clavicle.[27]

A third axis through the coronal plane permits anterior tilting of the superior angle, causing the inferior angle to lift posteriorly[73] (see Fig. 2-9c). Anterior tilting is restricted by the anterior acromioclavicular and trapezoid ligaments, while posterior tilting is restricted by the thorax as well as the posterior acromioclavicular and conoid ligaments.[27]

Inman et al[49] demonstrated that approximately 10 degrees of motion occurs at the acro-

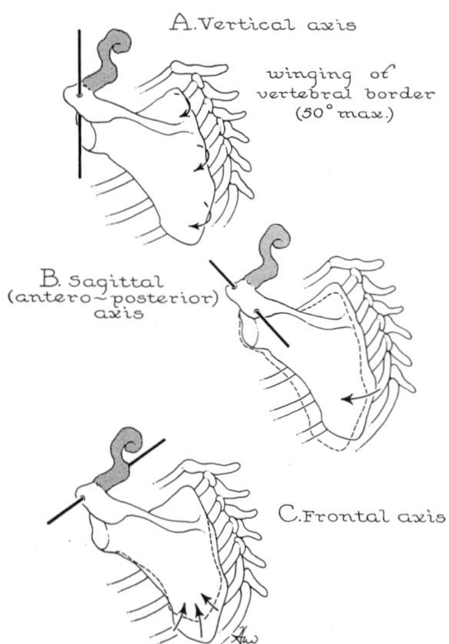


**Figure 2-9.** Three axes of motion shown through the acromioclavicular joint. (a) Vertical axis allows the glenoid to face toward the sagittal or coronal planes. (b) Sagittal axis allows slight medial and lateral rotation. (c) Coronal axis allows anterior and posterior tilting. (From Moseley HF. The clavicle: its anatomy and function. Clin Orthop 1958;58:24.)

mioclavicular joint during the first 30 degrees of flexion and abduction and then again in the last 45 degrees of motion. The acromioclavicular joint contributes greater motion at end range of elevation.[6] When irritation of this joint exists, clinical findings reveal pain at all shoulder end ranges, particularly during horizontal adduction. Bateman[6] stated that the acromioclavicular joint compensates for lost motion in the presence of glenohumeral joint restriction. This is important to keep in mind when dealing with restricted glenohumeral elevation, since repetitive forcing of end-range elevation causes scapular substitution and hence increased acromioclavicular compression, resulting in premature degenerative joint changes. Based on this concept, does the acromioclavicular joint require joint mobilization in the patient presenting with a "frozen shoulder"? Typically, these patients attempt to elevate the arm by performing scapular substitution; here, the acromioclavicular joint, as well as the scapulothoracic and sternoclavicular joints, compensates with excessive motion secondary to deficient glenohumeral motion. Therefore, it is inaccurate to equate restricted glenohumeral motion with lost acromioclavicular motion as such; joint mobilization of the acromioclavicular joint (for lost motion) is not always required in a patient with a "frozen shoulder."

Inman[49] warned against screw fixation negating acromioclavicular joint motion. Several investigators found screw fixation or coracoclavicular ossification to have little or no effect on shoulder elevation.[59,89] In fact, when Kirschner wires were attached to the clavicle of a patient whose distal clavicle was fixated to the corcoid by a screw, full clavicular rotation was observed[57] (Fig. 2-10). Kennedy and Cameron[59] reported that patients over 50 years of age had less satisfactory results and painful end-range abduction with screw fixation. They concluded that this group relied more on coracoclavicular ligamentous "play" than did the younger patients.

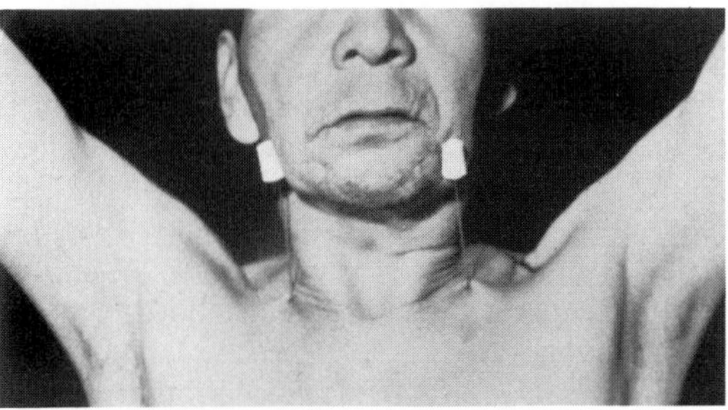

**Figure 2-10.** Clavicular rotation still present on left even though a screw fixes the distal clavicle to the base of the coracoid. (From Kennedy JC, Cameron H. Complete dislocation of the acromioclavicular joint. J Bone Joint Surg 1954;36B:202.)

## Scapulothoracic Joint

The scapulothoracic joint is not considered a true anatomic joint because it lacks qualifying characteristics. The scapula's concave ventral surface is filled by the subscapularis and conforms to the posterior thoracic convex wall. Between these structures is the powerful serratus anterior muscle. The scapula is suspended by the sternoclavicular ligaments (indirectly through the clavicle),[8] descending axioscapular muscles,[6,82] coracoclavicular ligaments, atmospheric pressure,[102] and fascia.[82] Scapulothoracic joint function enhances arm-trunk motion and glenohumeral stability. Glenohumeral joint stability is maximized as the glenoid adjusts to support the humeral head.[92] Another considerable task the scapulothoracic joint performs is to serve as a protective recoil mechanism[92] (Fig. 2-11). When an individual falls on an outstretched arm, force is translated through the arm. The body will "spring" forward on the scapula as supporting muscles absorb the energy. When the force is too great, glenohumeral joint stability and associated structures can be compromised.

The scapula lies in the scapular plane. Move-

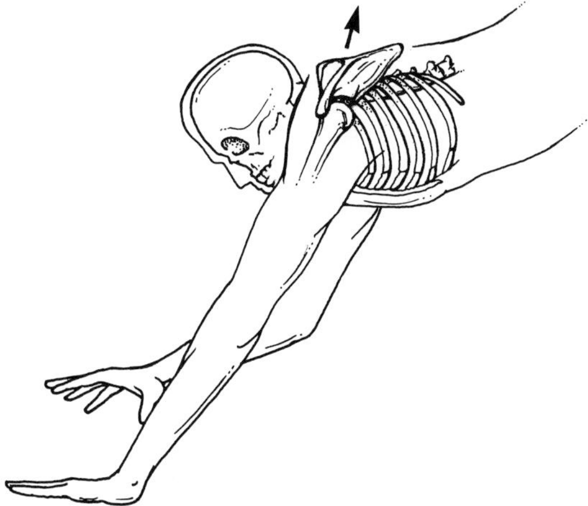

**Figure 2-11.** Recoil mechanism demonstrating protective shock-absorbing ability of the scapulothoracic muscles. (Adapted from Rowe CR, Sakellavides HT. Factors related to recurrences of anterior dislocations of the shoulder. Clin Orthop 1961;20:41.)

ment is mediated primarily through translation over the thoracic wall driven by the oblique attachment of the axioscapular muscles. Synchronous clavicular and scapular movement results because of the acromioclavicular ligaments and the claviscapular joint in addition to sternoclavicular joint motion. In fact, scapular and clavicular motion requires involvement of the sternoclavicular joint. Patients having a glenohumeral arthrodesis are completely dependent on scapular and clavicular movement.

## ELEVATION/DEPRESSION

Although gliding occurs between the scapula and thorax, the true fulcrum for motion is the sternoclavicular joint. Elevation is mediated primarily through the upper trapezius[102] and levator scapulae[25] action; when combined with retraction, the rhomboid becomes active.[25] Normal range of elevation has been measured from 4 to 6 cm,[6] although Duchene[33] reported 2 to 3.5 cm. Clinically, we have found the former estimate to be more accurate (Fig. 2-12a).

Scapular depression from a supine, sitting, or standing position is minimal, 1 to 2 cm[55] (see Fig. 2-12A). The lower trapezius, pectoralis minor, and serratus anterior muscles are responsible for true depression.[102] Depression occurs in conjunction with scapular anterior or posterior tilting. Contraction of the pectoralis minor and serratus anterior muscles (without humeral elevation) causes depression and anterior tilting, while depression and posterior tilting are mediated by the lower trapezius muscle. When a patient assumes the prone position, the shoulder girdle falls into a relatively elevated and protracted state. This is why muscle testing of the middle and lower trapezius requires manual "setting" of the scapula into anatomic position.

## ABDUCTION/ADDUCTION

These motions are defined by the vertebral scapular border moving laterally (abduction) and medially (adduction). Here again, we see the contri-

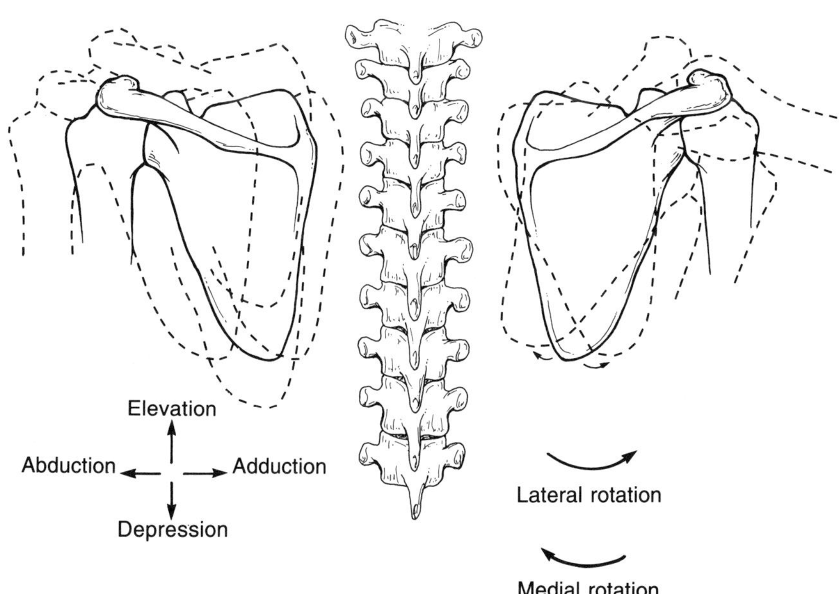


**Figure 2-12.** Motions of the scapulothoracic joint.

bution of the sternoclavicular joint providing a fulcrum for scapulothoracic motion.

Abduction is powered by the serratus anterior and pectoralis minor muscles.[6] The pectoralis major contribute to abduction by pulling on the fixed humerus, which then moves the scapula. Excursion of 7.5 to 10 cm is normal,[6] but this is dependent on resting position. Clinically, we have found 4 to 6 cm to be normal when true abduction is isolated from elevation (see Fig. 2-12a).

The rhomboids,[25] middle trapezius,[6] and lower trapezius[33] are responsible for adduction.[58] The levator scapulae is inactive unless elevation is performed.[25] Between 4 and 5 cm of excursion is considered normal,[6] but individuals having a resting scapula in abduction will demonstrate greater migration (see Fig. 2-12a).

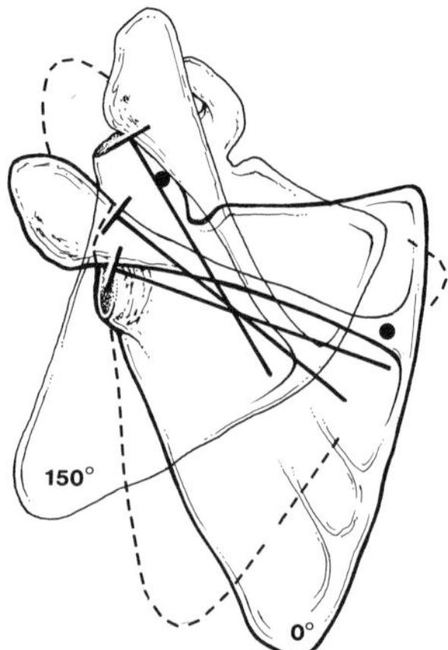

**Figure 2-13.** Change in the scapula's rotation axis during arm elevation, moving from the base of the scapular spine toward the glenoid.

## MEDIAL ROTATION (DOWNWARD)

Active scapular rotation is predominantly dependent on glenohumeral motion; however, acromioclavicular and sternoclavicular joint motion also enable the scapula to rotate. Medial rotation is sparsely discussed in the literature, probably because it rarely is lost. Movement is defined by the inferior angle rotating toward the spine and is mediated by the rhomboids, levator scapulae, and pectoralis minor[102] (see Fig. 2-12b).

## LATERAL ROTATION (UPWARD)

Lateral rotation is critical to optimize shoulder performance. The scapula's axis of rotation is not a fixed point but lies approximately at the root of the scapular spine (RSS).[34] Poppen and Walker[84] place it at the scapula's "lower midportion" (Fig. 2-13). During the first 30 to 60 degrees of elevation, scapular movement is quite irregular until a stable position is found.[34,49,64,93] Rotation of the glenoid approximately 10 degrees anteriorly ensues through the vertical acromioclavicular joint axis. The scapula continues to rotate laterally subsequent to 60 degrees, about the RSS, in an area confined to a certain region on the thoracic wall.[34] This demonstrates the stable clamping effect against the thoracic wall with little superior or inferior migration. During the first 90 degrees of motion, significant superior acromioclavicular joint migration occurs, corresponding to the clavicular elevation.[34] At approximately 100 degrees of elevation, the coracoclavicular ligament begins to tighten, pulling on the posterior lip of the clavicle and producing clavicular upward rotation.[34,49,93] Because the scapula continues to rotate, the RSS can no longer maintain its previous area on the thoracic wall. The center of rotation shifts toward the glenoid, resulting in medial and continued superior movement of the glenoid and lateral migration of the scapular inferior angle.[84] Along with lateral rotation, the scapular orients the glenoid fossa anteriorly toward the sagittal plane. The scapula tilts posteriorly as the superior angle moves away from the thoracic wall, while the inferior angle moves into it (Fig. 2-14). Radiographic tracing of the acromion and coracoid demonstrates this tilting.[64,84] Ten more degrees of acromioclavicular contribution occurs after 135 degrees.[49] In all, the scapula rotates approximately 60 degrees.[6,31,34,49,84,93]

Assessment of scapular rotation during arm elevation is essential. The scapula should begin to migrate into lateral rotation by 60 degrees of

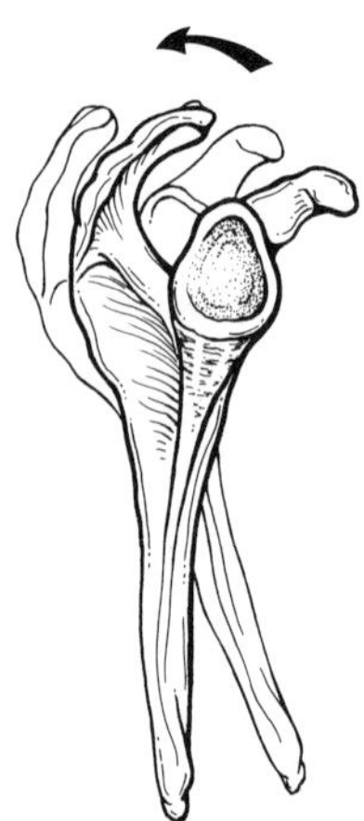
**Figure 2-14.** Scapular posterior tilting during arm elevation as the superior angle moves away from the thoracic wall while the inferior angle moves toward the thoracic wall.

elevation. If delayed, abnormal scapulohumeral rhythm may exists. In this situation, rotator cuff and bursa impingement is inevitable, since the glenoid and the acromion have not begun their superior travel as the greater tuberosity and associated rotator cuff tendon-bursa complex approach.

## Glenohumeral Joint

The glenohumeral joint is the most mobile of the four shoulder girdle articulations. Because of its inherent mobility, the associated restraints are constantly challenged. This joint is an intricate complex with a sometimes fragile system of checks and balances. Vulnerability is demonstrated by the number of patients seen with pathology of associated static and dynamic components.

The glenohumeral joint is the articulation between the larger spherical convex humeral head and the smaller concave glenoid fossa. Only 25 to 30 percent of the humeral head is covered by the glenoid surface in any given anatomic position.[19] The average humeral head diameter is 44 mm, compared with a glenoid diameter of 25 mm. The fossa is deepened by a 2-mm ridge of labral fibrocartilage tissue.[46]

The concept of glenohumeral motion occurring with a certain degree of rotation (spin), roll, and glide is well accepted. *Rotation* or *spin* is defined as multiple points on the humerus contacting one point on the glenoid surface. *Rolling* is defined as multiple humeral contact points articulating with multiple points on the glenoid. *Gliding* or *translation* is described as one humeral contact translating over multiple glenoid points (Fig. 2-15).

MacConnail[67] developed the term *roll-gliding* to describe joint motion between incongruent, concave and convex surfaces. The direction of rolling and gliding components is dependent on whether the concave or convex surface is moving. The convex/concave theory of arthrokinematics dictates that if a convex surface moves on a concave surface, then gliding occurs in the opposite direction to the rolling; if a concave surface moves on a convex surface, then rolling and gliding occur in the same direction (Fig. 2-16). The more congruent the surfaces are, the more gliding occurs, and the more incongruent, the more rolling takes place.[56] The disproportion between the glenohumeral articular surfaces would then dictate that rolling dominates. In recent investigations, however, this finding does not hold true.

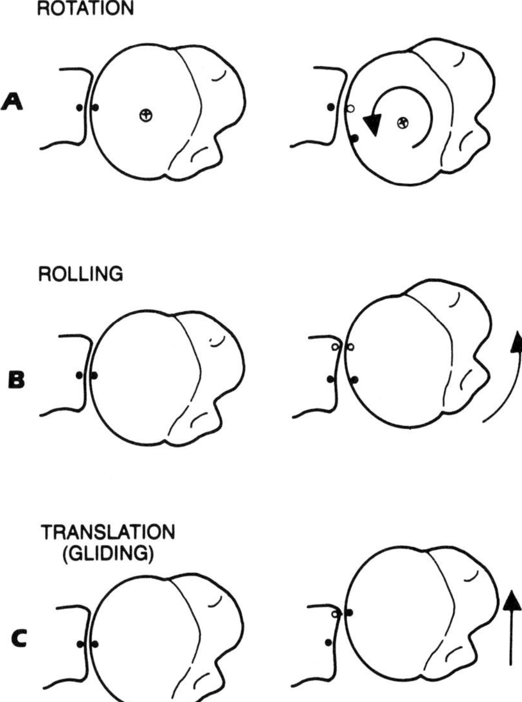


**Figure 2-15.** Three types of articular movement occur at the glenohumeral joint: (a) rotation, (b) rolling, (c) gliding. (From Matzen FA III, Zuckerman J. Biomechanics of the shoulder. In Frankel VH, Nordin M, eds. Basic biomechanics of the musculoskeletal system. 2nd ed. Philadelphia: Lea & Febiger, 1989: 231.)

Calliet[14] and Saha[94,96] agree that humeral head rolling on the glenoid is the predominate motion. They also agree that this is accompanied by some amount of gliding. Perry[82] states that rolling is not significant to glenohumeral motion other than during the initial 3 mm of superior excursion. She feels that gliding is the dominate component motion.[82] Howell et al.[47] advocate rotation as the predominate movement but disagree with Perry that the initial 3 mm of upward motion is due to rolling; instead, they feel that gliding governs this initial movement. Poppen and Walker[84] concisely demonstrated in a radiographic study that rolling does not prevail. They determined that during the initial 30 degrees of elevation in the scapular plane and often from 30 to 60 degrees, the humeral head glides upward on the glenoid fossa approximately 3 mm. After that point, the humerus center of rotation remains constant, moving 1 to 2 mm upward or downward relative to the glenoid center (Fig. 2-17). They concluded that after the initial rise, the humeral head will rotate or spin on a more or less fixed center with little, if any, excursion.[84]

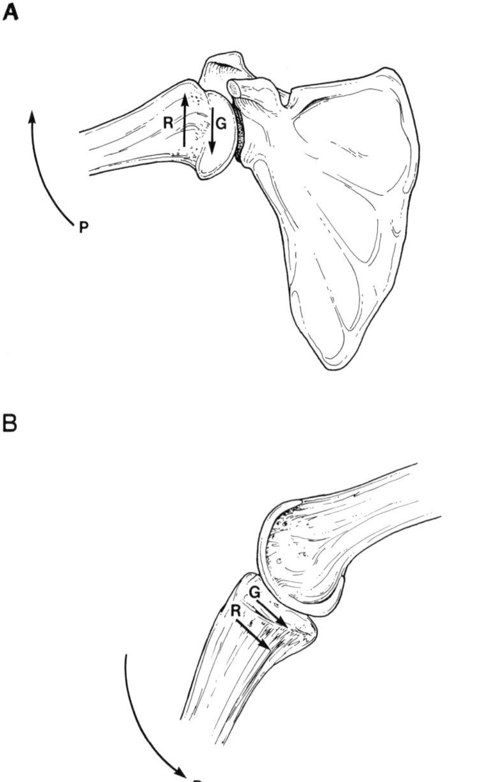


**Figure 2-16.** Traditionally accepted convex/concave rule as it applies to (a) the shoulder and (b) the knee.

Harryman et al.[40,41] found an average superior migration of 0.7 and 0.8 mm during abduction and flexion, respectively. Most recently, Kelkar et al.,[57a] using an extremely accurate three-dimensional technique of stereophotogrammetry on cadaver shoulders, found an average vertical excursion of 1.29 mm occurring through an arc of 180 degrees of scapular plane abduction. They found an average of 0.94 mm of superior glide in the first 30 degrees of motion (Fig. 2-18). They, as did Poppen and Walker, concluded that the initial superior rise was due the dependent (inferior) state of the humerus when in the unloaded condition. They strongly felt that after 30 degrees, pure rotation (spin) occurred at the glenohumeral interface.

What is important for the clinician to realize is that the humeral head does not truly "depress" with elevation and that gliding is superior and may be slightly inferior. The humeral head center of rotation remains relatively constant with the center of the glenoid. What changes, through rotation and subtle gliding of 1 to 2 mm (roll-glide), is the humeral articular contact point, which moves inferiorly to superiorly on the humeral head[57a, 76, 84] (Fig. 2-19). One must not mistake palpating "depression" of the greater tubercle (as the humerus elevates) as a sign of humeral head inferior gliding. Instead, greater tubercle movement represents medial migration beneath the acromion.

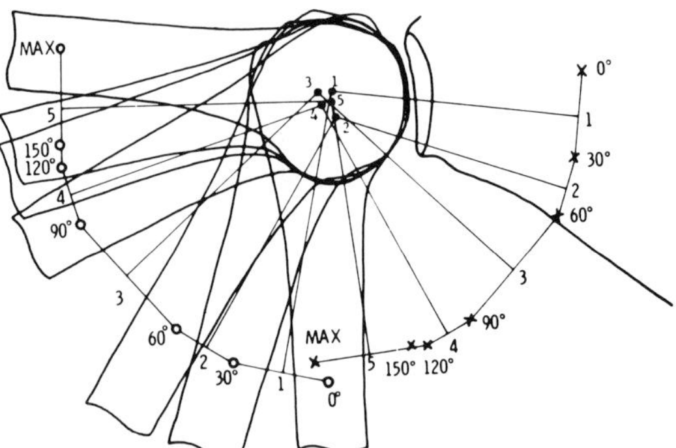


**Figure 2-17.** Vertical translatory excursion of the humeral head geometric center measured relative to the center of the glenoid. Measurements were taken at 30-degree intervals from zero to maximum scapular plane abduction. The X represents glenoid position, and the O represents humeral position. (From Walker PS. Human joints and their artificial replacements. Springfield, Ill.: Charles C Thomas, 1977.)

Controversy also exist about traditionally accepted concepts regarding translation or gliding in the anterior and posterior directions. Howell et al.[47] radiographically evaluated anterior and posterior translation with the arm positioned in various degrees of horizontal adduction/abduction and rotation. They concluded that the humeral head normally translates 4 mm posterior when in a position of 90 degrees of abduction, full external rotation, and maximal horizontal

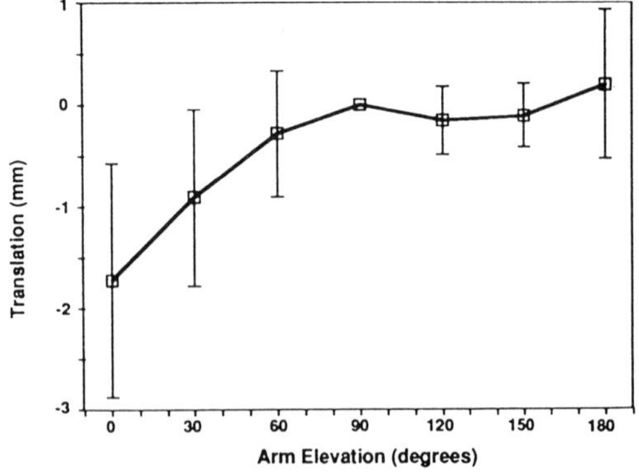


**Figure 2-18.** Normal humeral superior glide followed by rotation (spin) during plane of the scapula abduction. (From Kelkar R, Flatow EL, Bigliani LU et al. A sterophotogrammetric method to determine the kinematics of the glenohumeral joint. Adv Bioeng 1992;19:143.)

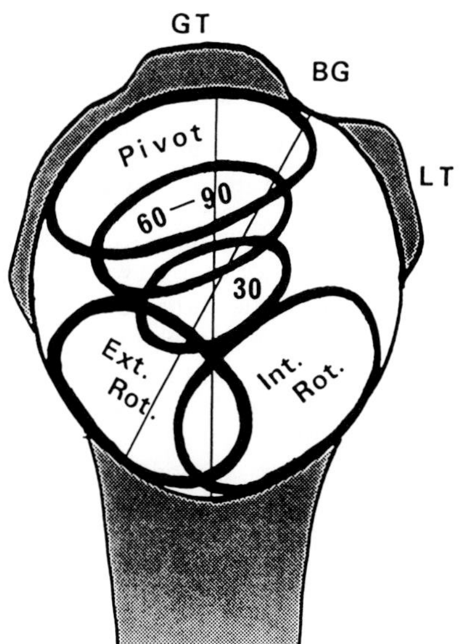


**Figure 2-19.** An inferior to superior change in humeral head contact with the glenoid at different positions of scapular plane abduction. Internal and external rotation contact points are also shown. (From Nobuhara K. The shoulder: its function and clinical aspects. Tokyo: Igaku-Shoin, 1977.)

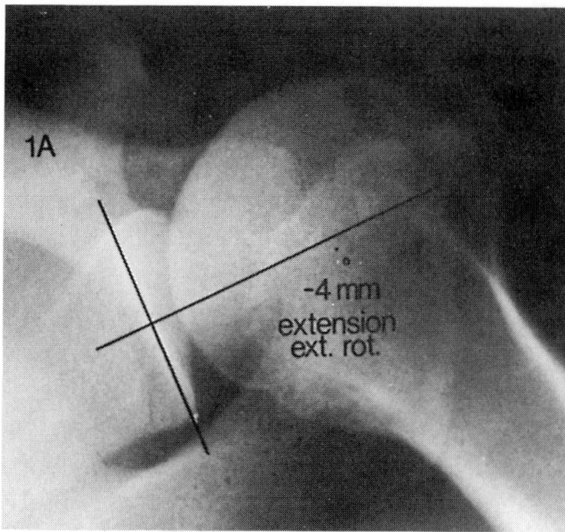


**Figure 2-20.** Axillary view (inferior through the glenohumeral joint) in 90 degrees of abduction, full external rotation, and horizontal abduction. The geometric center of the humeral head is 4 mm posterior to the center of the glenoid fossa, demonstrating normal posterior, not anterior translation. (From Howell SM, Galinat BJ, Renzi AJ, Marone PJ. Normal and abnormal mechanics of the glenohumeral joint in the horizontal plane. J Bone Joint Surg 1988;70A:230.)

abduction (Fig. 2-20). Patients with known anterior instability demonstrated anterior, not posterior, translation when placed in the same position. Harryman et al.[41] performed biomechanical analysis on cadavers, finding approximately 3.8 mm of anterior translation with flexion and 5 mm of posterior translation with extension. Tightening the posterior capsule significantly increased anterior translation and to some extent superior humeral head translation (Fig. 2-21). Additionally, they found that external rotation and internal rotation performed with the humerus at the side produced posterior and anterior gliding, respectively.

These studies concluded that the direction of translation is dictated by the tautening of the capsuloligamentous complex opposite the side of translation. As movement occurs and the static restraints tighten, they serve not only to counteract but also to reverse the humeral head movement. If the static restraints are stretched or their attachments are compromised, abnormal translation occurs. For example, in the presence of a Bankart lesion or a pachulous anterior and inferior capsule, the humeral head would translate anteriorly when placed in abduction and external rotation as opposed to posteriorly.

The old and new literature concerning humeral head translation has a significant impact on the clinician's concepts of joint mobilization. The idea of performing joint glides to reestablished proper joint mechanics based on traditionally accepted ideas of joint motions is seriously in question. For instance, the idea of performing anterior glide mobilization to reestablish *normal* anterior gliding during external rotation is not correct, since the humeral head *normally* glides posteriorly during external rotation. We feel that joint mobilization is essential in

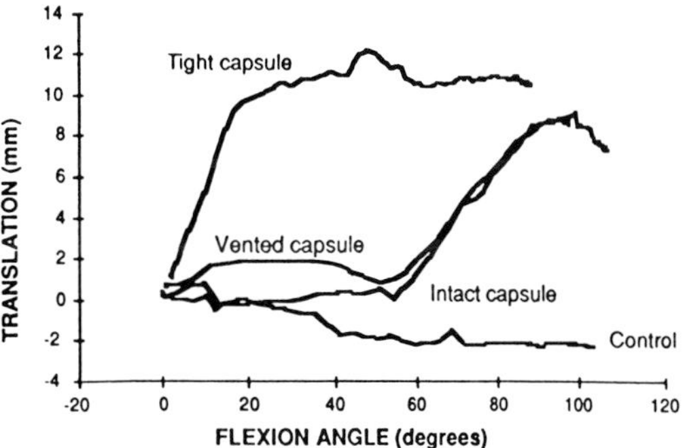


**Figure 2-21.** Normal anterior translation beginning at approximately 60 degrees of flexion in the intact capsule. Venting of the capsule leads to minimal changes in contrast to posterior capsular tightening, which causes early and increased anterior translation. (From Harryman DT, Sidles JA, Clark JM, et al. Translation of the humeral head on the glenoid with passive glenohumeral motion. J Bone Joint Surg 1990;72A:1339.)

relieving pain and increasing joint range of motion, but it is effective because directional mobilizations "stretch" isolated portions of the capsuloligamentous complex. By improving capsuloligamentous pliability in any portion of the CLC, regardless of the directions the humeral head translates during motion, proper joint mechanics and range of motion are restored in all ranges of motion and planes.

## STABILITY

The dilemma of stability or instability has been studied extensively through cadaver and operative investigations. Focus has been on anterior instability, since this is seen most commonly, followed by posterior instability and inferior instability. Discussion has centered around the primary stabilizing structures. Bankart[2] felt that the primary lesion was separation of the capsuloligamentous-labral complex from the glenoid rim. Saha[96] stressed the importance of the articular architecture, while DePalma et al.[29] proclaimed the subscapularis as the main stabilizing force. Rowe[92] felt it was multifactorial but acknowledged the preponderance of the Bankart lesion. Most investigators, orthopedic surgeons, and therapists would agree that intactness of the anterior capsuloligamentous mechanism is paramount to anterior stability. Recent studies confirm the need for an intact capsuloligamentous complex (CLC), as well as the role of the posterior capsular mechanism in anterior and posterior stability.[81,108] Therefore, four general structures are considered the main factors in stability: articular, labrum, capsuloligamentous complex, and rotator cuff. Related factors also will be discussed.

### ARTICULAR

Initial examination of the glenohumeral articular design leads one to question the architect. Surely they must have run out of materials. Saha[93] did extensive radiographic studies on cadavers and felt that he discovered the subtle nuances that provide greater articular stability. He determined that the normal glenoid was retroverted approximately 7.4 degrees, serving to discourage anterior humeral translation (see Fig. 2-3). In 80 percent of 21 shoulders studied, which were known to suffer anterior instability, 2 to 10 degrees of glenoid anteversion was found. A corresponding increase in humeral retroversion was felt to predispose the joint to anterior instability. Basmajian and Bazant[4] found a similar mechanism to Saha's retroversion influencing vertical stability. He discovered that a 5-degree superior tilt of the glenoid helped to prevent inferior humeral migration (see Fig. 2-3). Saha went on to advocate the glenohumeral index, which was basically an anthropomorphic measurement:

$$\text{Glenohumeral index} = \frac{\text{max diameter of glenoid}}{\text{max diameter of humeral}} \times 100$$

The anteroposterior indices were calculated as 57.6, while the inferosuperior indices were 75.3. Expansion of the former dimension would naturally result in greater horizontal stability. In fact, this is found in our brachiating primate ancestors. A reduction of this ratio due to hypoplasia leads to global instability.[93]

Separate yet related to the dimensions of the glenoid fossa is the apparent disparity between "sphericity" of the humeral head and the glenoid. Traditional orthopedic thought is that these two articular surfaces are completely incongruent; results from recent investigations using sterophotogrammetry contradict this concept. Soslowsky et al.[100a] used this three-dimensional technique to quantify the articular surface geometry in 32 fresh-frozen cadavers. Their results demonstrated excellent congruency between the glenoid and humeral head, with an average ratio of the radii of curvature between the two surfaces of 0.99 + 0.05. This conformity of surfaces dictates that pure rotation with minimal translation occurs at this joint.[57a,100a] The disagreement with previous research regarding articular conformity appears to be based on the fact that past investigations used radiographs that did not take into account the effect of the articular cartilage and labrum on radii of curvature.

A built-in safeguard promoting articular stability that is often forgotten is the effect of scapular motion. Scapular mobility allows the glenoid to adjust, providing a stable osseous platform for the humeral head.[90] This movable base compensates for articular deficiencies.

### LABRUM

Probably no smaller structure has caused greater controversy over its function than the glenoid labrum. This wedge-shaped ring of differentiated connective tissue encircles the bony glenoid, serving to bridge bone to the glenohumeral ligaments and biceps tendon (Fig. 2-22). The labrum is the weak link and tears (<30 years of age) when a continuous, progressive, low load is exerted across the anterior capsular mechanism.[87] Clinically, vulnerability of the labral attachment is demonstrated frequently, since the anterior labrum disassociates from the glenoid rim in most traumatic anterior dislocations. This is called the *Bankart lesion*.

Bankart[2] and Rowe,[91,92] proponents of the in-

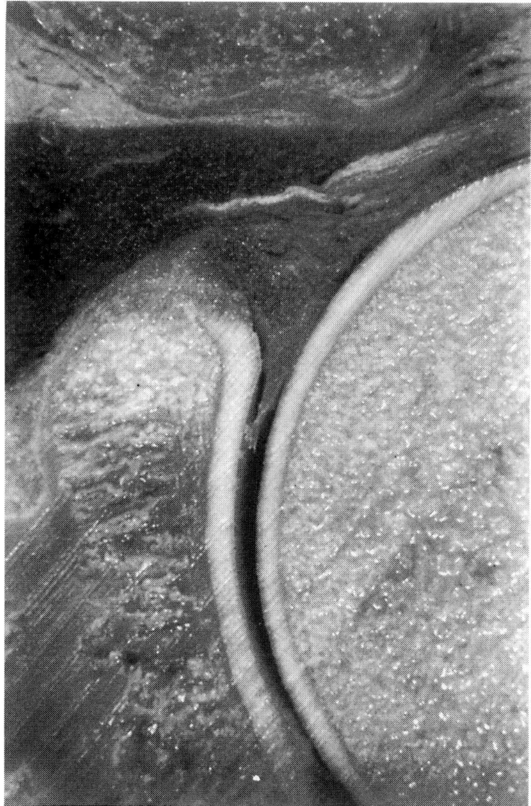

**Figure 2-22.** Labral insertion to the glenoid rim. (From O'Brien SJ, Arnoczky SP, Warren RF, Rozbruch RA. Developmental anatomy of the shoulder and anatomy of the glenohumeral joint. In Rockwood CA, Matzen FA, eds. The shoulder. Philadelphia: WB Saunders, 1990:14.)

fluence of labral stability, emphasized the importance of the labrum linking the capsule to the glenoid bony rim, as opposed to a buttress effect, in which the labrum acts as a physical block to humeral head displacement. Those who opposed the notion of labral stability[28,74,107] appear to do so based on the labrum's isolated effectiveness as a physical block. Removal of this structure through posterior dissection leads to no greater instability.[29,30,107] Then the question remains, "Was all the labrum removed?" Some of the confusion may arise from inherent labrum variation, as noted by Detrisac and Johnson,[30] who arthroscopically identified five types of labrums based on attachment.

If we accept the labrum as an intermediary between the capsuloligamentous complex and the bony rim, whether the glenohumeral ligaments and capsule completely or incompletely utilize the labrum in this manner, then the labrum must be important to the anterior stabilizing mechanism.

## CAPSULOLIGAMENTOUS COMPLEX

The glenohumeral joint capsule is thin and redundant and contributes little to stability.[72] The glenohumeral and coracohumeral ligaments reinforce the capsule to serve as the major static restraints[72,79–81,106–108] (Fig. 2-23). Ligaments, by nature, attach bone to bone and act to guide and limit motion. Their constraining function is evident only as the structures become taut. Essentially, ligaments fulfill a dual stabilizing role: (1) to provide a barrier against translation[107] and (2) to increase articular compressive forces as they tighten[27] (Fig. 2-24). The extreme of this function is seen in the presence of capsular adhesions. In the presence of fibrotic capsuloligamentous tissue, glenohumeral articular compression can be so oppressive that normal rotation is obliterated.

### Coracohumeral Ligament

The presence of the coracohumeral ligament (CHL) is the most consistent of those about the glenohumeral joint[28] (see Fig. 2-23). This ligament has two defined bands extending from the coracoid base to the greater and lesser tuberosities.[38,57] The ligament is intimately related to the rotator cuff and actually reinforces the supraspinatus superiorly and inferiorly[16a] (Fig 2-25a). The CHL and the superior glenohumeral ligament join to make up the rotator cuff interval that bridges the supraspinatus and subscapularis[33,41] (see Fig. 2-25b). In fact, the rotator cuff interval (the CHL[4,108] and superior glenohumeral[108]) is the primary restraint against inferior and posterior translation of the adducted shoulder.[41] Sectioning the interval essentially increased both anterior and posterior translation, while imbricating it significantly reduced translation in both directions. Harrymann et al.[41] found that tightening the rotator cuff interval lead to an 8-degree loss of flexion and a 18-degree loss of extension. This is consistent with the findings of Terry et al.,[106] who noted the CHL to be a primary restraint in both flexion and extension. Harryman et al.[41] also found that external rotation performed with the arm adducted decreased by 38 degrees and adduction decreased by 8 degrees when the interval was imbricated. In addition to maintaining vertical stability, the CHL restricts external rotation and extension.[40,60,80,106]

The coracohumeral ligament is important not only in stability but also in the presence of supraspinatus pathology. In light of the intimate relationship between the CHL and the supraspinatus muscle, and because the CHL limits external rotation when the arm is adducted, exercising into external rotation while adducted, whether it

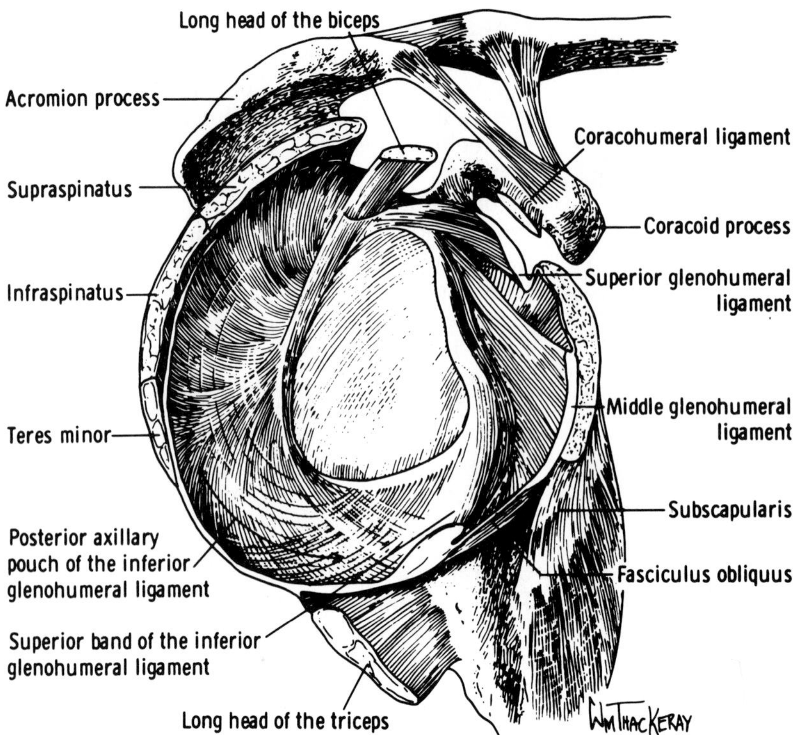


**Figure 2-23.** Lateral view of the glenoid showing the capsuloligamentous complex attachments in relation to the deep muscles and tendons. (From Turkel SJ, Panio MW, Marshal JL. Stabilizing mechanisms preventing anterior dislocation of the glenohumeral joint. J Bone Joint Surg 1981;63A:1209.)

be passively, actively, or with resistance, should be done with caution in the presence of a supraspinatus lesion. The passive tension developed in the CHL translates directly to the comprimised supraspinatus, causing pain or further disruption. This is important following a rotator cuff repair, particularly if the rotator cuff was retracted and required lateral mobilization of the retracted cuff tissue for repair.

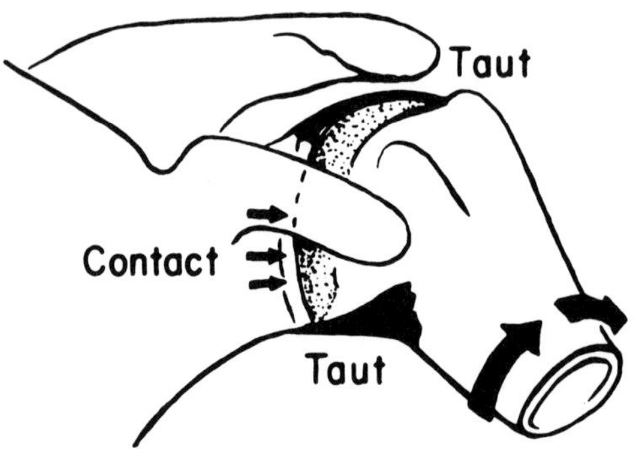


**Figure 2-24.** Capsuloligamentous complex tightening restricts abnormal translation and increases compressive forces across the joint. (From Dempster WT. Mechanisms of shoulder movement. Arch Phys Med Rehabil 1965;46:49.)

### Superior Glenohumeral Ligament

The superior glenohumeral ligament (SGHL) originates from the supraglenoid tubercle, labrum, and base of the coracoid process, inserting laterally just superior to the lesser tubercle (see Fig. 2-23). This structure, along with the coracohumeral ligament, prevents inferior humeral head subluxation. The SGHL also limits external rotation at 0 degrees of rotation[80,106,108] and is a restraint during extension.[106] Both the SGHL and the coracohumeral ligament have been implicated as the source of "fatigue" pain when a mild downward load is placed on the arm.[3] Following shoulder surgery and in the presence of reflex inhibition, tension that develops in these ligaments may explain, to some extent, postoperative pain. Once these ligaments have stretched, as in hemiplegia, it is difficult to regain stability.[3,4]

### Middle Glenohumeral Ligament

The middle glenohumeral ligament (MGHL) has a wider origin, extending from the inferior SGHL to the middle/inferior third of the anterior glenoid rim and scapular neck (see Fig. 2-23). This thicker ligament attaches to the anterior aspect of the anatomic neck.

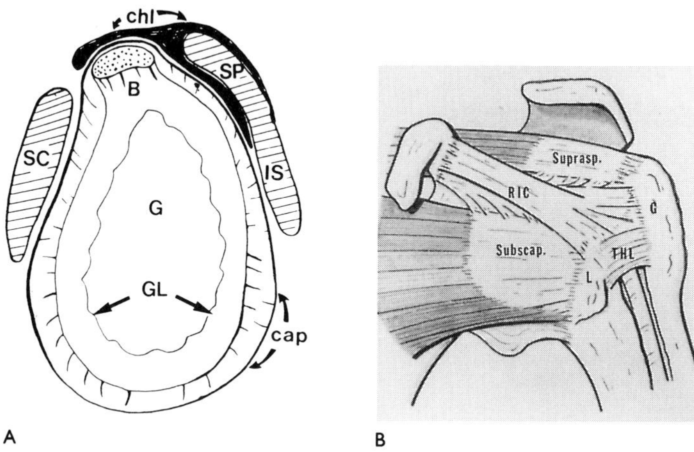


**Figure 2-25.** (a) CHL reinforces the supraspinatus superiorly and inferiorly. (From Clark JC, Harryman DT. Tendons, ligaments, and capsule of the rotator cuff. J Bone Joint Surg 1992;74A:713.) (b) Relationship of the rotator cuff interval (RIC) to the rotator cuff tendons and tubercles. L, lesser tuberosity; G, greater tuberosity; THL, transverse humeral ligament. (From Harryman DT, Sidles JA, Harris SZ, Matzen FA III. The role of the rotator internal capsule in passive motion and stability of the shoulder. J Bone Joint Surg 1992;74A:53. Clark JC, Harryman DT. Tendons, ligaments, and capsule of the rotator cuff. J Bone Joint Surg 1992;74A:713.)

The MGHL was found to have stabilizing effects at 0 and 45 degrees of abduction. External rotation at these positions caused tightening of the MGHL, providing a barrier against anterior displacement.[80, 108] This ligament was loose at 90 degrees of abduction and full external rotation,[108] although it was found to tighten during flexion combined with external rotation.[106]

#### Inferior Glenohumeral Ligament

The inferior glenohumeral ligament (IGHL) is the thickest of the glenohumeral ligaments. It has been reported to have two or three portions. Turkel et al.[108] described a superior band and axillary pouch (see Fig. 2-23). The superior band attaches along the upper half of the glenoid.[30] O'Brien et al.[79] performed a gross dissection and histologic study and found an axillary pouch bordered both anteriorly and posteriorly by defined thickened bands. The anterior band attached between 2 and 4 o'clock on the glenoid and labrum (consider the glenoid as the face of a clock). The posterior band was found to attach between its 7 and 9 o'clock positions, with the axillary pouch interposed between.[79] The IGHL inserts on the inferior anatomic and surgical necks of the humerus.

Controversy over this ligament arises from cadaver dissections, in which the structure was frequently ill-defined.[28] Others consistently identify this structure and give great credence to its stabilizing effect.[74, 79, 80, 106, 108]

As with the other glenohumeral ligaments, the IGHL's ability to restrict motion depends on humeral elevation and rotation. The superior band tightens when the humerus is rotated externally at neutral position and when the humerus is abducted without external rotation. When external rotation is performed at 90 degrees of abduction, the whole IGHL tightens, while the superior or anterior band wraps snugly across the humeral head, checking anterior displacement[79, 106, 108] (Fig. 2-26). O'Connell et al.[80] also found the greatest amount of strain through the IGHL at 90 degrees of abduction and full external rotation. Internal rotation performed at 90 degrees of abduction caused the posterior band and axillary pouch to fan out and "cradle" the humeral head posteriorly. The IGHL appears to be a single identifiable complex that stabilizes against abnormal anterior and posterior humeral head translation.[79] Conversely, one can appreciate how adhesions or contracture of this structure could limit external rotation, internal rotation, and elevation.

Turkel and coworkers[108] sequentially incised the glenohumeral anterior and posterior soft-tissue structures. The subscapularis was cut initially, followed by the SGHL, MGHL, and IGHL. Anterior dislocation occurred at neutral with external rotation, but at 90 degrees of abduction and full external rotation, the joint remained stable. It was not until the posterior cuff was cut that anterior dislocation occurred (note that this study did not introduce horizontal abduction or

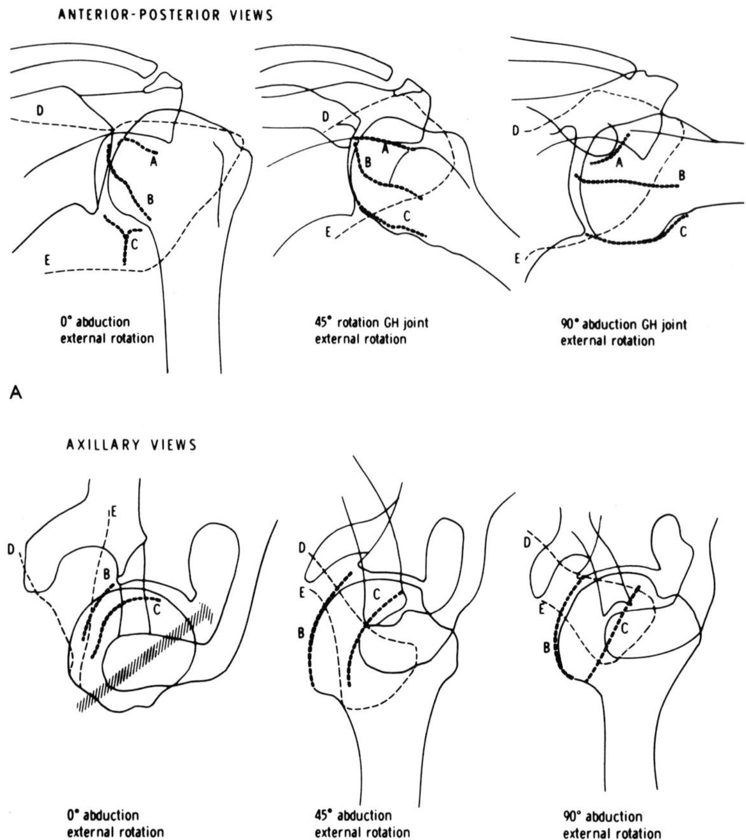


**Figure 2-26.** An anterior view (a) and an axillary (inferior) view (b) of the glenohumeral joint in three positions of abduction and full external rotation. The stabilizing relationship between the ligaments, subscapularis, and humeral head can be appreciated. Note how the IGHL, represented by b and c, acts as a barrier against anterior/inferior humeral head displacement. Also note in 90 degrees of abduction, the subscapularis's inferior border exposes the humeral head. A, superior margin of the MGHL; B, superior margin of the superior band of IGHL; C, inferior margin of the IGHL; D, superior border of the subscapularis; E, inferior border of the subscapularis. (From Turkel SJ, Panio MW, Marshal JL. Stabilizing mechanisms preventing anterior dislocation of the glenohumeral joint. J Bone Joint Surg 1981;63A:1208.)

apply any anterior force).* Oversen and Neilsen[81] found that when the capsule's anterior half, including the IGHL, was cut and an anterior force was applied, significant anterior displacement occurred between 70 and 90 degrees. Scapular fixation was similar to that in the study by Turkel et al.

To summarize, it appears that the MGHL, subscapularis, and superior band of the IGHL primarily provide stability from neutral position to midabduction, whereas the axillary pouch and superior or anterior band act together to prevent anterior displacement at greater ranges of abduction.[80,81,106,108] This is consistent with arthroscopic findings.[30]

Not only is anterior displacement influenced by sectioning the posterior cuff and capsule, but anterior structures also help to maintain posterior integrity.[81,98,108] Increased posterior displacement resulted after incising the upper half of the anterior capsule and subscapularis muscle.[81] Increased posterior translation also was demonstrated when the rotator cuff interval was sectioned.[41]

When the arm is flexed, internally rotated, and adducted, not only does the posterior capsule form a sling about the humeral head, but the anterior capsuloligamentous complex also "winds up," acting as a tether, preventing posterior subluxation or dislocation.[98] This phenomenon of the anterior and posterior static restraints assist-

* The study by Turkel et al. was done by fixating the scapula to a board while abducting the humerus to 90 degrees. This position does not take into account scapular rotation. Turkel's 90 degrees corresponds to approximately 120 to 135 degrees of true shoulder elevation.

ing in stabilizing against abnormal humeral head translation in the opposite direction gives us insight about multidirectional instability and the effectiveness of the inferior capsular shift procedure.

Expectedly, sectioning of the entire posterior capsule led to increased significant posterior displacement between 70 and 90 degrees.[74,81] Incising the posterior cuff along with the posterior capsule led to subluxation through the middle part of abduction.[81]

In summary, understanding the unique position-related constraining characteristics of the glenohumeral ligaments at *end range* provides the clinician with insight into capsuloligamentous pathology and anatomic appreciation of the unstable shoulder. The interdependency of the capsuloligamentous-labral complex becomes evident when examining the literature, leading us to conclude that the complex should be considered a functional unit. The IGHL appears to have a dual role of being the main restraint against anterior humeral head displacement when in external rotation at 90 degrees of abduction while also forming a substantial posterior barrier when the arm is internally rotated in the abducted position. The posterior rotator cuff and capsule are the primary restraints against posterior instability, yet the anterior capsuloligamentous complex assists with posterior stability, while the posterior structure assists with anterior stability.

Although the preceding studies focus on instability, they also provide insight regarding patients who have restricted or contractured soft tissue, as in adhesive capsulitis. No longer should the therapist consider isolated regions of the "capsule" as limiting a particular motion but should regard the restricted capsuloligamentous complex as a unit that requires stretching and mobilization in all directions.

## DYNAMIC EFFECT

The glenohumeral joint dynamic system is the fourth line of defense to be discussed against instability. The musculotendinous units surrounding the glenohumeral joint assist the static restraints in stabilizing responsibilities at end rages of motion *but* are probably the main stabilizers when movement occurs away from the end ranges or in midrange. In midrange, the CLC is relatively lax and thus is less effective as a barrier or in generating glenohumeral compression.

Under normal circumstances, the force transmitted by the supraspinatus, infraspinatus, teres minor, and subscapularis muscles provides significant stability. This is achieved several ways:

1. Contraction of these muscles centralizes the humeral head in the glenoid by increasing compressive forces[19,49,72,85,86,96] (Fig. 2-27).
2. The tension developed across the cuff tendons during a contraction squeezes the humeral head, preventing anterior and posterior displacement[96] (see Fig. 2-27).
3. Passive tension of the tendons provides some stability.[81,108]

Although all the cuff muscles, along with the deltoid, are considered stabilizers, the subscapularis is considered important for anterior integrity. DePalma and associates[29] were great advocates of the subscapularis "dynamic buttress" effect. Morrey and Chaos[72] calculated forces at the glenohumeral joint during 90 degrees of coronal plane abduction in external rotation. They determined the anterior shear force to increase from 12 to 42 kg in the unloaded upper extremity when the arm moved into 30 degrees of horizontal abduction from the coronal plane. The combined tensile strength of the subscapularis and capsuloligamentous complex was calculated as 120 kg.[87] Therefore, stability would be maintained. Anterior shear increases under higher speeds and greater loads, and when the force exceeds the tensile strength of the anterior structures, dislocation occurs. In the presence of an incompetent capsuloligamentous complex, the subscapularis is primarily responsible for impeding translation at lower positions of abduction (<90 degrees). This becomes increasingly difficult for the subscapularis with subsequent dislocations because evidence of tendon lengthening has been reported.[29,70,104] Inherent lengthening of this structure leads to inefficient translation of tension from the muscle to bone, and the "buttress effect" is lost.[29]

Turkel and coworkers[108] presented a sequential incising study that revealed a significant increase (an average 18 degrees) in external rotation in the neutral position once the subscapularis was cut. No significant increase in anterior translation was noted at 45 and 90 degrees of

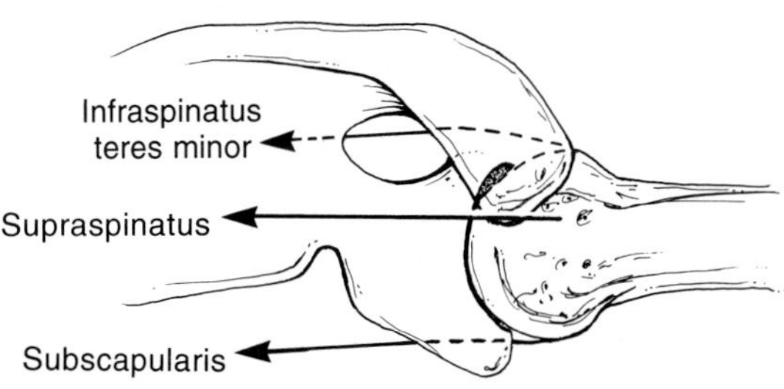


**Figure 2-27.** Dynamic effect of the rotator cuff causing compression as well as anterior and posterior barrier effect.

abduction, and the joint was unable to be dislocated.[81, 108] Interestingly, the inferior border of the subscapularis was noted to rise above the inferior humeral head at 90 degrees of abduction and external rotation; thus the subscapularis was an ineffective barrier against dislocation in this position[108] (see Fig. 2-26). This finding gives insight as to why patients with a deficient CLC and/or Bankart lesion recurrently dislocate in the abducted and externally rotated position even though they possess significant subscapularis strength.

The hypothesis that posterior cuff structures dynamically assist in anterior integrity has been discussed. Cain and coworkers[13] demonstrated by strain gauge that the posterior cuff, particularly the infraspinatus and teres minor, pulls the humeral head posteriorly when contracting, therefore reducing the anterior shear. This type of activity, in conjunction with the known decreased tensile strength of the rotator cuff,[87] explains the high incidence of rotator cuff tears in individuals older than age 45 when they anteriorly dislocate[43]; excessive translation in the presence of an aging, less elastic rotator cuff causes tearing.

Posterior stability is also dependent on the posterior cuff's dynamic effect.[13, 98] When the infraspinatus and teres minor muscles are incised, significant posterior displacement occurs.[81] One could logically conclude that if passive tension of these muscles maintains significant stability, then active contraction would further enhance stability. Saha[96] concluded that the infraspinatus and teres minor were horizontal steerers maintaining stability. The importance of the posterior rotator cuff and deltoid to posterior stability is seen clinically in that patients with posterior instability respond well when strengthening of the external rotators is emphasized.[98] This is particularly true if the patient is a subluxator as opposed to a dislocator.[30, 98]

## RELATED STABILIZING FORCES

Other forces that influence shoulder stability are atmospheric pressure and the "adhesion/cohesion" mechanism.[70] Steinler[102] recognized the role of atmospheric pressure but felt it was of minimal consequence. Recently, Kumar and Balasulramaniam[63] demonstrated the effect of atmospheric pressure. Cadaver shoulders were punctured before and after the overlying musculature was reflected off. These authors radiographically demonstrated inferior subluxation following joint invasion without dependence on muscle suspension. Harryman[40] evaluated humeral head translation and the effect of capsular venting and found a slight increase in anterior translation during flexion and horizontal adduction. Matzen et al.[70] described this phenomenon as disruption of "finite joint volume":

> When one pulls on the plunger of a plugged syringe, a relative vacuum is created that resists displacement of the plunger. Anatomical studies, surgical findings, attempts at aspiration, and magnetic resonance images all confirm that there is minimal (less than 1 cc) free fluid in the normal shoulder joint. The normal shoulder is sealed by the capsule so that outside fluid cannot enter it. Thus, like the syringe, the shoulder joint is stabilized by its limited joint volume. As long as the joint is a closed space containing minimal free fluid, the joint surfaces cannot be easily distracted or subluxated. Small translations of the humerus on the glenoid can be balanced by fluid flow in the opposite direction, allowing a nonuniform gap to open in the joint space. This gap can increase until all available fluid has been mobilized, at which point further motion of the joint is resisted by negative fluid pressure in the joint. This negative pressure pulls the capsule inward toward the joint space, putting its fibers "on the stretch." Individuals with more stretchy capsules will allow greater translation than those with stiff joint capsules.

Finite joint volume combined with the adhesion/cohesion mechanism enhances joint stability. *Adhesion* is described as fluid holding to a surface. *Cohesion* is the joining of two surfaces by fluid. Adhesion/cohesion is best demonstrated by wet microscope slides that stick together yet are able to slide on one another. The glenohumeral joint mimics this phenomenon at the contact area between the humerus and glenoid.

## SUMMARY

From the preceding discussion on contributors to stability, one should gain respect for the interplay of the related components. In summary, the IGHL appears to be the primary structure in providing anterior stability. The labrum is significant, being the weak link in the chain attaching the IGHL to the bony glenoid rim. Orthopedic surgeons are attempting to perform surgical procedures that reattach the labrum when a Bankart lesion exist, thus establishing the normal anatomic environment to the capsuloligamentous-labral complex. Accepting the capsuloligamentous-labral complex as a functional unit explains why global laxity of this complex leads to multidirectional instability and why a capsular-shift surgical procedure is required to address global laxity. Finally, atmospheric pressure and the adhesion/cohesion mechanism contribute to joint integrity. The subscapularis is important to anterior stability through the compressive forces imparted on the joint and through the buttress effect. Some question arises as to the true barrier effect at greater degrees of abduction. The posterior cuff provides a profound effect on posterior stability and assists in anterior stability. Regardless of the direction of instability, proper, efficient control of the rotator cuff is essential. The anterior capsule and structures are important to posterior stability.

The clinician needs to be aware of all components related to instability so that safe and effective treatment is performed during conservative and postoperative rehabilitation.

## Mechanical Joint Forces

Although the glenohumeral articulation is not a weight-bearing joint, significant force is transmitted through this articular interface. Compressive stress across the glenohumeral joint has been estimated at 1.2 N/mm$^2$.[109] The progressive repetitive and degenerative effect of these forces has been visualized in anatomic cadaver studies.[28]

Discussing joint and muscle forces will require explanation of mechanical terms. *Torque* is a term indicating a tendency to produce motion such as rotation. Simply, torque is

$$T = F \times D$$

where *F* equals force and, in the case of holding an extended arm at 90 degrees in space, will equal the mass of the upper extremity. Mass of the arm is accepted as 5 percent of body weight.[32] In this case, *D* equals the upper extremity moment arm, this being the perpendicular distance from the center of rotation, the humeral head, to the direction of force (Fig. 2-28). This distance is generally accepted as 31.8 cm based on normal anthropomorphic measures, although it will vary depending on limb length.[32] Therefore, at approximately 31.8 cm or approximately 1 ft from the humeral head, 5 percent of the body weight (BW) is creating a torque or moment in a counterclockwise direction:

$$T = 0.05\text{BW} \times 1 \text{ ft}$$

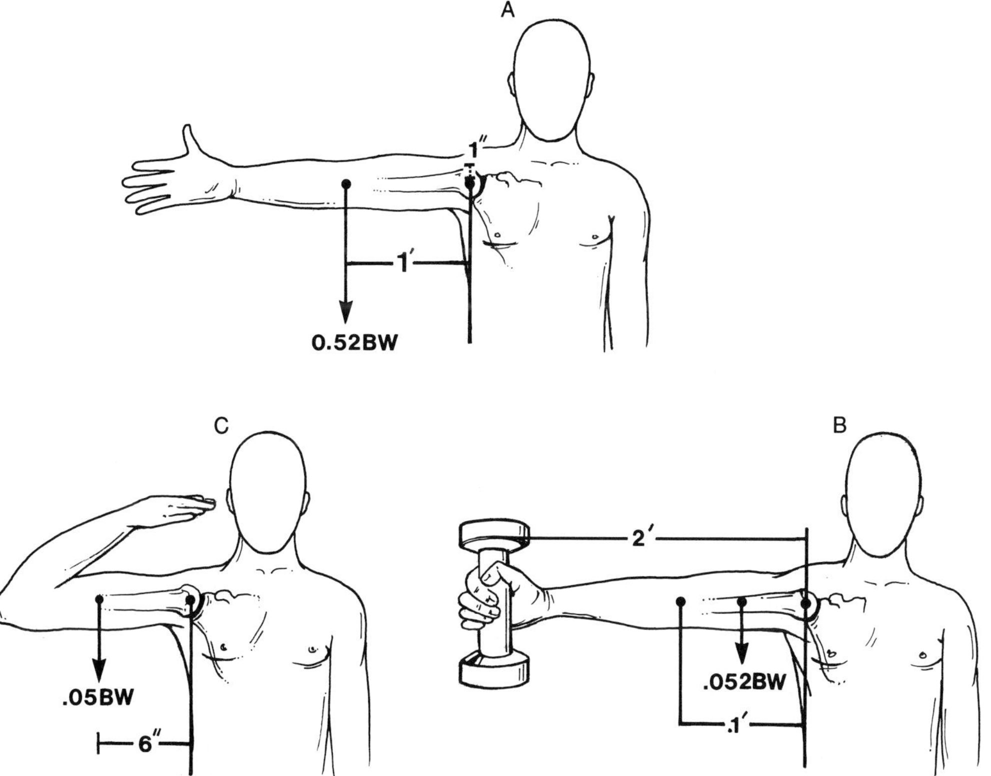


**Figure 2-28.** Free body diagram at 90 degrees demonstrating (a) effect of limb weight (b) when a 5-lb dumbbell is held in the hand and (c) when the elbow is fully flexed.

To maintain the arm in space, an equal amount of torque is needed in the opposite direction. This comes from torque created by muscle. As the arm is elevated away from the side of the body, the center of gravity moves further from the point of rotation, or fulcrum. Torque increases, reaching maximum at 90 degrees of abduction, since the center of gravity is furthest from the rotation point. If a 5-lb weight were added to the hand at a distance of 2 ft from the center of rotation, an additional torque would be created tending to rotate the arm down (see Fig. 2-28b):

$$T = 0.05 \text{ (body weight)} \times 1 \text{ ft} + 5 \text{ lb} \times 2 \text{ ft}$$

In a 150-lb person a 5-lb weight produces a 133 percent increase in torque, requiring a 133 percent increase in muscle demand to maintain the arm in space. Clinically, by using this equation and having a patient lift a designated weight in his or her hand, a quick determination of torque output for the shoulder abductors can be made which is consistent with data retrieved using an isokinetic dynamometer. To find peak torque, the patient is asked to slowly lift the maximum weight to 90 degrees of scapular plane abduction. Using this weight and distance, torque is calculated. In the preceding example, if the patient could lift the 5 lb to 90 degrees, the calculation would be 10 ft · lb (negating limb-weight). Muscle demand can be reduced by changing the center of gravity of the upper extremity. If the shoulder is maintained at 90 degrees of elevation and the elbow is bent, the center of gravity moves toward the shoulder, thus reducing the rotating moment by 30 percent[85] (see Fig. 2-28c). This is an important concept when educating shoulder patients about lifting and working positions.

Muscles create their own torque. The greater the moment arm of the muscle, the better is the mechanical advantage. The *moment arm* of the muscle is the perpendicular distance between the muscle line of pull and the point of rotation.

Typically, a moment arm is not constant because of varying joint motion and muscle movement. This is particularly true of the deltoid muscle. Muscle force is imparted along all structures where the muscle attaches and transverses, the latter being the joint. These forces can be quite significant. The resultant force, or joint-reaction force, is the magnitude sum of force vectors transmitted about the joint. Direction of forces are described by vectors that change as the line of pull of the muscles varies. The vectors are either of a shear or a compressive nature, with the former translating force parallel and the latter translating force perpendicular to the joint surface (Fig. 2-29).

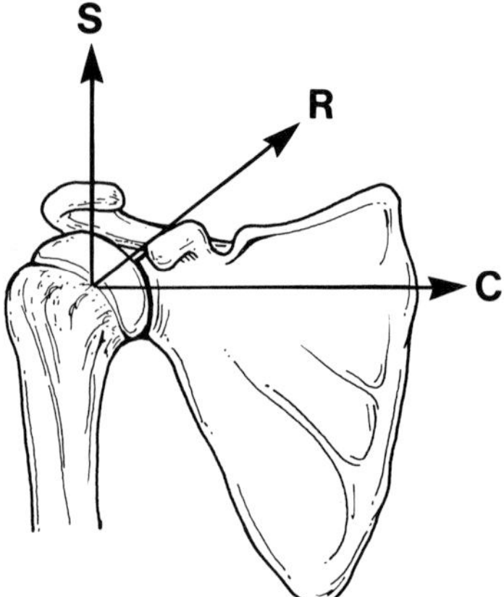


**Figure 2-29.** The resultant force *R* at the glenohumeral joint depends on the direction and magnitude of compressive (*C*) and shear (*S*) forces.

Inman et al.[49] scientifically investigate glenohumeral joint forces. They empirically determined three forces generated when abducting the arm: (1) the abductor musculature, predominantly the deltoid, (2) the weight of the arm, and (3) the combined force of (a) joint compression and friction and (b) the humeral depressors (i.e., the subscapularis, teres minor, and infraspinatus muscles). They estimated the weight of the upper extremity to be 9 percent of body weight, which is almost twice that accepted today. The total muscle torque required to elevate the arm generated by the three separate forces was found to peak at 90 degrees and was 8.2 times the weight of the limb, or approximately 70 percent of body weight. This force falls to zero at 180 degrees, where the limb is vertically overhead. The compressive and friction force (joint-reaction force) at the glenohumeral interface was calculated at 10.2 times the weight of the extremity, or 90 percent of body weight, and also peaked at 90 degrees of elevation. This is logical, since muscular demand is greatest when the center of gravity of the upper extremity is furthest from the center of rotation.

Poppen and Walker's results[85] were similar to those of Inman et al.[49] regarding force magnitude equaling 90 percent of body weight at 90 degrees of abduction. They calculated not only force requirements but also the resultant vector direction during active scapular plane abduction. At 60 degrees of abduction in neutral rotation, the resultant force was directed toward the superior aspect of the glenoid rim (Fig. 2-30). Elevation above this level lead to greater compressive

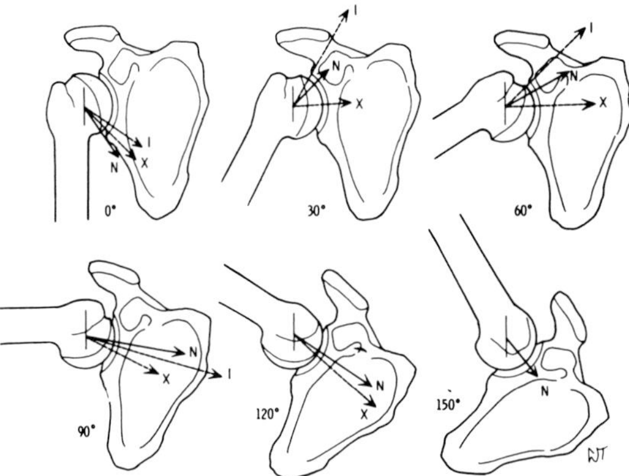


**Figure 2-30.** Approximate direction of resultant forces during scapular plane abduction in different positions of abduction and rotation. N, neutral; X, external rotation; I, internal rotation. (From Poppen NK, Walker PS. Forces at the glenohumeral joint in abduction. Clin Orthop 1978;135:169.)

forces, in which the resultant vector was centrally located through the glenoid. This change in vector direction occurs as a result of the constantly changing muscle moment arms and direction of fiber pull, particularly the deltoid.

Poppen and Walker[85] went on to determine direction of the resultant vector with internal and external rotation in the scapular plane. When the arm was externally rotated, the resultant vector was directed much more centrally into the glenoid. When it was internally rotated, the magnitude of the resultant increased, but more important, the vector was directed more superiorly, leading to greater shear forces from 0 to 60 degrees (see Fig. 2-30). The deltoid's orientation with respect to the glenoid face caused this change, increasing with external rotation and decreasing with internal rotation.

This is an important concept to grasp when performing a commonly used strengthening exercise of abduction in the plane of the scapula with full internal rotation, or "scaption" with internal rotation. Electromyographic (EMG) studies have demonstrated this position to isolate the supraspinatus.[51] In a young patient with a strong, intact rotator cuff, this exercise may be helpful in strengthening the supraspinatus, but in the older individual with a compromised rotator cuff, increased shearing forces are hazardous. This position initially stretches the supraspinatus and posterior cuff tendons and then requires maximal work to reduce excessive shear forces. We have found this exercise to only irritate the over 40-year-old rotator cuff patient and frequently the younger individual with reactive rotator cuff pathology.

# Muscle Properties

Muscles have two basic fiber alignments, longitudinal and oblique. This inherent orientation determines the function of muscle. The longitudinal fibers enable speedy contractions, whereas oblique fibers allow more fibers per area and less overall change in length, thus providing greater force. Estimates have been placed on muscle force production and work by determining the total cross-sectional area of all fibers. This is considered the *physiologic cross section*.[35]

One of the most important determinants of muscle force is the length of the muscle and associated fibers. This phenomenon is called the *length-tension relationship*.

Sarcomeres contain actin and myosin filaments forming cross-bridges. Their optimal resting length is accepted at 2.2 μm (Fig. 2-31). At this length, the peak number of cross-bridges is assembled, thus maximizing efficiency and force from the muscle. Excessive shortening and lengthening can lead to active and passive insufficiency, respectively. A muscle fiber stops producing tension when it shortens approximately 60 percent of its resting length.[35] This explains why one joint muscles are composed of fibers three times as long as the distance through which they have to shorten to achieve full range of motion.[35]

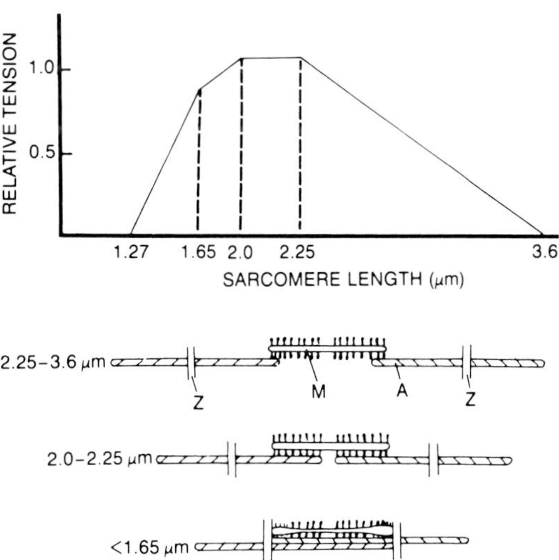


**Figure 2-31.** Length-tension concept demonstrated by change in sarcomere length and effect on relative tension. (From Pitman M, Peterson L. Biomechanics of skeletal muscle. In Frankel VH, Nordin M, eds. Basic biomechanics of the musculoskeletal system. 2nd ed. Philadelphia: Lea & Febiger, 1989:100.)

The type of muscle contraction is another major determinant of maximum force or torque created. An *isometric contraction* takes place without a change in muscle length. This will produce maximum output secondary to maximizing motor unit recruitment and tension development. A *concentric contraction* is defined as a shortening of the muscle. The third type, *eccentric contraction*, occurs when the muscle lengthens while being loaded. Eccentric contractions can develop force that is greater than both concentric and isometric contractions[23,61] (Fig. 2-32). This is due in part to passive tension developed by elastin and collagen fibers in the muscle tissues. When moving against gravity, all muscles contract concentrically, and if they maintain the corresponding plane, they are lowered eccentrically. Many of the tendinous injuries we see occur because of excessive or uncontrolled eccentric loading.[22] This concept of eccentric loading requires caution when rehabilitating the shoulder, particularly if isokinetics are used.

The speed of contractions also affects torque output. Muscles generating force at slower speeds, 60 degrees/s, have greater torque output than those moving at 180 degrees/s. Motor units are speed-dependent; therefore, fewer units are recruited at faster speeds, reducing maximum torque output. Slower speeds also allow the tension developed by the contractile elements to be transmitted through collagen and elastin components to the tendon. Speed and concentric activity output have an inverse relationship, but a linear effect appears to occur in eccentric activity[61] (see Fig. 2-32).

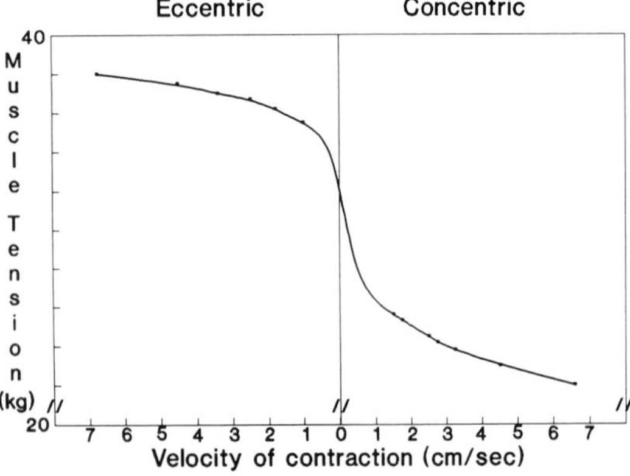


**Figure 2-32.** Relationship between velocity and muscle tension during eccentric and concentric work. (Data from Komi PV. Relationship between muscle tension, EMG and velocity of concentric and eccentric work. In Desmedth E, ed. New developments in electromyography and clinical neurophysiology. Vol. 1. Basel: S Karger AG, 1973:596.)

# Deltoid

The deltoid muscle has become increasingly important in human beings since they have attained an upright posture. This is due to an increase in relative size, comprising approximately 40 percent of the scapulohumeral muscle mass[28,49] and having a cross-sectional area of 18.2 cm$^2$.[5] Acromial widening and lateral migration have markedly enhanced the deltoid's efficiency. Widening allowed for an expansive surface to pull from, while lateral migration improved the moment arm, magnifying torque capabilities.[28,86]

The deltoid's three large heads—anterior, middle, and posterior—give contour to the shoulder. The arrangement of the middle head differs from those of the anterior and posterior heads. DePalma[28] described the middle fibers as being pennate with oblique fibers arising from four or five tendinous bands. As discussed previously, this type of oblique fiber orientation significantly multiplies muscle power.

At rest, the middle deltoid's line of pull with respect to the glenoid face is approximately 27 degrees.[82] Contraction predominately produces a shear force, attempting to sublux the humeral head superiorly. Initial abduction force has been estimated at 89 percent shear compared with 45 percent compressive[82] (Fig. 2-33). As the

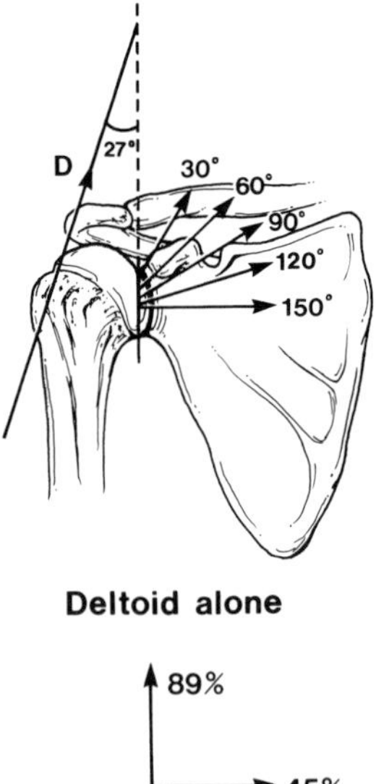


**Figure 2-33.** Deltoid angle of inclination at rest as well as percentage compressive and shear force generated at neutral position. The direction of the resultant force produced by the deltoid during abduction is depicted from 30 to 150 degrees. (Adapted from Morrey BF, An KN. Biomechanics of the shoulder. In Rockwood CA, Matzen FA III, eds. The shoulder. Vol. 1. Philadelphia: WB Saunders, 1990:241.)

arm is abducted in the scapular plane, the shear force is reduced and the compressive force is increased due to the changing orientation of deltoid fibers. At 60 degrees of abduction, the shear and compressive force are equal.[82] At 90 degrees, the line of pull of all three deltoid heads is 60 degrees to the glenoid face. This improves to almost 80 degrees at maximum abduction[85] (Fig. 2-34b).

Poppen and Walker[85] found that as the line of pull improves, so does the deltoid moment arm (see Fig. 2-34A). At 30 degrees of abduction, the middle deltoid moment arm is 1.6 cm, compared with 0.5 cm for the anterior deltoid. Their moment arms increase with further abduction and at 60 degrees are approximately equal, being 2.6 cm. The posterior deltoid moment arm is still insignificant at 60 degrees. The middle deltoid moment arm plateaus at 150 degrees of abduction, while the anterior and posterior deltoid moment arms climb to 4.2 and 2.2 cm, respectively.

The improvement in line of pull and increase in moment arm during abduction would be meaningless to the deltoid if the scapula did not rotate, functionally lengthening the deltoid. Without scapular rotation, the deltoid would excessively shorten by 90 degrees of abduction, and the arm could not actively raise past this point; this is called *active insufficiency*.[49,66] The action of the deltoid is not as simple as one would have suspected. It maximizes function by a complex interplay of mechanical adjustments as the insertion raises overhead and the scapula rotates.

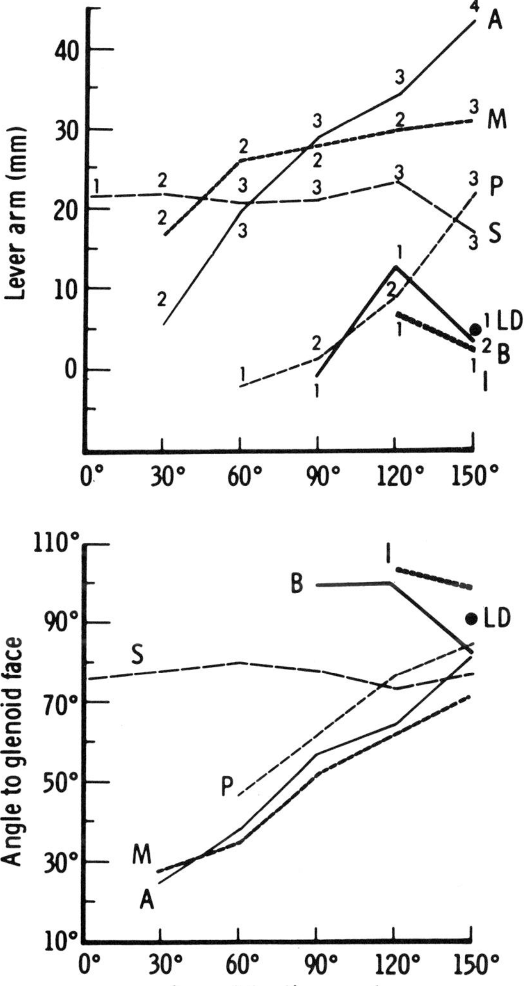


**Figure 2-34.** Moment (lever) arm length (a) and angle to the glenoid (b) of some abducting muscles as the arm is elevated in the scapular plane. A, anterior deltoid; M, middle deltoid; P, posterior deltoid; S, supraspinatus; B, biceps; LD, latissimus dorsi; I, infraspinatus. (From Poppen NK, Walker PS. Forces at the glenohumeral joint in abduction. Clin Orthop 1978;135:168.)

## Rotator Cuff

The rotator cuff muscles are the core of dynamic control about the glenohumeral joint. Comprised of four muscles and associated tendons, the rotator cuff dynamically maintains articular congruity, thus allowing the larger, more powerful shoulder muscles to move against great resistance.

The supraspinatus is a relatively small muscle with respect to cross-sectional area, 5.72 $cm^2$.[5] It arises from the supraspinatus fossa, inserting on the superior facet of the greater tuberosity. The supraspinatus has a resting moment arm of 2.2 cm, which does not change except at maximum elevation[85] (see Fig. 2-34A) The muscle's lever arm is improved by insertion onto the prominent greater tuberosity. The resting angle to the face of the scapula has been estimated at both 70 degrees[82] and 80 degrees.[85] Consequently, the dynamic effect centrally locates the humeral head in the glenoid fossa.[19,49,72,82,85,86,96] Force has been estimated at 93 percent compressive and 4 percent shear[82] (Fig. 2-35). This muscle also imparts a depressive force due to tendon compression of the superior humeral head.[69,111] Loss of supraspinatus function unleashes the deltoid's upward shear, impairing shoulder function and leading to impingement of the supraspinatus tendon and subacromial bursa against the coracoacromial arch[19,49,85] (Fig. 2-36). This is the most likely mechanism leading to humeral head superior migration in patients having chronic rotator cuff tears.[42,110]

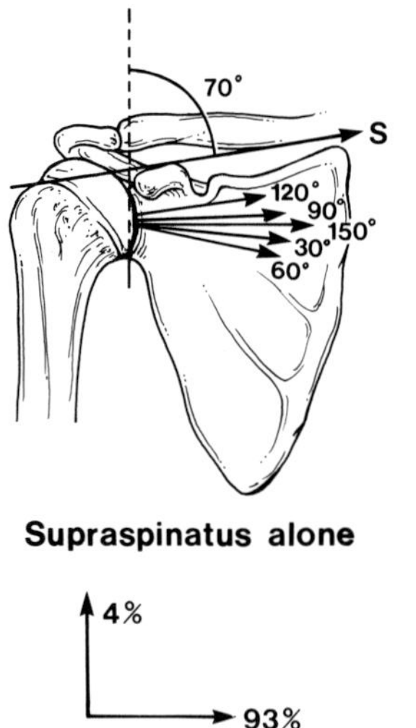


**Figure 2-35.** Angle of supraspinatus at rest as well as percentage compressive and shearing force generated at neutral position. The direction of the resultant force produced by the supraspinatus during abduction is depicted from 30 to 150 degrees. (Adapted from Morrey BF, An K-N. Biomechanics of the shoulder. In Rockwood CA, Matzen FA III, eds. The shoulder. Vol. 1. Philadelphia: WB Saunders, 1990:241.)

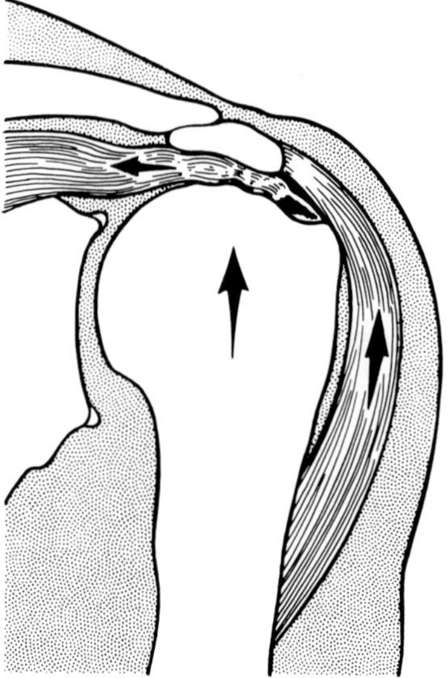

**Figure 2-36.** Proper functioning of the supraspinatus produces abduction but, more important, results in glenohumeral compression, since the deltoid also abducts. The loss of supraspinatus function causes increased vertical translation and impingement. (From Matzen FA III, Arntz CT. Rotator cuff tendon failure. In Rockwood CA, Matzen FA III eds. The shoulder. Vol. 2. Philadelphia: WB Saunders, 1990:649.)

# Glenohumeral Force Couple

When considering the actions of the deltoid, supraspinatus, infraspinatus, teres minor, and subscapularis muscles, one can appreciate the force-couple concept (Fig. 2-37). A *force couple* is defined as equal forces producing a rotation by pulling in opposite direction. We have seen the abducting forces of the deltoid and supraspinatus muscles and their corresponding shear and compressive qualities. We now need to complete the picture with the depressive forces of the infraspinatus, teres minor, and subscapularis muscles.

The line of pull to the glenoid face of the infraspinatus and subscapularis muscles has been estimated at 45 degrees, and the teres minor, at 55 degrees.[82] These three muscles have a negligible moment arm as abductors.[26] Their responsibility in the force couple is to exert a predominate downward shear, which peaks at 60 degrees of elevation, as well as a compressive load.[6,49,96] As the deltoid draws the humeral head upward, the depressors tug downward, allowing humeral rotation yet maintaining glenohumeral joint conformity. Compromise of these humeral head depressors by any means results in an imbalanced struggle against the opposing deltoid shear, leading to superior humeral head displacement.

# Muscle Activity

Basic EMG research has established a proportional relationship between action-potential count and muscle tension.[4,18,65] As tension develops through the contracting muscles, action potentials rise.[18,65] Determining the level of EMG activity can indicate contribution of the muscle

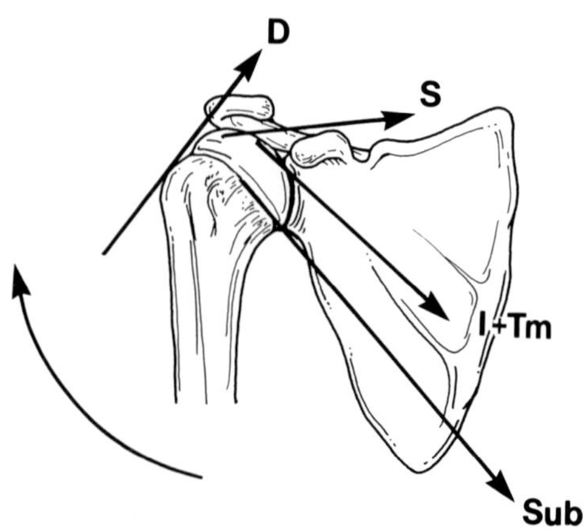


**Figure 2-37.** Deltoid and rotator cuff force couple.

during a specific motion. Most studies have evaluated muscle action during single-plane motion. Care must be taken when correlating results from these studies to functional movements because functional movement can be much more complicated than single-plane motion.

# Elevation

## DELTOID

In the normal shoulder, the middle deltoid is active in all planes of elevation,[64,77,85,99,103] while the anterior and posterior heads command flexion and extension, respectively. The middle and anterior heads elevate in the scapular plane with less contribution from the posterior deltoid.[64,77] Celli and coworkers[16] found that the contribution of the posterior head did not occur until 60 degrees, while others found activity at 45 degrees.[82] These findings correlate well with the moment-arm determination of Poppen and Walker.[84] The posterior deltoid does commit more to coronal plane abduction[64] because the muscle is required to move the humerus into relative extension from the scapular plane.

Although the anterior fibers dominate motion in flexion, the middle fibers become more involved at 60 degrees.[50] This occurs because of relative humeral realignment toward the scapular plane as the scapula translates forward over the thoracic wall. Also, one must remember the obligatory internal rotation that swings the deltoid insertion forward, giving the middle deltoid a more efficient line of pull.

Without deltoid contribution in flexion, 35 to 80 percent isometric torque deficits were found at 0 and 150 degrees, respectively.[21] Extension reduced by 60 percent at neutral,[21] while others found only a 38 percent deficit in extension in patients having their deltoid excised secondary to tumors.[68]

## SUPRASPINATUS

The supraspinatus and deltoid are in optimal alignment in the scapular plane.[54] The supraspinatus is active in all planes of elevation,[49,50,64,77,103] contrary to original views as the isolated initiator of abduction. This has been clearly disprovened by EMG studies,[49,50] induced nerve palsy studies,[20,21,48] and clinical observation.[68,101] In fact, 40 to 60 percent of elevation torque output has been attributed to the supraspinatus and infraspinatus muscles.[20,21,48,62] There remains some controversy over the stabilizing effect versus "abducting effect." Celli et al.[16] defined a *stabilizer* as a muscle demonstrating constant activity by EMG compared with a *mover*, whose activity increased with motion. They found the deltoid to be the abducting force (mover), while the supraspinatus was a stabilizer. Ito[50] found a linear progression of electrical activity in the supraspinatus and deltoid during abduction. Laumann[64] noted significant early activity of all the rotator cuff muscles and deltoid, however, this was quite apparent in the supraspinatus.

The most interesting evidence of supraspinatus and deltoid dependence comes from quantitative torques studies and clinical observations. Colachis[20,21] found that by inducing an axillary nerve palsy, thus paralyzing the deltoid and teres minor, a 40 to 75 percent isometric torque deficit was produced when abducting in the scapular plane. This deficit increased progressively through the abduction range. Similar deficits were seen in flexion and coronal plane abduction (Fig. 2-38). Although deficits were produced, all subjects could abduct their arm through the range, indicating that the supraspinatus, infraspinatus, and subscapularis muscles were effective abductors. Since the infraspinatus and subscapularis have poor moment arms for abduction, the supraspinatus was considered the prime abductor. When a suprascapular nerve palsy was induced, a 30 percent deficit was noted at 0 degrees, increasing to 65 percent at 30 degrees, only to reduce to 35 percent at 150 degrees (Fig. 2-39). Because the supraspinatus and infraspinatus were inactive, the deltoid was considered the prime abductor. Colachis[21] concluded that the deltoid was of greater importance to arm motion above 60 degrees. This agrees with our isometric data on subjects who demonstrated a reduced torque deficit at higher ranges of abduction compared with lower ranges after a suprascapular nerve block[62] (Fig. 2-40). This correlates well with increasing mechanical efficiency of the deltoid as abduction increases.[85]

Howell et al.[48] supported the work of Colachis[20,21] by determining isokinetic torque in the scapular plane at 60 degrees. They also induced axillary and suprascapular nerve palsies and found approximately 50 percent torque reduction in each condition. Thus the deltoid and supraspinatus produced equivalent torque for scapular plane abduction. Markhede et al.[68] found 0, 29, and 40 percent deficits at 0, 45, and 90 degrees of coronal plane abduction, respectively, in patients having an excised deltoid. Others have noted the adequacy of the intact

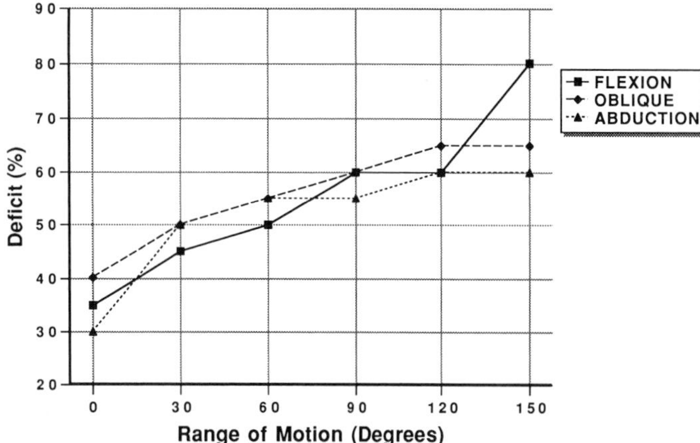


**Figure 2-38.** Percent muscle-force deficit created by an induced axillary nerve palsy during varying degrees of elevation in three different planes. (Data from Colachis SC, Strohm BR, Brechner VL. Effects of axillary nerve block on muscle force in the upper extremity. Arch Phys Med Rehabil 1969;50:647.)

rotator cuff muscles producing abduction without deltoid function.[9,16,101]

Care must be taken when extrapolating information from these studies into the clinical setting, particularly when relating to rotator cuff disease. The above-mentioned studies are dealing with an intact capsuloligamentous-tendinous envelope. Disruption of the envelope can have a significant effect on the deltoid–rotator cuff relationship, either directly through a breach in the tendon reducing compressive force and torque production or indirectly creating

1. The loss of uninvolved rotator cuff muscles to efficiently translate tension from their origin to insertion, which may in part insert into the torn fibers. This results in reduced depressive and compressive forces.
2. Pain from tension on the torn fibers and subacromial impingement. This can lead to muscle reflex inhibition causing further shutdown of activity.[24]
3. The loss of passive integrity normally provided by tension from the contiguous capsuloligamentous-tendinous envelope.

## INFRASPINATUS AND TERES MINOR

The infraspinatus and teres minor muscles have a combined cross-sectional area of 13.74 cm$^2$.[5] They are active throughout elevation,[49,64,77,103] fulfilling two responsibilities: (1) force-couple requirements and (2) serving as a posterior barrier against translation.

The infraspinatus demonstrates a linear pro-

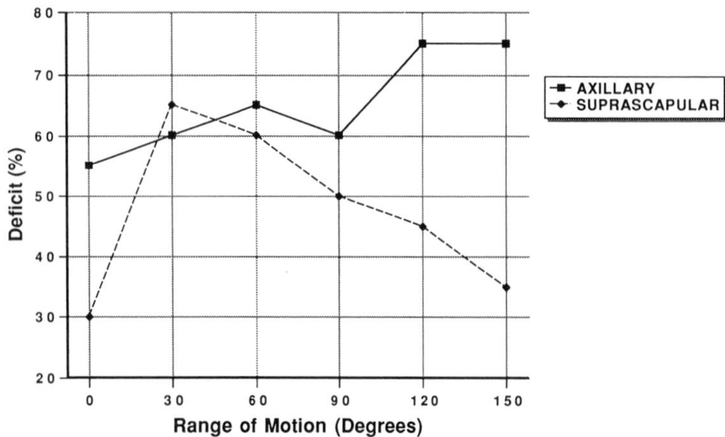


**Figure 2-39.** Percent muscle-force deficit created by an induced suprascapular and axillary nerve palsy at varying degrees of scapular plane abduction. (Data from Colachis SC, Strohm BR. Effect of suprascapular and axillary nerve blocks on muscle force in the upper extremity. Arch Phys Med Rehabil 1971;52:22.)

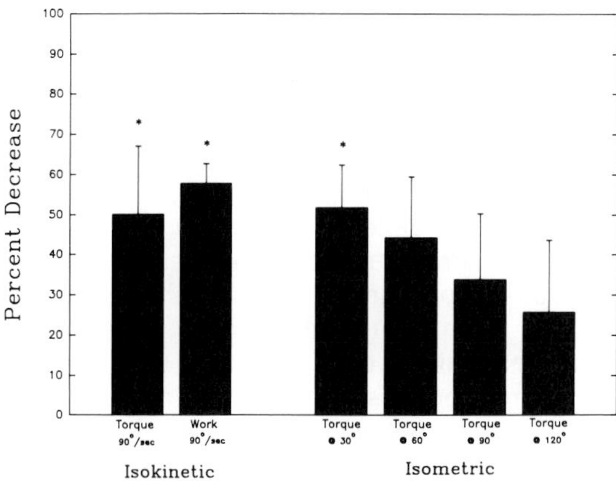


**Figure 2-40.** Percent abductor-force deficit created by an induced suprascapular nerve palsy. (From Kuhlman JR, Iannotti JP, Kelley MJ, et al. Isokinetic and isometric evaluation of the shoulder: implications for clinical assessment of rotator cuff strength. J Bone Joint Surg 1992;74A:1320.)

gression in activity throughout coronal[49] and scapular plane abduction.[50,96] Activity differs somewhat in flexion, being higher and peaking at 60 and 120 degrees.[49] Activity is enhanced due to the muscle demand created when the elbow is flexed to 90 degrees, producing a moment toward internal rotation. The role of the infraspinatus may be more than just a stabilizer. Ito[50] found increasing activity at flexion and abduction end range, demonstrating a strong possibility of abducting capabilities. Celli et al.[16] performed EMGs on a group of patients having axillary nerve lesions who had only the supraspinatus (sopraspinoso), infraspinatus (sottospinoso), and scapulothoracic muscles intact (Fig. 2-41). They found that these individuals had full abduction and that the infraspinatus acted as a "mover" (electrical activity increase through the range), while the supraspinatus was the "sta-

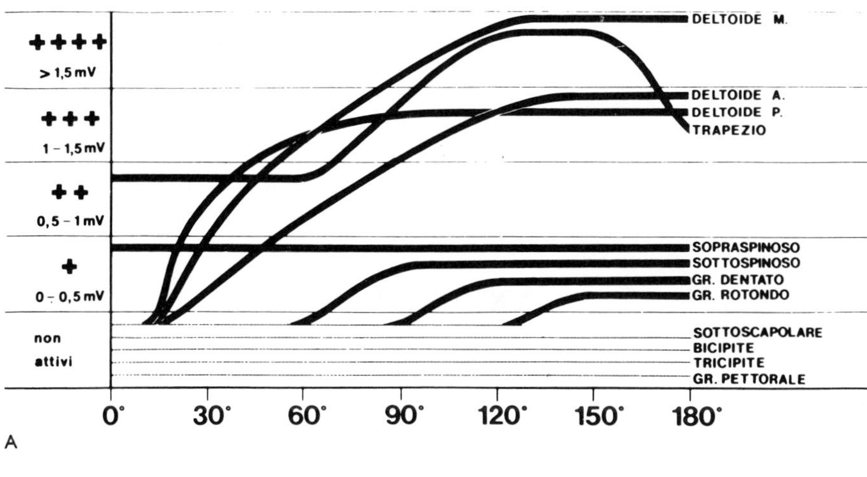


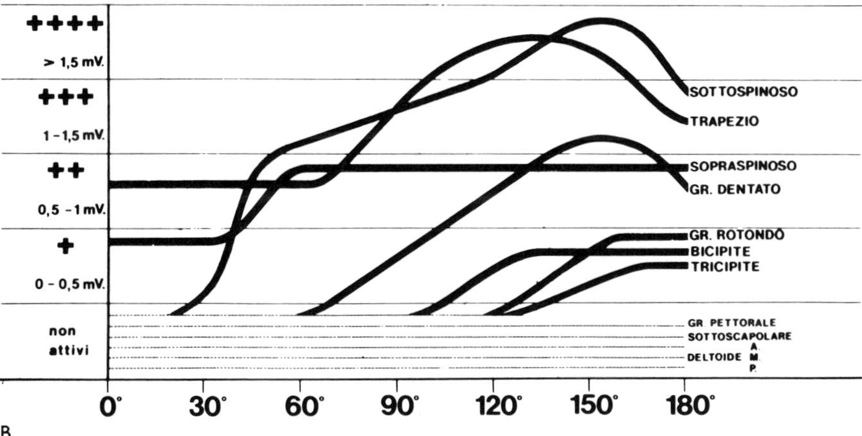


**Figure 2-41.** (a) A normal EMG. (b) An EMG of a patient with deltoid paralysis. Note the significant activity of the infraspinatus (sottospinoso) in part B. Sopraspinoso = supraspinatus. (From Celli L, Balli A, DeLuise G, Rovesta C. Some new aspects of the functional anatomy of the shoulder. Ital Trans Othop Traumatol 1985;11:83.)

bilizer." The teres minor acts similarly to the infraspinatus but to a lesser degree.[49] Clinically, emphasis on strengthening these posterior cuff muscles is essential in rehabilitating the nonoperative and postoperative rotator cuff lesion.

### SUBSCAPULARIS

The subscapularis acts synergistically with the posterior cuff muscles to depress and compress the humeral head. This muscle is endowed with a substantial cross-sectional area of 16.3 $cm^2$; only the deltoid is larger.[5]

The subscapularis is more active in abduction than in flexion. Peak activity in the coronal plane abduction is between 90 and 120 degrees, after which it falls to coincide with flexion activity.[49] Saha[96] found increasing activity up 150 degrees, followed by a rapid decline. Saha felt that the infraspinatus, teres minor, and subscapularis muscles were "steerers" at the glenohumeral joint. This information is in conflict with that of others, who found a progressive rise in activity at end range.[16,50]

### BICEPS

The biceps, although predominantly an elbow flexor and forearm supinator, can be an effective elevator. In anatomic position, the biceps has no abducting moment through which it can work. Humeral external rotation places the long head laterally, causing it to act like a pulley, assisting in arm elevation. The long head tendon is capable of stabilizing the humeral head through a compressive action.[60,66] Perry[82] feels that since the biceps cross-sectional area is only 9 $cm^2$ and only half the muscle corresponds to the long head, stabilizing force effecting the humeral head is minimal.

### PECTORALIS MAJOR

Inman and coworkers[49] found a contribution from the clavicular and manubrial portions of the pectoralis major only in flexion. The clavicular head initially peaks at 75 degrees and then rises again at 115 degrees. Manubrial head contribution was minimal.

This muscle can become synergistically essential in peripheral nerve lesions compromising deltoid and supraspinatus function. In conjunction with the scapulothoracic muscles, the pectoral clavicular head flexes and adducts the arm, allowing the hand to be brought to the mouth.

In summary, the predominate elevators are the supraspinatus and deltoid muscles, yet studies suggest that the contribution from the infraspinatus is significant. Clinically, we see remarkable compensatory ability of the shoulder musculature to elevate the arm. This is clearly demonstrated in patients with the deltoid excised,[68] but most recently by Rockwood et al.[88] Their follow-up study of patients with massive rotator cuff tears demonstrated good to excellent results in pain relief and function. In patients who had an irreparable infraspinatus and supraspinatus tendon tear, the tear was debrided along with an appropriate subacromial decompression. These authors concluded that as long as the decompression was good and the anterior deltoid strong, the patient did well, even though the rotator cuff was deficient.

## Extension

Shoulder extension is accomplished by the posterior deltoid, latissimus dorsi, teres major, infraspinatus, teres minor, and triceps muscles. The middle deltoid also contributes to extension.[103] Colachis[20,21] found 60 percent deficits in extension when the axillary nerve was anesthetically blocked. The majority of the deficit was recognized as posterior deltoid dysfunction opposed to teres minor involvement. Markhede[68] found 38, 21, and 29 percent extension deficits at 0, 45, and 90 degrees of flexion, respectively, in patients with the deltoid removed.

## External Rotation

External rotation is powered by the infraspinatus, posterior deltoid, and teres minor muscles. External rotation torque deficits of 55 percent were found when an axillary nerve palsy was induced and 60 percent with the suprascapular nerve blocked.[20,21] This is in agreement with our finding of a 67 percent deficit of external rotation torque output in the presence of a suprascapular nerve palsy.[62] It is difficult to quantify percentage contribution of just the infraspinatus and teres minor muscles in the preceding conditions, but approximately 80 percent of torque output is attributed to them. Significant activity of the teres minor and infraspinatus was noted in full external rotation and horizontal extension.[52,55,83] This is the late cocking-phase position in throwing and is advocated for strengthening the posterior cuff muscles.[10] Celli et al.[16] examined external rotation at the neutral position with the elbow flexed. They found that motion up to 30 degrees is purely glenohumeral, and only the infraspinatus was contracting (they did not examine teres minor function). Further external rotation lead to adduction of the scapula through activity of the scapular adductors.

We have noted this type of synergy between the scapular adductors, particularly the middle trapezius, during external rotation. When resisting shoulder external rotation at the neutral position, the trapezius and rhomboids stabilize the vertebral border of the scapula. This is needed because the infraspinatus, teres minor, and posterior deltoid all pull from their origins, producing "medial winging" of the scapula. This is quite evident in individuals having peripheral nerve disruption of the trapezius and rhomboids (Fig. 2-42).

## Internal Rotation

Internal rotation is powered by the subscapularis, teres major, pectoralis major, latissimus dorsi, and anterior deltoid muscles. Studies quantifying muscles involved in internal rotation are lacking. The anterior deltoid was found to contribute to internal rotation, demonstrating a 6 percent[21] and 27 percent[20] deficit when an axillary nerve palsy was induced. Strong eccentric activity occurs in the subscapularis during the late cocking phase of throwing.[52,53] Controversy exist regarding activity of the latissimus dorsi, teres major, and pectoralis muscles in unresisted rotation. There is agreement that all three are active during forced internal rotation.[3]

## Functional Activities

Studies investigating functional overhead use have been performed to determine EMG activity and fatigue levels.[39,44,45,55,100] Localized muscle fatigue was found in the supraspinatus, but only in experienced welders, whereas inexperienced welders demonstrated fatigue of other muscles as well.[55] Herberts et al.[45] found that supraspinatus fatigue was significantly reduced when overhead activities were performed at 45 degrees of abduction compared with 0 and 90 degrees. Sigholm et al.[100] investigated several parameters: hand load, arm position, elbow angle, and arm rotation. Three static positions were examined, neutral and 45 and 90 degrees, for both flexion and abduction. They found that the supraspinatus was heavily loaded at 45 degrees but was not further loaded at 90 degrees. Although the anterior deltoid did show increased activity, it was not significant.

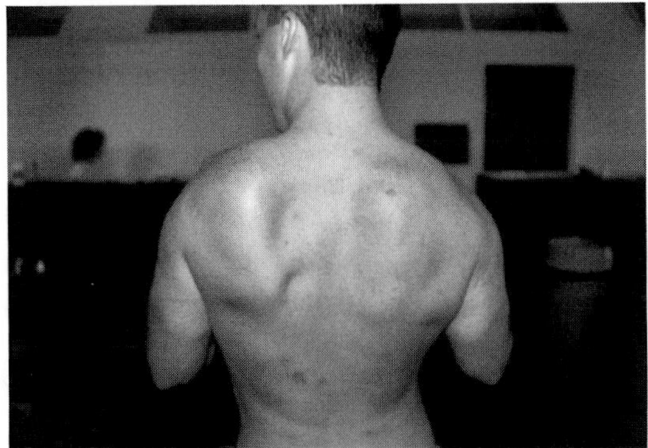

**Figure 2-42.** Patient with trapezius paralysis attempts to externally rotate against resistance. Apparent scapular winging is noted, demonstrating a strong synergy between the glenohumeral external rotators and the middle and lower trapezius.

Interesting findings regarding the infraspinatus were made by EMG studies. This muscle demonstrated the highest level of fatigue[45] and was found to have the greatest hand-load dependence.[100] High fatigue levels were found in other studies.[44] Elbow flexion and arm rotation had little affect on muscle load.[100]

The upper trapezius showed increased fatigue when the arm was raised from 45 to 90 degrees of abduction.[45] Sigholm et al.[100] and Hagberg[39] found that weight in the hand increased the load of the upper trapezius.

In summary,

1. All muscles, particularly the supraspinatus, infraspinatus, and upper trapezius, demonstrate fatigue during overhead work. A direct cause and effect therefore exist between this finding and rotator cuff pathology in the overhead working force.
2. Ideally, work should be done below shoulder level, but if overhead activity must be done, a slight degree of abduction is recommended.
3. There is a direct correlation between the weight of the tool and the muscle load in overhead work. Therefore, tools should be supported, or care to select lighter tools is recommended.

## Scapulothoracic Muscles

These muscles incorporate the trapezius (upper, middle, and lower), serratus anterior (upper and lower digitations), levator scapula, rhomboids, and pectoralis minor (Fig. 2-43). Because of their action on the scapula, they provide a stable yet mobile base from which the glenohumeral joint and associated muscles can function. Loss of the these muscles, particularly the trapezius or serratus anterior, seriously hampers scapulohumeral rhythm and shoulder function.

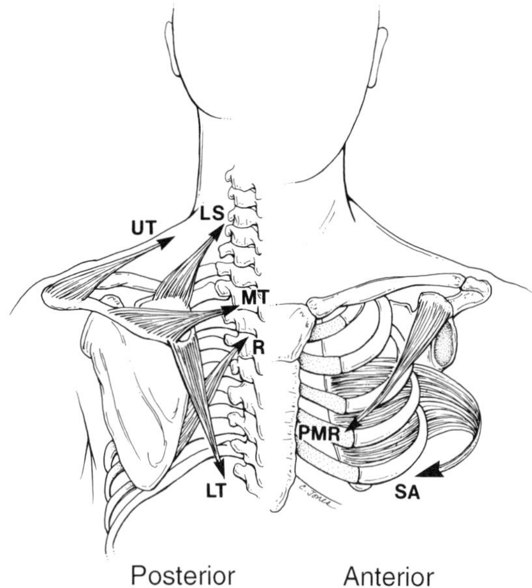


**Figure 2-43.** Scapulothoracic muscles.

## POSTURAL SUPPORT

The upper trapezius and levator scapula provide passive suspension for the shoulder girdle.[6,82] Fascia overlying these muscles and the sternocleidomastoid are also felt to provide significant support.[82] The rhomboids and serratus anterior contribute less to direct scapular suspension.

Activity was found in the upper trapezius fibers at rest,[7,16,;49] but EMG silence was noted when encouraging relaxation. Relaxation of the upper fibers could be promoted even with 10 lb of weight held in the hand, but adding a load elicited activity from the levator scapulae.[7] Both the levator scapulae and upper trapezius are important in supporting the head on the body. There is a high incidence of postural strain and trigger-point formation because of their dual role.[6] These muscles are also typically involved in periscapular pain associated with rotator cuff pathology. When chronic upper trapezius weakness is present, such as in an accessory nerve palsy or facioscapulohumeral muscular dystrophy, gravity slowly prevails, causing stretching of the secondary restraints. The clavicle's lateral end sinks and drops forward to the point of a downward orientation with respect to the horizontal. The scapula follows the clavicle and abducts with respect to the uninvolved side (Fig. 2-44).

The forward shoulder posture commonly seen in the population can lead to two typical types of scapular migration, one being toward abduction and depression. This places excessive stretch and strain on all fibers of the trapezius as well as the levator scapulae and rhomboid. Kendall[58] refers to this stretching effect on muscle as "stretch weakness." Weakness can be easily demonstrated with proper manual muscle testing techniques. The second posture places the inferior angle in elevation with respect to the opposite inferior angle, yet the acromion is lower and the scapula is medially rotated (Fig. 2-45). This causes the contiguous scapula to fulcrum on its ventral midpoint over the curved thoracic wall. This anterior scapular tilting causes posterior displacement of the inferior angle from the thoracic wall. Depending on the extent of displacement, this positioning is often mistaken for a serratus anterior palsy. Commonly, an individual participating in a unilateral sport or activity demonstrates this type of orientation on the dominant side. Posturing of this sort can lead to adaptive shortening of the levator scapulae, rhomboid, and pectoralis minor and stretch weakness of the serratus anterior and lower trapezius.[56]

## SERRATUS ANTERIOR AND TRAPEZIUS FORCE COUPLE

The serratus anterior and trapezius force couple serves four paramount functions:

1. To orient the scapula, maintaining the glenoid surface in an appropriate position to support the humeral head and reduce tension across

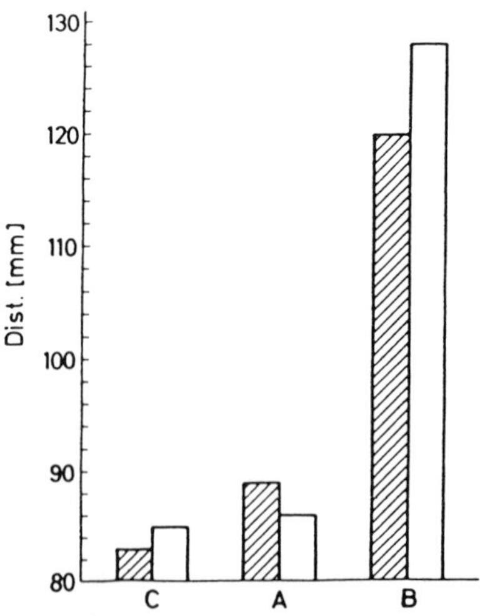


**Figure 2-44.** Mean distance of the spine to the medial scapular border with the arms at the side without weight (filled columns) and holding an 8-kg weight (empty columns). (A) Healthy subjects. (B) Trapezius paralysis. (C) Serratus anterior paralysis. (From Laumann U. Kinesiology of the shoulder joint. In Kolbel R, et al., eds. Shoulder replacement. Berlin: Springer-Verlag, 1987.)

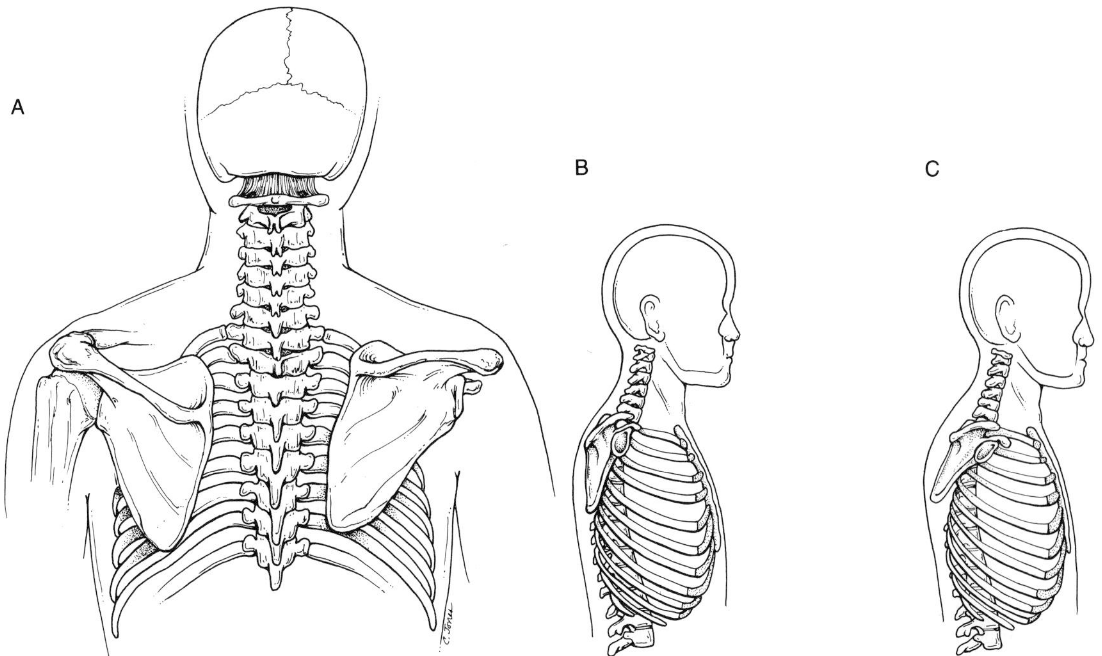


**Figure 2-45.** (a) Abnormal scapular position at rest noted on the right (scapular elevation and medial rotation) due to right hand dominance. (b) Normal scapular position noted on a lateral view. (c) Abnormal anterior tilting and elevation of the scapula on the thoracic wall noted on a lateral view. This is consistent with hand dominance.

the static stabilizers. Without this, potential instability arises.[92]

2. Through scapular rotation, maintaining efficient length of the deltoid fibers through the range, enhancing the power and stabilizing effect. Without scapular rotation, only 90 degrees of active abduction is available.[49, 66]
3. Preventing impingement of the subacromial structures (i.e., rotator cuff and bursa) on the corcoacromial arch.
4. Providing a stable base that enables the axiohumeral and scapulohumeral muscles to move the arm against resistance. Trying to move the humerus without the trapezius and/or serratus is like to trying to push against a solid wall while on roller skates.

The force couple is classically broken into upper and lower components. The former is composed of the upper trapezius, levator scapulae, and serratus anterior upper digitations. The lower component is composed of the lower trapezius and the lower serratus digitations.[49] This force couple functions in all planes of elevation (Fig. 2-46).

During the setting phase of scapular motion, between 30 degrees of abduction and up to 60 degrees of flexion, the upper and middle trapezius muscles demonstrate increased activity compared with the serratus anterior.[64] As the arm is elevated, the upper trapezius and levator scapulae elevate the scapula, being consistent with clavicular rise. Activity of the upper trapezius continues in a linear fashion as the scapula rotates about its axis[49, 50, 64] (Fig. 2-47a). Activity is fairly constant in both flexion and abduction. The upper trapezius fibers have a dual role as elevators and rotators, pulling at the acromial insertion. The upper serratus fibers also assist in upward rotation.

Members of the lower component act in assisting the upper fibers. The lower trapezius pulls inferiorly from its insertion at the scapular spine base, which is superior to the axis of rotation. This acts to direct the glenoid upward. The lower trapezius contribution is greater through the range of abduction. In flexion, activity plateaus between 70 and 120 degrees, after which activity significantly increases to coincide with the abduction curve (see Fig. 2-47c).

The lower fibers of the serratus are extremely important in rotating and abducting the scapula. This muscle enjoys the largest moment arm among the elevating muscles.[34] The activity of the fifth and sixth digitations is higher than that of the seventh and eighth digitations, demonstrating greater importance to the lower force-couple component. The force couple is now complete,

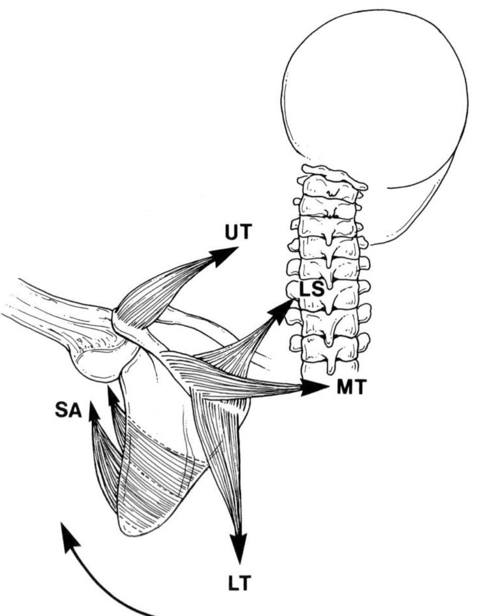


**Figure 2-46.** Serratus anterior and trapezius force couple generating scapular rotation.

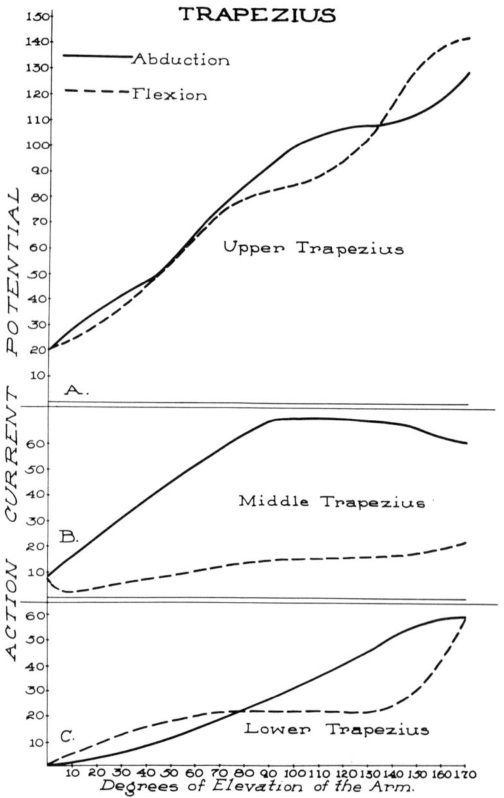


**Figure 2-47.** Differences in trapezius fiber firing during flexion and abduction. (B,C) Note significant differences in middle and lower trapezius during coronal plane abduction compared with flexion. (From Inman VT, Saunder JR, Abbott LC. Observations on the function of the shoulder joint. J Bone Joint Surg 1944;26A:1.)

as the serratus anterior lower fibers pull the inferior angle forward and laterally. Serratus activity is greater in flexion than in abduction in the fifth and sixth digits and after 90 degrees in the seventh and eighth fibers. At end range, all fibers are equally active. This is consistent with Laumann's[64] study demonstrating the direction of scapular rotation. The scapular $\gamma$ (gamma) angle between the medial end of the scapular spine and vertebral column increases with flexion (Fig. 2-48). The scapula translates forward on the thoracic wall, directing the glenoid toward the sagittal plane (Fig. 2-49a). For this to occur, the serratus is more active in pulling the scapula forward. The scapula always attains the same terminal position whether elevating in abduction or in flexion.[64] This would explain why EMG activity is equal for the scapular rotators at flexion and abduction end range. The differences in scapular migration between flexion and coronal plane abduction are explained by the differences in activity of the lower trapezius, middle trapezius, and rhomboids, all having greater action-potential counts in abduction. Laumann[64] found that coronal plane abduction lead to a decrease in the scapular angle $\gamma$ (gamma) (see Fig. 2-48), so the glenoid was directed more laterally, toward the coronal plane (see Fig. 2-49b). The scapular adductors draw the medial scapular border in (adduct), orienting the glenoid laterally toward the humerus. If the glenoid remains toward the sagittal plane due to weakness of the scapular adductors, tension is increased across the anterior-inferior CLC, jeopardizing stability. Maximizing scapular muscle strength to effectively position the glenoid is as important to glenohumeral stability as optimizing rotator cuff strength to centralize the humeral head. During flexion, "controlled relaxation" (eccentric activity) develops in these muscles to allow the scapula to migrate forward (see Fig. 2-47b).

Clinically, serratus anterior palsy is more common and results in greater functional impairment than trapezius palsy. This is somewhat dependent on return of innervation. The prolonged, particularly complete trapezius palsy can be debilitating due to loss of scapular suspension and subsequent depression of the shoulder girdle. The importance of mechanical effect can only be appreciated by examining a patient with this condition. When working with a patient having an isolated trapezius palsy, the individual can present with fairly good but weak sagittal plane movement, but abduction is significantly impaired. An individual burdened with a complete serratus palsy can neither flex nor abduct the arm fully. We also have seen up to a 25 percent reduction of internal and external torque

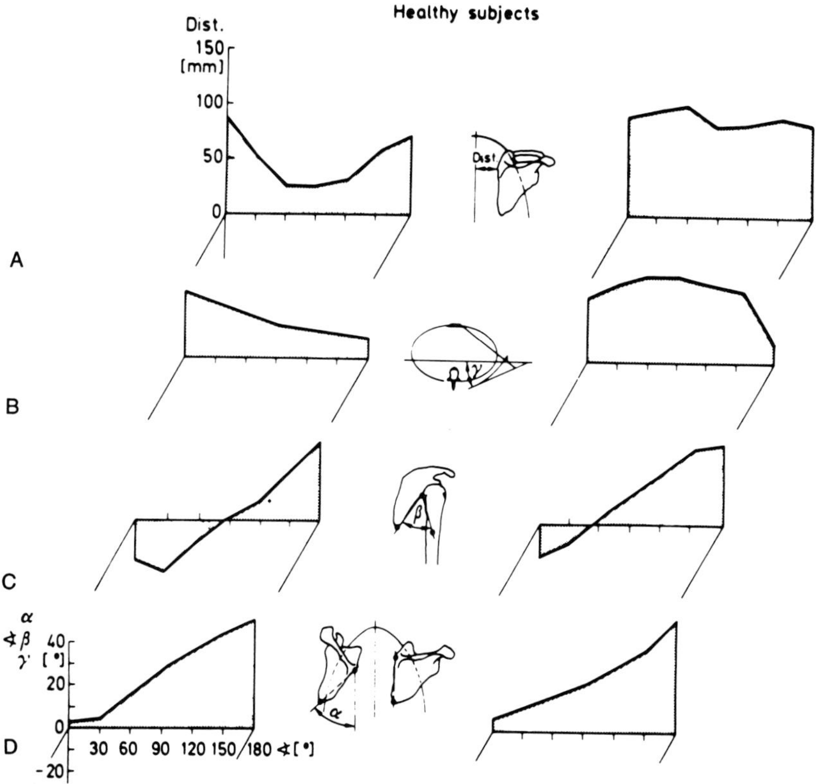


**Figure 2-48.** Scapular motion represented from three spatial axis during frontal (F) or coronal plane abduction and sagittal (S) plane elevation or flexion. Note the significant difference in $\gamma$ during sagittal plane motion due to anterior orientation of the glenoid. Also note that whether elevated in the coronal or sagittal plane, end-range excursions are identical. (From Laumann U. Kinesiology of the shoulder joint. In Kolbel R, et al., eds. Shoulder replacement. Berlin: Springer-Verlag, 1987).

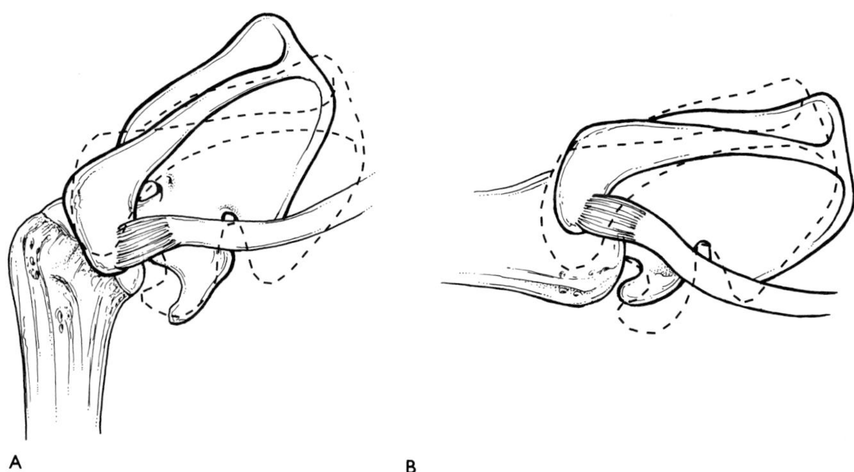


**Figure 2-49.** Significant change in glenoid orientation when moved in the sagittal plane (a) and coronal plane (b). This is an attempt of the glenoid fossa to maintain osseous support for the humeral head.

output in patients with a serratus or trapezius nerve palsy.

Recognition of the scapulothoracic contribution to shoulder function is imperative. A great deal of research and clinical effort have been directed toward the rotator cuff, yet the nuances of the scapulothoracic muscles have not been thoroughly investigated. The clinician must evaluate for scapulothoracic muscle dysfunction, particularly in the presence of apparent primary rotator cuff pathology and glenohumeral instability. Many times only the glenohumeral soft tissues are treated when significant dysfunction of the scapulothoracic muscles exist, resulting in continued shoulder symptomatology.

# Summary

In this chapter we have discussed the anatomic and biomechanical properties of the shoulder complex. An impressive interdependency can be appreciated between muscle action, ligament control, and osseous orientation. Understanding this relationship is paramount to successfully assessing and treating shoulder dysfunction.

# References

1. American Academy of Orthopaedic Surgeons. Joint motion: method of measuring and recording. Chicago: American Academy of Orthopaedic Surgeons, 1965.
2. Bankart ASB. The pathology and treatment of recurrent dislocation of the shoulder joint. Br J Surg 1938;26:23.
3. Basmajian JV. Muscles alive. 4th ed. Baltimore: Williams & Wilkins, 1979.
4. Basmajian JV, Bazant FJ. Factors preventing downward dislocation of the adducted shoulder joint. J Bone Joint Surg 1959; 41A:1182.
5. Bassett RW, Browne AO, Morrey BF, An KN. Glenohumeral muscle force and moment mechanics in a position of shoulder instability. J Biomech 1990;23:405.
6. Bateman JE. The shoulder and neck. Philadelphia: WB Saunders, 1971.
7. Bearn JG. An electromyographic study of the trapezius, deltoid pectoralis major, biceps and triceps muscles during static loading of the upper limb. Anat Rec 1961;140:103.
8. Bearn JG. Direct observation on the function of the capsule of the sternoclavicular joint in clavicular support. J Anat 1967;101:159.
9. Bechtol CO. Biomechanics of the shoulder. Clin Orthop 1980; 146:37.
10. Blackburn TA, McLeod WD, White B, Wofford L. Analysis of posterior rotator cuff exercise. Athletic Train 1990;25:40.
11. Blakely RL, Palmer ML. Analysis of rotation accompanying shoulder flexion. Phys Ther 1984;64:1214.
12. Boone DC, Azen SP. Normal range of motion of joints in male subjects. J Bone Joint Surg 1979;61A:756.
13. Cain PR, Mutschler TA, Fu FH, Lee SK. Anterior stability of the glenohumeral joint: a dynamic model. Am J Sports Med 1987; 15:144.
14. Calliet R. Shoulder pain. Philadelphia: FA Davies, 1977.
15. Cave AJE. The nature and morphology of the costoclavicular ligament. J Anat 1961;95:170.
16. Celli L, Balli A, deLuise G, Rovesta C. Some new aspects of the functional anatomy of the shoulder. Ital Trans Othop Traumatol 1985;11:83.
16a. Clark JC, Harryman DT. Tendons, ligaments, and capsule of the rotator cuff. J Bone Joint Surg. 1992;74A:713.
17. Clarke GR, Willis LA, Fish WW, Nichols PJ. Assessment of movement at the glenohumeral joint. Orthopedics 1974;7:55.
18. Close JR, Nichel ED, Todd AB. Motor unit action potential counts. J Bone Joint Surg 1960;42A:1207.
19. Codman EA. The shoulder. Boston: Thomas Todd, 1934.
20. Colachis SC, Strohm BR. Effect of suprascapular and axillary nerve blocks on muscle force in upper extremity. Arch Phys Med Rehabil 1971;52:22.
21. Colachis SC, Strohm BR, Brechner VL. Effects of axillary nerve block on muscle force in the upper extremity. Arch Phys Med Rehabil 1969;50:647.
22. Curwin S, Standish WD. Tendonitis: it's etiology and treatment. Lexington, Ky.: The Collamore Press, 1984.
23. Davies GJ. A compendium of isokinetics in clinical usage. 3rd ed. Onahaska, Wisc.: S and S Publishing, 1987.
24. de Andrade JR, Grant C, Dixon A St J. Joint distension and reflex muscle inhibition in the knee. J Bone Joint Surg 1965;47A:313.
25. De Freitas V, Vitti M, Furlani J. Electromyographic study of levator scapulae and rhomboideus major muscles in movements of the shoulder and arm. Electromyogr Clin Neurophysiol 1980;20:205.
26. de Luca CJ, Forrest WJ. Force analysis of individual muscles acting simultaneously on the shoulder joint during isometric abduction. J Biomech 1973;6:385.
27. Dempster WT. Mechanisms of shoulder movement. Arch Phys Med Rehabil 1965;46:49.
28. DePalma AF. Surgery of the shoulder. Philadelphia: JB Lippincott, 1973.
29. Depalma AF, Cooke AJ, Prabhakar M. The role of the subscapularis in recurrent anterior dislocations of the shoulder. Clin Orthop 1967;54:35.
30. Detrisac DA, Johnson LL. Arthroscopic shoulder anatomy: glenohumeral capsular ligaments. Thorofare, N.J.: Slack, 1986.
31. Doody MS, Freedman L, Waterland JC. Shoulder movements during abduction in the scapular plane. Arch Phys Med Rehabil 1970;51:595.
32. Drillis R, Contini R, Bluestein M. Body segment parameter: a survey of measurement techniques. Artif Limbs 1964;8:329.
33. Duchenne GB. Physiology of motion. Trans. EB Kaplan. Philadelphia: JB Lippincott, 1949.
34. Dvir Z, Berme N. The shoulder complex in elevation of the arm: a mechanism approach. J Biomech 1978;11:219.
35. Elftman H. Biomechanics of muscle. J Bone Joint Surg 1966; 48A:363.
36. Freedman L, Munro RH. Abduction of the arm in the scapular plane: scapular and glenohumeral movements. J Bone Joint Surg 1966;48A:1503.
37. Germain NW, Blair SN. Variability of shoulder flexion with age, activity and sex. Am Corr Ther J 1983;37:156.
38. Williams PL, Warwick R, eds. Gray's anatomy. Philadelphia: WB Saunders, 1980.
39. Hagberg M. Work load and fatigue in repetitive arm elevation. Ergonomics 1981;24:543.
40. Harryman DT, Sidles JA, Clark JM, et al. Translation of the humeral head on the glenoid with passive glenohumeral motion. J Bone Joint Surg 1990;72A:1334.
41. Harryman DT, Sidles JA, Harris SZ, Matzen FA III. The role of the rotator internal capsule in passive motion and stability of the shoulder. J Bone Joint Surg 1992;74A:53.
42. Hawkins RJ, Bell RH, Hawkins RH, Kopper GJ. Anterior dislocation of the shoulder in the older patient. Clin Orthop 1986; 206:192.
43. Hawkins RJ, Misamore GW, Hobeika PE. Surgery of full thickness rotator cuff tears. J Bone Joint Surg 1985;67A(9):1349.
44. Herberts D, Kadefors R, Anderson G, Petersen I. Shoulder pain in industry: an epidemiological study in welders. Acta Orthop Scand 1981;52:299.
45. Herberts D, Kadefors R, Broman H. Arm positioning in manual tasks and electromyographic study of localized muscle fatigue. Ergonomics 1980;23:655.
46. Howell SM, Galinat BJ. The glenoid labral socket: a contained articular surface. Clin Orthop 1989;243:122.
47. Howell SM, Galinat BJ, Renzi AJ, Marone PJ. Normal and abnormal mechanics of the glenohumeral joint in the horizontal plane. J Bone Joint Surg 1988;70A:227.
48. Howell SM, Imobersteg AM, Seger DH, Marone PJ. Clarification of the role of the supraspinatus muscle in shoulder function. J Bone Joint Surg 1986;68A:398.
49. Inman VT, Saunder JR, Abbott LC. Observations on the function of the shoulder joint. J Bone Joint Surg 1944;26:1.
50. Ito N. Electromyographic study of shoulder joint. J Jpn Orthop Assoc 1980;54:53.

51. Jobe FW, Moynes DR. Delineation of diagnostic criteria and a rehabilitation program for rotator cuff injuries. Am J Sports Med 1982;10(6):336.
52. Jobe FW, Moynes DM, Tibone JE, Perry J. An EMG analysis of the shoulder in ptching: a second report. Am J Sports Med 1984; 12:218.
53. Jobe FW, Tibone JE, Perry J, Moynes D. An EMG analysis of the shoulder in throwing and pitching: a preliminary report. Am J Sports Med 1983;11:3.
54. Johnston TB. The movements of the shoulder joint: a plea for the use of the "plane of the scapula" as the plane of reference in movements occurring at the humero-scapular joint. Br J Surg 1937;25:252.
55. Kadefors R, Petersen I, Herberts P. Muscular reaction to welding work: an electromyographic investigation. Ergonomics 1976; 19:543.
56. Kaltenborn FM. Mobilization of the extremity joints: examination and basic treatment techniques. Oslo: Olaf Bokhandel, 1980.
57. Kapandji I. The physiology of joints. Vol 1. Baltimore: Williams & Wilkins, 1970.
57a. Kelkar R, Flatow EL, Bigliani LU, et al. A stereophotogrammetric method to determine the kinematics of the glenohumeral joint. Adv Bioeng 1992;19:143.
58. Kendall FP, McCreary EK. Muscle testing and function. 3rd ed. Baltimore: Williams & Wilkins, 1982.
59. Kennedy JC, Cameron H. Complete dislocation of the acromioclavicular joint. J Bone Joint Surg 1954;36B:202.
60. Kent B. Functional anatomy of the shoulder complex. Phys Ther 1971;51:867.
61. Komi PV. Relationship between muscle tension, EMG and velocity of concentric and eccentric work. In Desmedth E, ed. New developments in electromyography and clinical neurophysiology. Vol. 1. Basel: Karger, 1973.
62. Kuhlman JR, Iannotti JP, Kelley MJ, et al. Isokinetic and isometric evaluation of the shoulder: implications for clinical assessment of rotator cuff strength. J Bone Joint Surg 1992;74A:1320.
63. Kumar VP, Balasubramaniam P. The role of atmospheric pressure in stabilizing the shoulder: an experimental study. J Bone Joint Surg 1985;67B:719.
64. Laumann U. Kinesiology of the shoulder joint. In Kolbel R, Helbig, Blauth, eds. Shoulder replacement. Berlin: Springer-Verlag, 1987.
65. Lippold OC. The relation between integrated action potentials in a human muscle and its isometric tension. J Physiol (Lond) 1952;117:492.
66. Lucas DB. Biomechanics of the shoulder joint. Arch Surg 1973;107:425.
67. MacConail MA, Basmajian JV. Muscles and movements: a basis for human kinesiology. Baltimore: Williams & Wilkins, 1969.
68. Markhede G, Monastyrski J, Stener B. Shoulder function after deltoid muscle removal. Acta Orthop Scand 1985;56:242.
69. Matzen FA III. Biomechanics of the shoulder. In Frankel VH, Nordin M, eds. Basic biomechanics of the skeletal system. Philadelphia: Lea & Febiger, 1980.
70. Matzen FA, Thomas SC, Rockwood CA. Anterior glenohumeral instability. In Rockwood CA, Matzen FA, eds. The shoulder. Philadelphia: WB Saunders, 1990.
71. McGregor L. Rotation at the shoulder: a critical injury. Br J Surg 1937;1524:425.
72. Morrey BF, Chao EY. Recurrent anterior dislocation of the shoulder. In Dumbleton J, Black J, eds. Clinical biomechanics. London: Churchill Livingstone, 1981.
73. Moseley HF. The clavicle: its anatomy and function. Clin Orthop 1958;58:17.
74. Moseley HF, Overgaard D. The anterior capsular mechanism in recurrent anterior dislocation of the shoulder. J Bone Joint Surg 1962;44B:913.
75. Murray MP, Gore DR, Gardner GM, Mollinger LA. Shoulder motion and muscle strength of normal men and women in two age groups. Clin Orthop 1985;192:268.
76. Nobuhara K. The shoulder: its function and clinical aspects. Tokyo: Igaku-Shoin, 1977.
77. Nuber GW, Bowman ID, Perry JP, et al. EMG analysis of classical shoulder motion. Trans Orthop Res Soc 1986;11:
78. Nuber GW, Jobe FW, Perry JP, et al. Fine wire EMG analysis of the shoulder during swimming. Am J Sport Med 1986;14:7.
79. O'Brien SJ, Neves MC, Arnoczky SP, et al. The anatomy and histology of the inferior glenohumeral ligament complex of the shoulder. Am J Sports Med 1990;18:449.
80. O'Connell, PW, Nuber GW, Mileski RA, Lautenschlager E. The contribution of the glenohumeral ligaments to anterior stability of the shoulder joint. Am J Sports Med 1990;18:579.
81. Ovesen J, Nielsen S. Anterior and posterior shoulder instability. Acta Orthop Scand 1986;57:324.
82. Perry J. Biomechanics. In Rowe C, ed. The shoulder. New York: Churchill Livingstone, 1988.
83. Perry J. Anatomy and biomechanics of the shoulder in throwing, swimming, gymnastics and tennis. Clin Sports Med 1983;2:247.
84. Poppen NK, Walker PS. Normal and abnormal motion of the shoulder. J Bone Joint Surg 1976;58A:195.
85. Poppen NK, Walker PS. Forces at the glenohumeral joint in abduction. Clin Orthop 1978;135:165.
86. Radin EL. Biomechanics and functional anatomy. In Post M, ed. The shoulder: surgical and nonsurgical management. 2nd ed. Philadelphia: Lea & Febiger, 1988.
87. Reeves B. Experiments on the tensile strength of the anterior capsular structures of the shoulder in man. J Bone Joint Surg 1968;50B:858.
88. Rockwood CA, Williams GR, Birkhead WZ. The long-term results of acromioplasty and debridement of irreparable degenerative lesions of the rotator cuff. Accepted for publication. J Bone Joint Surg 1994.
89. Rockwood CA, Young DC. Disorders of the arcomioclavicular joint. In Rockwood CA, Matzen FA, eds. The shoulder. Philadelphia: WB Saunders, 1990.
90. Rowe CR. The shoulder. New York: Churchill Livingstone, 1988.
91. Rowe CR, Pajel D, Southmayd WW. The Bankart procedure. J Bone Joint Surg 1978;60A:1.
92. Rowe CR, Sakellarides HT. Factors related to recurrences of anterior dislocations of the shoulder. Clin Orthop 1961;20:41.
93. Saha AK. Mechanism of shoulder movements and a plea for the recognition of "zero position" of glenohumeral joint. Ind J Surg 1950;12:153.
94. Saha AK. Theory of shoulder mechanism: descriptive and applied. Springfield, Ill.: Charles C Thomas, 1961.
95. Saha AK. Anterior recurrent dislocation of the shoulder. Acta Orthop Scand 1967;68:479.
96. Saha AK. Dynamic stability of the glenohumeral joint. Acta Orthop Scand 1971;42:491.
97. Sarrafian SK. Gross and functional anatomy of the shoulder. Clin Orthop 1983;173:11.
98. Schwartz E, Warren RF, O'Brien SJ, Fronek J. Posterior shoulder instability. Orthop Clin North Am 1987;18(3):409.
99. Shelvin MG, Lehman JF, Lucci JA. Eleclomyographic study of the function of some muscles crossing the glenohumeral joint. Arch Phys Med Rehabil 1969;50:264.
100. Sigholm G, Herberts P, Almstrom C, Kadefors R. Electromyographic analysis of shoulder muscle load. J Orthop Res 1984; 1:379.
100a. Soslowsky LJ, Flatow EL, Bigliani LU, Mow VC. Articular geometry of the glenohumeral joint. Clin Orthop (in press). 1992; 285:181.
101. Staples OS, Watkins AL. Full active abduction in traumatic paralysis of the deltoid. J Bone Joint Surg 1943;25:85.
102. Steindler A. Kinesiology of the human body under normal and pathologic conditions. Springfield, Ill.: Charles C Thomas, 1955.
103. Sugahara R. Electromyographic study of shoulder movements. Jpn J Rehab Med 1974;11:41.
104. Symenoides PO. The significance of the subscapularis muscle in the pathogenesis of recurrent anterior dislocation of the shoulder. J Bone Joint Surg 1972;54B:476.
105. Technical Manual Air Force Manual. Washington: Department of the Army and the Air Force, 1968.
106. Terry GC, Hammon D, France P, Norwood LA. The stabilizing function of the passive shoulder restraints. Am J Sports Med 1991;19:26.
107. Townley CO. The capsular mechanisms in recurrent dislocation of the shoulder. J Bone Joint Surg. 1950;32A:370.
108. Turkel SJ, Panio MW, Marshal JL. Stabilizing mechanisms preventing anterior dislocation of the glenohumeral joint. J Bone Joint Surg 1981;63A:1208.
109. Walker PS. Human joints and their artificial replacements. Springfield, Ill.: Charles C Thomas, 1977.
110. Weiner DS, MacNab I. Superior migration of the humeral head. J Bone Joint Surg 1970;52B:524.
111. Zuckerman JD, Matzen FA. Biomechanics of the shoulder: basic biomechanics of the musculoskeletal system. 2nd ed. Philadelphia: Lea & Febiger, 1989.

# Chapter 3

# Shoulder Pathology

**Terry R. Malone**
**Gwendolyn Waser Richmond**
**Jill L. Frick**



## Tissue Response

### Macrotrauma and Microtrauma

The inherent compromise of mobility for stability presented by the shoulder complex plays a key role in the appreciation of shoulder pathologies. No other major joint has such minimal trunk anchorage, thus presenting the requirement of muscular action to provide function. This process places tremendous demands on the neuromuscular system to enable coordinated actions. High-demand distal muscle function is superimposed on proximal muscular stabilization involving a variety of muscle activation modes.

Our thanks to Joel Henry for his contribution on the section entitled Thoracic Outlet Syndrome.

Minimal alteration in any part of this coordination sequence may lead to abnormal function and compensatory action. Frequently, this altered sequence will result in what is termed *microtrauma* (repetitive functional demands) as opposed to *macrotrauma*, which involves a single overt event resulting in a definable injury with a very specific acute onset.

These terms, *microtrauma* and *macrotrauma*, provide a framework to view shoulder pathology. The role of medical intervention/rehabilitation is quite different in each and requires a team approach if optimal outcomes are to be achieved. This team must be composed of medical and rehabilitative specialists. Interestingly, macrotrauma is often a clearly defined, discrete lesion, with the resulting damage able to be seen with appropriate medical evaluation. Unfortunately, microtrauma is not as easily evaluated or treated as the aforementioned specific lesion. The use of the arthroscope, ultrasound, and magnetic resonance imaging (MRI) has led to a better appreciation of these differences and hopefully better treatment regimens.

Specific lesions will be discussed in detail in the latter portions of this chapter, while the following general concepts and recommendations serve as a framework for the treatment of selected tissues and pathologies.

## INFLAMMATION, REPAIR SEQUENCE

Macrotrauma injuries result in an acute inflammation, repair, remodeling response pattern. This is predictable and consistent, as outlined in Table 3-1. The modulators of this sequence involve a host of cellular characters, as seen in Table 3-2. Much of what is accomplished in rehabilitation may be linked directly to these modulators. In fact, rest and specific exercise sequences are modifiers in and of themselves, as well as influencing these aforementioned factors.

**Table 3-1**

**The Sequence of Inflammation, Repair, and Remodeling**

| | |
|---|---|
| Inflammation | Circulatory response<br>Exudate/phagocytic actions<br>Fibrin clot/localization |
| Repair | Epithelialization (wound closure)<br>Scar formation |
| Remodeling | Along lines of stress (Wolff's law revisited)<br>Long-term process |

**Table 3-2**

**Modulation of the Inflammation, Repair, and Remodeling Sequence**

| | |
|---|---|
| Enzymes | Collagenase, acid hydrolases |
| Arachidonic acid | Prostaglandins, leukotrienes |
| Circulatory | Prothrombin, thrombin, complement |
| Multiple growth factors | Fibroblast growth factor, interleukins, interferons, macrophage factors |

Although a great deal is known regarding macrotrauma and the resulting injury, inflammation, repair, remodeling sequence, much less well appreciated is the body's response to microtrauma. The shoulder is a prime model of repetitive use, which demands considerable neuromuscular integrity of all its functioning parts to provide synchronous actions. Minimal alterations result in a "robbing Peter to pay Paul" phenomenon or adaptive postures to allow continued function. Clinicians often see these patients with rotator cuff symptoms that are related to what may be termed a *tendinopathy*. Cellular evaluation demonstrates that these problems are not a part of the usual macrotraumatic sequence because no inflammatory cells are present. However, the patient presentation is one of inflammation, and treatment directed appropriately within the rehabilitation sequence focusing on minimizing the painful response often linked to the inflammatory sequence is successful.

It is vital for clinicians to recognize the importance of the aging process and the resulting decreased adaptabilities seen in the aging individual. Specific problems of aging are presented with the individual pathologies in the later portions of this chapter. Suffice it to say that long-term adaptive processes may play a role in the development of shoulder pathology related to athletic or employment demands. These changes frequently involve the neuromuscular system, leading to what rehabilitative specialists refer to as "dysfunction."

It is interesting to note that many shoulder pathologies carry monikers that may not be reflective of the actual physiologic process. *Capsulitis* is often not a true inflammatory condition of that tissue, yet it conveys a message of the tissue reactivity; i.e., the capsule is altered, resulting in decreased range of motion. In fact, the causative tissue may in actuality be the synovium (Dr. Kevin Speer, Duke University Orthopaedics, personal communication), yet the overall treatment may not be altered by the more specific diagnosis.

## TISSUE INTERACTION AND STRUCTURE

Synchronous shoulder function demands specific recruitment sequences and the interaction of neural drive, active muscular tension, passive ligamentous restraint, and inherent bony/articular orientation. Alteration of any component can have a profound influence on the overall function of the shoulder complex.

### NEURAL ACTIONS

The shoulder is more dependent on neural control than any other major joint in the body. Without neural drive, the inherent lack of stability of the glenohumeral joint emerges rapidly (i.e., chronic subluxation following a cerebral vascular accident). Alteration of drive is seen with pain (inhibition) and injury (neural or muscular tendinous/soft tissue). Abnormal firing patterns (attempts to substitute) are common with many shoulder pathologies, including macrotrauma, microtrauma, and problems of restricted range of motion. Rehabilitation must allow normal, pain-free patterns if physiologic function is to evolve.

### MUSCLE

Muscle per se should be viewed as a connective tissue composed of contractile and noncontractile elements. The contractile fibers may be subdivided as to aerobic or anaerobic functional composition, which is reflective of both use (training) and genetics (predetermined limits). Noncontractile tissues envelope and link contractile elements and are important in providing inherent stiffness to the muscle mass.

The effects of aging on muscle must be reviewed carefully, because many changes may be related to disuse rather than aging alone. Lack of stress (demand) leads to a decrease in tissue mass in a metabolically active tissue. Thus many of the previously held beliefs regarding aging are being challenged. Research has documented a decrease in both mass and strength with aging.[53,54,76] A small linear decrease in strength is seen in the decades 20 to 70, but a much greater decrease is seen in the population of 70-year-olds and above.[159,163]

The number of sarcomeres may decrease with age and thus present a decrease in general mobility.[63] Some selective changes may occur in fiber area, since type II motor units may be more affected than their type I counterparts.[8] Muscle response to training appears to be similar across decades, but with neural factors becoming more important in the later decades.[45,92,93,141] To summarize the effects of aging on muscle: (1) it is difficult to differentiate the changes seen from the effects of aging versus functional demands, (2) a linear decrease in strength occurs from 20 to 70 years, with a more significant decrease thereafter, and (3) muscle tissue responds to training similarly but with neural factors becoming more important in later life.

### TENDON

Tendon serves as a very special connective tissue. Discussion of this structure must include its special "junctions" to both muscle and bone, where it serves as a transitional tissue (Fig. 3-1).

The myotendinous junction involves an intricate, extensive folding membrane that allows an interdigitation of muscle and connective tissue.[5,157] It appears that the muscle tendon junction plays a major role in force transmission.[112] In fact, the specialized appearance of the structure is in keeping with that of a load-bearing structure.[50] The folding pattern allows much greater stress dissipation, since stress is a function of cross-sectional area, and the oblique angulation provides more shear force rather than direct stress.[50,155]

Although quite useful, the special adaptations render the junctional sarcomeres less extensible[72] and result in tendon being the frequent site of macrotrauma (indirect muscle injury—related to stretching or lengthening of muscle as opposed to direct injury such as laceration or contusion) strain injury.[79]

The tendon itself is composed of dense connective tissues with parallel collagen fibers. Type I collagen predominates, and this material is the principal restraint to tension.[171] Individual components serve as stress controllers at different levels of stress, thus presenting an interesting nonlinear stress/strain curve.[171] Viscoelastic responses are seen in normal physiologic loading.

A blood supply for the tendon is from interspersed vessels that are relatively sparse, primar-

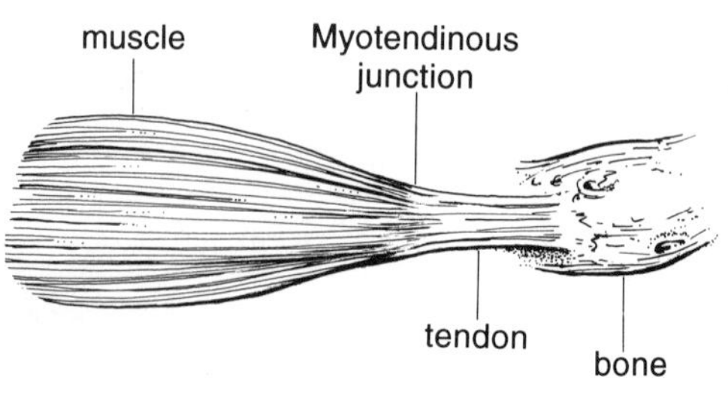

Myotendon junction

ily from the paratendon, thus pointing toward some level of diffusion for cellular nutrition. Specific areas of tendon may possess a lessened blood supply due to function or structure (such as sites of friction, compression, or torsion).[29,49,77,87,128] The supraspinatus tendon demonstrates a specific critical area of relative avascularity that is the site of most rotator cuff ruptures.[77,94,128] This critical zone is considered to be representative of the anastomoses of the muscular and tendinous vessels.[114] Other authors disagree with the concept of avascularity, since recent investigations, using modern technology, have revealed adequate vascularization of the rotator cuff.[23,25]

Tendon-bone interfaces/insertions are typically either direct or indirect. Direct fiber insertions, as seen in the supraspinatus tendon, characteristically demonstrate a four-zone tissue transition (tendon, fibrocartilage, mineralized fibrocartilage, bone), resulting in the tendon inserting at a right angle (Fig. 3-2). Indirect insertions involve a broader periosteal blending, allowing a greater dissipation area (i.e., less concentration of force per unit area).[172] The presence of fibrocartilage in the transition zone and the 90-degree angle of insertion may serve as a "tension buffer," playing a key role in reducing stress concentration.[14]

Injury classification with regard to the muscle-tendon unit has been a difficult challenge. Macrotraumatic injuries are represented by a distinct onset and follow the traditional inflammation, repair cycle. However, microtraumatic overuse or accumulation/repetitive-stress reactions that present as injuries do not exhibit the typical healing response. Apicitis, apophysitis, and tendinitis may thus be appropriate in specific conditions, while tendinosis is probably a better descriptor in repetitive-stress reactions.

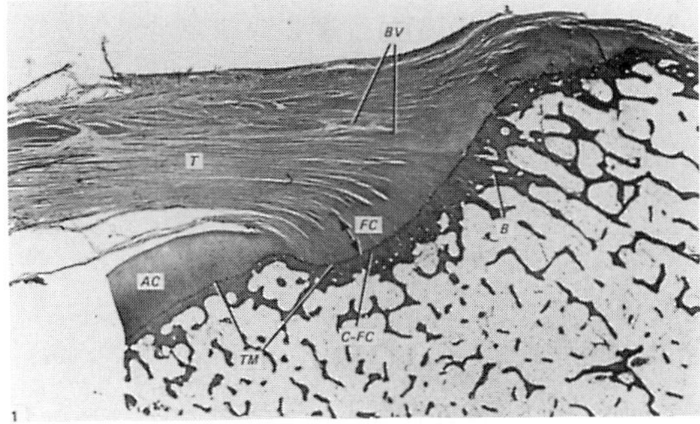


**Figure 3-2.** Transitional zone of insertion. Tendon characteristically demonstrates a four-zone tissue transition (tendon, T; fibrocartilage, FC; mineralized fibrocartilage, C-FC; bone, B), resulting in the tendon inserting at a right angle and possessing a mechanical buffer that effectively reduces stress at the point of insertion. (Reproduced with permission from Benjamin M, Evans EJ, Copp L. The histology of tendon attachments to bone in man. J Anat 1986;89:100.)

To demonstrate and clarify these complex interactions, we will discuss the suprahumeral/subacromial space. This constrained "area" presents both structural (bony/soft-tissue enlargement) and functional (pain, neuromusculature compromise) challenges to the involved tissues. The clinical dilemma is frequently to differentiate the primary and secondary factors that cause symptoms and thus to enable appropriate intervention. Our clinical suspicion is often not definitive but operational, such as the clinical syndrome of cuff tendinopathy/impingement. This allows communication between patient and medical providers but should be viewed in this special context.

This rigidly defined space is bordered superiorly by the acromion and coracoacromial ligament. The humeral head forms the mobile inferior surface and allows the interposed tissues (bursa and biceps tendon atop the rotator cuff) to be compressed or compromised when inadequate space or muscular control is present.

Primary impingement may be related to trauma, enlargement/reactive tissue, and abnormal structure (bony orientation, changes, or size). Conversely, secondary impingement may be seen following the development of abnormal muscular control and is frequently intermixed with other glenohumeral lesions including the labrum or capsuloligamentous complex. Thus shoulder conditions frequently present in a very complicated clinical pattern of dysfunction and pain.

Neer[97] described impingement as a progressive pattern involving a distinct three-stage process. Stage one lesions were described as those which involved edema, hemorrhage, and inflammation and were reversible with conservative treatment. Stage two lesions involved fixed fibrotic changes and did not necessarily allow successful treatment with conservative measures. Stage three lesions involved bony changes and cuff ruptures necessitating surgical management. Other authors question the "absolute" progressive process and espouse a more interrelated schema.[83,161] Our experience points toward acceptance of the latter, particularly when viewing the population as a whole.

Bursal involvement in this process is a given but often is of a secondary nature. Unfortunately, once enlarged or thickened, the bursa is extremely pain sensitive. Thus the bursa is likely to be an innocent victim—an unfortunate bystander who is compressed either by loss of muscular depression or decreased relative space due to tissue enlargement.

The sequence of pathology associated with the tendon itself is quite difficult to assess because only an end-stage "disease" or process is observed at surgery. The majority of these end-stage lesions are seen within the "critical zone."[161] This portion of the supraspinatus tendon is often seen to have relatively poor vascularity, particularly with the arm in an adducted position. Some authors believe that this area is the junction of osseous and muscular vessels and may be relatively underperfused in certain positions.[94, 128, 135] It should be noted that the vascularity of this critical zone may or may not have a cause-and-effect role in cuff pathology, since tendon nutrition may be more related to the diffusion of tissue fluids.[80] However, for the clinician, when applying modalities or mechanical forces, it is recommended to avoid the adduction/side-arm position and enhance vascular perfusion during treatment.

Increased age (>40 years) is strongly correlated with rotator cuff pathology. The incidence of rotator cuff tendonopathy appears related to excessive mechanical demands placed on the capsuloligamentous cuff envelope, tendon structure alteration, decreased tendon tensile strength, and poor vascularity. When considering these factors, a vicious cycle emerges, making one wonder if the sequence of these cumulative effects is responsible for the manifestation of rotator cuff pathology during the fifth and sixth decades.

Impingement syndrome can thus be seen as a primary or secondary process with a variety of causes. Definitive treatment must be directed toward the primary factor and frequently involves multiple tissues and interventions. We hope that this example is helpful in viewing the context of the shoulder as the reader examines the individual entities discussed in the remainder of this chapter.

# Specific Pathologies

## Impingement Syndrome

The subacromial space is formed superiorly by the coracoacromial arch, which is comprised of the coracoacromial ligament and acromion and inferiorly by the humeral head. The contents of the subacromial space include the rotator cuff tendons, the long head of the biceps tendon, and the subdeltoid bursa.

### PATHOGENESIS

Impingement occurs when there is encroachment of the acromion, coracoacromial ligament, or acromioclavicular joint on the rotator cuff tendons and subdeltoid bursa that lie beneath them.[83] Impingement can also occur on the coracoid process (Fig. 3-3). Although many equate impingement syndrome and rotator cuff pathology, it is helpful to distinguish the two. Rotator cuff pathology can exist without true mechanical impingement being the primary causative factor, for example, when repetitive tension on the cuff results in inflammation. Also, others believe true impingement syndrome is reserved for those individuals with osseous alterations in the subcoracoacromial structures. The important point to understand and agree on is that primary cuff pathology can exist in the absence of mechanical impingement.

Certainly mechanical impingement does occur and can be the result of several different factors. The primary culprit is an abnormal structure of the acromion. Other contributing or causative factors include rotator cuff pathology, weakness of the rotator cuff and/or the scapulathoracic musculature, glenohumeral instability, or tightness of the posterior glenohumeral joint capsule. The question of true etiology is what came first—the rotator cuff changes or the bony changes.

Several variations of acromial shape are seen in the population. These include flat, curved, and hooked acromions. Variations in structure of the acromion also may be due to abnormal ossification at the three centers of ossification.[83] A close

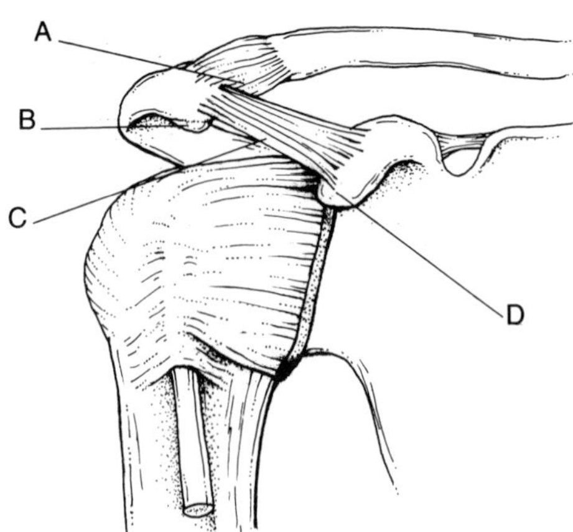


**Figure 3-3.** Sites of impingement: (a) the acromioclavicular joint, (b) undersurface of the acromion, (c) the coracoacromial ligament, and (d) the coracoid process.

association has been made between individuals with curved or hooked acromions (type III) and those suffering from impingement syndrome. In addition, a relationship exists between the presence of an unfused or malfused acromial epiphysis and individuals suffering from impingement syndrome.[83]

One of the main functions of the rotator cuff is stabilizing the humerus in the glenoid fossa. If weakness exists in the rotator cuff, there is a loss of this depression/compression mechanism and a subsequent superior shifting of the humeral head, resulting in a decrease in subacromial space. This is primarily a problem with flexion and abduction (elevation), since the depressor mechanism is needed to counterbalance the upward pull of the deltoid.[83] Disruption of this force couple leads to impingement of the rotator cuff, resulting in inflammation and scarring with a subsequent decrease in subacromial space and perpetuation of the impingement problem. In addition, tendon damage perpetuates weakness in the rotator cuff, and a vicious cycle begins.

Glenohumeral instability also may contribute to impingement. Compromise of the capsuloligament-labral complex results in abnormal humeral head translation either immediately or following fatigue of the dynamic stabilizers, causing superior displacement of the humeral head.

Finally, tightness in the posterior glenohumeral joint capsule is seen commonly in individuals suffering from impingement syndrome (Fig. 3-4). Clinically, this tightness is seen as a loss of motion with respect to internal rotation and horizontal adduction. Posterior capsule tightness also manifests as pain at the end range of shoulder flexion (elevation) as superior displacement of the humeral head causes the head to strike against the anteroinferior acromion during this motion.[83]

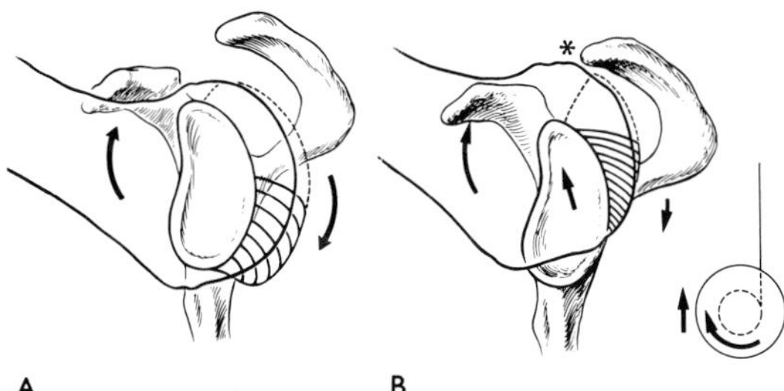


**Figure 3-4.** (a) Normal posterior capsular elasticity allows the humeral head to stay centralized during shoulder flexion. (b) Posterior capsule tightness results in superior humeral head migration causing impingement between the soft tissues that cover the humeral head and anteroinferior acromion. (Reproduced with permission from Matsen FA, Arntz CT. Subacromial impingement. In Rockwood CA, Matsen FA, eds. The shoulder. Vol. 2. Philadelphia: WB Saunders, 1990.)

### CLASSIFICATION

Impingement syndromes are found most commonly in individuals who repeatedly bring the upper extremity into an elevated position for recreation or vocation.[146] Repetitive microtrauma is more often the causative factor than one incident of macrotrauma.[130] Thus impingement syndrome can be viewed as a progressive degenerative process.[1] Neer[97] has developed a classification system for impingement syndrome based on this idea (Fig. 3-5).

In stage I, edema, inflammation, and hemorrhage can be identified in the subacromial contents, particularly the bursa and tendons. Swelling of these structures is responsible for impingement. Stage I is generally seen in individuals less than 25 years of age, and the symptoms generally can be reversed if repetitive overhead causative activities are discontinued or if adjustments are made to improve shoulder biomechanics (i.e., achieve proper muscular balance). In stage II, aggravation of subacromial contents has progressed to cause, thickening of the bursa and fibrosis of the tendons. This is most commonly seen between the ages of 25 and 40 years and is more difficult to reverse. However, symptoms can be reversed if treated with appropriate rest, anti-inflammatories, and progressive pain-free strengthening. Stages I and II are also classified as uncomplicated, since they are amenable to treatment, as opposed to stage III, which is considered complicated impingement. In the third and final stage, there may be partial- or full-thickness tendon tears and changes in bony configuration of the humeral head and acromion. This final stage is generally identified in individuals greater than 40 years of age, and if tendon fiber failure has progressed to a full-thickness tear, surgery most often will be required.[1,97,161]

For simplicity, we will discuss tendinitis and calcific tendinitis separately but realize its relationship to Neer's classification scheme.

## Rotator Cuff Tendinitis

*Rotator cuff tendinitis* refers to inflammation of any of the four rotator cuff tendons. The role of the rotator cuff is to provide humeral rotation and abduction and, more important, to secure the head of the humerus into the glenoid fossa so that more powerful axiohumeral and scapulohumeral muscles may produce desired motions.[1,146] The most common area of the rotator

**Stage I:** **Edema and Hemorrhage**

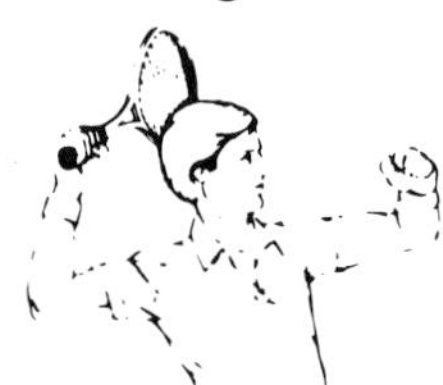

| | |
|---|---|
| typical age | <25 |
| diff. diagnosis | subluxation, A/C arthritis |
| clinical course | reversible |
| treatment | conservative |

**Stage II:** **Fibrosis and Tendinitis**

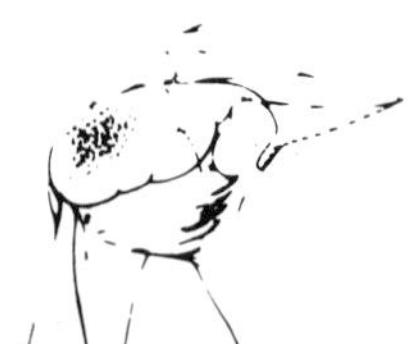

| | |
|---|---|
| typical age | 25–40 |
| diff. diagnosis | frozen shoulder, calcium |
| clinical course | recurrent pain with activity |
| treatment | consider bursectomy; C/A ligament division |

**Stage III:** **Bone Spurs and Tendon Rupture**

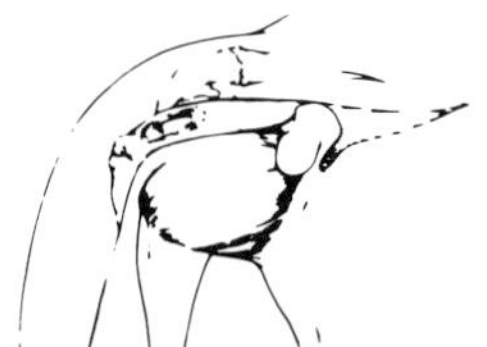

| | |
|---|---|
| typical age | >40 |
| diff. diagnosis | cervical radiculitis; neoplasm |
| clinical course | progressive disability |
| treatment | anterior acromioplasty; rotator cuff repair |

**Figure 3-5.** Neer's classification system for impingement. (Reproduced with permission from Neer CS II. Impingement lesions. Clin Orthop 1983;173:70.)

cuff to undergo pathologic and advanced degenerative change is the supraspinatus tendon.[28,30,31,41,146] The supraspinatus originates from the supraspinous fossa of the scapula and inserts into the superior facet of the greater tubercle of the humerus. It forms the floor of the subacromial bursa and the roof of the glenohumeral joint space. Its primary function is to stabilize the position of the humeral head during glenohumeral motion by preventing abnormal upward displacement of the humeral head and thus decreasing the likelihood of impingement by counteracting the deltoid force.[28,146] It is thought to be particularly susceptible to degeneration, tendinitis, and rupture in part because of the avascularity of the distal portion of the tendon.[128] This distal 1-cm area is commonly referred to as the *critical zone* because it is poorly perfused when the tendon is under tension (Fig. 3-6). In addition to stabilization of the humeral head during glenohumeral motion, the supraspinatus tendon is continually under tension to prevent downward subluxation from the pull of gravity.[146]

Tendinitis of the rotator cuff, most commonly the supraspinatus, can result from overuse and eccentric overload, with repetitive overhead activities leading to tendon fiber failure. Failure or fatigue of the supraspinatus can result in superior translation of the humeral head, causing a decrease in the subacromial space and increasing the potential for impingement.[1] Disruption of the tendon fibers themselves results in swelling and inflammation, which in turn decrease the subacromial space, and the vicious impingement cycle described above is underway.

As mentioned earlier, shoulder instability also can lead to rotator cuff (primarily supraspinatus) tendinitis. The static stabilizers of the glenohumeral joint include the capsule, labrum, coracohumeral ligament, and glenohumeral ligaments. If there is a lesion or laxity in any of these structures, the rotator cuff must compensate by preventing abnormal translation of the humeral head. This increased concentric and eccentric loading may result in overuse tendinitis, fatigue, and abnormal superior gliding.

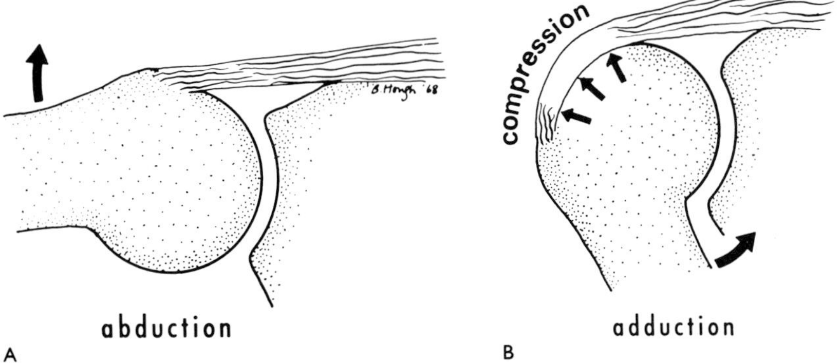


**Figure 3-6.** Mechanical causes of disruption in vascularity. The tendon can undergo significant tension/compression during abduction (a) and adduction (b). (Reproduced with permission from Rathbun J, MacNab I. The microvascular pattern of the rotator cuff. J Bone Joint Surg 1970;52B:540.)

## HISTORY AND PRESENTATION

Patients with supraspinatus tendinitis often will relate a history without a specific injury. They will frequently be athletes involved in sports with repetitive overhead activity, however, such as swimming, baseball, or tennis, or will be involved in an occupation requiring prolonged overhead activity. They may describe their pain as acute and excruciating at times but will more often than not report a chronic low-grade aching pain and fatigue sensation. This will most often be localized to the lateral aspect of the upper arm or the deltoid insertion.[83] They also may report difficulty sleeping on the involved upper extremity as well as a catching sensation in their shoulder when their arm is in flexion or internal rotation.[83,146]

Physical examination will reveal pain with active abduction and external rotation. Such patients may present with a "painful arc" at 70 to 120 degrees of active elevation as the inflamed subacromial tissue passes beneath the coracoacromial arch and is compressed. Passive motion is generally full and pain free, but internal rotation and abduction may occasionally be limited and produce pain.[46] An impingement sign described by Neer[97] and Hawkins[57] is of diagnostic value when rotator cuff irritation or tearing is suspected (Fig. 3-7a). Neer's impingement sign is elicited as the examiner stands behind the

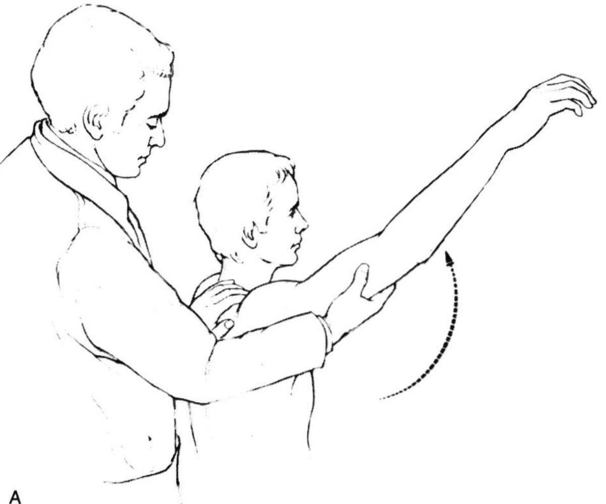


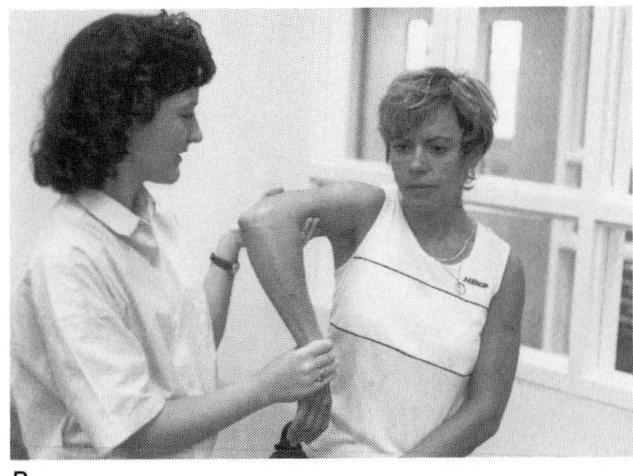


**Figure 3-7.** Impingement signs. (a) Neer's impingement sign is elicited as the examiner stands behind the patient and prevents scapular rotation with one hand and uses the other hand to raise the involved arm in forced forward elevation. (b) Hawkins impingement sign has been described as forced elevation with the arm in internal rotation. (Reproduced with permission from Neer CS II. Impingement lesions. Clin Orthop 1983;173:70.)

patient and prevents scapular rotation with one hand and uses the other hand to raise the involved arm in forced forward elevation. Hawkins' impingement sign has been described as forced elevation with the arm in internal rotation (see Fig. 3-7b). These maneuvers cause pain as the inflamed tendon and bursa are compressed against the acromion. It should be noted that presence of the impingement sign does not always indicate a primary etiology of "impingement"; remember that rotator cuff inflammation can occur without mechanical impingement. Thus the presence of the impingement sign indicates *what* tissues (location of irritation) are involved but does not indicate *why* they are irritated (etiology).

These maneuvers also will cause pain in patients with many other shoulder conditions, including adhesive capsulitis, instability, arthritis, calcific tendinitis, and bone lesions. However, a differential diagnosis for rotator cuff involvement can be made when pain on this maneuver is eliminated or significantly reduced with an injection of 10 cc of 1.0% lidocaine into the subacromial space; this is called the *impingement test* (Fig. 3-8). Other areas can be injected to determine a change in symptoms, these include the acromioclavicular joint, biceps tendon, glenohumeral joint, and subscapular bursae.

Manual muscle testing of the supraspinatus will result in pain and/or weakness depending on the extent of tissue involvement. Weakness and pain with resisted motion are reliable signs of tendon inflammation. Significant weakness without pain suggests a complete tear, pain without weakness suggests an active tendinitis, and weakness with pain suggest a partial tear.[83] Assessment of strength should be performed following the impingement test to determine if the pre-injection weakness noted is due to pain. If the weakness is related to inhibition from pain, then strength should be better following the injection; if it is not any better, then one should suspect either a tear and/or involvement of some other structure.

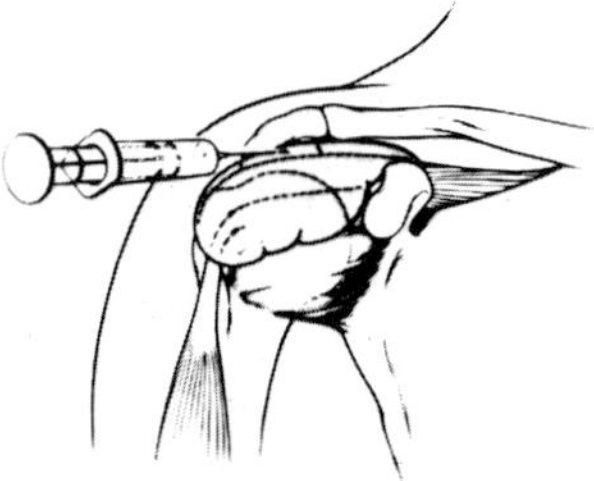

**Figure 3-8.** The impingement test. Differential diagnosis for cuff involvement can be made when pain on this maneuver is eliminated or significantly reduced with an injection of 10 cc of 1.0% lidocaine into the subacromial space. (Reproduced with permission from Neer CS II. Impingement lesions. Clin Orthop 1983;173:70.)

Results of joint mobility testing may or may not be positive. As mentioned previously, glenohumeral instability may be contributing to impingement. If this is the case, one should expect to see an increase in joint mobility, particularly with anterior, posterior, or inferior glides. In this situation, anterior and posterior apprehension tests also may be positive. Patients will generally report localized tenderness to palpation of the supraspinatus tendon insertion at the greater tuberosity. It is imperative that the stability status of the glenohumeral joint be determined so as to rule this in or out as being a potential causative factor.

## MANAGEMENT

Management of supraspinatus tendinitis will depend on how far the degenerative changes have progressed. However, conservative management should always be attempted. Initial treatment consists of rest from aggravating activities and an anti-inflammatory course. A prudent, selective choice of useful anti-inflammatory therapies is initiated. If this is ineffective in relieving symptoms, corticosteroid injections may be considered. However, these injections should be performed with significant caution because of their tendency to promote degeneration and rupture in an already compromised structure. Injections have been shown to produce tendon atrophy and reduce the ability of a damaged tendon to heal.[83] If performed, the subacromial space is injected. Pain-free passive range-of-motion exercises should be initiated early in order to maintain normal or improve limited range of motion. Direct treatment of the tendon through friction massage and soft-tissue mobilization techniques is advocated. Once the anti-inflammatory course has taken effect and near-full active and passive pain-free range of motion has been achieved, progressive resistive exercise can be added with advancement to pain-free isokinetics and sport-specific training. Eccentric exercise should be included in the strength-training program, since deficits in eccentric force production may be responsible for tendinitis. If conservative management fails, acromioplasty, release of the coracoacromial ligament, and bursectomy may be required to increase the amount of subacromial space. Such measures may be necessary in cases of chronic tendinitis or in cases where tendon degeneration has progressed to large partial- or full-thickness tendon tears. The presence of such tears can be determined by arthrogram, ultrasonography, or MRI if conservative treatment is unsuccessful.

The goals of postoperative physical therapy following an acromioplasty or partial decompression, are the same as with conservative treatment: rest, reduce inflammation, recover full range of motion, selective strengthening exercises, and pain-free function. Initially, treatment consists of gentle active assistive range-of-motion exercises and pain-free isometrics. Functional pain-free use of the extremity is encouraged. When adequate pain-free range of motion is recovered, the patient can begin progressive resistive exercises with an emphasis on the rotator cuff musculature. Once range of motion, flexibility, and strength have been normalized, analysis and modification of athletic and occupational demands should be performed prior to the patient's return to activity in order to prevent recurrence of symptoms.

## Bicipital Tendinitis

The second most common site of tendinitis in the shoulder is in the long head of the biceps tendon. This tendon may be affected at its intraarticular portion, at or close to its site of origin, or as it passes through the bicipital groove (Fig. 3-9). Intraarticular bicipital tendinitis most commonly occurs in conjunction with supraspinatus tendinitis. In fact, Simmonds and Burkhead[147] propose that changes in the biceps tendon occur in response to changes in the supraspinatus tendon. This may be related to the synovial lining of the biceps tendon being continuous with the synovium of the shoulder joint.[109] Bicipital tendinitis also may be caused by an eccentric overloading, which is frequently seen in athletes who must use their biceps to decelerate elbow extension and pronation during the follow-through phase of a throw or swing. As with the supraspinatus tendon, repetitive overhead use can result in biceps tendon irritation.[46]

Irritation of the tendon is also common as it passes through the intertubercular groove under the transverse humeral ligament. The mechanism is most commonly due to subluxation of the biceps tendon secondary to laxity of the transverse humeral ligament or a poorly developed lesser tuberosity. Subluxation results in fraying and swelling of the tendinous fibers and the tendon sheath. A decrease in the depth of the intertubercular groove is an anatomic anomaly predisposing an individual to subluxation and subsequent tendinitis.[161] A direct blow to the tendon or tendon sheath also may result in inflammation of the tendon.

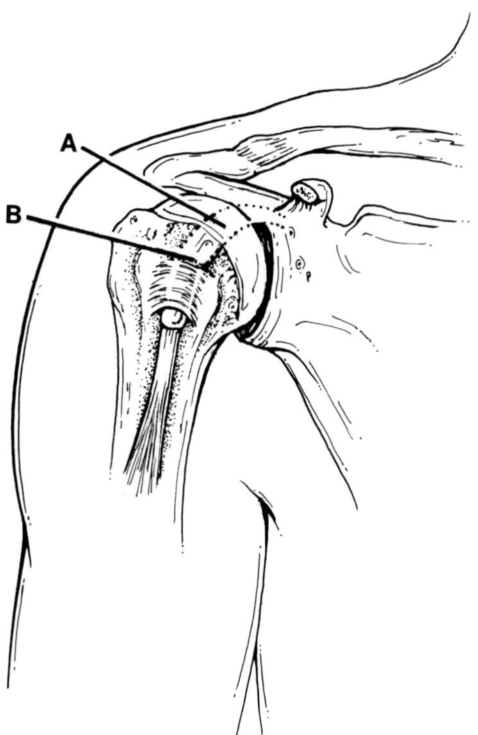


**Figure 3-9.** The long head of the biceps. This tendon may be affected at its intraarticular portion (a), at or close to its site of origin, or as it passes through the bicipital groove (b).

### HISTORY AND PRESENTATION

Individuals suffering from bicipital tendinitis may not recall a specific injury. As with supraspinatus tendinitis, they will be involved in repetitive overhead activities. Occasionally, a severe strain of the upper extremity in a position of abduction and external rotation will result in medial displacement of the biceps tendon out of the bicipital groove. This will most often be reduced spontaneously.[105]

Physical examination will reveal full active and passive range of motion, with the possible exceptions of slight limitations in passive abduction and internal rotation secondary to pain.[105] Patients will exhibit pain and/or weakness with resisted forward shoulder flexion, elbow flexion, supination, and abduction with external rotation.[105, 146] They will report pain with activity that is relieved by rest. They will usually demonstrate significant tenderness to palpation of the biceps tendon as it passes through the bicipital groove. The impingement sign is positive, and the impingement test, by injecting into the biceps groove or intraarticularly, indicates biceps involvement. Other special tests that are sometimes positive include Yergason's, Lippman's, Ludington's, and the straight arm raise test.[46]

Radiographs may reveal a shallow or irregular bicipital groove. An arthrogram will demonstrate a thickened tendon sheath and may reveal a shifting of the tendon toward the lesser tuberosity causing friction and irritation.[105]

### MANAGEMENT

Management of bicipital tendinitis is quite similar to that of supraspinatus tendinitis. Activities that exacerbate the patient's symptoms are eliminated. Rest and an anti-inflammatory course are initiated as described previously. If corticosteroid injections are deemed necessary, they are done within the tendon sheath rather than into the tendon. Again, in many instances, friction massage has been proven to be successful in reducing the patient's complaints of pain on resisted muscle testing and palpation. Once inflammation has subsided, near-full pain-free active and passive range of motion has been achieved, tenderness to palpation has decreased, and resisted isometric testing is pain free, progressive resistive exercise can be initiated. If indicated, progression to isokinetics and patient-specific functional training is the final step in rehabilitation. If conservative management fails, surgery is indicated, which usually consists of acromial arch decompression and excision of the transverse humeral ligament.[109] After excision of the ligament, the tendon is evaluated for fraying. If damage is minimal, the surgery is complete. If significant damage has occurred, the biceps tendon is sutured to the surrounding soft-tissue structures or fixated to the upper humeral shaft, and the intraarticular portion of the tendon is removed.[105, 109]

## Calcific Tendinitis

Calcific tendinitis consists of the deposition of calcium into the substance of the tendon. It may occur in any tendon but is seen most commonly in the shoulder and is located most frequently at the point of attachment. The calcium deposits may consist of calcium phosphate, oxalate, carbonate, or calcium hydroxyapatite.[139] Within the shoulder, the most common location of calcific tendinitis is the supraspinatus tendon, where it may appear as one large deposit or several smaller deposits (Fig. 3-10). Deposits are found most commonly in the avascular portion of the supraspinatus tendon. Initiation of this pathology is not fully understood, but it is thought that deposits may be a result of pressure at the avascular region or a decrease in oxygen supply to this region. These factors result in a transformation of tenocytes into chondrocytes, resulting in dense, homogeneous calcium deposits.[160] This disease process may be silent for long periods of time. Symptoms are usually the result of deposits that are large enough to cause impingement under the acromial arch with abduction or flexion.[139] Fortunately, calcific tendinitis is a self-healing condition that will cycle through deposition to resorption. Resorption of deposits may occur when there is development of new vessels to the previously avascular region. Calcific tendinitis may be divided into acute and chronic phases. The chronic phase is the time when deposition is occurring, while the acute phase occurs with resorption of the deposits. The acute phase begins when the deposit ruptures into the bursa or is absorbed into the tendon. Pain generally occurs during absorption. The acute phase generally lasts 3 to 4 days, but pain may be excruciating during this time.

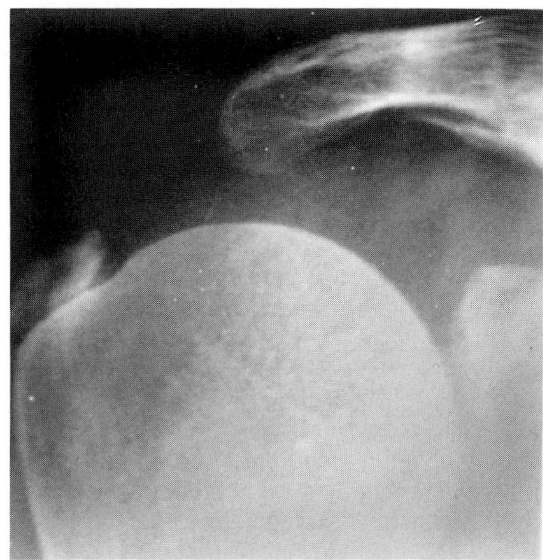

**Figure 3-10.** The most common location of calcific tendinitis is the supraspinatus tendon, where it may appear as one large deposit or several smaller deposits. (Reproduced with permission from Caspari RB, Jackson RW, Poehling GG. Operative arthroscopy. New York: Raven Press. 1991:467.)

### MANAGEMENT

Management consists of ice and pain medication. If discomfort is persistent, corticosteroid injections into the subacromial space may be indicated. In severe cases of the disease, surgical resection of the calcium deposits may be necessary, but in general it is better to let the disease process progress full cycle independently.[109] Typically, calcium deposits will last for several months before resorption begins.[160] Physical therapy management consists of modalities to decrease pain (TENS, ice), maintenance of range of motion, and strengthening without aggravation of symptoms.

# Bursitis

Although bursitis is a common clinical diagnosis describing specific shoulder pain, it is rare for the bursa to be a primary source of pain.[111,160] Very often an older patient who has had recurrent episodes of nonspecific shoulder pain will report that he or she suffers from "bursitis". In many situations, these patients have been incorrectly diagnosed as having this condition, or they have assumed this from having heard or read about it as a common cause of shoulder pain. Bursitis is found as a primary condition of pain in patients with rheumatoid arthritis, tuberculosis, gout, and pyogenic infections[111] or direct insult in contact injuries. More often than not bursitis is associated with an irritation of the rotator cuff or biceps tendon or calcific tendinitis.

There are several bursae found in the shoulder region; however, in most cases, only the large subacromial or subdeltoid bursa is clinically significant.[120,146] This bursa lies between the undersurface of the deltoid muscle and the outer surface of the supraspinatus tendon and rotator cuff. Normally, the roof of the subacromial bursa adheres to the coracoacromial ligament and acromion superiorly, and the floor blends with the superficial surface of the rotator cuff. The subacromial bursa does not communicate with the glenohumeral joint. However, in the presence of a complete rotator cuff tear, a communication between the glenohumeral joint and the bursa does occur and can be demonstrated by arthrography.[119,146] (see Fig. 4-9). The primary function of the subacromial bursa is to reduce friction in the suprahumeral space, notably on the supraspinatus tendon as it passes under the coracoacromial arch.[119]

## CLASSIFICATION

Bursitis can be acute or chronic. The following discussion of bursitis will be related to the subacromial bursae. Acute subacromial bursitis is distinguished by spontaneous onset without precipitating factors. Chronic bursitis is believed by most to be the result of repetitive microtrauma with episodes of impingement against the coracoacromial arch and is thought to be more prevalent in patients aged 25 to 40 years of age. Neer described this abnormal response in the bursa occurring during stage II impingement: fibrosis and tendinitis. When the rotator cuff tendons become inflamed, there is a reduction of subacromial space causing impingement and irritation of the overlying bursa. The bursa becomes inflamed and fibrotic with repeated episodes of mechanical impingement. The shoulder usually functions adequately for light activities but becomes significantly aggravated with vigorous overhead use in sports or vocation. At this stage, the lesion is not usually reversible.[97] Codman[28] described the subacromial bursa as "an absolutely necessary part of the shoulder joint. When its surfaces are inflamed so that they cause painful friction, the arm cannot be rotated or abducted. Their complete adhesion has the same effect."

## HISTORY AND PRESENTATION

In acute subacromial bursitis, the pain can be extreme and associated with a speedy onset. The patient will have significant difficulty in actively or passively elevating the arm. Palpation of the bursae may reveal thickening and exquisite tenderness.

Chronic bursitis is almost always associated with tendinitis; therefore, the patient presents with many symptoms resembling rotator cuff tendinitis. The patient may present with nagging, aching pain in the area of insertion of the deltoid. This pain can become especially severe at night and will frequently refer down the lateral aspect of the humerus.[15,168] The subacromial bursa can be palpated through the deltoid, but tenderness on palpation cannot be differentiated from the underlying tendon.[146] Often the tenderness on palpation is diffuse rather than specific, as in the case of a tendinitis. Both active and passive abduction usually will result in a painful arc of motion between 80 to 120 degrees of abduction. As the greater tuberosity of the humerus passes under the acromion, the sensitive bursa is compressed, resulting in pain. If the subacromial bursa is the primary source of shoulder pain, testing specific resisted movements to incriminate the contractile elements should be relatively pain free. However, compressive forces caused by the muscular contraction can result in shoulder pain due to inflammation of the bursa yet it must be remembered that the bursa is rarely the primary source of pain.[21] The impingement sign described by Neer is a classic sign of bursitis. As the scapula is stabilized and the shoulder is forced into elevation, the patient will experience pain in the area of the subacromial bursa. Injection of lidocaine into the subacromial bursa will relieve the pain.[97]

## MANAGEMENT

Treatment of bursitis consists primarily of relative or selective rest, avoiding overhead and other aggravating activities. Physical therapy is implemented to maintain pain-free passive range of motion, while active exercise is minimized to only pain-free regions because it can cause further microtrauma and pain.[168] Pain-free range of motion is advocated because it can promote gliding within the subcoracoacromial space and prevent fibrotic adhesion formation. Soft-tissue mobilization techniques specific to the subdeltoid region are often beneficial. Ice, oral anti-inflammatories, and/or judicious use of corticosteroid injections may be beneficial to decrease pain and swelling of the bursa and adjacent tendons. Local injections of corticosteroids should be limited to not more than three per year.[22,97,111] Phonophoresis with hydrocortisone cream or iontophoresis can be a helpful therapeutic treatment to diminish inflammation of the bursa and subsequent pain. As pain subsides, the patient is instructed in passive range-of-motion exercises, active pain-free range-of-motion exercises, and pain-free resistive exercises with an emphasis on the rotator cuff musculature. The objective of nonoperative care is to regain pain-free range of motion, strength, and function and to instruct the patient in activity modification in order to avoid future repetitive microtrauma and injury.[57]

Surgery is considered when the pain and disability of bursitis persist despite an adequate course of conservative treatment. Surgery consists of debridement of the thickened and fibrotic subacromial bursa and excision of the coracoacromial ligament. Neer[97] does not promote performing an anterior acromioplasty for simple impingement problems in patients younger than age 40 unless an overhang or prominence of the undersurface of the anterior acromion is evident at the time of surgery. Neviaser[106] suggests that the bursa be incised and dissected free from the rotator cuff and deltoid but that it is preferable to retain the bursa if possible because it helps to protect the rotator cuff tendons.

## Rotator Cuff Tears

Lesions affecting the rotator cuff are the most common problems affecting the shoulder.[31] For this reason, treatment of rotator cuff disorders and related problems is more frequent than any other type of problem in the shoulder region. The rotator cuff consists of the supraspinatus, infraspinatus, teres minor, and subscapularis muscles (Fig. 3-11). As discussed earlier, the rotator cuff acts to dynamically stabilize and balance the humeral head in the glenoid while the major muscle groups (deltoid and pectoralis major) act to move the humerus. The rotator cuff also assists in producing internal rotation and elevation and provides the majority of external rotation torque. Disruption of the rotator cuff can and often does lead to a significant loss of shoulder function.

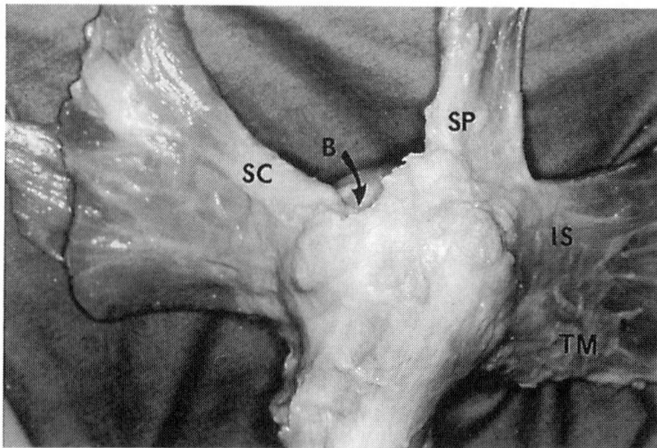


**Figure 3-11.** The rotator cuff. The rotator cuff consists of the supraspinatus, infraspinatus, teres minor, and subscapularis muscles. (Reproduced with permission from Clark JC, Harryman UT. Tendons, ligaments, and capsule of the rotator cuff. J Bone Joint Surg 1992;74A:713.)

### PATHOGENESIS

As mentioned previously, disorders of the rotator cuff are usually classified under Neer's[97] three stages of progressive degeneration. Stages I and II are detailed in the section on impingement. This section will deal with the lesions in stage III, tears of the rotator cuff.

The supraspinatus tendon is the most commonly injured of the rotator cuff tendons due to one or more of a combination of mechanical, vascular, traumatic, and degenerative factors.[107] Because of its anatomic position, the supraspinatus tendon is prone to impingement against the coracoacromial arch.[97] The questionable vascular nature in the critical zone, 1 cm from the tendon insertion, is believed to be a contributing factor in the prevalence of rotator cuff pathology. Positioning of the arm can result in increased pressure of the humeral head on the supraspinatus tendon, tending to "wring out" the vessels in this area[25,128] (see Fig. 3-6).

Rotator cuff tears are believed to be the end result of a degenerative process. This degenerative process may in fact be the summation of catabolic factors that lead to dysfunction in the over 40-year-old age group. Although true mechanical impingement is believed to contribute to tendon attrition, it cannot explain the higher incidence of articular-side tears compared with bursal-side tears of the supraspinatus tendon. A possible scenario related to rotator cuff tendon pathology is microtendon failure occurring early in one's life that results in scarring and more load to neighboring fibers. This "micro" failure produces temporary symptoms that "may" respond to rest or palliative modalities. With continued stress, further failure and scarring result.[82] This cycle leads to progressive degeneration of the rotator cuff tissue, terminating in partial- or full-thickness tears. When considering the incredible mechanical demands the rotator cuff tendons are burdened with, i.e., excessive tensile loading at or near end ranges, the significant increased incidence of lesions to this structure can be appreciated.

## CLASSIFICATION

Tears of the rotator cuff are usually classified according to thickness and etiology. Terms used to describe the tears include *partial-* or *full-thickness tears, acute* or *chronic*, and *traumatic* or *degenerative*. Tears usually begin in the area of the critical zone in the supraspinatus tendon approximately 1 cm from its humeral insertion. If the defect extends from the articular surface through to the bursal surface of the rotator cuff, the lesion is classified as a full-thickness tear (Fig. 3-12). Partial-thickness tears are more common and include those lesions which involve only the superficial or bursal surface, midsubstance, or deep or articular surface of the tendon, the latter being the most common and perhaps the most difficult to detect early on.

Most rotator cuff tears occur in individuals older than 40 years of age with previous shoulder symptoms.[82,97] Although patients may relate their pain to a specific recent incident, further questioning often reveals a previous history of shoulder complaints. The most recent or "acute" injury was more likely an incidental degree of trauma superimposed on a progressive degenerative lesion. This is appropriately referred to as an *acute extension of a tear.*[97]

Acute tears, those occurring in a person without a previous history of cuff pain but associated with trauma, are rare, accounting for only 5 to 8 percent of rotator cuff tears.[82,97,99] When a rotator cuff tear occurs in the younger patient, 20 to 30 years old, they are usually the result of repetitive, forceful use of the arm overhead (microtraumatic) or are the result of a sudden, definite injury to the glenohumeral joint of sufficient magnitude to rupture the tendons and capsule (macrotraumatic).

Other descriptions of rotator cuff tears include the specific tendons involved and whether the detached tendons are retracted, atrophic, or absent.[82] The tears may be divided into various sizes according to the measurement of the longest diameter; a small tear is less than 1 cm, a medium-sized tear is less than 3 cm, a large tear is less than 5 cm, and a massive tear is more than

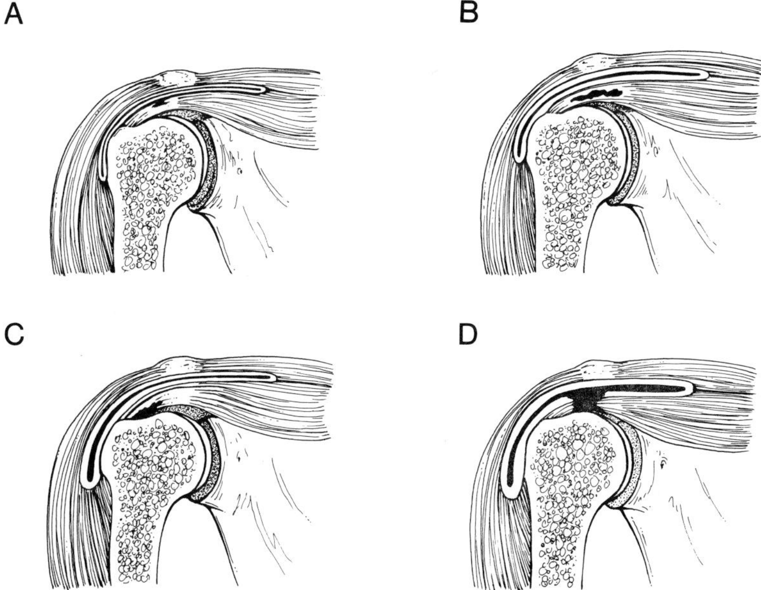


**Figure 3-12.** Rotator cuff tears. Partial-thickness tears are more common and include those lesions which involve either the bursal side (a), midsubstance (b), or articular side (c). If the defect extends from the articular surface through the bursal surface of the rotator cuff, the lesion is classified as a full-thickness tear (d).

5 cm in diameter. In massive tears, the torn cuff edge is usually retracted.[126]

Spontaneous healing of the torn rotator cuff tendon is very infrequent secondary to retraction of the torn fibers from one another or from their bony insertion.[173] It is also speculated that healing is limited due to continuous washing of synovial fluid disallowing hematoma formation. However, in small, partial-thickness tears, vascular proliferation and granulation have been observed in the area of the tear; this is particularly true in the distal stump. These findings support the notion that spontaneous healing may occur occasionally.[173]

## HISTORY AND PRESENTATION

Patients who present with a rotator cuff tear report an event, many times of an insignificant nature, followed by persistent shoulder pain, especially with use in the overhead position or with external rotation. The pain is usually in the lateral aspect of the shoulder and may radiate down the arm in the region of the biceps tendon but rarely extends below the elbow. Night pain and the inability to sleep on the involved shoulder are classic symptoms of the lesion.[22,57,82,106] The patient may experience difficulty in elevating the arm and often relates symptoms of shoulder weakness and early fatigue in activities of daily living or recreation.

Physical examination may or may not demonstrate atrophy of the spinati muscles depending on the length of time since the actual tear and the size of the tear. Tenderness may be present on palpation of the tuberosities and bicipital groove, and the acromioclavicular joint may be prominent and tender. The anterior region of the acromion, often with associated spurring, may be tender as well. A full-thickness cuff tear occasionally can be palpated through the deltoid. Subacromial crepitus frequently can be palpated as the patient elevates the arm.[22,82,106]

Although the patient with a rotator cuff tear may be able to elevate the arm, passive range of motion is usually greater than active. Loss of active motion is frequently due to pain and/or weakness. Inability to lift the arm or a positive drop-arm test is suggestive of a massive tear.[82,106] A painful arc between 70 and 120 degrees of elevation is indicative of rotator cuff involvement due in part to a strong supraspinatus contraction in this position[15,22] and also in part to the fact that in this position the lesion is mechanically compressed. The impingement sign and test discussed earlier are of diagnostic value when a rotator cuff tear is suspected.

Strength of the major muscle groups must be tested, but the presence of pain can make assessment difficult due to inhibition. The impingement test will help to clarify whether weakness is due to pain or a rotator cuff tear. A significant increase in abductor and external rotator strength following the subacromial injection indicates rotator cuff involvement[74] but not a complete tear. Weakness of the external rotation in the absence of pain and without radicular or peripheral nerve involvement is the most significant sign of a rotator cuff tear.[22,57] Weakness of external rotation and abduction without pain usually correlates with a chronic nonreactive full-thickness tear of the supraspinatus, whereas weakness and pain indicate a partial-thickness or reactive full-thickness tear.

## DIAGNOSTIC TESTS

Shoulder arthrography has been used as the standard technique for diagnosing rotator cuff tears. Contrast material is injected into the shoulder, and brief exercise is performed to increase dye perfusion. If radiographs following exercise demonstrate intravasation of the dye into the tendon, a partial-thickness tear is suspected. Extravasation of the dye from the glenohumeral joint into the subacromial space is diagnostic of a full-thickness tear.[57,82] Ultrasonography is a noninvasive technique that is gaining acceptance in the diagnosis of rotator cuff tears. In recent studies, the accuracy, sensitivity, and specificity obtained with ultrasonography were each greater than 90 percent.[40] Magnetic resonance imaging (MRI) has become the "gold standard" in the diagnosis of rotator cuff tears, although at this time the technique is considerably more expensive than arthrography. The ability to differentiate rotator cuff degeneration and partial-thickness cuff tears from chronic tendinitis was excellent, with a sensitivity and specificity of 82 and 85 percent, respectively.[40]

Plain radiographic abnormalities often lag behind the degenerative course of rotator cuff pathology. Stages I and II impingement lesions often exhibit normal radiographs. The more significant radiographic changes are seen in late stage II and in patients with stage III lesions and include cystic changes around the greater tuberosity, sclerotic changes and osteophytes under the anterior third of the acromion often associated with the coracoacromial ligament, acromioclavicular joint changes, and narrowing of the subacromial space.[57] Superior migration of the humeral head is considered a telltale sign of significant rotator cuff weakness and is highly suspicious for rotator cuff tearing, especially when the other signs are also present.

## MANAGEMENT

The majority of patients with stage I and stage II impingement lesions respond well to conservative treatment, as addressed in the section on rotator cuff tendinitis. For the patient with stage III impingement lesions resulting in rotator cuff tears or for acute tears of the rotator cuff, conservative management, including rest, immobilization, physical therapy, analgesics, and anti-inflammatory medications, may fail to relieve the symptoms.[42] Most tears are likely to increase in size over time with a subsequent decrease in function. In this situation, repair within 3 to 6 months of the diagnosis is recommended. If conservative treatment is chosen, reassessment of external rotator strength and shoulder function should be performed at least every 6 months. Regression of or no change in strength coupled with a further decrease in function and/or an increase in pain will serve as an indicator of tear progression and assist in the decision making for surgical intervention.[22] The high-demand athlete in his or her early twenties or thirties with a proven rotator cuff tear is a good candidate for early surgical repair. Early intervention is indicated because the cuff tissues are healthier in terms of blood supply and healing capacity.[74]

The goal of surgical treatment of the rotator cuff tear is to restore functional anatomy by reestablishing continuity of the rotator cuff and to reduce the potential for repeated impingement.[42] An anterior acromioplasty and subacromial decompression with release of the coracoacromial ligament is indicated in patients requiring surgical intervention unless the cause of the tear was shoulder instability.[22,31,42] The most common technique used for rotator cuff reconstruction is the direct repair. First, all torn and degenerative marginal tissue must be debrided back to healthy-appearing tendon. Full-thickness vertical tears are closed by suturing tendon to tendon. In the case of horizontal tears, the cuff edges are mobilized laterally and inserted into a bony trough placed near the original attachment between the articular margin and the greater tuberosity. Sutures placed through drill holes into the bone ensure firm fixation.[40,106] Partial-thickness tears are repaired with the same basic principles used for repair of full-thickness tears. Other techniques for repairing massive tears include incorporation of the biceps tendon, superior mobilization of the subscapularis, pectoralis muscle fascia transfers, allographic fasciae latae grafts, freeze-dried cadaver rotator cuff grafts, and synthetic materials such as carbon fiber grafts.[22,106]

### Postoperative Management

A carefully supervised physical therapy program must be implemented in order to attain optimal surgical benefit. The postoperative rehabilitation program will vary according to the technique of repair and the type of pathology; it must be individualized. More often than not, the patient is placed in a sling or abduction splint immediately following surgery and will continue to utilize the shoulder support for approximately 3 to 6 weeks. Gentle pendulum exercises are initiated during the first postoperative week, as well as early passive range of motion in flexion (elevation) and external rotation in order to prevent adhesions and to avoid disruption of the repair caused by delayed mobilization.[22,31,42,82] The limit of these motions should be determined at surgery following completion of the repair and should be communicated to the therapist by the surgeon. Some patients will progress quicker than others with respect to passive glenohumeral motion. Those patients in whom progress is slower will require more assertive manual techniques, but care and caution need to be exercised so as not to overstretch or challenge the repair. At approximately 6 weeks postoperatively, the patient can be instructed in gentle isometrics and allowed to use the arm for light-duty daily activities.[74,82] In performing light daily activities, the elbow should remain flexed and at the side in order to avoid strain of the shoulder and the repair.[74] The patient is allowed to begin active elevation of the arm against gravity in the supine position and progresses to elevation in the sitting position. Active assistive stretching is continued and gradually intensified to eliminate residual tightness.[41]

As revascularization and healing occur, tendon to bone repair will be at its strongest immediately after surgery and at its weakest 3 weeks postoperatively.[82] The surgeon must offer recommendations in rehabilitation because he or she is knowledgeable as to the quality of the tissue, the repair, and the fixation. Active resistive exercises that stress the repaired tissues are not initiated for approximately 2 months (depending on the patients' size and quality of repair, 6 weeks may be appropriate) in order to provide adequate time for soft-tissue to bone healing.[22,82] Therapeutic pool exercises emphasizing range of motion and light resistive strengthening patterns with the arm elevated less than 90 degrees may be implemented early (6 to 8 weeks postoperatively) in the rehabilitation program. Manual resistive exercises of the scapula may be initiated, provided that the glenohumeral joint is well supported. Resistive exercises are begun conservatively, and the patient is advised to avoid sudden, jerky movements and lifting of heavy weights.[82] Manual resistive exercises in the scapular plane are advocated. Preoperative range-of-motion deficits and the degree of weakness and atrophy will affect postoperative results. Progressive resistive strengthening exercises should be implemented to regain the strength of all muscle groups of the involved shoulder. The patient should be instructed that the repair should be protected from heavy loads (i.e., carrying 15 lb in the operated hand) for 6 months to 1 year after surgery.[99] Although recreational activities are generally well tolerated by 6 months after surgery, full recovery of muscle strength can take many months.[22,41] It is frequently helpful to educate the patient to a 6-month/12-month concept: 6 months to comfortable 90-degree positions and 12 months to powerful use of the arm at a 90-degree angle.

# Fractures

Fractures of the shoulder complex may include fractures of the acromion, scapula, clavicle, and proximal humerus, with fractures of the proximal humerus being the most common.[4] In fact, proximal humerus fractures account for 45 percent of all humeral fractures.[17]

## PROXIMAL HUMERAL FRACTURES

### CLASSIFICATION

The large variation in location and extent of proximal humeral fractures requires a universal classification system. The most widely accepted classification was developed by Neer in 1970 with a consideration of anatomy, displacement, and biomechanics[96] (see Table 3-3). Neer's classification system is based on the status of the four parts of the proximal humerus: head, lesser tuberosity, greater tuberosity, and shaft. There are six major classifications of proximal humeral fractures. *One-part fractures* occur when one of the preceding four anatomic structures is minimally displaced. *Minimal displacement* is defined as displacement of less than 1 cm or angulation less than 45 degrees. *Two-part fractures* occur when one fragment is displaced in reference to the other three and the displacement is greater than 1 cm or angulated more than 45 degrees. *Three-part fractures* are defined as displacement of two of the four structures in relation to each other and the other two structures, while *four-part fractures* occur when there is displacement of all four fragments and the humeral head is out of contact with the glenoid fossa (Fig. 3-13). The final two categories in Neer's classification system are fracture-dislocations and compression/impression fractures. *Fracture-dislocations* are characterized by displacement of the humeral head outside the joint space in combination with a fracture. These fractures are named according to the number of fracture fragments and the direction of dislocation, such as two-part anterior fracture-dislocation. *Impression fractures* involve compression of the humeral head and are classified according to the percentage of articular surface affected. There are three subclassifications of impression fractures: less than 20 percent surface involvement, 20 to 45 percent surface involvement, and greater than 45 percent surface involvement[96] (Fig. 3-14).

Fortunately, 85 percent of proximal humeral fractures are minimally displaced or nondis-

**Table 3-3**

**Neer's Classification Scheme for Proximal Humerus Fractures**

| Category | Characteristic |
|---|---|
| I. One-part fracture | One of four anatomic structures* is displaced less than 1 cm or angulated more than 45° |
| II. Two-part fractures | One of four structures is displaced more than 1 cm or angulated more than 45° from the other three |
| III. Three-part fractures | Displacement of two of four structures in relation to each other and other two structures |
| IV. Four-part fractures | Displacement of all four fragments and humeral head out of contact with glenoid fossa |
| V. Fracture-dislocations | Displacement of humeral head outside of joint space in combination with a fracture |
| VI. Impression/compression fractures | Compression of humeral head |

*Four anatomic structures: head, shaft, lesser tuberosity, greater tuberosity

Adapted from Neer CS II. Displaced proximal humeral fractures: I. Classification and evaluation. J Bone Joint Surg 1970;52A(6):1077.

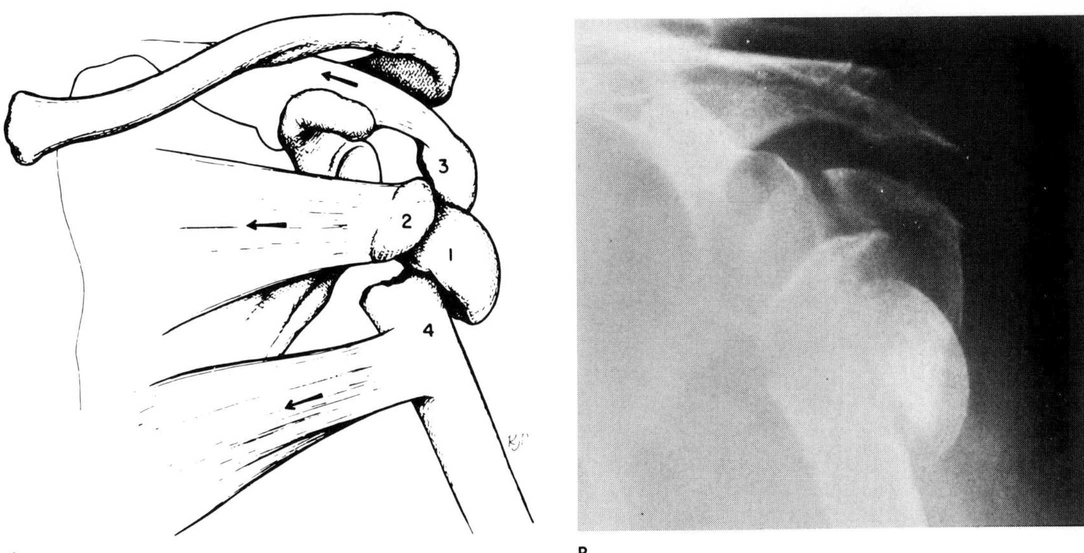


**Figure 3-13.** Four-part fracture. Four-part fractures occur when there is displacement of all four fragments and the humeral head is out of contact with the glenoid fossa. (a) Radiograph. (b) Schematic. (Reproduced with permission from Rockwood CA Jr, Green DP, eds. Fractures in adults. 2nd ed. Philadelphia: JB Lippincott, 1984:696.)

placed or one-part fractures, according to Neer's classification.[58] The remaining 15 percent are significantly displaced. Most proximal humeral fractures occur in older individuals with demineralized bone and are the result of violent forces, such as from a fall. The demineralization of bone is a normal age-related change characterized by a decrease in trabecular bone density and a thinning of cortical bone. The decrease in trabecular bone density produces cavitation in the humeral head and tuberosities, which in conjunction with the advancement of the medullary cavity toward the epiphysis results in weakening of the proximal humerus.[58,124] In some elderly individuals, the extent of this demineralization is amplified by osteoporosis. Therefore, despite a decrease in activity in the elderly, the frequency of proximal humeral fractures is greatest in this population because of a higher incidence of falls and a decreased resiliency of bony structure.

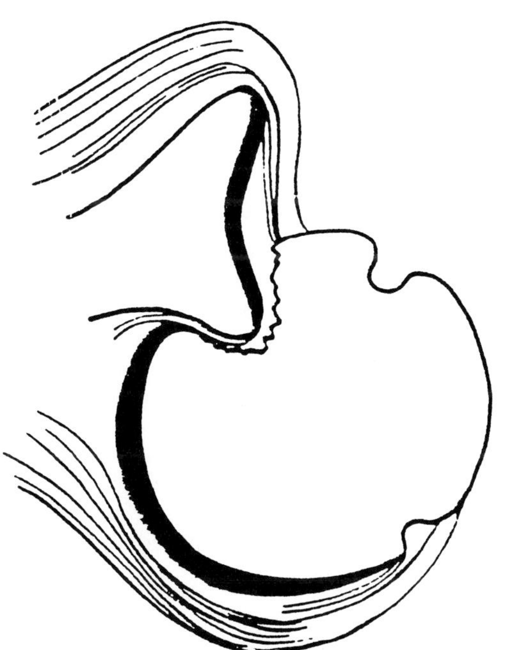

**Figure 3-14.** Impression fracture. Impression fractures involve compression of the humeral head and are classified according to the percentage of articular surface affected. (Reproduced with permission from Rockwood CA Jr, Green DP, eds. Fractures in adults. 3rd ed. Philadelphia: JB Lippincott, 1991:1073.)

## HISTORY AND PRESENTATION

Patients suffering from proximal humeral fractures will most commonly recall the following mechanisms of injury: direct trauma to the shoulder, axial loading through the elbow, or an indirect force from a fall on an outstretched arm.[17,58] By far, the most common injury is a fall on an outstretched arm. In this situation, the forearm is generally pronated, limiting external rotation at the shoulder. This limitation prevents clearance of the greater tuberosity under the acromion and frequently results in a fracture, a dislocation, or both.[58]

Patients will complain of significant pain in the shoulder, with a subsequent loss of motion. They frequently present to the emergency room with their arm in an adducted position. In addition, they may present with tenderness to palpation, crepitus with shoulder motion, and possible deformity and ecchymosis.[17,58] Fracture-dislocations are frequently characterized by deformity (i.e., an anterior fracture-dislocation will result in an anterior bulge and posterior flattening, with the opposite resulting from a posterior fracture-dislocation).[17]

Physical examination does not generally lend itself to strength testing because pain and loss of normal joint mechanics significantly limit force production and motion. If a fracture is suspected or detected by x-ray, neurologic and vascular evaluations are mandatory prior to attempting reduction. Any paresthesias, decrease in sensation, or decrease in pulses warrants further evaluation.[17] Neurologic injury, particularly to the axillary nerve, is most often associated with anterior fracture-dislocation and displaced surgical neck fractures.[58] Trauma to the vascular system may isolate the head of the humerus from its blood supply, leading to avascular necrosis.

The definitive diagnosis of fracture is accomplished with multiple-plane radiographs. Other soft-tissue injuries that frequently occur in conjunction with proximal humeral fractures include inflammation of the subacromial bursa and rotator cuff tears. The signs and symptoms of these injuries are detailed elsewhere in this chapter.

## MANAGEMENT

There are many different methods of management of proximal humeral fractures. Selection of the appropriate management is determined by the classification of the fracture, the age and activity level of the patient, the patient's motivation and compliance, and the general health of the patient.[58] In some instances with elderly patients, it is wiser to accept a functional loss than to risk surgery.[124]

### Conservative

Since most proximal humerus fractures are minimally displaced, there is no need for reduction. In these cases, an initial rest period is necessary to allow for initiation of callus formation. This period lasts for 3 weeks, during which time patients are usually placed in a sling. While immobilization can have deleterious effects on cartilage, ligament, muscle, and tendon, some form of immobilization is necessary to stabilize fracture fragments.[71] Assisted motion exercises are initiated once the fragments have approximated, which usually occurs between 3 and 6 weeks and should be confirmed by x-ray. At 6 weeks, fracture union is nearly complete, and gentle active resistive exercise and stretching may begin and progress gradually until the patient has obtained functional range of motion and strength.

Two-part fractures normally require some form of reduction, and in most cases, closed reduction is successful. Closed reduction may be obtained by manipulation or traction and is usually successful only with two-part fractures or grade I impression fractures. Repeated attempts at closed reduction may cause displacement, fragmentation, or neurologic damage and therefore should not be performed. If closed reduction does not provide a stable approximation of fragments, surgical stabilization will be necessary.[17] The difficulty with closed reduction involves muscular forces on fracture fragments. With fractures of the humeral shaft, the pectoralis major tends to produce a strong medial and anterior pull. Fractures of the lesser tuberosity may be displaced into internal rotation by the subscapularis, while fractures of the greater tuberosity may be displaced into external rotation by the pull of the supraspinatus, infraspinatus, and teres minor muscles. Therefore, frequent radiographs are necessary to ensure maintenance of fracture approximation after closed reduction.[58] Once closed reduction is obtained, a brief period of immobilization (3 to 4 weeks), followed by the gradual addition of active and resistive exercises (4 to 6 weeks), is performed as described above for minimally displaced fractures. However, the clinician must be sure that the fracture fragments are approximated and moving in unison before exercise is initiated. This is most frequently determined by the examiner grasping the humeral head in one hand and rotating the elbow with the opposite hand. Absence of movement between the humeral head and shaft suggests clinical continuity.[58] This also may be determined by observation of the fracture site in radiographs taken with the arm in various positions.

If closed reduction is unsuccessful for two-part fractures, percutaneous pinning may be employed. This involves the stabilization of fracture fragments by introducing pins through the skin. It provides more stabilization than closed reduction alone but is not as invasive as open reduction. Since this form of fixation is not rigid, sling immobilization is generally used for approximately 4 weeks. Pins are removed after clinical union has been achieved.[58]

### Surgical

Open reduction and internal fixation (ORIF) is indicated for most three-part fractures, grade II impression fractures, and two-part fractures not approximated with the preceding methods. The goal of open reduction and internal fixation is to secure fracture fragments with minimal hardware and allow for early mobilization of the extremity.[17] ORIF is generally successful for two- and three-part fractures. Because of the stability of this fixation, active exercises in pain-free range of motion may be initiated 7 to 10 days after surgery. At approximately 6 weeks after surgery, progressive resistive exercise, passive stretching, and joint mobilization techniques are indicated.[58]

Hemiarthroplasty is the most extensive form of management of proximal humeral fractures and is usually indicated only in severe three-part fractures, most four-part fractures, and grade III impression fractures. Hemiarthroplasty is generally mandatory if the blood supply to the humeral head has been interrupted, resulting in avascular necrosis, or the fragments are displaced to the degree that malunion or nonunion will result even with attempts at open reduction and internal fixation.[17,58] Hemiarthroplasty will generally result in adequate pain relief and return of function. Rehabilitation may begin early, with active assisted exercise beginning 2 to 3 days after surgery and progressive resistive exercise, stretching, and joint mobilization beginning at 6 weeks. Failure of hemiarthroplasty will usually be secondary to adhesions in the surrounding soft tissues, particularly the rotator cuff. If this occurs, the only remaining option for the patient is to undergo a total shoulder replacement or shoulder fusion.[124]

In summary, rehabilitation following proximal humerus fracture is not so much dependent on the type of fracture as it is on the stability of the fracture fragments. Once the fracture fragments are approximated (approximately 3 to 4 weeks with closed reduction and 3 to 7 days with open reduction), active pain-free exercises may be initiated. When clinical union is achieved (approximately 6 weeks after fracture barring any complications), resistive exercises, passive stretching, and joint mobilization techniques may begin. Clinicians must be sure to closely monitor the patient's response to manual techniques, since an increase in pain or a decrease in function may signal a problem that requires further medical evaluation. Frequent communication between the therapist and the physician is also important. Radiographs must be taken periodically to document the stability of the reduction and provide guidelines for progression of rehabilitation.

### COMPLICATIONS

It is important that the clinician be familiar with common complications following proximal humeral fractures. These include nonunion, malunion, avascular necrosis, vascular injury, neurologic injury, and joint stiffness.[17,58,124] Nonunion is generally the result of unstable closed reduction, an insufficient period of immobilization, or poor bone quality.[17] If a patient begins to demonstrate a loss of normal mechanics of the shoulder or begins experiencing intolerable pain, the clinician should suspect a poor union and have this evaluated on radiographs. Malunion is typically associated with three- and four-part fractures where there is severe deformity. Malunion can only be treated with ORIF, bone grafting, or hemiarthroplasty. In addition to malunion, avascular necrosis is a common complication of four-part fractures. Because of the retrograde blood supply to the proximal humerus, there is a high incidence of avascular necrosis with fractures involving the articular segment.[58] In fact, 80 to 90 percent of four-part proximal humeral fractures result in avascular necrosis.[58] Symptoms of avascular necrosis include pain and a dramatic loss of motion; unfortunately, these symptoms usually become evident after collapse and resorption of the humeral head has begun. This is a process that is not reversible, and the patient will require a total shoulder replacement.[17] Vascular injury is usually associated with fractures that result from blunt trauma. Any vascular injury that is identified should be repaired in conjunction with stabilization of the fracture. Finally, joint stiffness is usually secondary to adhesions in the soft tissue surrounding the fracture site or to a loss of space in the glenohumeral joint secondary to an increase in size of the humeral head because of callus formation. These soft-tissue restrictions generally can be overcome with massage/soft-tissue mobilization, joint mobilization, passive stretching, and exercise.[124] The extent of restricted motion may be greater given the degree of involvement in the fracture. Clinicians should be aware of early signs of these complications so that they may be reversed if at all possible.

## MIDSHAFT FRACTURES

In addition to proximal humeral fractures, the humerus may be fractured in the midshaft region. Injury in this region is usually the result of a direct blow to the shaft resulting in a transverse-comminuted fracture or a fall on an outstretched arm resulting in a spiral fracture.[143] In the presence of a midshaft fracture, the physical examination will reveal a flail arm that the patient will attempt to support with a sling or the opposite upper extremity. If a midshaft fracture is suspected, a thorough neurovascular examination should be performed because there is a high incidence of radial nerve injury associated with these fractures. However, the radial nerve is rarely completely severed, and recovery usually occurs.[143] The midshaft of the humerus is also a common site for metastases in the elderly with resultant frequent fractures.

Closed treatment for midshaft fractures is usually successful in obtaining alignment without clinical deformity. This may be secondary to the thickened periosteum of this region. Transverse fractures are typically reduced under anesthesia, while gravity provides alignment of spiral fractures.[143] In both cases, a U-shaped splint is applied in conjunction with a sling for 4 to 6 weeks. Clinical union is typically achieved at 6 weeks, at which time active and passive exercises are initiated and continued until the patient has regained motion, strength, and function of the arm. If nonunion does occur at this site, intramedullary nailing with bone grafting is indicated.[143]

## ACROMIAL FRACTURES

Acromial fractures are rare, but if they occur, it is usually in response to direct trauma to the shoulder or a fall on the shoulder.[4] Diagnosis is made by careful palpation and localization of the exact site of the majority of the discomfort and is confirmed with radiographs. Management is determined by the degree of fracture displacement. If the fracture is undisplaced or minimally displaced (less than 1 cm), the patient is treated symptomatically by limiting activity and providing a sling for comfort. If the fracture is significantly displaced, open reduction and internal fixation are often indicated.[4] If acromial fractures remain unrecognized for 3 or more weeks, union may only be achieved by open reduction, internal fixation, and bone grafting.[4]

## SCAPULAR FRACTURES

Scapular fractures are also rare and generally are undisplaced. As with acromial and clavicular fractures, the mechanism of injury for a scapular fracture is typically a direct blow or fall on the outstretched arm. Scapular fractures are treated symptomatically by a decrease in activity and the temporary use of a sling. Clinical union usually occurs in 6 to 8 weeks.[4] A common complication following scapular fracture is the adherence of the musculature overlying the scapula. These adhesions may result in a decrease in scapular mobility and an alteration in normal scapulohumeral rhythm. The formation of adhesions may be limited by deep tissue mobilization during the healing phase (0 to 6 weeks), followed by passive stretching and joint mobilization, including scapulothoracic mobilization, after clinical union has been achieved.

Fractures of the glenoid fossa are a specific type of scapular fracture that is typically associated with dislocations of the glenohumeral joint. These fractures are generally treated symptomatically unless they involve more than 25 percent of the glenoid surface. In this case, open reduction and internal fixation are generally indicated to obtain union and reduction of dislocation.[4] A specific fracture of the glenoid is an avulsion fracture associated with the Bankart lesion, which is discussed elsewhere in this chapter.

## CLAVICULAR FRACTURES

Clavicular fractures are probably second in incidence to proximal humeral fractures and have been classified into three categories depending on the location of the fracture. Group I clavicular fractures are of the middle third of the clavicle or diaphysis and are the most common type of clavicular fracture.[3, 103] The mechanism of injury for a diaphyseal clavicular fracture is typically a fall on the point of the shoulder or outstretched arm.[3, 103] Such a fall results in buckling and fracture of the middle third of the clavicle, with the proximal fragment being elevated and the shoulder and distal fragment being displaced inferiorly. Patients generally present with localized pain and swelling as well as crepitation at the fracture site. Closed treatment is almost always successful and consists of a splint or a figure 8 bandage that pulls the shoulder superiorly and posteriorly into its anatomic position.[3, 103] Splinting and limitation of active motion to 30 degrees of flexion, abduction, and extension are maintained for 6 to 8 weeks to allow for complete union.[103] Once union is achieved, stretching and strengthening exercises are performed to allow a gradual return to functional activities. Though rare, if nonunion occurs, open reduction and internal fixation with bone grafting will be required.[103]

Group II clavicular fractures are those which occur in the distal portion of the clavicle between the coracoclavicular ligaments and the acromioclavicular joint. These fractures often occur in conjunction with an acromioclavicular joint sprain or separation.[4] The mechanism of injury for distal clavicular fractures is typically a force or fall on the point of the shoulder resulting in a downward force to the humerus and scapula.[3] This category of clavicular fractures consists of three subclassifications. Type I fractures involve a fracture of the clavicle at some point between the coracoclavicular ligaments and the acromioclavicular joint, with both these boundary structures remaining intact. The coracoclavicular ligaments and the acromioclavicular joint serve as an internal splint for closed reduction.

Treatment of these fractures is symptomatic, with the use of a sling for comfort and a decrease in activity for 3 to 6 weeks. Type II distal clavicle fractures are the same as type I with the added characteristic of a torn coracoclavicular ligament, which results in a significant posterior and superior displacement of the proximal fragment. These fractures are treated with splinting in the same manner as for a grade III acromioclavicular joint separation, namely, the Kenny Howard sling. Approximation is often difficult to achieve with this sling, and thus there is a high rate of nonunion.[3,4] Type III fractures consist of fractures of the clavicular surface of the acromioclavicular joint. Treatment of these fractures consists of excision of the distal portion of the clavicle in order to diminish the likelihood of degenerative joint disease of the acromioclavicular joint.

Type III clavicular fractures consist of fractures of the proximal third of the clavicle. These fractures are extremely rare and are very seldom displaced. The mechanism of injury is typically a direct blow from the lateral side, and management almost always consists of figure 8 splinting for comfort.[3]

## Dislocations and Subluxations

The glenohumeral joint is the most mobile joint of the body; this is at the expense of joint stability. For this reason, the glenohumeral joint is the most commonly dislocated joint, with a rate of incidence of 1 to 2 percent.[90] The rate of recurrence of dislocations is very high, at 80 to 95 percent in younger patients.[24,137] *Shoulder dislocation* is defined as the "complete separation of the articular surfaces of the glenohumeral joint, due to either direct of indirect forces applied to the shoulder."[115] *Subluxations* are often associated with dislocations and may be defined as "increased humeral head translation on the glenoid."[115] Subluxations may or may not be associated with pain, apprehension, or disability.[115,165] The degree of trauma associated with dislocation will depend on the forces involved, previous injuries, and the patient's general ligamentous laxity.[115]

### CLASSIFICATION

Classification of shoulder instability includes the type: dislocations, subluxations, or dislocation-subluxations. The direction of instability is also considered: anterior, posterior, inferior, or multidirectional.[165] Dislocations of the shoulder are also classified as traumatic (primary and recurrent dislocations, chronic dislocations, transient dislocations) and atraumatic (spontaneous primary and recurrent dislocations and recurrent voluntary dislocations)[137] (see Table 3-4). Traumatic dislocations account for approximately 95 percent of all dislocations. Atraumatic dislocations are much less common and can be voluntary or involuntary. Voluntary dislocators often have a long history of dislocating the shoulder with minimal pain or apprehension. Some patients with normal muscular development and no increased ligament laxity also can voluntarily dislocate the glenohumeral joint and often will try to gain attention or sympathy by performing this act. These patients must be sorted out when considering surgical treatment options. Other patients may eventually lose control of the voluntary ability to dislocate and cannot perform normal activities of daily living without incidences of recurrent dislocations.[149] Atraumatic dislocations are seen primarily in the hypermobile patient with excessive ligament laxity or in one with a generalized connective-tissue disorder (i.e., Ehlers-Danlos).[61] This patient is differentiated from the primary traumatic dislocator who has multiple subsequent episodes resulting in eventual atraumatic dislocation episodes. Matsen[81] has simplified instability considerations with two acronyms, TUBS and AMBRI; these are shown in Table 3-5. These will prove helpful to the clinician when attempting to determine appropriate treatment plans for the patient presenting with a history of shoulder instability.

**Table 3-4**

**Classification of Shoulder Instability**

- Type
  - Dislocations
  - Subluxations
  - Dislocation-subluxations
- Direction
  - Anterior
  - Posterior
  - Multidirectional
- Etiology
  - Traumatic
  - Atraumatic
    - Spontaneous primary and recurrent dislocations
    - Recurrent voluntary dislocations and subluxations

### DISLOCATIONS

Dislocation occurs when the humeral head becomes completely dissociated from the glenoid fossa (Fig. 3-15). The mechanism of injury causing instability at the shoulder is usually trauma of either a direct or indirect force nature placed on the stabilizing structures. In the case of anterior

**Table 3-5**

**Matsen's Classification of Instability**

| | |
|---|---|
| **TUBS** | **T**raumatic etiology<br>**U**nidirectional<br>**B**ankart lesion<br>**S**urgical Bankart repair |
| **AMBRI** | **A**traumatic etiology<br>**M**ultidirectional<br>**B**ilateral<br>**R**ehabilitation<br>**I**nferior capsular shift is the preferred surgical treatment[81] |

instability, the force can be applied to the posterior aspect of the joint, pushing the humeral head anteriorly over the glenoid fossa. An indirect force, such as a vigorous positioning into hyperextension, abduction, and external rotation, can cause anterior instability. Indirect forces such as those described are frequently encountered in many athletic activities (football, volleyball, basketball, baseball pitching, swimming, tennis, and gymnastics). These stresses can cause weakening or failure of the capsuloligamentous-labral complex (CLLC), resulting in stretching of the soft-tissue envelope and frequently detachment of the labrum or Bankart lesion. A glenohumeral subluxation or dislocation may result depending on the amount of humeral head displacement from the glenoid fossa.[84] The less frequent posterior instability is most often the result of either a direct blow to the anterior aspect of the shoulder, a fall onto an outstretched hand with the elbow locked into extension, or seizures or electric shock.[85, 144, 145] Subluxation in either direction may be the result of previous dislocation or may progress to a recurrent dislocation pattern.[165, 149]

Other lesions are often associated with a dislocation, including stretch injuries of the brachial plexus (frequently involving the axillary nerve), Bankart lesions (detachment of the labrum from the glenoid rim), Hill-Sachs lesions (depression fractures of the posterolateral humeral head), fractures of the glenoid rim, and stretching or rupture of the axillary or posterior humeral circumflex artery.[90] The Bankart lesion incidence in traumatic anterior dislocations is 87 percent and is considered the most common reason for recurrent instability[138] (Fig. 3-16). Stability is lost due to avulsion of the labrum and capsuloligamentous complex (CLC) from the glenoid rim resulting in loss of the barrier and compression effect. Hill-Sachs lesions occur at the posterolateral humeral head, since this area is relatively soft cancellous bone and is compressed against the anterior glenoid rim. The presence of this lesion is considered to be one of the causative factors in recurrent dislocations,

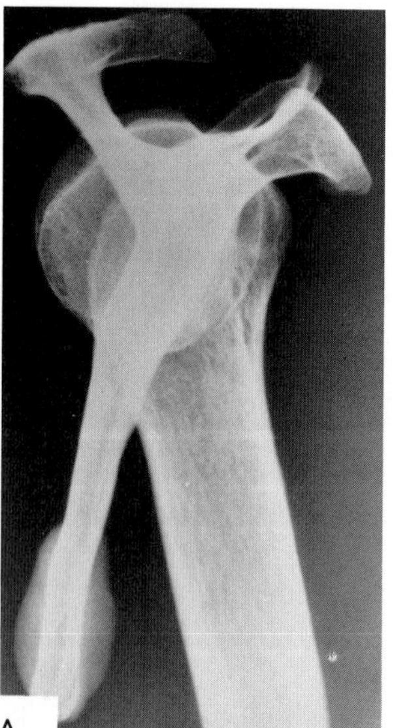


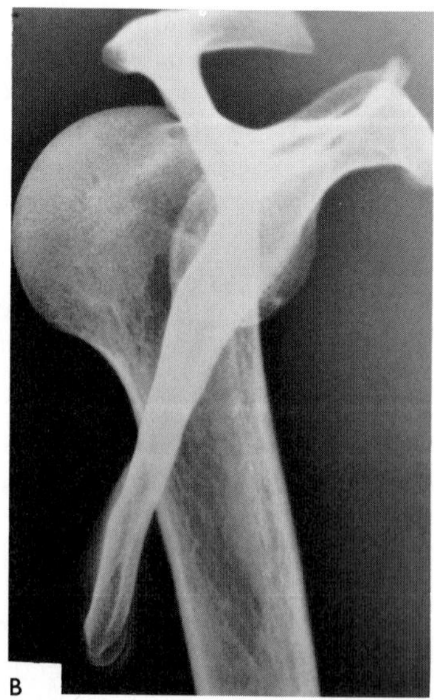


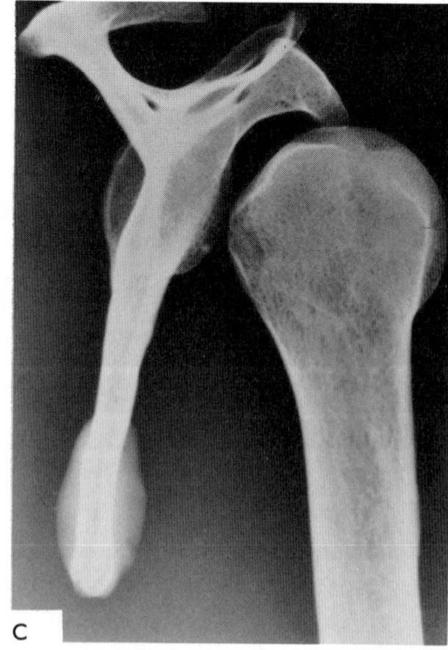


**Figure 3-15.** Glenohumeral dislocation occurs when the humeral head becomes completely dissociated from the glenoid fossa. (a) Normal. (b) Posterior dislocation. (c) Anterior dislocation. (Reproduced with permission from Thomas SC, Matsen FA III. Subluxations and dislocations about the glenohumeral joint. In Rockwood CA Jr, Green DP, Bucholz RW, eds. Fractures in adults. 3rd ed. Vol. 1. Philadelphia: JB Lippincott, 1991:1066.)

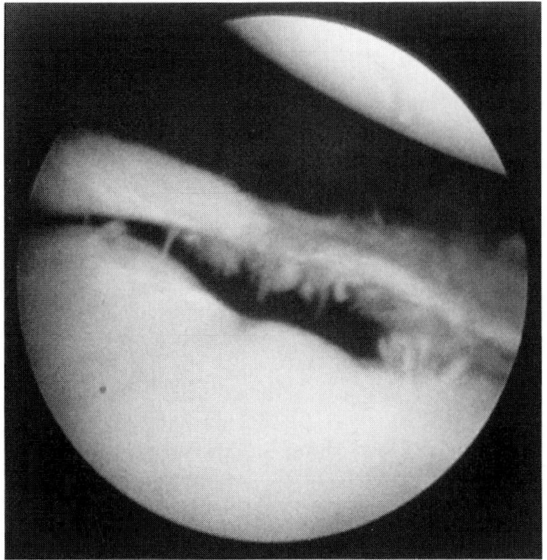

**Figure 3-16.** The Bankart lesion. The Bankart lesion is considered the most common reason for recurrent instability. (Reproduced with permission from Caspari RB, Jackson RW, Poehling GG. Operative arthroscopy. New York: Raven Press, 1991:510.)

and this lesion was found in 77 percent of traumatic dislocations[24] (Fig. 3-17). Fractures and damage to the glenoid rim are common in traumatic dislocations; injuries from mild chip fractures to severe fractures were noted in 73 percent of traumatic dislocations in a study performed by Rowe.[138]

## SUBLUXATIONS

Subluxation at the glenohumeral joint represents increased humeral head translation on the glenoid due to compromise or inherent laxity of the CLLC. Based on anatomic studies, *subluxation* has been defined as "head translation greater than one-half the width of the glenoid but less than the sum of one-half the glenoid and one-half the humeral head."[149] Subluxations tend to be the more problematic classification of shoulder instabilities due to the clinical symptom overlap of subluxations and impingement syndrome. Symptoms of both conditions frequently occur, with the patient's main complaint being shoulder pain. Subluxation can start suddenly or gradually through repetitive use in sports. Participation in certain sports such as throwing and swimming can lead to progressive joint laxity. Initially, the patient may be asymptomatic, but repetitive stresses to the CLLC at the end range of motion will lead to pain and overloading. These stresses can lead to labral damage varying from small tears to detachment (Bankart lesions).[115] If labral injury affects the inferior glenohumeral ligament, repeated injury can lead to clinical subluxations.[149] Patients may often complain of pain on the posterior aspect of the shoulder with anterior instability. This is due to repetitive traction placed on the rotator cuff and posterior capsule during subluxation.[115,165] Repeated subluxations can progress to recurrent dislocations.[149]

A complete understanding of the mechanisms of arm motion that produce pain is required. This will help in the diagnosis of the direction of instability. For example, if pain is experienced in cocking phase of throwing, anterior subluxation is considered. Conversely, pain in the follow-through phase during humeral adduction and internal rotation of the shoulder is suggestive of posterior instability or weakness.[115,165]

## DIRECTION OF INSTABILITY

### Anterior

Anterior instability is by far the most common, accounting for approximately 95 percent of all shoulder dislocations.[90] The most common type of anterior dislocation is the subcoracoid dislocation, where the humeral head is anterior to the glenoid fossa and inferior to the coracoid process. The second most common is the subglenoid dislocation, where the head of the humerus is anterior to and below the glenoid fossa. Other types are much more rare, including the subclavicular dislocation, in which the head of the humerus lies medial to the coracoid process and inferior to the clavicle; the luxatio erecta dislocation presents with the arm fixed in a position of complete elevation as the humeral head

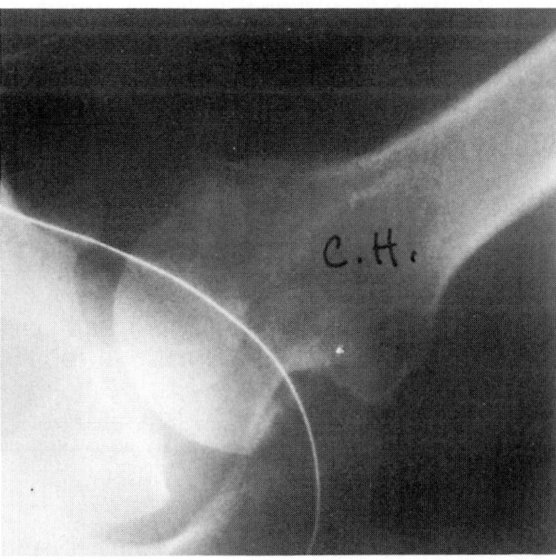


**Figure 3-17.** Hill-Sachs lesion. (Reproduced with permission from Rockwood CA Jr, Green DP, eds. Fractures in adults. 2nd ed. Philadelphia: JB Lippincott, 1984:740.)

dislocates anteriorly and inferiorly; and finally, the most rare of dislocations is the intrathoracic dislocation, in which the head of the humerus is driven between the ribs into the thoracic cavity.[84]

**Posterior**

Posterior dislocations are relatively infrequent, accounting for only 1 to 4 percent of all dislocations.[20,85,144,145] Approximately 98 percent of all posterior shoulder dislocations are subacromial; other classifications include subglenoid and subspinous.[145]

**Multidirectional**

*Multidirectional instability* (MDI) has been defined as shoulder instability occurring in more than one plane of motion. It can be present in two or three directions but usually has a significant component of inferior laxity combined with increased anterior or posterior translation, in the absence of labral detachments.[113,149] Patients suffering with MDI can range from those with excessive ligament laxity (atraumatic), to those who perform repetitive activities at extremes of motion (microtraumatic), to one who sustains a traumatic injury to the shoulder (macrotraumatic).[149] Repetitive microtrauma often has a cumulative effect, causing an increase in the magnitude of the MDI.[113,149] Patients with MDI are more likely to be "continuously disabled for any given activity than those with simpler instability patterns."[149] Secondary rotator cuff tendinitis and radiating pain and paresthesia are frequently associated with MDIs. Treatment is usually nonsurgical, and patients with generalized ligament laxity tend to do better with a conservative rehabilitation program than those with MDI due to traumatic insult. If they are willing to modify their activities, approximately 50 to 70 percent of patients with MDI and ligament laxity respond positively to a nonsurgical rehabilitation program. If the conservative approach fails, an inferior capsular shift is recommended.[81,149]

## HISTORY AND PRESENTATION

In an acute traumatic dislocation, the patient presents to the clinician, trainer, or emergency room in obvious painful distress. The history and mechanism of injury, along with radiographs and physical examination, will usually reveal the problem. In an anterior dislocation, the shoulder is usually held in a position of moderate abduction, and any attempt to produce further abduction or movements of adduction and internal rotation are severely limited due to pain. The lateral contour of the shoulder is flattened, and anterior prominence of the humeral head may be palpated and visualized (Fig. 3-18). The patient suffering an acute posterior dislocation usually presents with the arm adducted and internally rotated. The coracoid process will appear prominent with an empty anterior glenoid fossa, and the humeral head will be noted as a posterior bulge beneath the posterior margin of the acromion.[145]

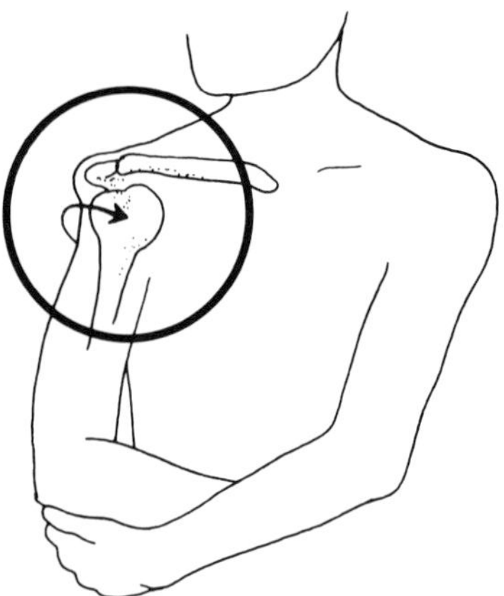

**Figure 3-18.** Clinical impression of anterior dislocation. The lateral contour of the shoulder is flattened, and an anterior prominence of the humeral head may be palpated and visualized. (Reproduced with permission from Arnheim D. Modern principles of athletic training. St. Louis: Times Mirror/Mosby, 1989: 706.)

Acute dislocations should be reduced as quickly and gently as possible to minimize stretching of neurovascular structures, muscle spasm, and compression damage to the humeral head.[84] Ideally, x-rays should be taken prior to reduction in order to rule out associated fractures, but on the playing field, a seasoned team physician or licensed trainer may attempt an immediate reduction. However, one should keep in mind the likelihood of axillary nerve damage and posterior humeral circumflex artery damage. If one suspects that these important structures are significantly traumatized, then reducing the dislocated shoulder probably should take place in an emergency room setting. X-rays are required after reduction to confirm the relocation of the head of the humerus and to rule out any resulting fractures.[115,137]

When the patient presents following an unstable event, either dislocation or subluxation, and it is reduced, physical examination includes an accurate assessment of shoulder motion, strength, and stability. Internal and external rotation should be assessed with the arms at the side and abducted to 90 degrees. Patients with anterior instability are frequently unwilling to fully externally rotate with the arm abducted to 90 degrees due to apprehension. Patients with posterior instability may have a posterior apprehension test. Stress testing should be performed anteriorly, posteriorly, and inferiorly; apprehension would be suggestive of instability in that direction. A positive sulcus sign is indicative of multidirectional instability. To elicit a sulcus sign, the patient sits with the arms relaxed at the side, traction is placed in an inferior direction at the wrist. A positive sign is noted when a prominent depression, a sulcus, is noted anteriorly beneath the acromion.[115,165]

The "load and shift" test is used to document passive translation of the humeral head. With the patient in a sitting position, the examiner grasps the humeral head between the thumb and index finger. A compressive force is gently loaded to the glenoid with the humeral head, and an attempt is made to translate the humeral head anteriorly, posteriorly, and inferiorly. Translation is classified into three grades: grade I is demonstrated by translation of up to 50 percent of the diameter of the humeral head or translation up to the rim of the glenoid, grade II allows the humeral head to be pushed over the rim greater than 50 percent of the diameter of the humeral head with spontaneous reduction of the humeral head, and grade III results in dislocation of the humeral head. The affected arm must be compared with the opposite side, since the amount of normal variation is as yet undetermined. Associated grinding and clicking, suggesting damage to the labrum, also should be noted.[13,90]

## DIAGNOSTIC TESTS

Radiologic evaluations can be beneficial in assessing the direction of instability, since fractures, new bone formation, and rounding of the anterior glenoid lip correspond with the direction of instability. Defects of the posterolateral humeral head also may be detected, and these are associated with anterior instability. During examination under anesthesia, stress radiographs can be helpful in documenting the presence and direction of instability.[84] The computed tomographic (CT) scan and magnetic resonance imaging (MRI) are helpful in detailing labral lesions.

Arthroscopy greatly assists with further assessment of shoulder pathology and can be used to identify intraarticular lesions associated with shoulder instability. The expected lesions would include fraying of the labrum, separation of the labrum from the glenoid (Bankart lesion), compression fracture of the posterolateral humeral head (Hill-Sachs lesion), and capsular rents, strains, or redundancy.[84,165]

## MANAGEMENT

Following dislocation and reduction, the patient is immobilized in adduction and internal rotation. The ideal period of immobilization is somewhat controversial. Because of the higher incidence of recurrent dislocations, longer immobilization is advocated in the younger population (under 20 years old) compared with the older population (over 40 years old). Therefore, some physicians recommend the younger population be immobilized for a 6-week period and the older patient 2 to 3 weeks. Others do not believe the period of immobilization to be a factor in recurrence and use immobilization as dictated by pain. A rehabilitation program emphasizing strengthening of the internal rotators and anterior shoulder musculature follows the immobilization phase. The rationale for this aspect of rehabilitation is that ligament and capsular healing requires 6 weeks and that adequate muscular rehabilitation of the stabilizing structures is necessary before return to full activity. Typically, patients over age 40 are immobilized for short time periods (only 1 week to 10 days) due to concern over loss of motion and their low recurrence rate.[115]

Following an acute subluxation, the shoulder may be immobilized for a short interval to allow tightening and healing of damaged or traumatized tissues. The patient is advised against performing activities which aggravate or reproduce symptoms. Following either dislocation or subluxation, once the direction of instability is determined, an appropriate rehabilitation program is initiated to strengthen the supporting musculature on the side of the instability. For anterior instability, the emphasis is on strengthening internal rotators/shoulder depressors. Conversely, external rotators are strengthened when the direction of instability is posterior.[47] However, it is very important to achieve proper muscle balance between the internal and external rotators, and a strengthening program incorporating both, without undue stress to the affected supporting tissue, is the most appropriate format regardless the primary direction of instability. It will be important to progress the patient through rotational strengthening exercises in a variety of planes of shoulder flexion and abduction. Adequate functional strengthening and proprioceptive training will not occur if the patient performs all rotational exercises with the arm in an adducted or protected position. Therefore, rehabilitation is eventually progressed to more provocative functional positions when it is determined that it is safe to do so. Strengthening exercises of the scapular stabilizing muscles is also critical because the scapula serves as a stable platform for all humeral motion.[65,84] It is also important to regain any loss of motion (external or internal rotation) prior to returning to throwing. With loss of motion, abnormal stresses are placed on the joint in order to compensate for the loss of power; this will inevitably lead to inflammation of the rotator cuff and shoulder pain.[115,165] Two caveats to conservative treatment of the unstable shoulder are to restrict swimming or diving into waves and to be very certain to prevent side-arm sleeping postures and prone sleeping with the arms elevated overhead or under the pillow early in the rehabilitation program.

If the patient continues to experience glenohumeral instability despite an appropriate trial of conservative therapy, operative treatment must be considered.[115,165] Generally, those patients who suffer recurrent traumatic dislocations respond well to reparative surgery. However, in patients with voluntary recurrent dislocations, the response is much less favorable, and most surgeons are reluctant to operate.[137]

**Surgical Management**

Several different surgical procedures have been described to manage the unstable shoulder. The Bankart repair appears to be one of the most popular choices because it is an anatomic repair without deformation of tissue; the tissues are taken down layer by layer with adequate and separate exposure of the subscapularis muscle, the capsuloligamentous complex (CLC), and the joint. All pathologic lesions can be identified and repaired. If a Bankart lesion is found, the labrum and associated CLC are reattached to the rim of the glenoid. If there is not a Bankart lesion, the medial capsule is double-breasted over the lateral capsule to securely reinforce its attachment to the glenoid rim and to reduce the size of the capsule. The muscles are reattached to their normal anatomic position without transplantation or shortening.[137] A reverse type of Bankart repair is commonly used on the posterior capsule in the case of posterior instability. Capsular shifts are also used frequently to eliminate a large, redundant capsuloligamentous complex, which is typically characteristic of the MDI patient. (Specifics of surgical techniques are discussed in Chap. 4.) Arthroscopic treatment by debridement of labral lesions also proves to be valuable.[90] Reconstructive surgery can sometimes be delayed or avoided, since symptoms of pain, catching, and clicking in the shoulder will improve following arthroscopic debridement and rehabilitation, allowing desired participation in functional and recreational activities.[165]

**Postoperative Management**

The postoperative rehabilitation course varies with the type of procedure performed and is tailored to the individual patient. Following repairs for anterior shoulder instability, the shoulder is usually immobilized in a conventional sling for 3 to 6 weeks.[65,84,115] The patient is allowed to come out of the sling for daily range-of-motion exercises, taking care not to stretch the capsular repair. Recognition and consideration must be given to patient apprehension and/or complaints of pain. Appropriate exercises include pendulum exercises, gentle passive flexion and scapular plane abduction (elevation), and minimal external rotation. Isometrics with the arm at the side of the body are allowed. Shoulder shrugs, protraction, and retraction help to maintain mobility of the scapulothoracic, sternoclavicular, and acromioclavicular joints. After the immobilization period, active and active assistive exercises are performed. Flexion and abduction (elevation) to 90 to 100 degrees should be possible, as well as 35 to 40 degrees of external rotation. Resistive exercises for internal rotation, flexion, abduction, and horizontal adduction are performed. Strengthening in external rotation should be performed with the elbow flexed to 90 degrees and the arm at the side in a comfortable range of motion only.[65] Exercise performed in the scapular plane is advantageous postoperatively owing to less stress placed on the suture lines (Fig. 3-19). Gradual progressive strengthening for all the major muscle groups of the glenohumeral joint and the scapulothoracic joint are performed. Again, it will be important to progress the athlete through rotational strengthening exercises in a variety of planes in order to achieve neuromuscular control and strength appropriate for functional and athletic demands. Moreover, recognition and consideration should be given to the patient's response to each exercise, and modifications in forces should be applied or limits to range of motion utilized to protect the repair. Proprioceptive activities as well as functional drills should be performed prior to the patient's return to throwing and sports participation at approximately 6 months after surgery. The goal of the rehabilitation program is the recovery of full, pain-free range of

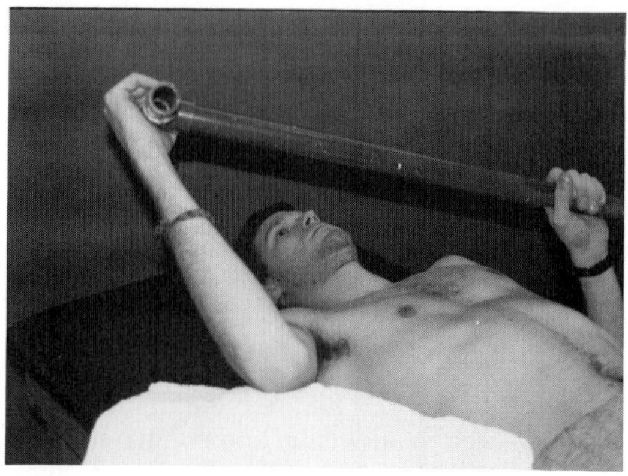

**Figure 3-19.** External rotation in the scapular plane.

motion and strength of the shoulder in order to prevent recurrent injury.

The rehabilitation program for the repair of posterior instability follows approximately the same guidelines as for anterior instability but with awareness of protecting stress on the repair by limiting movements of internal rotation, horizontal adduction, and elevation. Following 4 to 6 weeks of immobilization in neutral rotation and slight extension, rehabilitation is initiated with passive exercises to recover comfortable range of motion. Strengthening exercises should emphasize internal and external rotation.[145] Once again, functional drills should be performed prior to return to sports participation.

In those patients with generalized ligamentous laxity and resulting multidirectional instability, the surgical procedure of choice is frequently the inferior capsular shift. Rehabilitation with these patients can be "slower" because many patients with multidirectional instability will recover motion rapidly. These patients typically have very little trouble regaining motion; rather, the emphasis of their program is placed on strengthening the dynamic stabilizers. One year after surgery, it is ideal for the involved shoulder to have approximately 10 degrees less flexion (elevation) and 20 degrees less rotation than the other shoulder.[98]

With expertise in the surgical management of shoulder instability, coupled with skillful postoperative rehabilitation and good patient compliance, the incidence of recurrent problems will diminish. However, it is important to recognize that even with great surgical expertise, the very best rehabilitation program, and complete patient compliance, there will still be patients who are not permitted to return to previous levels of activity. Realizing this should not prevent clinicians from attempting to return patients to the highest level of function as possible. However, it is also a responsibility of clinicians to make their patients aware of the risks and dangers inherent in returning to specific activities.

## Glenoid Labrum

The glenoid labrum is a fibrocartilaginous annular lip that is attached to the margin of the articular surface of the glenoid. It is triangular in cross section, similar to the meniscus in the knee, with the base attached to the circumference of the glenoid and its free end being thin and sharp. The labrum is also continuous with the long head of the biceps tendon; this anatomic relationship may contribute to labral tears.

There are several theories regarding the function of the glenoid labrum. The most common theories of its function include deepening the articular cavity, protecting the edges of the glenoid, serving as the attachment point for the glenohumeral ligaments, and providing lubrication to the joint. The configuration of the glenohumeral joint allows for minimal bony restraint, since only one-quarter of the humeral head is in contact with the glenoid fossa at any one time. Therefore, stability demands are placed on surrounding soft-tissue structures, including the labrum, glenohumeral ligaments, and musculature.[117]

The labrum and glenohumeral ligaments are connected anatomically, which allows them to function as a stronger stabilizing force. The inferior glenohumeral ligament is attached to the anteroinferior labrum, and the middle glenohumeral ligament inserts on to the labrum adjacent to the glenoid fossa. The superior glenohumeral ligament is attached to the superior labrum after it passes inferior to the tendon of the long head of the biceps, which is also attached to the superior labrum.[1] In addition to linking the glenohumeral ligaments to the glenoid rim, the glenoid labrum itself deepens the glenoid cavity by approximately 2 to 3 cm.

### CLASSIFICATION

Several different types of labral damage are seen clinically. These include radial tears, longitudinal tears, bucket-handle tears, avulsion injuries, and labral fraying or degenerative tears.[6] The mechanism of injury that results in these labral pathologies may be either a repetitive-use injury or an acute injury, microtrauma or macrotrauma.[130]

Repetitive overhead activity frequently results in an increase in translation of the humeral head, causing labral fraying and wearing down of the rim of the glenoid fossa. Extended trauma may include stretching of the glenohumeral ligaments and joint capsule.[6] These minor degenerative changes can be progressive to the point where a labral detachment (Bankart lesion) occurs, resulting in frank instability of the glenohumeral joint.[1,6]

Macrotrauma to the labrum is usually the result of an episode of instability that is short of dislocation, a sudden avulsion injury, or forceful entrapment of the labrum between the glenoid rim and humeral head. Glenohumeral instability that is short of dislocation causes shearing forces on the labrum, resulting in labral tears.[1] Disruption of the glenoid labrum is the most common injury seen in recurrently subluxating or dislocating shoulders.[117] (Fig. 3-20).

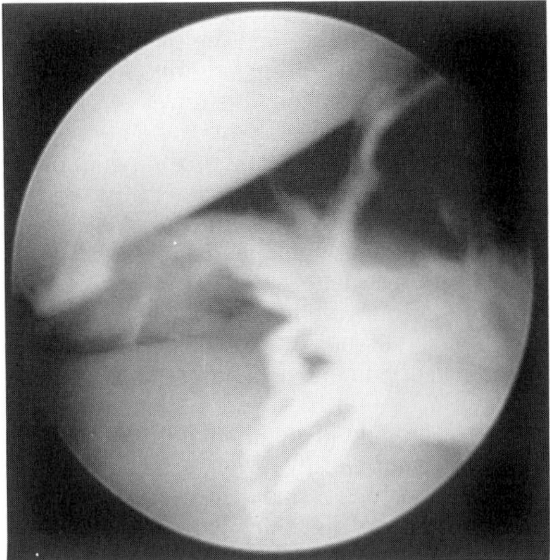

**Figure 3-20.** Labral fraying. (Reproduced with permission from Caspari RB, Jackson RW, Poehling GG. Operative arthroscopy. New York: Raven Press, 1991:494.)

Sudden superior labral avulsion injuries are usually secondary to a forceful eccentric contraction of the biceps. This is seen most often in individuals involved in racquet or throwing sports. Large, eccentric forces of the biceps are involved in the deceleration of throwing and may result in avulsion of the superior labrum at the biceps attachment.[1,6,117] In the acceleration phase of throwing, horizontal adduction and internal rotation may produce a humeral grinding force on the anterior and superior glenoid labrum. Individuals with weak posterior stabilizing musculature may be more susceptible to this mechanism of injury.[19]

Finally, entrapment of the labrum between the humeral head and glenoid fossa may occur secondary to a fall on an outstretched abducted arm. This results in a shearing injury to the labrum.[6] A common labral injury is referred to as the *SLAP lesion*. This lesion consists of damage to the *s*uperior *l*abrum that extends from *a*nterior to *p*osterior. It may be the result of any of the macrotrauma mechanisms of injury: superior labral entrapment after a fall on the outstretched arm, forceful eccentric biceps contraction, or glenohumeral instability that results in detachment of the labrum from the glenoid rim, the Bankart lesion. In general, anterior labral damage is associated with forceful abduction, extension, and external rotation. Superior lesions appear to be more degenerative in nature, whereas inferior lesions are associated with instability. Posterior labral damage occurs when a strong posterior force is applied in the direction of the long axis of the humerus when the shoulder is in a position of 90 degrees of flexion and minimal adduction.[117]

## HISTORY AND PRESENTATION

Damage to the glenoid labrum may manifest functionally by allowing the shoulder to subluxate or dislocate recurrently. It also may cause the shoulder to click, catch, or lock secondary to partially attached fragments being interposed between articular surfaces. Patients with labral damage are generally able to accurately localize their pain anteriorly or posteriorly. This pain may be constant or intermittent and may be a general ache or sharp pain in the shoulder and arm. Patients will typically complain of a clicking, locking, or catching sensation in their shoulder similar to that described with a meniscal tear in the knee. These patients also will report feelings of shoulder instability. Typically symptoms will improve with rest and will increase with return to activity.

On physical examination, passive and active range of motion will be full and pain free, with the possible exception of a painful click at some point in the range. There will not usually be any noticeable strength deficits. Special tests that are valuable in diagnosing labral tears include anterior and posterior apprehension tests due to the related instability and the clunk or grind tests. The anterior apprehension test is positive if the patient has a look or reports a feeling of apprehension when the examiner slowly abducts and externally rotates the shoulder. In the posterior apprehension test, the examiner forward flexes and medially rotates the shoulder and applies a posterior force on the patient's elbow. This test also may cause pain as the labral attachments are strained. Again, the test is positive if the patient is apprehensive.[78] The clunk test is performed with the patient's arm in full abduction while supine (Fig. 3-21). The examiner provides an anterior force to the posterior aspect of the humeral head with one hand while passively rotating the humerus with the other hand. A tear in the labrum may produce a clunk or grinding sound when hit by the humeral head.[46] Palpation of the shoulder may produce generalized tenderness that is usually accurately localized to anterior or posterior regions. Joint mobility may be increased as compared with the uninvolved shoulder, particularly with anterior and posterior glides. Many times a painful click is present during respective glides.

## DIAGNOSTIC TESTS

X-rays will be negative unless the labral tear has occurred in conjunction with a dislocation causing a Hill-Sachs lesion (posterolateral defect of

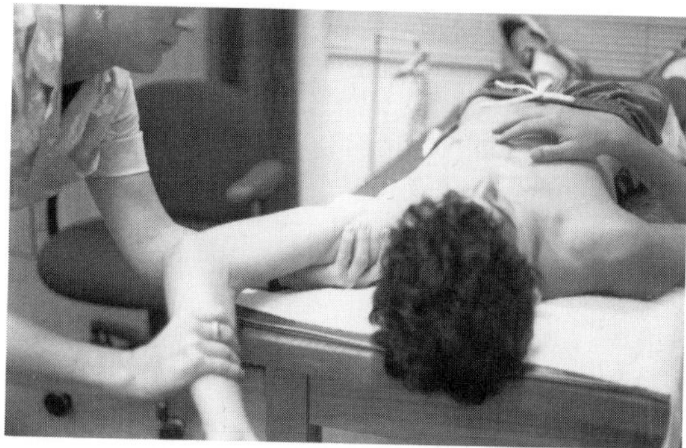

**Figure 3-21.** The clunk/grind test. This test should be performed at multiple angles of abduction as the arm is internally and externally rotated.

the humeral head) or a bony Bankart lesion (detachment of the glenoid labrum with avulsion fracture of the glenoid rim). Arthroscopy can be used for diagnosis of labral tears and subsequent resection of the torn piece. Examination under anesthesia (EUA) is helpful to determine the extent of shoulder instability. If subluxation is present, a capsulorrhaphy may be suggested in addition to partial labral resection. Otherwise, functional glenohumeral instability will continue. Anterior subluxation is often associated with an anteroinferior labral tear, while posterior subluxation is often associated with a midposterior labral tear. If the EUA is negative for subluxation, simple resection of the torn labral piece is all that is needed. Capsulorrhaphy should be avoided in the absence of anatomic instability because it causes needless contracture of anterior or posterior shoulder structures.[117]

Glenohumeral CT arthrography is the most definitive and reliable test for detecting labral pathology. An arthrogram with axillary views of the glenohumeral joint is necessary to obtain a profile view of the labrum including both anterior and posterior portions. Subtle labral changes seen with arthrography consist of irregular margins and indicate general degeneration. However, the arthrogram is quite sensitive in detecting the movement of contrast material into complete or incomplete labral tears. If a tear is incomplete, the labrum will appear notched. If the tear is complete, contrast material will accumulate, and only a small remainder of the anterior or posterior labrum will be seen.[117] It is possible that a patient will present with defects in both the anterior and posterior labrum, but injury is more commonly isolated to only one region.

### MANAGEMENT

Conservative management of labral tears simply consists of ice, relative rest (especially from overhead activities), and strengthening to balance shoulder musculature and prevent further injury. Despite strengthening efforts, the patient may continue to complain of functional instability, and a painful click will remain as long as a fragment of the labrum is lodged between articular surfaces. Therefore, arthroscopic surgery is most often required to alleviate symptoms. Postoperative management for labral resection generally consists of a brief immobilization period (2 to 4 days), followed by strengthening, stretching, and a gradual return to functional activities. In general, full range of motion should be obtained in 4 weeks, and patients should be able to return to sports within 3 months.[19] Long-term follow-up reveals excellent recovery after labral resection.[117] If glenohumeral instability is present and a capsulorrhaphy is required in addition to labral resection, postoperative management will be dictated by the rehabilitation parameters of the capsular reconstruction performed. This will involve a longer period of immobilization (3 to 6 weeks), followed by active/active assisted range of motion, joint mobilization, and passive stretching within the parameters of the surgical reconstruction. Strengthening will progress from isometrics to progressive resistive exercise to isokinetics and functional training. Return to sports generally occurs at about 6 to 9 months after surgery.

## Acromioclavicular Separation

The acromioclavicular joint is a diarthrodial joint formed by the junction of the medial aspect of the acromion and the distal end of the clavicle. In approximately 50 percent of the population, these joint surfaces are separated by a disc or meniscus.[169] The bony configuration of the acromioclavicular joint does not provide inherent stability. Stability of this joint must be derived from the surrounding ligaments and musculature. Superiorly, the joint capsule is thickened by the superior acromioclavicular ligament, and inferiorly, the capsule is strengthened by the thin inferior acromioclavicular ligament.[52] The superior ligament provides two-thirds of the force necessary to prevent superior and posterior displacement.[136] This ligament is considered the most important stabilizer of the joint for normal activities of daily living.[104] In addition, there are two coracoclavicular ligaments. The trapezoid ligament passes from the coracoid process to the anterior clavicle and functions to prevent anterior subluxation.[52] The conoid ligament originates on the base of the coracoid process and passes superiorly and anteriorly to attach to the inferior surface of the clavicle just medial to the trapezoid ligament.[169] Muscular stabilization of the acromioclavicular joint is provided by the deltoid and trapezius muscles, which envelope the joint.

## MECHANISM OF INJURY

Injury to the acromioclavicular joint resulting in separation accounts for only 12 percent of dislocations of the shoulder complex (glenohumeral, acromioclavicular, and sternoclavicular joints).[169] Injury is almost always related to a traumatic event. Most often the mechanism of injury is a direct blow to the shoulder or an indirect injury caused by a fall on an outstretched hand. It is estimated that approximately 70 percent of acromioclavicular dislocations are the result of a direct blow to the shoulder.[136] This injury is more frequent in sports such as football, lacrosse, ice hockey, and wrestling secondary to violent contact of the shoulder with the playing surface, lacrosse sticks, or another player. Often the forces applied to the shoulder are twofold: the weight and force of one player contacting another and the shoulder striking a fixed surface such as the ground. These two forces drive the acromion and humerus inferiorly, leaving the clavicle behind and resulting in rupture of some or all of the supporting ligaments of the joint. The consequence is an apparent superior or posterior displacement of the clavicle.[104,169] Typically, the superior acromioclavicular ligament is strained and/or ruptured first. With more violent forces, this is followed by rupture of the two coracoclavicular ligaments. Trauma to the deltoid and trapezius musculature, such as detachment or contusion, is likely to occur if the forces applied to the joint are overly excessive.[122,169]

## CLASSIFICATIONS

Injury to the acromioclavicular joint has been classified according to the extent of damage to the supporting structures of the joint. One of the most widely accepted classification schemes was described by Allman[3] (Fig. 3-22). Grade I injury or sprain is secondary to a mild force and involves only partial tearing of some of the fibers of the acromioclavicular ligament and capsule. Grade II injury, known as *separation* or *subluxation*, results from a moderate force and involves complete rupture of some of the fibers of the capsule and acromioclavicular ligament. Finally, grade III injury, known as *complete acromioclavicular dislocation*, is the result of a very violent force causing complete rupture of the acromioclavicular and coracoclavicular ligaments. This type of injury also may involve damage to supporting musculature.[3,103] In severe grade III injuries, the clavicle may be locked pos-

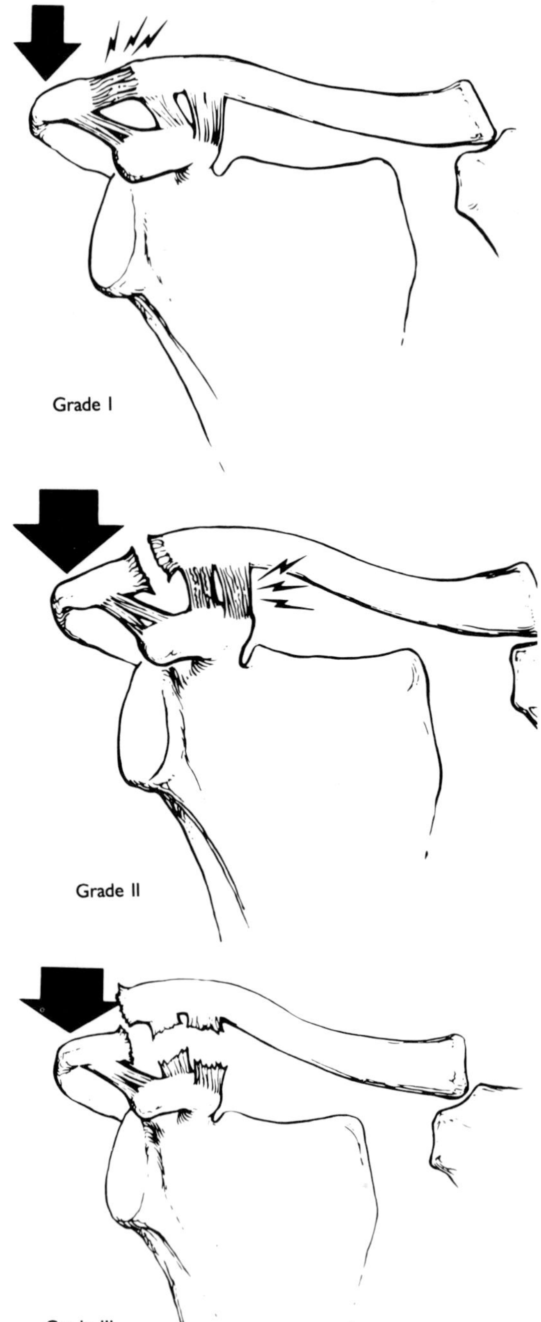


**Figure 3-22.** Classification of acromioclavicular separations. (a) Grade I injury or sprain tears some of the fibers of the acromioclavicular ligament and capsule. (b) Grade II injury involves complete rupture of some of the fibers of the capsule and acromioclavicular ligament. (c) Finally, grade III injury causes complete rupture of the acromioclavicular and coracoclavicular ligaments. (Reproduced with permission from Rockwood CA Jr, Thomas SC, Matsen FA III. Subluxations and dislocations about the glenohumeral joint. In Rockwood CA Jr, Green DP, Bucholz RW, eds. Fractures in adults. 3rd ed. Vol. 1. Philadelphia: JB Lippincott, 1991:1193.)

teriorly and superiorly on top of the acromion or may actually "buttonhole" through the trapezius so that it is palpable under the skin.[104]

## HISTORY AND PRESENTATION

Diagnosis of acromioclavicular injury is based on radiographs (x-rays), history, and physical examination. With a grade I injury, physical examination will reveal minimal pain, minimal point tenderness at the acromioclavicular joint, possible soft-tissue swelling, and perhaps a slight decrease in active range of motion, particularly end-range abduction and horizontal adduction.[3, 103, 169] X-rays are negative. In grade II injuries, all the preceding findings will be seen with the addition of a joint deformity confirmed on x-ray. This deformity may be seen with the naked eye as either a superior or posterior prominence of the distal clavicle. With grade II injuries there will almost always be pain with active range of motion. In sequence, grade III injuries include the preceding findings with the joint deformity being obvious and x-rays confirming the diagnosis. The clavicle "appears" to be displaced superiorly, although it is actually the scapula that is displaced inferiorly. This deformity occurs because the coracoclavicular ligaments are the scapula's "bridge" to the clavicle, which attaches to the axial skeleton. Without these ligaments, the weight of the arm displaces the scapula and humerus inferiorly, giving the appearance of a superiorly migrated clavicle.

Because most clinicians refer to the clavicle as superior, we will use this direction, keeping in mind the preceding discussion. The displacement can be appreciated on physical examination by a "ballottable" clavicle, a clavicle that can be manually depressed inferiorly but will bounce back superiorly.[3, 122] The high-riding clavicle is a significant cosmetic deformity, and many patients are unhappy with this appearance.[122, 167] Active range of motion will be very painful, and the patient will often hold the arm in an adducted position for protection and comfort.[103]

Radiographs are a key element of diagnosis and classification of acromioclavicular injury. Grading is based on two different sets of osseous landmarks. The first is the displacement between the distal clavicle with respect to the articulating acromion, and the second is the widening between the coracoid and inferior distal clavicle. In grade I sprains, no abnormalities are identified on x-ray. This is the case even when radiographs are taken with the patient holding weights. A grade II injury, or subluxation, will result in a widening of the acromioclavicular joint or coracoclavicular space on radiographs with or without the holding of weights. The increase in joint space will be less than or equal to the width of the clavicle. In grade III injuries, or dislocation, the radiograph will reveal displacement of the clavicle that is greater than the width of the clavicle or an increased coracoclavicular space of 25 to 100 percent greater than the normal side.

## MANAGEMENT

The appropriate management of acromioclavicular joint injuries is somewhat controversial; however, the controversy is centered on the management of grade III injuries, or complete dislocations. It is commonly thought that grade I and II acromioclavicular sprains are best treated conservatively, nonoperatively, and symptomatically. Grade I injuries are treated with rest and a sling for the patient's comfort for a brief period, usually a few days. Ice may be used acutely for management of pain and swelling. Pain-free range-of-motion exercises are advocated early on, especially in an athlete. Progressive resistive exercises are initiated within the patient's tolerance, with a focus on the deltoid and trapezius. The patient may return to regular recreational activities when symptom-free.[3, 34, 104, 136, 169]

Grade II injuries are treated similarly, with increased importance placed on the use of a sling. In this situation, the sling is used to provide comfort as well as some reduction of the subluxation. The sling will typically be worn 2 to 3 weeks. Some physicians prefer the Kenny-Howard sling (Fig. 3-23). While this sling can achieve reduction, it requires constant care and frequent adjustments to maintain an appropriate clavicular position.[104, 169] In a study of 164 acromioclavicular injuries, Cox[34] determined that the use of an acromioclavicular immobilizer (Kenny-Howard sling) resulted in improved position on

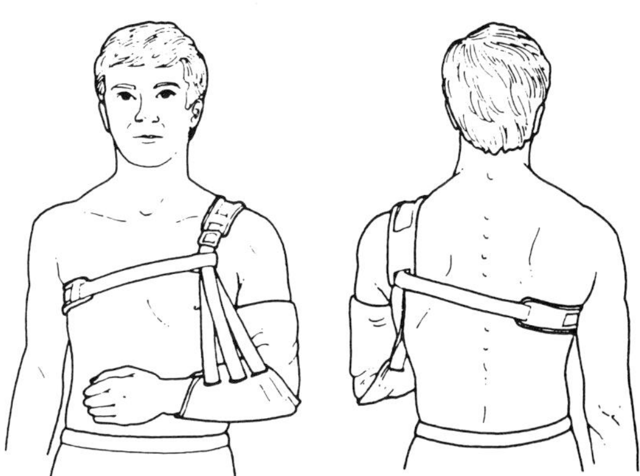

**Figure 3-23.** The Kenny-Howard sling. (Reproduced with permission from Rowe C. The shoulder, acromioclavicluar-sternoclavicular joints. New York: Churchill Livingstone, 1988:299.)

radiographs and fewer symptoms than were experienced by individuals not immobilized. However, patient compliance is very difficult to ensure with this device. In an athlete or overhead laborer, compliance should be strongly encouraged because this may reduce the likelihood of developing traumatic arthritis or at least retard the rate at which arthritic changes occur.

The management of grade III injuries is extremely controversial, with two distinct schools of thought. Advocates of closed treatment, or "skillful neglect," feel that nonoperative, symptomatic management and appropriate rehabilitation are quite successful. Symptomatic treatment again consists of rest, ice, and immobilization. The immobilization period is generally extended to 4 to 6 weeks, followed by rehabilitation for range of motion and strengthening using active exercise, appropriate isokinetics, and sport-specific training focusing on the deltoid and trapezius muscles.[3,34,136,169] Rowe[136] reported that 80 percent of patients treated conservatively were satisfied to the point where they desired no further intervention. In a recent study by Tibone et al.,[154] it was determined that no significant loss of strength was noted with conservative care of grade III injuries. The most frequent complications of closed treatment include residual pain, weakness, cosmetic deformity, and subluxation.

In contrast, open treatment is advocated by some to ensure appropriate reduction. Many operative techniques, repair or reconstruction of torn stabilizing structures, joint excision, and internal fixation, have been used, with the goal joint stability.[3] The most frequent surgical interventions employed include stabilization of the clavicle to the coracoid process by fixation wire or screw, fixation of the acromioclavicular joint with transfer of the coracoacromial ligament to form a new superior acromioclavicular ligament, or resection of the distal end of the clavicle. Partial clavicular resection is usually indicated only with old symptomatic dislocations and should only involve the distal 1 cm of bone.[136] Open reduction is followed by a period of immobilization and then rehabilitation in the form of range of motion and strengthening in the same manner as for closed management. The most frequent complications encountered with open reduction include wound infection, migration of fixation devices, degenerative arthritis, and residual pain and weakness.

In addition to being a complication of open reduction, degenerative arthritis may be a sequela of closed treatment. Degenerative changes seem to occur frequently in acromioclavicular joints, even after minor trauma, but are particularly common with grade II and III injuries.[3] The degeneration is thought to be secondary to uneven contact of joint surfaces, unrecognized fractures, or articular derangement and is progressive as one ages.[3,136] Aggressive overhead use of the arm, also may escalate the arthritic processes. The pain associated with chronic symptomatic dislocations is generally thought to be secondary to these arthritic changes and can only be relieved with resection of the distal end of the clavicle.[136] For this reason, nonoperative symptomatic treatment may eventually require operative intervention. In most cases it is wiser to avoid surgical intervention if at all possible.

# Arthritis

Severe shoulder pain and disability caused by arthritis are relatively uncommon, occurring in only 5 to 10 percent of all patients complaining of shoulder pain.[15,43] Of the specific arthritic entities that may cause shoulder disability, rheumatoid arthritis is by far the most frequent.

## RHEUMATOID ARTHRITIS

Rheumatoid arthritis is a systemic disease, affecting many joints, but the shoulder is infrequently the focus of treatment. When the shoulder is affected, the inflammatory and destructive process involves the entire shoulder girdle, including the bursa, rotator cuff, scapula, and musculature.[44] These structures may be involved to varying degrees. Rheumatoid arthritis usually presents bilaterally, but its effect in the dominant side is generally more significant.[43] Neer[99] assigns three classifications to rheumatoid arthritis of the shoulder: dry, wet, and resorptive. In *dry* rheumatoid arthritis, there is a tendency for loss of joint space, periarticular sclerosis, bone cysts, and stiffness. *Wet* rheumatoid arthritis is characterized by proliferative synovial disease with marginal erosions and intrusion of the humeral head into the glenoid. Finally, *resorptive* rheumatoid arthritis is demonstrated by significant resorption of the humeral head or the glenoid.[30] Other characteristics of rheumatoid arthritis at the shoulder include a primary subdeltoid-subacromial bursitis, bicipital tenosynovitis and tendinitis, isolated rotator cuff tendinitis, and reflex sympathetic dystrophy.[30,35]

### HISTORY AND PRESENTATION

Pain is the most common complaint of the patient with symptomatic rheumatoid arthritis of the shoulder. Patients will complain of pain in the activities of daily living as well as at rest. In the course of this disease, the patient experiences episodes of acute pain as well as periods of relative symptomatic remission. In the acute phase, the patient frequently splints the shoulder in a position of adduction and internal rotation. This results in capsular tightening and loss of motion.[35]

On physical examination, muscular wasting is evident, and there is occasional bulging over the anterior proximal humerus, which may be due to joint effusion and bursitis. Range of motion is decreased in all directions actively as well as passively, and passive motion can prove to be quite painful due to inflammation of the synovium.[168] Early in the disease, strength is usually good in the limited range of motion, but over time, progressive loss of strength accompanies the loss of motion. In the acute phase, there is tenderness and warmth to palpation over the anterior and posterior aspects of the joint and superiorly over the acromion. After the acute episode has subsided, specific tenderness to palpation is not frequently identified.[35]

## MANAGEMENT

### Conservative

Because of the systemic nature of rheumatoid arthritis, therapeutic management consists primarily of drug therapy. However, physical therapy is vital to maintain functional range of motion, assist with pain control, and educate the patient in joint protection and long-term management of this chronic disease.[168] During the acute phase, gentle range-of-motion activities are indicated to the point of the patient's tolerance. Isotonic strengthening exercises are often contraindicated because they tend to exacerbate the inflammatory process, but isometric exercise may be implemented. Palliative measures such as transcutaneous electrical stimulation (TENS), ice, heat, phonophoresis, and iontophoresis are frequently used, while some physicians occasionally provide an intraarticular steroid injection because this may be an effective adjunctive treatment to help control localized inflammation.[35,43,44] The patient must be taught to modify activities of daily living to prevent stress or overload on the acutely swollen joint. When symptoms subside, isotonic strengthening exercises using light forms of resistance such as elastic bands, manual resistance, or 1- to 2-lb cuff weights are initiated as well as stretching exercises in an attempt to regain lost motion. Finally, maintenance exercises consisting of range of motion, strengthening, and endurance are advised for optimal long-term function.[51]

### Surgical

When conservative management fails to give the patient adequate relief of pain, surgical measures are considered. The surgical procedures that are performed most frequently include synovectomy, bursectomy, acromioplasty, and arthroplasty.[88] The goal of physical therapy following these surgical procedures is to facilitate recovery of range of motion, strength, and function while reducing pain. When a synovectomy, bursectomy, or acromioplasty is performed, a progressive range-of-motion and strengthening program is implemented with attention to joint effusion. Rehabilitation activities should not increase effusion, and appropriate modalities may be used to help control swelling.

Total shoulder arthroplasty or replacement (TSR) is the operative choice in a patient with chronic pain and loss of functional range of motion due to severe articular damage. The prosthesis most frequently used is the Neer prosthesis. It consists of a metal humeral head with an intermedullary fixation stem and a polyethylene glenoid component. (See Chap. 4 for a full explanation of surgical technique.) The function of the shoulder following arthroplasty depends on the reconstruction and rehabilitation of supporting musculature, specifically the deltoid and rotator cuff muscles.[88] Rehabilitation following a total shoulder arthroplasty should be guided and supervised by the physical therapist. The prognosis of a person with rheumatoid arthritis following a TSR depends on the extent of rotator cuff involvement. If poor-quality cuff tissue is present at the time of surgery, limited goals are expected. The physical therapist must have an appropriate understanding of the surgical procedure to allow for healing constraints. The main emphasis of physical therapy is protection of the arthroplasty.[7] There are many different postoperative regimens depending on the surgeon's interpretation of the stability of the implant, the quality of the soft-tissue or bone repair, and the surgeon's belief or disbelief in the benefits of early motion.[30]

### Postoperative Care

Neer[99] describes a three-phase postoperative rehabilitation program for total shoulder arthroplasty. Phase one begins 2 to 5 days following surgery. Passive and gentle active assistive range-of-motion exercises including supine flexion and external rotation with the elbow bent at the side of the body are initiated. Range-of-motion exercises are progressive over the next 6 weeks. Pendulum exercises, assisted extension, pulleys, active assistive internal rotation behind the trunk, and active assistive external rotation with hands clasped behind the head and performed. Isometric flexion, extension, abduction, and internal and external rotation exercises are begun at about 3 weeks postoperatively. The second phase of the rehabilitation program is begun at 4 to 6 weeks postoperatively. Active exercises including supine forward elevation, active assistive standing flexion, and rotational exercises with controlled self-stretching are performed. Isometric exercises in the five previously mentioned patterns are continued, and comfortable resistance is added to the active motion. When performing internal and external rotation exercises, the physical therapist must remember that the subscapularis muscle was released and reapproximated and must be allowed to heal without overstretching or overloading. The third phase of the rehabilitation program begins at about 3 months postoperatively. At this time, deficiencies in range of motion are addressed, with more assertive stretching and strengthening exercises being performed.[64, 100]

## OSTEOARTHRITIS

While osteoarthritis (degenerative joint disease) is the most common of all arthritic conditions, its presentation in the glenohumeral joint is less common compared with weight-bearing joints in the lower extremities.[43, 168] Degenerative changes can begin in the person as young as 20 years old, and these changes will usually peak in severity by the sixth decade.[51] Degenerative osteoarthritis in the relatively young patient also may be the result of anterior reconstructive shoulder procedures that have overconstrained the normal glenohumeral motions. In osteoarthritis, radiographs demonstrate joint space narrowing, subchondral sclerosis, peripheral osteophytes on both the inferior margin of the glenoid and the humeral neck, and cystic changes in the subchondral bone[43, 51, 168] (Fig. 3-24). There also may be degeneration in the surrounding soft tissues, primarily the rotator cuff, which will frequently result in partial- or full-thickness rotator cuff tears. Rupture of the long head of the biceps tendon is not uncommon with this condition. Typically, a patient with primary osteoarthritis with good rotator cuff function does well following a TSR. In contrast, primary damage to the rotator cuff causing weakness and abnormal biomechanics may in time lead to deterioration of the glenohumeral joint. This sequence of events, known as *rotator cuff arthropathy*, is treated in a similar fashion as osteoarthritis of the glenohumeral joint, except that the rotator cuff must be addressed.

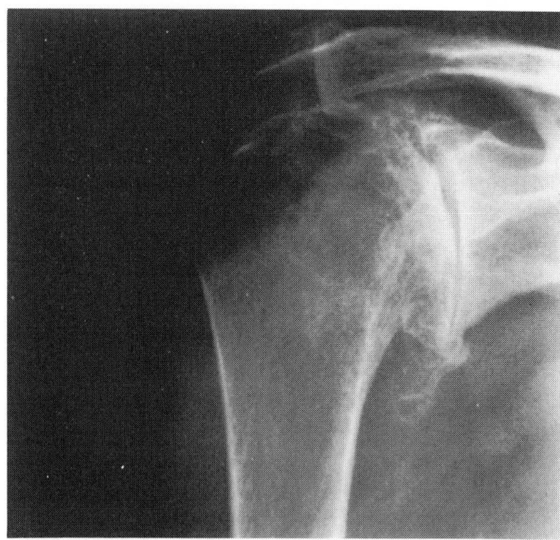

**Figure 3-24.** Osteoarthritis. In osteoarthritis, radiographs demonstrate joint space narrowing, subchondral sclerosis, peripheral osteophytes on both the inferior margin of the glenoid and the humeral neck, and cystic changes in the subchondral bone. (Reproduced with permission from Cofield RH. Degenerative and arthritic problems of the glenohumeral joint. In Rockwood CA Jr, Matsen FA III, eds. The shoulder. Philadelphia: WB Saunders, 1990:678.)

### MANAGEMENT

Conservative treatment of osteoarthritic disease will include anti-inflammatory medications, range-of-motion exercises, and moderate strengthening exercises, avoiding overuse or repetitive overhead work. Biomechanical studies have demonstrated that the resultant forces providing stability of the humerus on the glenoid reach their peak of at least 10.2 times the weight of the extremity at 90 degrees of elevation.[123] The physical therapist should keep in mind that elevation and abduction of the arm to 90 degrees place a significant stress on the glenohumeral joint. Once again, when conservative management fails to provide adequate relief of pain, surgical treatment must be considered.

## OSTEOARTHRITIS OF THE ACROMIOCLAVICULAR JOINT

Degenerative disease of the acromioclavicular joint is not uncommon.[168] It is one of the joints that demonstrates early degenerative change. Osteophytic proliferation can begin in a middle-aged person and progress with age; this can compromise the supraspinatus outlet, causing impingement.[166] The disease process is usually due to previous traumatic injury or generalized osteoarthritis. Degenerative disease of the acromioclavicular joint presents in two ways on clinical examination. The first is associated with impingement of the rotator cuff, demonstrated by a painful arc of abduction between 60 and 120 degrees. This presentation frequently coincides with radiologic evidence of a large bone spur on the inferior aspect of the acromioclavicular joint. Other patients will present with diffuse shoulder pain and a high painful arc with arm elevation between 120 and 180 degrees of abduction. Pain in this pattern is caused as the acromion is compressed against the clavicle, and there is frequently localized tenderness on palpation of the acromioclavicular joint. Radiographs will often demonstrate acromioclavicular joint narrowing and sclerotic changes. Treatment of the degenerative acromioclavicular joint depends on the patient's presenting symptoms. In the presence of a degenerative spur associated with a painful arc, medical therapy and activity modification are the first treatments of choice. If these fail, subacromial decompression will often be performed. Localized acromioclavicular joint pain also will be treated with activity modification and analgesic therapy. A long-acting corticosteroid injection into the joint space can greatly reduce the pain.[168] If conservative treatment of localized acromioclavicular joint pain fails, the surgeon may choose to perform a distal clavicle resection or arthroplasty.

### OTHER OSTEOARTHRITIC DISORDERS

Many other arthritic diseases can affect the shoulder joint, but none as frequently as rheumatoid arthritis. These include juvenile rheumatoid arthritis, osteonecrosis, neuropathic arthritis, ankylosing spondylitis, crystal-induced arthritis (gout and pseudogout), and polymyalgia rheumatica, to name just a few. Diseases of the connective tissues are by no means completely understood, and it is likely that some subtle forms of arthritis affecting the shoulder joint are not easily recognizable. Differential diagnosis is made through performance of laboratory testing of blood and joint aspirates. A careful history must be taken and clinical examination performed in conjunction with these studies for an accurate diagnosis to be made.[43] Although the etiology of arthritic disease of the shoulder can be quite different, the outcome is similar—a variable degree of destruction of the articular surfaces as well as the soft tissue of the shoulder. Treatment is directed at the symptoms and generally follows the same guidelines as those discussed for rheumatoid arthritis. The goal of physical therapy is to decrease pain and inflammation and to recover and maintain as much range of motion as possible, allowing the patient maximal function in necessary daily activities.

## Adhesive Capsulitis

Frequently referred to as "frozen shoulder," adhesive capsulitis affects women more frequently than men and most often occurs during their fourth, fifth, or sixth decade of life.[32,70,101,164] Controlled studies also have demonstrated increased incidence of adhesive capsulitis in patients with diabetes. In these patients, symptoms often occur at a younger age and are very frequently bilateral. The prognosis may be worse in the diabetic patient with a longer duration of symptoms and more residual limitation of motion.[59] The reasons for this are as yet undetermined. Adhesive capsulitis is one of the most common orthopedic complaints of the shoulder. Despite its frequency, its etiology remains unknown and controversial.

### PATHOGENESIS

The pathology was first described by Duplay in 1872 as "periarthrite scapulohumerale," with the onset attributed to subacromial bursitis.[59] In 1934, Codman[28] described "frozen shoulder" as "essentially a tendinitis, with only secondary involvement of the bursa. . . . a history of trauma is absent, vague or not clearly associated with the onset of symptoms." J. Neviaser[102] introduced the term *adhesive capsulitis* in 1945 when he discovered dense thickening of the shoulder with intraarticular adhesions, especially in the dependent axillary fold. DePalma[39] reported that frozen shoulder syndrome was caused by bicipital tenosynovitis, and Simmonds[147] reported that "vascular reactions around areas of degeneration" in the supraspinatus tendon were the essential cause of the frozen shoulder. Reeves[129] defined frozen shoulder as "an idiopathic condition of the shoulder characterized by the spontaneous onset of pain in the shoulder with restriction of every movement in every direction." T. Neviaser[108] went on to describe the stages of this pathology as seen by arthroscopy. Despite years of research and treatment of these patients, most would concur with Codman's opinion[28] in 1934: "This is a class of cases which I find difficult to define, difficult to treat and difficult to explain from the point of view of pathology."

It is generally accepted that the glenohumeral capsule becomes inflamed, thickened, fibrotic, and adherent to the humeral head.[101,108] Primary and secondary classifications have been proposed. In *primary* adhesive capsulitis, the onset is spontaneous with no particular trauma, whereas *secondary* adhesive capsulitis is frequently due to a previous, perhaps minor trauma, immobilization, or systemic disorder.[60,110] The disease process primarily affects the loose, redundant axillary fold, causing progressive shoulder pain and a severe restriction of both passive and active range of motion.

Regardless of the etiology, the clinical picture presents three consecutive stages in the disease process, each one of which usually lasts 3 to 4 months: pain (freezing), stiffness (frozen), and recovery (thawing).[129,140,164] The stiffness stage is frequently related to the recovery stage; the longer the stiffness, the longer is the recovery.[129] This pathology tends to be self-limiting but can last anywhere from 6 months to 3 years.[110,129,131,153,164] Although no treatment has been shown to be consistently effective, it does seem that the recovery process can be accelerated with such therapeutic measures as heat, joint mobilization, stretching, and anti-inflammatories.

T. Neviaser[108] describes four stages in the disease process which are identifiable by arthroscopy. In stage I, the patient has mild signs and symptoms mimicking an impingement syndrome, where restriction of motion is minimal and it appears that pain could be due to a rotator cuff tendinitis. Typical conservative treatments for the rotator cuff in these specific patients fail. Arthroscopy at this time would demonstrate "erythematous fibrinous pannus over the synovium" in the axillary fold. In the second stage, arthroscopy would show the synovium to be "red, angry, and thickened," with adhesions growing across the fold onto the humeral head. The normal space between the humeral head and the glenoid is lost. In this stage the physical examination would demonstrate a loss of motion in all planes as well as pain in all parts of the range of motion. Stage III typically shows only a "pink synovitis" not as abundant as in the second stage. By now, the axillary fold is approximately half its original size, and the humeral head continues to be compressed into the glenoid even with traction. Finally, in stage IV, synovitis is no longer apparent, but the axillary fold is severely contracted and range of motion is at its most restricted level.[108]

Clinical diagnosis of adhesive capsulitis can become quite frustrating because of other conditions present with similar signs and symptoms. Arthrography has been the standard diagnostic technique, although the history and clinical presentation typically suffice to make the diagnosis. The affected shoulder demonstrates a significant loss of joint volume. Where the normal joint would hold 20 to 30 ml of dye, the shoulder with adhesive capsulitis can only accommodate 5 to 10 ml of fluid. A loss of the redundant axillary fold is also noted[18,101,108,129,131] (Fig. 3-25). However, these classic arthrographic changes will not be apparent during the early stage ("freezing") or late in the resolution phase ("thawing"), when normal arthrograms are often seen.[59]

## HISTORY AND PRESENTATION

The patient presents to the clinician with shoulder pain referring to the region of the deltoid insertion.[32] Frequently, pain will radiate down

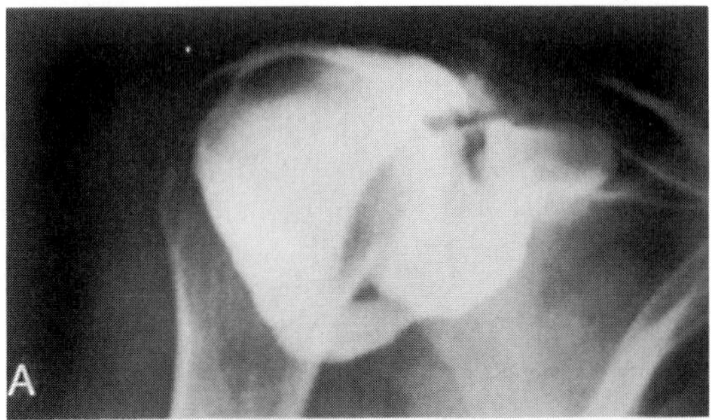


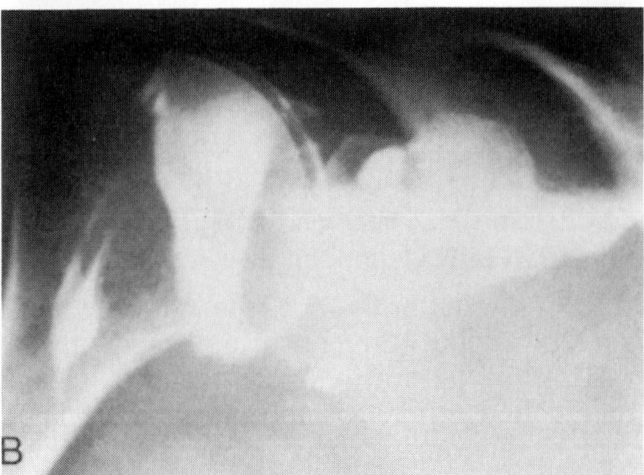


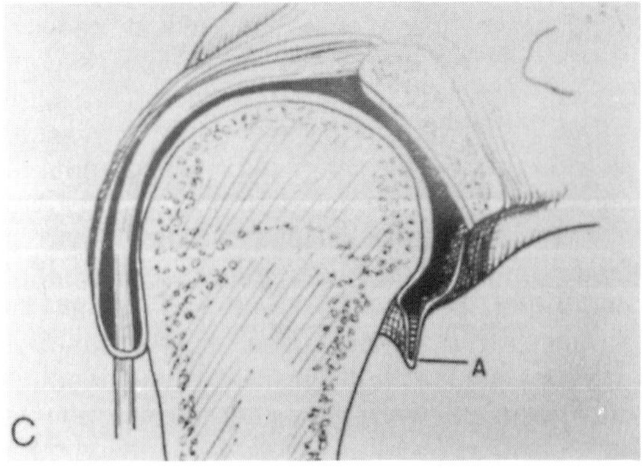


**Figure 3-25.** Arthrography. Arthrography has been the standard diagnostic technique for adhesive capsulitis. The affected shoulder will demonstrate a significant loss of joint volume. In addition, one often notices loss of the redundant axillary fold. (Reproduced with permission from Neviaser TJ. Adhesive capsulitis. Orthop Clin North Am 1987;18:439.)

the lateral aspect of the upper arm (C5 dermatome) and possibly into the forearm.[131] Patients typically complain of difficulty with the activities of daily living, particularly those motions requiring end-range elevation, internal rotation, or external rotation. Patients also experience pain at night when attempting to sleep on the affected side. The symptoms are usually gradual in onset, and reports of pain vary from mild to severe. More often than not these patients initially report their complaints to a clinician several weeks to several months after onset. Occasionally, the patient presents with a passive, timid personality who tends to dismiss his or her own health issues, being preoccupied with spouse, children, or occupation. This psychological profile is important to understand in one's approach to these patients. They often need firm reassurance that their condition will improve. They also need to understand that they must play an important role in their rehabilitation. The treating clinician needs to realize that the success of clinical care is very dependent on not harming or hurting these patients, since this will often cause them to withdraw from treatment. Gaining the trust of such patients is critical to success. An important part of earning such patients' trust takes place during the initial evaluation. By being thorough, reassuring, and gentle in one's approach, each clinician improves his or her chances of being instrumental in improving such patients' condition.

On physical examination, patients demonstrate increased compensatory scapulothoracic motion. Mild atrophy of the deltoid and supraspinatus may be apparent.[131] Their active and passive ranges of motion are both limited by end-range pain. The true end feel with passive range-of-motion testing is capsular, although there is often protective muscle guarding masking the true limitation to passive motion. The clinical test of most value in diagnosing adhesive capsulitis is limitation of motion which follows a typical capsular pattern; external rotation is most limited, followed by abduction and then internal rotation. All planes of motion are affected to some degree, and all accessory motions of the glenohumeral joint are limited, including inferior, anterior, and posterior glides and lateral distraction.[164] All these patients present with a significant limitation of less than 90 degrees of passive glenohumeral coronal plane abduction. Often, scapulothoracic motion compensates for decreased glenohumeral movement and is easily noted during active elevation. Elevation of the arm is typically performed with significant shoulder girdle hunching.[131] Strength testing in the available motion is usually strong and asymptomatic, although pain with resisted motions can be present during the freezing phase. Palpation often reveals a diffuse tenderness, but identification of an area of point-specific tenderness is difficult.[59,101,131]

Certainly, several other pathologic conditions can create painful restriction of glenohumeral motion and should not be confused with adhesive capsulitis. As stated earlier, the arthrogram can be of value to help rule out other conditions, including "arthritides, neglected dislocations (particularly posterior), calcific tendinitis, local tumors, stroke shoulder, cerebral and pulmonary lesions, referred pain (cervical or abdominal), rotator cuff tears, and immobilization of shoulder following fracture."[140]

## MANAGEMENT

Management of adhesive capsulitis consists primarily of a passive stretching program.[32,108,164] This should be initiated with heat, either superficial or deep, applied to the axillary area, allowing for relaxation and/or an increase in the extensibility of collagen fibers within the connective tissues. Joint mobilization primarily consisting of inferior glides and distraction should precede stretching. Passive stretching is preferred over active stretching because it allows greater mechanical advantage than the patient's muscle power alone. However, it is important that forceful stretching be avoided, particularly in the freezing phases. The patient must complement the physical therapy program with diligent adherence to a home exercise program, including pendulum exercises and passive and active assistive stretching activities. In independent stretching activities, as well as with clinical treatment, the principles of low-load, long-duration techniques should be utilized because these forces are more likely to induce permanent connective-tissue changes and are less likely to harm the patient or increase the patient's apprehension. Infrequently, during the application of these techniques, an audible sound can be heard or felt by the patient and/or the clinician. Often, following this response to passive treatment, the patient and clinician appreciate an improvement in passive and active range. When this takes place without any adverse reactions such as pain, swelling, or more limited range, it is speculated that an intra- or extraarticular adhesion has been ruptured. It is reassuring to both patient and clinician if the likelihood of this type of response is explained ahead of time. The importance of the patient adhering to a regular home exercise program cannot be overemphasized. In addition to stretching exercises, strengthening exercises should be performed through available and improving range of motion. These patients need frequent contact with the treating therapist to ensure compliance with their home program. One of the best ways to accomplish this is to monitor their knowledge of their program by having them frequently repeat their exercises in the clinic. The frequency of clinical treatment can be reduced as the patient progresses with range of motion. One helpful guideline is that when the patient reaches 165 degrees of passive elevation and 90 degrees of passive glenohumeral abduction, then in most cases the emphasis shifts to a home program. When patients reach this goal, there seems to be less likelihood of them regressing, and they can be monitored weekly, biweekly, or perhaps monthly. Functional use of the extremity for activities of daily living is encouraged. Oral anti-inflammatories may help in the reduction of pain and the inflammatory process, while the use of corticosteroid injections is somewhat controversial, with inconsistent results.[164]

When all conservative measures fail, if progress plateaus without an acceptable amount of motion, or if the condition worsens, surgery may need to be performed in an attempt to restore lost motion. In some cases, manipulation under general anesthesia followed by physical therapy will be adequate to regain motion. With the scapula stabilized, the arm is taken into 90 degrees of pure abduction. After manipulation into external rotation is performed, further abduction can be obtained. Finally, the arm is rotated internally. The operator can usually hear and feel adhesions tear.[32,108] Care must be taken during manipulation because overaggressiveness can result in complications, including "fractures and dislocations of the humerus, ruptures of the rotator cuff, increased inflammation and scarring, and even radial palsy."[140] Contraindications for manipulation include a history of instability or dislocations, fractures, or neoplasms. It is important to recall these possible consequences and contraindications when choosing to performing manual therapy in the clinical setting as well. If full range of motion is not achieved with manipulation, arthrotomy may be necessary. The arthrotomy is performed in the anteroinferior portion of the axillary fold. The capsule is incised, and the wound is closed without suturing of the capsule.[108] Distension of the capsule by infiltration debrisement[70,140,164] or arthroscopy[131] also has been reported to be of value in the treatment of adhesive capsulitis. Following surgery, the patient must follow a strict stretching regimen, as described earlier.

As a note of caution, adhesive capsulitis should not be referred to as a *frozen shoulder*, which is an all-inclusive term for many pathologies limiting motion of the shoulder. This error may result in improper treatment, since the specific pathology has not been identified. Diagnostic tests can often rule out other causes of limited passive range of motion. Once these other causes have been ruled out, one can proceed with a certain degree of assurance that one is dealing with adhesive capsulitis. Patients should respond to clinical treatment, although their response is often slow. Any improvement in passive range of motion is considered a positive response to treatment. If patients demonstrate no response to clinical care in 3 to 4 weeks, they should be referred for further diagnostic workup.

## Infection

Infection of the shoulder joint is an uncommon pathology. This is due primarily to the normal defense mechanisms, excellent blood perfusion, and antibiotic prophylaxis.[55] However, the rapid morbidity of shoulder sepsis requires that the signs, symptoms, disease progression, and treatment options be familiar to all clinicians.

Susceptibility of a joint to infection is determined by the adequacy of one's defense mechanisms.[55] With this in mind, it follows logically that sepsis is found most commonly in older individuals (over 60 years) with other major medical problems or individuals with some degree of suppression of their immune system.[75]

The focus of pathology in the infected shoulder appears to be the articular cartilage. The acellular surface of hyaline cartilage consisting of collagen fibers and proteoglycans serves as a target for bacterial adhesions. Here, there is a receptor-specific cell-to-bacteria interaction that propels infection.[55]

The three major pathways by which infection will enter a joint include hematogenous spread from the synovial blood supply or sepsis, spread from adjacent osteomyelitis, and penetration due to trauma or exposure at the time of surgery.[55] Of these, the most common pathway is trauma or surgical intervention. Introduction of infection by medical intervention is usually associated with surgery, arthroscopy, aspiration, or injections.

In the presence of a rotator cuff tear, it is possible to have an extensive communication between the joint synovium, joint space, and bursal system. In addition, the joint capsule is open where the tendon of the long head of the biceps enters the joint. Because of these anatomic relationships, injection or trauma to any of these structures can lead to extensive infection of the shoulder joint[55] (Fig. 3-26).

## SEPSIS

Approximately 3 to 12 percent of joint sepsis occurs in the shoulder. and will most often be limited to the glenohumeral joint.[75] The acromioclavicular and sternoclavicular joints are usually only involved when infection is secondary to extensive trauma or a specific injection. The most frequent causal organism is *Staphylococcus aureus*.[55]

### HISTORY AND PRESENTATION

Individuals suffering from intraarticular sepsis will typically complain of joint pain, swelling, decreased range of motion, and occasional fever. Patients will typically report that joint motion increases their pain, and they therefore hold their upper extremity splinted against their body. Diagnosis of septic arthritis is based on positive blood cultures, positive cultures of aspirated joint fluid, a fever of unknown etiology, increased white blood cell count, and increased erythrocyte sedimentation rate.[55,125] Radiographs and bone scans are not particularly helpful because bone destruction and deposition are not usually evident until approximately 2 weeks after onset.[125]

Prompt diagnosis is crucial in septic arthritis because patients diagnosed late rarely respond positively to treatment. Leslie and Harris[75] performed a retrospective study that indicated that only patients diagnosed and treated within 4 weeks of the onset of symptoms respond well. This is quite unfortunate, since septic arthritis is often incorrectly diagnosed as bursitis, tendinitis, or adhesive capsulitis.[75]

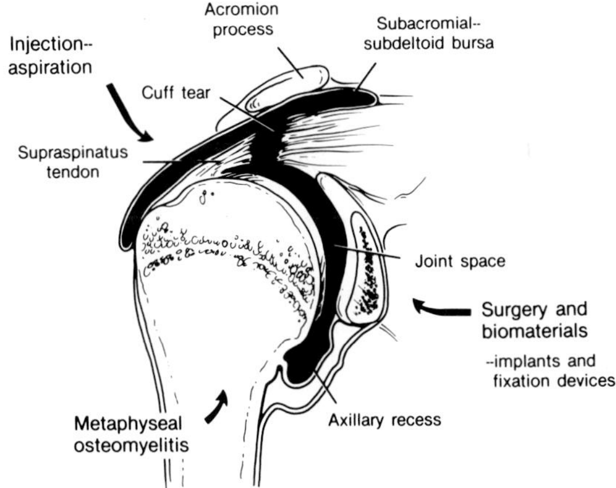


**Figure 3-26.** Routes of infection. (Reproduced with permission from Gristina AG, et al. Sepsis of the shoulder: molecular mechanisms and pathogenesis. In Rockwood CA Jr, Matsen FA III, eds. The shoulder. Vol. 2. Philadelphia: WB Saunders, 1990:922.)

### MANAGEMENT

Treatment of sepsis must be specific and prompt, because inadequate treatment may result in further spread of infection, septic shock, or death. Other sequelae of delayed treatment include joint destruction and contractures.[55] Selection of treatment is based primarily on the status of the individual's immune system and the type of bacterial organism. Once the causal organism is identified by cultures, specific systemic antibiotics are initiated. The next step in management of septic arthritis is somewhat controversial. Either repeated needle aspirations or open surgical debridement will be performed. It appears that the most successful management occurs with immediate surgical debridement. If aspirations are initiated but are not successful within 7 days, surgery is indicated.[55] In retrospect, Leslie and Harris[75] concluded that patients treated with surgery had a better outcome than those treated with aspiration followed by debridement, who in turn had a better outcome than those treated with aspiration alone.

Surgical debridement consists of the removal of all toxic products, foreign bodies, and damaged tissues, followed by closed suction and irrigation.[55] Intravenous antibiotics are typically employed for approximately 4 weeks, followed by oral antibiotics. Evaluations of white blood cell count, fever, and erythrocyte sedimentation rates guide antibiotic therapy.[55]

Little research has been done to determine the most beneficial physical therapy intervention for septic arthritis, but it appears that maintenance of active and passive range of motion is the primary goal.[55] However, it may be necessary to limit range of motion if the bone structure has been weakened in order to prevent fracture. Unfortunately, long-term follow-up of patients with septic arthritis reveals a significant loss of glenohumeral joint motion and residual pain.[75] Physical therapy is needed to maximize function of the glenohumeral joint.

## OSTEOMYELITIS

Unlike septic arthritis, osteomyelitis is usually introduced into a joint by hematogenous spread. This spreading is most often due to surgery, direct inoculation, or spreading from adjacent osteomyelitis. Areas of decreased blood flow serve as a medium for bacterial growth.[125] The infection will generally spread up and down the medullary canal and eventually penetrate the periosteum. While osteomyelitis is more rare in adults than in children, it is more severe in adults, since it is usually the result of more than one infecting organism. However, like septic arthritis, the most common pathogen in osteomyelitis is *S. aureus*. (Fig. 3-27).

### MANAGEMENT

The main principles in management are to remove the infectious material, preferably with antibiotics but occasionally with surgical debridement, preserve articular cartilage, and prevent injury to the growth plate. Physical therapy management is generally limited, since the infected upper extremity is usually immobilized at the side of the body to prevent pathologic fracture.[125] Immobilization is more important with osteomyelitis than with septic arthritis because the periosteum of the long axis of the medullary canal may be altered, predisposing to fractures. Once the infection has been removed and radiographs reveal adequate bone stock, appropriate range-of-motion and strengthening activities are initiated.

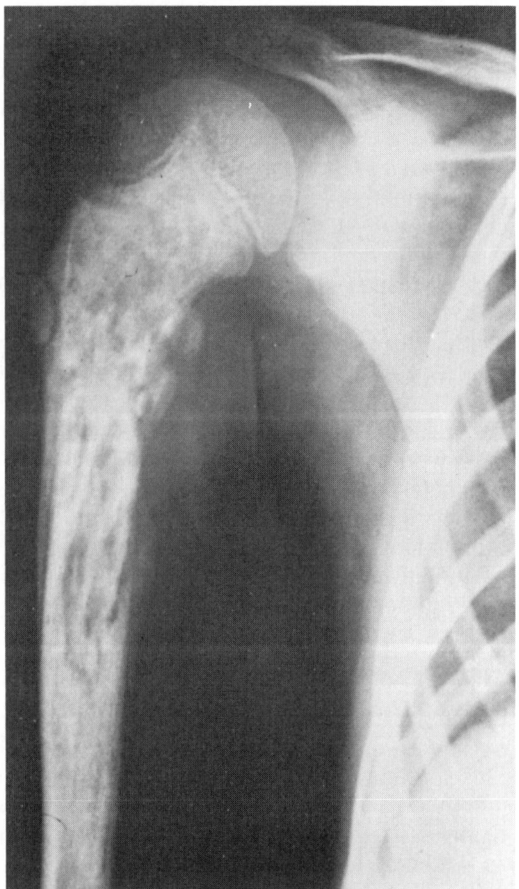

**Figure 3-27.** Osteomyelitis. Radiograph of a child with *Staphylococcus aureus* osteomyelitis. (Reproduced with permission from Post M. Orthopaedic management of shoulder infections. In Post M, ed. The shoulder: surgical and nonsurgical management. 2nd ed. Philadelphia: Lea & Febiger, 1988:141.)

## TRAUMA AND SURGERY

Clinicians should recognize that the introduction of a foreign body into the shoulder joint can predispose the joint to infection. Therefore, following surgery, injection, or open fracture with subsequent reduction, the joint should be closely monitored for signs of infection. The classic signs of infection are dolor (pain), rubor (redness), kalor (elevated temperature), and turgor (swelling). Close inspection of the postoperative or postinjection shoulder should be performed, looking for these signs. In addition to observation, the clinician should palpate for tenderness and increased skin temperature. For the first 3 to 4 days postoperatively, it is wise to assess body temperature several times a day in order to identify early signs of infection. If any of these signs are found, or if the incision begins draining pus or nonserous fluid, further medical evaluation and initiation of appropriate antibiotics are indicated.

### MANAGEMENT

In the case of traumatic open fractures, the wound will be cleansed thoroughly before the fracture is reduced and the wound closed. Drains are placed to prevent the accumulation of pus, and oral or intravenous antibiotics are used until all cultures are negative.

Risk of infection secondary to surgery is minimal because of the use of prophylactic antibiotics. Antibiotics are used preventively for most surgical interventions, and infection rates are 1 to 5 percent.[55] The most common antibiotics used prophylactically are Keflex and Ancef. However, once an infection occurs, it is often resistant to treatment. Implanted biomaterials such as fixation devices and prosthetic joints may be the focus of infection, and infections centered on foreign bodies are difficult to control with the host's natural defense mechanisms. Again, the most common pathogen is *S. aureus*, and it is generally persistent to the point where the foreign body must be removed. All infected tissue is removed, and resection or fusion of the joint is performed.[55] Following open reduction and internal fixation or total shoulder replacement, patients should be monitored for increases in pain or decreases in motion, which are the initial symptoms of a breeding infection. As discussed previously, prompt referral for further medical evaluation is imperative.

# Thoracic Outlet Syndrome

The diagnosis of thoracic outlet syndrome must be considered in all painful conditions of the shoulder that are accompanied by neurologic or vascular symptoms in the upper extremities.[133] Both osseous and soft-tissue components of the shoulder girdle have the potential to compromise the neurovascular bundle traversing it. *Thoracic outlet syndrome* can be defined as symptoms of arterial insufficiency, venous engorgement, or nerve dysfunction, either singularly or in combination, that are produced by compression or stretching of the subclavian artery, subclavian vein, or portions of the brachial plexus as they pass from the neck to the axilla.[69]

The designation *thoracic outlet syndrome* encompasses several neurovascular syndromes occurring at the shoulder girdle and superior aperture of the thorax. The *scalenus anticus syndrome*, the *costoclavicular syndrome*, and the *hyperabduction syndrome* represent subcomponents of the thoracic outlet syndrome, occurring at distinct anatomic locations[2,26,69,86,158] (Fig. 3-28). These subsyndromes are capable of isolated or combined influences sufficient to create and sustain neurovascular dysfunction.

## SCALENUS ANTICUS SYNDROME

The scalenus anticus syndrome is entrapment between the attachments of this muscle and a congenital cervical rib. Historically, the existence of cervical ribs received the earliest attention as the principal source of neurovascular compression.[69,151] Variations of congenital cervical ribs are present in less than 1 percent of the population; however, it is estimated that no greater than 10 percent of these go on to develop thoracic outlet syndrome.[69] Incomplete cervical ribs or elongations of the C7 transverse process occur with the anterior articulation absent or replaced by fibrous fascial bands.[26,158] The presence of a cervical rib can potentially alter the position of the brachial plexus by reducing the floor of the posterior triangle, relocating the plexus and subclavian artery forward and up against the posterior border of the scalenus anticus.[2,158] Adson[2] and Naffziger[95] reported cases of neurovascular irritation between the first rib and the scalenus anticus muscle and fascia or by myofascial compression alone in the absence of cervical ribs at the interscalene triangle. Adson's diagnostic maneuver attempts to increase neurovascular compression within the interscalene triangle by first positioning the scalenes on stretch and then inducing active contraction through deep inspiration. The radial pulse is monitored at the wrist for changes in volume, with the arm resting on the thigh. Adson's original description of this diagnostic maneuver does not call for traction on the arm, which could introduce nonspecific tissue tension at sites other than within the triangle.[2]

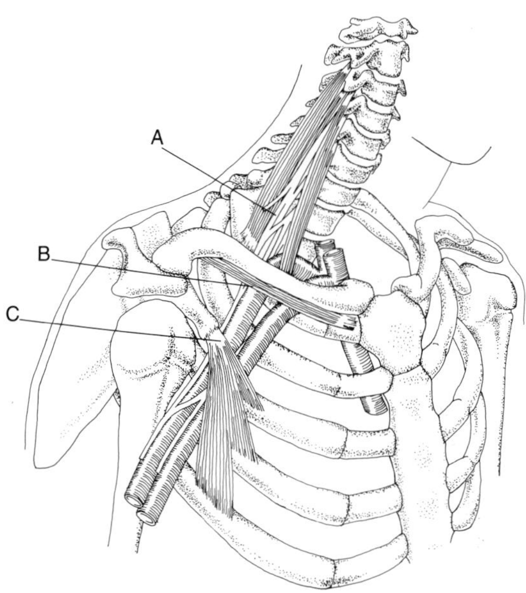

**Figure 3-28.** The three most common sites of neurovascular compression. (a) Scalenus anticus syndrome. Compression occurring between the anterior and middle scaleni muscles and their respective myofascial elements. (b) Costoclavicular syndrome. Compression occurring between the clavicle and first rib. (c) Hyperabduction syndrome. Compression occurring as a result of the neurovascular bundle being compressed against the undersurface of the coracoid process.

The normal anatomic placement of the subclavian vein is anterior to the scalenus anticus, not being present within the interscalene triangle. Other primary sites of compression should therefore be suspected with venous system involvement. Scalene shortening is commonly found to exist with forward head postural dysfunction involving straightening of the cervical lordosis and positioning of the cranium anteriorly (Fig. 3-29). Frequent recruitment of the scalenes for inspiration can occur with primary mouth breathing and upper chest breathing patterns. Soft-tissue and osseous neurovascular compression can result from scalene hyperactivity. Vessel and nerve constriction within the scalene myofascia is accentuated. Shortening can realign the first rib and superior fibers of the serratus anterior up and forward, reducing the dimensions of the posterior triangle.

Conservative management should emphasize correction of forward head posture and establishment of nasal-abdominal breathing for efficient respiration. Manual therapy is directed at stretching the scalenes and cervical fascia and mobilizing the first rib inferiorly and posteriorly to enhance excursion during exhalation.

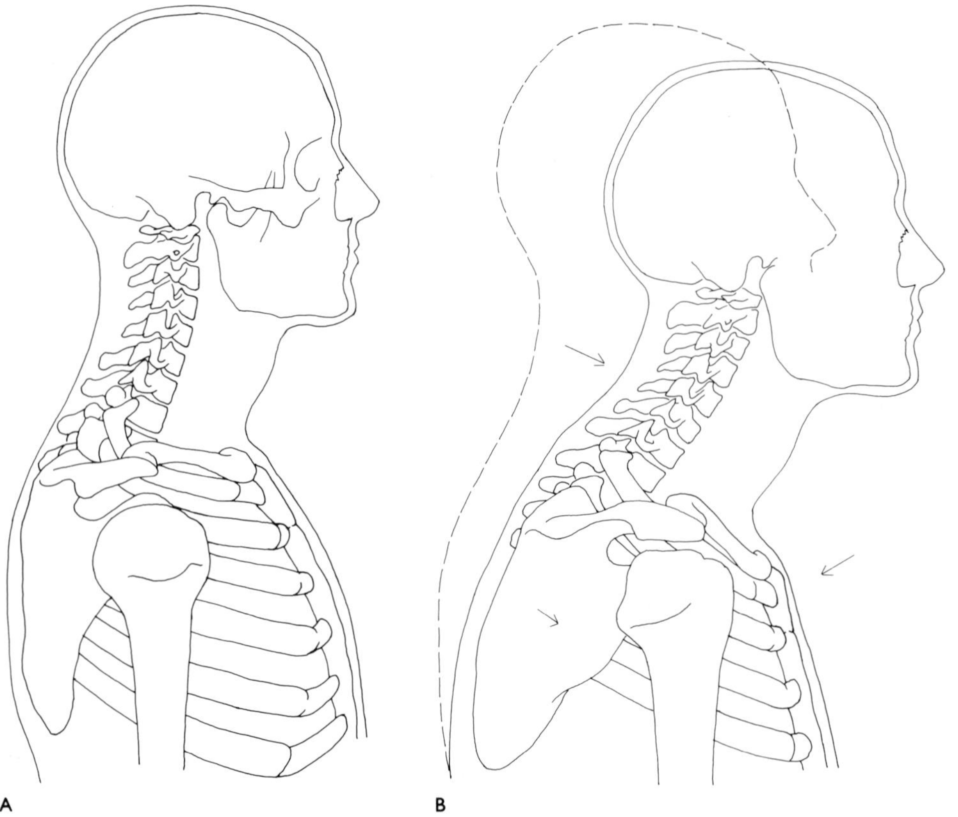


**Figure 3-29.** (a) Balanced postural relationships in the upper quarter. (b) Forward head postural dysfunction.

## COSTOCLAVICULAR SYNDROME

The primary mechanism of costoclavicular syndrome involves simultaneous depression of the shoulder girdle and fixation of the clavicle down and back toward the first rib, thereby reducing the retroclavicular free space containing the neurovascular bundle.[26,69,151,158] The descent of the shoulder girdle during midlife, the result of gradual weakening of the supporting musculature, and settling of the vertebral column are natural consequences of aging in many individuals, being more pronounced in females.[38,56] The resulting osseous realignment and myofascial adaptive shortening increase the likelihood for neurovascular entrapment in the costoclavicular spaces by permitting the shoulder girdle to sag on the thoracic cage, over which it is normally suspended.[26,38,132]

The so-called military bracing diagnostic position both approximates the clavicle to the neurovascular bundle and introduces some degree of traction. The subclavian vein is particularly vulnerable to compression, situated anterior to the scalenus anticus and closest to the clavicle in the narrow, proximal portion of the costoclavicular space. Rehabilitation requires shoulder girdle elevation exercises, postural strengthening, and functional stabilization of the clavicle and scapula in relation to the axial skeleton.

## HYPERABDUCTION SYNDROME

The potential for compression and stretch irritation can occur at two sites distal and lateral to those previously described and is identified as the hyperabduction syndrome.[26,69,158] The creation of an "anatomic scissors"[36] formed by the clavicle and first rib can produce shearing and compression in the retroclavicular free space during hyperabduction of the arm, the position imparted when performing Wright's diagnostic maneuver. Additional mechanical irritation can result in this position when the neurovascular bundle is stretched around the coracoid process and under the pectoralis minor tendon, which together act as a pulley to intensify the mechanical forces of tension and compression exerted along the course of the bundle.[26]

Other opportunities exist for compression and entrapment as the bundle and its branches pass through the subclavius muscle, clavipectoral fascia, costocoracoid membrane, and suspensory ligament of the axilla.[26,86,108] Management of the hyperabduction syndrome includes stretching tight pectoral myofascia, strengthening of antagonists, mobilization of the clavicle, and modification of activities requiring sustained or repetitive positioning in elevation or hyperabduction.

## ETIOLOGY OF THORACIC OUTLET SYNDROME

The etiology of thoracic outlet syndrome involves dynamic and static mechanical forces, anatomic predisposition, exposure to trauma, and the cumulative effects of aging.[26,69] The onset of symptoms typically may be seen to occur when the anatomically predisposed individual is exposed to environmental perpetrating factors, the combined effects of which exceed the existing potential for functional accommodation. Anatomic predisposition can be congenital or acquired. The conditions necessary for development of thoracic outlet syndrome vary considerably between subjects. The activation of symptoms may be insidious or posttraumatic, with spontaneous occurrence more common in adult females.[133] The obese or heavy-chested female need not be considered at increased risk on this basis singularly, without consideration of all potential perpetrating factors. The stereotypical individual with spontaneous onset thoracic outlet syndrome is an employed female between 20 and 45 years of age with asthma or active respiratory allergies and forward head posture.

## PERPETRATING FACTORS

Changes in myofascial tension and length as a result of sustained positioning or repetitive movements of the head, neck, shoulder girdle, and arm, scalene respiratory hyperactivity, muscle hypertrophy, acquired forward head posture, and habitual slouching have all been cited as factors capable of perpetrating or sustaining thoracic outlet syndrome.[2,26,38,69,133,134,151] Trauma, both singular and cumulative, can result in postinflammatory changes, including adhesion, fibrosis, and scarring, that can serve as a source of mechanical irritation. Splinting and guarding in response to pain can accelerate adaptive shortening in muscle, a nonpathologic process that normally occurs very slowly.[68] Metabolic disturbance affecting peripheral nerves can increase the susceptibility to mechanical irritation from compression and stretch that would otherwise be asymptomatic.

## CLINICAL SIGNS AND SYMPTOMS

Thoracic outlet syndrome can include any combination of neurologic, arterial, or venous system involvement. Neurologic thoracic outlet syndrome involving portions of the brachial plexus occurs in 95 percent or more of all cases.[69,134] Vascular complications occur much less frequently, involving the arterial system in 5 percent and the venous system in 2 percent of all reported cases.[36,69]

The severity, location, and nature of symptoms attributed to thoracic outlet syndrome vary considerably depending on the extent to which individual or combinations of nerves, arteries, and veins become affected. Signs and symptoms are typically position-sensitive and more or less intermittent in the developing stages of dysfunction. Provocation or relief of symptoms by selective positioning and alteration of mechanical forces at localized anatomic levels serves as the basis for clinical examination maneuvers for thoracic outlet syndrome described in detail in Chapter 5.

Neurogenic thoracic outlet syndrome affecting the brachial plexus creates symptoms and neurologic dysfunction similar to those produced at other sites, including cervical nerve root(s), ulnar nerve entrapment in the cubital tunnel at the elbow or Guyon's canal at the wrist, or median nerve compression at the carpal tunnel. Pain and paresthesia are the most universal complaints associated with neurogenic thoracic outlet syndrome.[26,151] Grip weakness and diminished dexterity are also reported commonly. Sleep disturbance with nocturnal exacerbation of upper extremity symptoms is typical, and inquiry as to its existence should always be included in the history. Lower brachial plexus components derived from C8, T1, and often C7 are typically implicated. Symptoms of pain, numbness, and tingling occur in the ulnar distribution most frequently but not exclusively; they are also commonly present in the median distribution. Upper extremity pain, when present, typically follows the anatomic pathway of the involved nerve trunks. The existence of concomitant involvement at more than one site, the so-called double crush injury, complicates the clinical presentation and must be considered in the differential diagnosis. Upton and McComas.[162] and Osterman[116] described the potential for increased distal nerve irritability when proximal compression of the same nerve trunk or contributing nerve root exists. Neurogenic thoracic outlet syndrome can be divided into true and nonspecific or disputed subclassifications.[36] True neurogenic thoracic outlet syndrome must correlate demonstrable electromyographic findings and radiographic abnormalities with a characteristic clinical presentation. The incidence is estimated to be as low as 1 in 1 million people.[36]

Nonspecific neurogenic thoracic outlet syndrome is the most common type and must be determined by clinical evaluation, often without supporting diagnostic findings. Symptoms of pain and paresthesia are typically intermittent and position-sensitive, brought on by mechanical irritation sufficient to cause transient nerve ischemia but insufficient to result in nervous tissue injury. Objective sensory and motor changes may not be demonstrable with electrodiagnostic or clinical examination in most cases. One study of 300 patients reported that pain and paresthesia were present in all subjects; however, only 16.6 percent demonstrated decreased sensation to pin prick, while motor weakness was present in 28.3 percent of cases.[15] Upper plexus involvement affecting C5, C6, or C7 occurs less frequently, often in combination with those of the lower segments. Peripheral nerve entrapment of the dorsal scapular, long thoracic, and suprascapular nerves at the level of the scalenus medius and cervical fascia can be contributory to cervical and shoulder dysfunction.[38,132,162] Shoulder ache and discomfort of varying degree may be present and distributed throughout the pectoral, axillary, and subscapular regions. Shoulder pain accompanying thoracic outlet syndrome may be primarily myogenic. Travell[156] identified myofascial trigger points in the scalene and pectoral muscles that contribute to both local and referred symptoms.

Symptoms associated with vascular system disturbances include complaints of cold intolerance, a feeling of heaviness in the arm, and easy fatigue or cramping in the hand or upper extremity during activity, improving with rest. Reports of pain may be absent other than that accompanying activity-related ischemia, improving with rest. Clinical observation may reveal increased limb circumference, skin tightness, and decreased skin temperature. Pallor in the distal extremity becoming more pronounced when moving from the dependant to overhead position can be indicative of arterial insufficiency. Diminished radial pulse volume or reduction in brachial blood pressure at rest may be detected in the involved extremity.[69,95] A bruit may be revealed upon auscultation at the supraclavicular level.[95] Retarded wound healing and skin ulceration occasionally occur in advanced cases; gangrene can occur in extreme situations. Cyanotic discoloration on the palmar surface and engorgement of the dorsal veins of the hand in the dependant position, decreasing with arm elevation, is indicative of venous system dysfunction. The absence of change from the dependant to the elevated position may be secondary to the presence of obstruction in the upper limb caused by venous thrombosis.[69]

## TREATMENT

Conservative management of thoracic outlet syndrome may include rest and appropriate anticoagulant therapy, analgesic and anti-inflammatory medications and modalities, modification of perpetrating occupational and recreational activities, stress-reduction measures, and correction of related musculoskeletal, breathing, and postural dysfunction by a physical therapist. Treatment planning must be tailored to individually address each component identified by systematic clinical evaluation. Caution must be given to the use of isometric exercises when a component of soft-tissue compression is contributory and range of motion with weights when repetitive movements are found to be a source of irritation. When respiratory hyperactivity is identified or inspiration is found to reproduce symptoms and signs during clinical testing, aerobic exercise should be deferred. Exercises must be closely monitored for reproduction of signs and symptoms and modified to tolerance. Given the diagnosis to be accurate, the success of conservative therapy demonstrates considerable variation among individuals. The length and extent of involvement and existing biologic potential for healing, the timeliness of intervention, the compliance and motivation of the patient, and the skill of the attending physicians and treating therapists are all factors.

Surgery frequently results in discovery of nerve and vessel injury and connective-tissue changes not appreciated with available diagnostic techniques and not amenable to prior therapeutic measures.[134] Postoperative management should address the same perpetrating factors previously identified.

## SUMMARY

Thoracic outlet syndrome presents multiple concerns to the clinician responsible for evaluation and treatment of shoulder pain and dysfunction. In many cases, the shoulder girdle is the primary site of neurovascular compromise, which produces symptoms that mimic those generated by other sources of dysfunction. Thoracic outlet syndrome routinely coexists with other musculoskeletal and neurologic dysfunction of the upper quarter such as carpal tunnel syndrome, subacromial impingement, and cervical nerve root pathology that can evolve concurrently as a consequence of exposure to common predisposing environmental factors and trauma. The differential diagnosis is complicated by the number of anatomic systems involved and the wide range of signs and symptoms attributed to them. Controversy is rampant concerning the existence of thoracic outlet syndrome as a distinct diagnostic entity and the long-term benefits of surgical treatment. The diagnosis should always be considered in painful conditions of the shoulder that are accompanied by upper extremity neurologic or vascular symptoms.

# Brachial Plexus and Peripheral Nerve Injuries

The brachial plexus, arising from C5–T1 nerve roots, provides sensory and motor innervation to the upper extremity. In some individuals, C4 and T2 may contribute to the plexus, creating a prefixed or postfixed plexus, respectively.[67] The nerve roots contributing to the brachial plexus combine to form three trunks which then divide into anterior and posterior divisions. The divisions combine to form cords that terminate in individual peripheral sensory, motor, and sensorimotor nerves of the upper extremity. The brachial plexus is frequently divided into two portions. The supraclavicular portion consists of the trunks, located near the subclavian artery, while the infraclavicular portion consists of the nerves, located near the axilla[67] (Fig. 3-30).

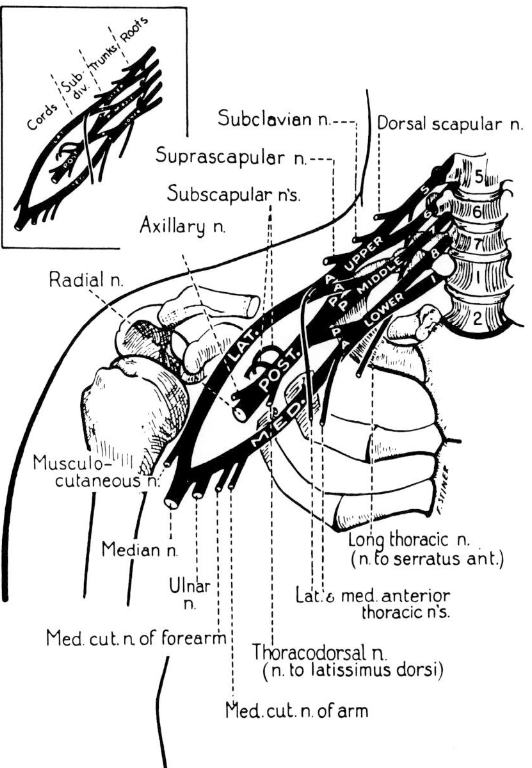


**Figure 3-30.** The brachial plexus. (Reproduced with permission from Haymaker W, Woodhall B. Peripheral nerve injuries. Philadelphia: WB Saunders, 1956:210.)

## CLASSIFICATION

In addition to varying mechanisms of injury, there are varying degrees of severity of injury to the plexus. Sunderland[152] classified nerve injuries based on the consequences of the injury. These variations have been classified into three main categories: neuropraxia, axonotmesis, and neurotmesis. *Neuropraxia* is the mildest form of nerve injury and is characterized by a transient loss of conductivity, which usually only lasts days to weeks. In this mild injury, wall degeneration (the breakdown of myelin sheaths) does not occur.[142,143] The next category is known as *axonotmesis* and is characterized by more severe damage to the axons, with the nerve distal to the injury undergoing wall degeneration.[143] Peripheral regeneration is possible along the intact neural tubes. Symptoms are typically present for weeks to months. Finally, in *neurotmesis*, the axons are destroyed, with damage of the neural tube in the proximal segment and wall degeneration of the distal segment. Regeneration is not possible, and recovery of function occurs only with surgical intervention, in which the damaged nerve is debrided and the viable ends sutured together.[143] The most severe injury to the plexus occurs when forces applied to the region are strong enough to result in avulsion of the nerve roots from the spinal cord. This is the one situation in which no recovery of function is possible.[11,67,73]

Nerve regeneration occurs very slowly (approximately 1 mm/day), and there is thus an extended period after injury during which recovery may occur. However, the maximal period is usually 20 to 24 months after injury.[67] After this time period, the area of myoneural junction has fibrosed to the point that the muscle is unable to accept a nerve.[67] Because of the slow rate of nerve regeneration, injuries to the supraclavicular plexus generally have a better prognosis than injuries to the infraclavicular portion.

## MECHANISMS OF INJURY

Fortunately, the brachial plexus is not frequently injured, but when nerve damage does occur, it is one of the most serious shoulder derangements.[12] There are several mechanisms of closed injury that may damage the brachial plexus, including compression, angulation, stretch or traction injuries, entrapment, or vascular compromise.[12,67,127] Open injury to the plexus is uncommon but may occur with severe trauma.

Gunshot wounds to the neck and shoulder, motorcycle accidents, industrial accidents, and stabbings often result in devastating injuries to the plexus. Compression injuries typically occur as a nerve passes through fibrous tissue or through an osseofibrous canal. They also may result from a direct blow to the nerve or improper positioning, particularly during surgery.[127]

Traction injuries result from any stretching of the plexus, particularly forces that cause an increase in the acromiomastoid angle, the angle between the shoulder and the head (Fig. 3-31a). Most brachial plexus injuries are traction injuries and involve the supraclavicular portion of the plexus. Traction injuries are frequently the result of motorcycle accidents, motor vehicle accidents, a fall on an outstretched arm, or athletic injuries.[11] In a traction injury, the area of the plexus that is injured will be determined by the position of the arm. If the arm is abducted, the infraclavicular portion of the plexus is involved, while the supraclavicular portion of the plexus is involved if the arm is adducted.[67]

The most common nerve injury in athletics is transient brachial plexopathy, more frequently known as a "burner" or "stinger." These injuries frequently occur in wrestlers, basketball players, and hockey players but are most common in football players.[142] They may be the result of either traction or compression of the supraclavicular portion of the plexus, particularly the C5–6 nerve roots. The mechanism of injury is typically a blow to the player's head, neck, or shoulder that results in lateral cervical flexion in conjunction with contralateral shoulder depression (a traction injury) (see Fig. 3-31a) or lateral flexion with ipsilateral rotation and extension (a compression injury)[142] (see Fig. 3-31b). An individual suffering from a burner will complain of a burning or numb sensation in the lateral aspect of the arm that usually extends down into the fingers. In addition, such a person will experience weakness of the upper extremity (particularly deltoid, biceps, supraspinatus, and infraspinatus) with a sensation of heaviness and difficulty in raising the involved extremity overhead.[142, 150] These symptoms are most often very transient and are generally gone within several minutes. An athlete should not be permitted to return to play unless he or she has regained full range of motion, full strength, and normal neurovascular function. In only 5 to 10 percent of individuals is damage more severe with symptoms lasting several hours or longer.[150] In general, rehabilitation of burners consists of maintaining range of motion (cervical and upper extremity) and normalizing the strength of the involved musculature. When the range of motion and strength are full, the individual should be ready to return to play. However, athletes with persistent pain or paresthesias should not return to play because nerve damage may be more extensive than originally thought. Electromyographic studies are indicated in the presence of persistent symptoms.

## HISTORY AND PRESENTATION

A thorough history and physical examination will reveal existing neurologic deficits. Subjective complaints consistent with nerve damage in-

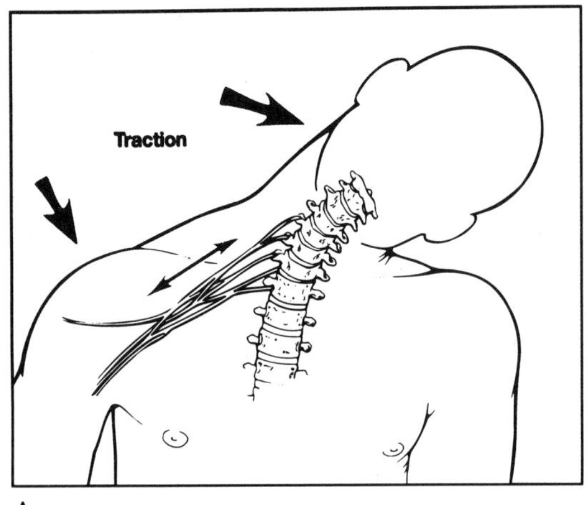


A

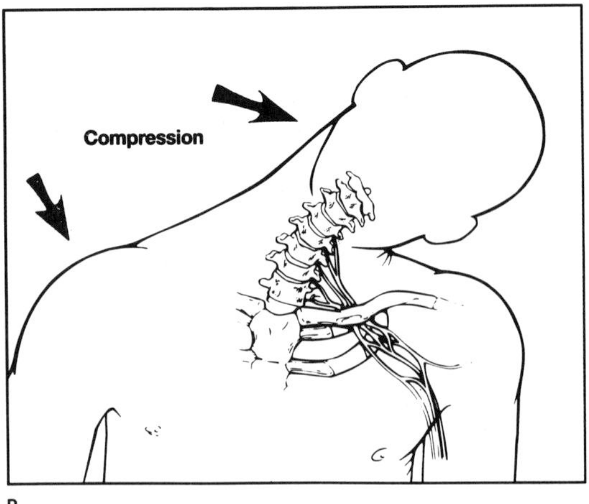


B

**Figure 3-31.** Burner's syndrome. The mechanism of injury is typically a blow to the player's head, neck, or shoulder that results in lateral cervical flexion in conjunction with contralateral shoulder depression (a traction injury or burner's syndrome) (a) or lateral flexion with ipsilateral rotation and extension (a compression injury) (b). (Reproduced with permission from Sallis RE, Jones K, Knopp W. Burners: offensive strategy for an underreported injury. Physician Sports Med 1992;20:47.)

clude sensations of burning, numbness, or radiating, shock-like pain.[11] However, if nerve injury is confined to a motor nerve, the patient will have no complaints of pain with the exception of pain arising from an accompanying injury.

Active and passive range of motion will be full in all directions except for motions whose primary musculature has been denervated. Manual muscle testing is helpful in determining the location of injury, particularly whether it is proximal in the plexus or localized to peripheral nerves. Most often injury is confined to the peripheral nerves.[11] If the patient is able to perform some motion with decreased strength or only through partial range, the prognosis for recovery is better than if one muscle is completely paralyzed.[73] In addition, sensory testing should be performed to help localize the nerve lesion. Damage to sensory nerves may result in a loss of cutaneous sensation and deep sensation as well as a loss of joint position sense.[143]

Radiographs of the cervical spine and shoulder should be performed whenever there is a significant upper quarter injury. If fractures or dislocations are identified, thorough evaluation should be performed to rule out nerve injuries that are closely correlated with certain dislocations or fractures. Finally, if nerve injury is highly suspected, electromyographic studies, including nerve conduction velocity testing, should be performed to obtain baseline electrical activity. This is helpful in forming a definitive diagnosis and for comparison at later dates to determine if and at what rate recovery is taking place.[67] If a muscle is responsive to interrupted current, the neuromuscular connection is intact, and recovery is likely. If the muscle only responds to direct or galvanic current, the prognosis is more guarded, but recovery is still possible.[11] Electromyographic studies are most valuable when performed 3 to 4 weeks after injury, since this is when signs of axonal disruption develop. The common signs of axonal disruption include fibrillation potentials and positive sharp waves.[142]

### MANAGEMENT

In general, nerve lesions are treated conservatively. Initially, this conservative treatment consists of some form of immobilization, usually a sling that is used to support the weight of the arm and to protect the denervated or weakened musculature.[11,12,67] Then passive or active assisted range of motion should be performed regularly to maintain joint mobility.[12,67,73] In addition, electrical stimulation may be beneficial to help minimize atrophy. Electrical stimulation of denervated muscle should be performed until there is a sign of reinnervation.[11,12] Conservative treatment has failed if there is no sign of progress or recovery clinically or by electrical studies in 3 to 4 months. If this occurs, surgical exploration is indicated.[11,12,67]

During surgery, the affected nerve root sheath will be opened and any scar tissue will be debrided back to the point of healthy nerve tissue, followed by suturing of the nerve ends together.[12,67] Occasionally, direct repair will not be possible, and an autograft will be used. Most frequently, the sural nerve will be used as the donor nerve.[73] Following surgery, physical therapy is indicated for range of motion and strengthening. If nerve repair is not possible, arthrodesis may be performed to allow the upper extremity to be used as an assist to the opposite upper extremity.[73] The most frequent position of arthrodesis for maximal function is 20 degrees of abduction, 30 degrees of flexion, and 30 to 40 degrees of internal rotation. This will allow the patient to reach to the midline, mouth, and opposite axilla.[73]

## ACUTE BRACHIAL NEUROPATHY

Injury to the brachial plexus may present as an acute brachial neuropathy. This condition has an unknown etiology, but possible predisposing factors include shoulder trauma, vigorous exercise, recent thoracic surgery, contact or noncontact sports, viral infections, allergic reactions, and immunizations.[62,67] Acute brachial neuropathy occurs twice as often in males as in females and generally occurs in the second or third decade.[67,73] Clinical presentation includes severe shoulder pain sometimes extending to the scapula, arm, and hand. This pain is generally present at rest and increases in intensity with an increase in activity.[62,67,73] In conjunction with the pain there is a loss of sensory and motor function. Loss of motor function generally occurs in proximal shoulder and scapular musculature, while sensory loss is generally over the lateral deltoid.[62,67] Bilateral involvement may occur, but most often the pathology is limited to the dominant arm.[62,73] The course of this pathology can generally be divided into two distinct phases. Phase I extends from the onset of pain until the resolution of pain and may last up to 4 weeks. Phase II is characterized by diminished pain but significant weakness.[62]

The prognosis of the patient with acute brachial neuropathy is fairly good, with approximately two-thirds of patients improving in the first several months after onset. Between 80 and 90 percent of patients will achieve full recovery in 2 to 3 years.[62,67,73] Treatment is primarily symptomatic. During phase I, the upper extremity is rested, with the exception of gentle range-of-motion exercises. A sling may be used for protection, and analgesics or modalities are employed for pain control. In phase II, range-of-motion exercises are continued with the addition of progressive resistive exercises.

## PERIPHERAL NERVE INJURIES

While peripheral injury may occur to any nerve of the plexus, some of the more common injuries include injuries to the suprascapular, axillary, and musculocutaneous nerves (Fig. 3-32).

### SUPRASCAPULAR NERVE

The suprascapular nerve arises from the proximal part of the upper trunk of the brachial plexus. It descends and crosses the superior border of the scapula through the scapular notch, which is bounded superiorly by the transverse scapular ligament. The nerve then sends branches to the supraspinatus and infraspinatus muscles and the shoulder joint.[127] There are several different mechanisms of injury to the suprascapular nerve. A projectile falling on the supraclavicular region may result in an increase in the acromiomastoid angle and a stretching of the suprascapular nerve.

In addition, fractures of the scapular notch may result in nerve damage.[12,148] However, the most common mechanism of injury is friction irritation of the nerve in the scapular notch. This is due to excessive scapular and glenohumeral motion, particularly scapular protraction with glenohumeral horizontal adduction.[12,148] This repetitive motion results in increased motion in the suprascapular foramen, causing increased friction on the nerve.

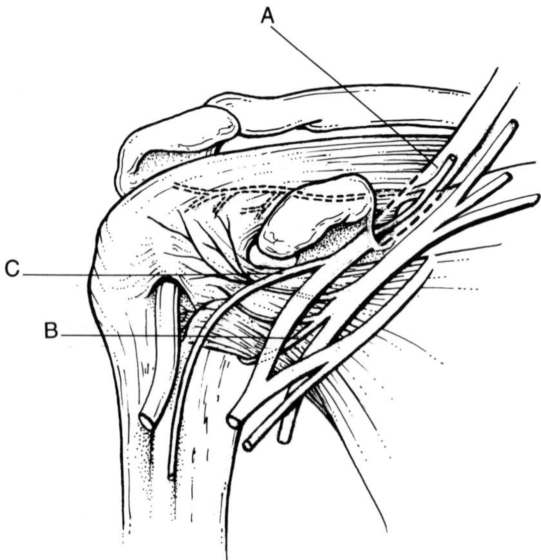


**Figure 3-32.** Peripheral nerve injuries. Peripheral injury may occur to any nerve of the plexus. Some of the more common injuries include injuries to the suprascapular, axillary, and musculocutaneous nerves, since these particular nerves lie in very close proximity to the glenohumeral joint.

Patients who have sustained injury to the suprascapular nerve will present with weakness of abduction and external rotation and atrophy of the supraspinatus and infraspinatus muscles. They will frequently complain of a deep achy pain in the shoulder and neck. There will be no cutaneous sensory deficits, since the suprascapular nerve does not provide cutaneous innervation. Electromyographic testing will show signs of partial or complete denervation of the supraspinatus and infraspinatus muscles. Specifically, there will be muscle fibrillation and a delay in conduction velocity at the site of the nerve entrapment.[67,127] Injury to the suprascapular nerve may mimic rotator cuff injury, and the differential diagnosis is very important. If clinical examination and history do not indicate a clear enough diagnosis, then diagnosis may be accomplished by advanced imaging techniques in MRI.

Conservative treatment includes the avoidance of protraction and adduction motions while performing pain-free resistive exercises for abduction and external rotation. Electrical stimulation may be performed to minimize atrophy.[11,12,148] As mentioned previously, if conservative treatment is unsuccessful in 2 to 3 months, surgical intervention is indicated. Surgery generally consists of neurolysis, removing scar tissue, or decompression of the scapular notch by dividing the transverse scapular ligament.[67] Following surgery, electrical stimulation may be continued until there are signs of reinnervation. This is done in combination with range-of-motion and strengthening exercises.[12,127] Various physical therapy modalities also may be beneficial in pain control.

### AXILLARY NERVE

The axillary nerve arises from the posterior cord of the brachial plexus and passes anterior and inferior to the shoulder joint. It wraps around the surgical neck of the humerus and divides to provide motor innervation to the deltoid and teres minor muscles and sensory innervation to the skin over the deltoid.[67,127] The axillary nerve is most frequently injured in conjunction with fractures or fracture-dislocations. Fractures of the surgical neck of the humerus frequently result in axillary nerve damage.[67] The nerve is particularly vulnerable to injury with an anteroinferior glenohumeral dislocation.[73,127] In addition, nerve damage may result from a direct upward force to the axilla. The patient with axillary nerve damage will complain of pain vaguely localized to the anterolateral shoulder region. Such patients will report decreased sensation at the lateral aspect of the shoulder and will demonstrate weakness in abduction and external rotation.[67,127] Atrophy of the deltoid and teres minor musculature may be evident. Conservative treatment, including splinting, electrical stimulation, and range-of-motion exercises, is usually successful, and most lesions heal spontaneously.[11,67] Once again, if recovery has not occurred in 2 to 3 months, surgical exploration is performed, with debridement and nerve repair as indicated.

### MUSCULOCUTANEOUS NERVE

The musculocutaneous nerve is the highest terminal branch of the brachial plexus arising from the lateral cord. This nerve is most frequently injured by a crushing blow directly to the nerve, forcing it against the lateral bicipital groove.[11,12] The patient will present with weakness of the biceps, coracobrachialis, and brachialis muscles. Such patients will often have significant pain presenting as a type of causalgia. In addition, patients will report numbness along the lateral border of the forearm.[11,12] Treatment is most often conservative, with surgical exploration indicated after 3 months without any signs of recovery.

## Multiple Injuries

Multiple injuries to the shoulder are usually the result of violent trauma suffered in an industrial accident, motor vehicle accident, or competitive sports participation. Because of its structure and the relative lack of muscular protection, damage to the shoulder joint and surrounding soft tissue, as well as the neurovascular system, can be severe. It is critical that a quick assessment of the injuries be made in order to preserve nerve, circulatory, and ultimately muscular function. Failure to assess and treat the injuries appropriately can lead to complications and significant disability.

When the patient presents to the emergency room, it is the responsibility of the emergency room physician to stabilize the patient and then prioritize the treatment for injuries of the shoulder. First, circulatory status must be addressed. Adequate perfusion is necessary to keep the tissues alive, and surgery will be performed, if indicated, to restore circulation. Nerve function is addressed early, and once again, if there has been damage to the nerve, a skillful surgical team should be summoned to address these concerns as early as possible. Soft-tissue injuries are repaired surgically or treated conservatively, depending on the extent of the damage. With respect to joint disruption and/or fractures, the orthopedic surgeon will determine the need for either open or closed reduction. Open reduction and internal fixation (ORIF) are performed if stability and proper realignment cannot be achieved conservatively. Given the fact that multiple injuries of the shoulder region often involve the vascular, neurologic, and musculoskeletal systems, the treatment approach also needs to establish priorities. The patient often progresses from in-hospital management to outpatient treatment. It is the responsibility of each clinician to investigate thoroughly all previous interventions and their effects on the patient. This requires extra effort on the part of the outpatient therapist, since this information may not always be readily available. Communication with the referring physician, the in-hospital departments (nursing, radiology, physical therapy, etc.), and the patient is important. Results of all previous diagnostic tests should be known. This information will assist the treating therapist in prioritizing treatment and in planning appropriate goals.

### MANAGEMENT

Initially, the shoulder will be placed in a protected position, whether in traction, a splint, a customized brace, or a sling. At the appropriate time, allowing for healing constraints, range-of-motion exercises will be implemented. When functional pain-free range of motion is achieved, progressive resistive strengthening exercises will be initiated. Finally, proprioceptive and functional drills will precede a return to work and recreational activities. All these activities will depend on the integrity of the surgical or conservative repair and should be directed by the primary orthopedist.

Multiple injuries to the shoulder imply several pathologic injuries. Constraints of healing must be considered in the treatment plan for the complicated shoulder. This chapter discusses a host of specific injuries inherent to the shoulder and the management plan for each. These can be used as a general guideline for the treatment of the shoulder with multiple injuries, but close communication with the primary orthopedist is mandatory for satisfactory rehabilitation results.

## Contusions

A *contusion* to the shoulder is the result of a traumatic compressive injury causing damage to supporting soft tissue or bones. A direct blow to a muscle causes capillary rupture and bleeding, resulting in an inflammatory reaction.[66] The extent of the damage will be affected by the force or frequency of the blow. Most contusion injuries around the shoulder are the result of sports participation, either from direct contact with opponents or from falling on the playing surface. In football, the shoulder joint is partially protected by pads. However, contusions are the most common injury of the shoulder, since direct blows beneath the shoulder pad can bruise soft tissues, including subcutaneous tissue, the deltoid, biceps, or triceps.[121,174] Lacrosse is another contact/collision sport that places the shoulder at risk, especially for attackers who frequently use their arm to ward off blows from the opponent's stick.[89]

## CLASSIFICATION

Contusions are graded in severity by the restriction of motion in the associated joints.[46,66] With a mild contusion, active or passive range of motion is decreased by less than one-third the normal joint range of motion. A moderate contusion results in limitation of joint range of motion to one-third to two-thirds normal. Finally, a severe contusion results in a dramatic loss of motion, allowing less than one-third the normal range (Table 3-6). Muscular pain and spasm can be associated with cellular muscle damage and bleeding in the fascial compartment.[27] Severe or repetitive blows can result in traumatic myositis ossificans or exostosis of the bone.[27,89,121] Contusions to the lateral portion of the acromion or clavicle can produce bone bruising and an associated periosteal reaction. Soft tissues covering the acromion are injured as well. These injuries, known as *shoulder pointers*, may be difficult to differentiate from grade I acromioclavicular separations and should be treated as such.[9,46] Most shoulder pointers and contusions directly affecting the glenohumeral joint can be prevented in sports with protective padding. Presently, those sports which put the shoulder most at risk, such as football and hockey, require the use of shoulder pads. In addition to the traditional shoulder pads, athletes also have the option of wearing pads that cover the lateral aspect of the upper arm in the area of the deltoid tubercle, which is a common area for contusions. However, protective shoulder padding remains optional in other sports (rugby, lacrosse), but use should be encouraged, especially in a player with a history of shoulder injury.

**Table 3-6**

**Classification of Contusions**

| | |
|---|---|
| *Mild* | Joint range of motion limited by less than one-third normal range of motion |
| *Moderate* | Joint range of motion limited to one-third to two-thirds normal range of motion |
| *Severe* | Joint range of motion limited to less than one-third normal range of motion |

## HISTORY AND PRESENTATION

The patient will usually present with a history of soft-tissue injury caused by trauma. Often this injury will go unattended because in the excitement of play the athlete does not bring it to the attention of the trainer and later dismisses it as incidental bruising. Edema and discoloration due to resultant hemorrhage may or may not be apparent.[91] Active and passive motion will be limited by pain and spasm depending on the severity of the contusion, and there will be point-specific tenderness to palpation at the site of the injury. The patient suffering a shoulder pointer will present with point tenderness at the distal clavicle as well as pain during active or passive arm movement.[46]

## MANAGEMENT

Proper early treatment for soft-tissue contusions or shoulder pointers prevents permanent disability from the injury and will be directed toward reduction of hemorrhage, inflammation, and pain. Application of ice will cause vasoconstriction and limit bleeding as well as help to control effusion and pain.[10,27,46] Heat, both superficial and deep, forceful stretching, vigorous massage, and weight lifting are contraindicated and should be avoided because they can aggravate pain, increase blood flow, and may cause myositis ossificans.[10,66] Gentle stretching and massage, however, should be implemented early in order to avoid inelastic scarring of the disrupted muscle tissue and the subdeltoid bursa. Soft-tissue damage can lead to altered biomechanics and primary and secondary trigger points. After the acute injury has subsided, whirlpool, massage, and joint mobilization will prove helpful in regaining full range of motion. Persistent soft-tissue pain despite appropriate rest must be managed with soft-tissue mobilization and treatment of trigger points; also, scapular isometrics, resistive exercises using scapular stabilization, and modalities including TENS and phonophoresis should be performed.[91] As pain subsides, active motion and progressive strengthening exercises may be performed. Return to activity is dependent on symptomatic improvement and full passive range of motion, allowing for adequate and pain-free performance of sport-specific skill and agility drills.[46]

The development of ectopic bone in the múscle (myositis ossificans) or as an outgrowth of the underlying bone (exostosis) is a somewhat uncommon complication resulting from hemorrhage caused by contusions. Clinical presentation of pain, effusion, and diminished range of motion is the same as that seen in a contusion. As the ectopic bone develops, radiographic changes may be noted in 2 to 3 weeks, and a hard mass may be palpated within 4 weeks. Once again, initial treatment is conservative, avoiding vigorous stretching, massage, and exercise. Treatment is the same as with soft-tissue contusion, but the injury will now take longer to resolve, and the athlete should not be pushed to return to activity before it has been determined it is safe to do so. Spontaneous resorption of ectopic bone has been reported. If the ectopic bone growth remains symptomatic or predisposes the athlete to further injury, it may be surgically removed when mature.[46]

# References


1. Abrams JS. Special shoulder problems in the throwing athlete: pathology, diagnosis, and nonoperative management. Clin Sports Med 1991;10(4):839.
2. Adson AW. Cervical ribs: symptoms, differential diagnosis for selections of the insertion of the scalenus anticus muscle. J Int Coll Surg 1951;16:546.
3. Allman FL. Fractures and ligamentous injuries of the clavicle and its articulation. J Bone Joint Surg 1967;49(4):774.
4. Anderson T. Difficult sports-related shoulder fractures. Clin Sports Med 1990;9(1):31.
5. Andreev DP, Wassilev WA. Specialized contacts between sarcolemma and sarcoplasmic reticulum at the ends of muscle fibers in the diaphragm of the rat. Cell Tissue Res 1986;243:415.
6. Andrews JR, Kupferman SP, Dillman CJ. Labral tears in throwing and racquet sports. Clin Sports Med 1991;10(4):901.
7. Andrews L, Gunnels C. Total shoulder replacement. In Donatelli R, ed. Physical therapy of the shoulder. New York: Churchill Livingstone, 1991.
8. Aniansson A, Headberg M, Henning GB, et al. Muscle morphology, enzymatic activity, and muscle strength in elderly men: a follow-up study. Muscle Nerve 1986;9:585.
9. Arnheim D. Modern principles of athletic training. St. Louis: Times Mirror/Mosby, 1989.
10. Bassett FH. Basketball. In Schneider R, et al., eds. Sports injuries: mechanisms, prevention, and treatment. Baltimore: Williams & Wilkins, 1985.
11. Bateman JE. Nerve injuries about the shoulder in sports. J Bone Joint Surg 1967;49(4):785.
12. Bateman JE. Nerve lesions about the shoulder. Orthop Clin North Am 1980;11(2):307.
13. Bell R, Noble J. An appreciation of posterior instability of the shoulder. Clin Sports Med 1991;10(4):887.
14. Benjamin M, Evans EJ, Copp L. The histology of tendon attachments to bone in man. J Anat 1986;89:100.
15. Bennett R. The painful shoulder. Postgrad Med 1983;73(5):153.
16. Bergfeld JA, Andrish JT, Clancy WG. Evaluation of the acromioclavicular joint following first- and second-degree sprains. Am J Sports Med 1978;6(4):153.
17. Bigliani LU. Fractures of the proximal humerus. In Rockwood C, Matsen F, eds. The shoulder. Vol. 2. Philadelphia: WB Saunders, 1990.
18. Binder AI, Bulgen DY, Hazleman BL, et al. Frozen shoulder: an arthrographic and radionuclear scan assessment. Ann Rheum Dis 1984;43:365.
19. Blackburn TA. Throwing injuries to the shoulder. In Donatelli RA, ed. Physical therapy of the shoulder. 2nd ed. New York: Churchill Livingstone, 1991.
20. Blasier R, Burkus K. Management of posterior fracture-dislocations of the shoulder. Clin Orthop 1988;232:197.
21. Bowling R, Rockar P, Erhard R. Examination on the shoulder complex. Phys Ther 1986;66(12):1866.
22. Brems J. Rotator cuff tear: evaluation and treatment. Orthopedics 1988;11(1):69.
23. Brooks CH, Revell WJ, Heatley FW. A quantitative histological study of the vascularity of the rotator cuff tendon. J Bone Joint Surg 1992;74B:151.
24. Calandra J, Baker C, Uribe J. The incidence of Hill-Sachs lesions in initial anterior shoulder dislocations. Arthroscopy 1989; 5(4):254.
25. Chansky H, Iannotti J. The vascularity of the rotator cuff. Clin Sports Med 1991;10(4):807.
26. Thoracic outlet syndrome. CIBA, 1971.
27. Ciullo JV, Jackson DW. Track and field. In Schneider R, Kennedy JC, Plant NL et al, eds. Sports injuries: mechanism, prevention, and treatment. Baltimore: Williams & Wilkins, 1985.
28. Codman EA. The shoulder. 2nd ed. Boston: Thomas Todd, 1934.
29. Codman EA, Akenson JB. The pathology associated with rupture of the supraspinatus tendon. Ann Surg 1931;93:348.
30. Cofield R. Degenerative and arthritic problems of the glenohumeral joint. In Rockwood C, Matsen F, eds. The shoulder. Vol 2. Philadelphia: WB Saunders, 1990.
31. Cofield R. Rotator cuff disease of the shoulder. J Bone Joint Surg 1985;67 A(6):974.
32. Connolly J, Regen E, Evans OB. The management of the painful, stiff shoulder. Clin Orthop 1972;84:97.
33. Cotton RE, Rideout DF. Tears of the humeral rotator cuff. J Bone Joint Surg 1964;46B:314.
34. Cox JS. The fate of the acromioclavicular joint in athletic injuries. Am J Sports Med 1981;9(1):50.
35. Cruess R. Rheumatoid arthritis of the shoulder. Orthop Clin North Am 1980;11(2):333.
36. Cuetter AC, Bartoszek DM. The thoracic outlet syndrome: controversies, overdiagnosis, overtreatment and recommendations for management. Muscle Nerve 1989;12:410.
37. Cummings G, Crutchfield R, Barnes M. Orthopedic physical therapy series, Vol. 1: Soft tissue changes in contractures. Atlanta: Stokesville Publishing Company, 1983.
38. Darnell MW. A proposed chronology of events for forward head posture. J Craniomandib Pract 1983;1:4.
39. DePalma AF. Loss of scapulohumeral motion. Ann Surg 1952;135:193.
40. Ellman H. Diagnosis and treatment of incomplete rotator cuff tears. Clin Orthop 1990;254:64.
41. Ellman H. Surgical treatment of rotator cuff ruptures. In Watson M, ed. Surgical disorders of the shoulder. New York: Churchill Livingstone, 1991.
42. Ellman H, Hanker G, Bayer M. Repair of the rotator cuff. J Bone Joint Surg 1986;68A(8):1136.
43. Ellman M. Arthritis of the shoulder. In Post M, ed. The shoulder: surgical and nonsurgical management. 2nd ed. Philadelphia: Lea & Febiger, 1988.
44. Ellman M, Brown N, Curran J. Shoulder arthritis. Postgrad Med 1983;73(5):158.
45. Enoka RM: Muscle strength and its development: new perspectives. Sports Med 1988;6:146.
46. Falkel JE, Murphy TC. Common injuries of the shoulder in athletes. In Malone T, ed. Sports injury management: shoulder injuries. Vol 1. Baltimore: Williams & Wilkins, 1988.
47. Flax H. Differential diagnosis of lesions producing stiff shoulder. Am J Phys Med 1981;60(1):20.
48. Foster C. Multidirectional instability of the shoulder in the athlete. Clin Sports Med 1983;2(2):355.
49. Frey C, Shereff H, Greenidge N. Vascularity of posterior tibial tendon. J Bone Joint Surg 1990;72A:884.
50. Garrett WE Jr, Tidball JG. Myotendinous junction: structure, function, and failure. In Woo S L-Y, Buckwalter JS, eds. Injury and repair of the musculoskeletal soft tissues. Park Ridge, Ill.: AAOS, 1988.
51. Gibson K. Rheumatoid arthritis of the shoulder. Phys Ther 1986;66(12):1920.

52. Glick JM, Milurn JJ, Haggerty JF, et al: Dislocated acromioclavicular joint: follow-up study of 35 unreduced acromioclavicular dislocations. Am J Sports Med 1977;5(6):264.
53. Green HJ. Characteristics of aging human skeletal muscle. In Sutton JR, Brock RM, eds. Sports medicine for the mature athlete. Indianapolis: Benchmark Press, 1986.
54. Grimby G, Saltin B. The aging muscle. Clin Physiol 1983;3:209.
55. Gristina AG, Kammire G, Voytek A, et al. Sepsis of the shoulder: molecular mechanisms and pathogenesis. In Rockwood C, Matsen F, eds. The shoulder. Vol. 2. Philadelphia: WB Saunders, 1990.
56. Haber EC, Storey MD. Effort thrombosis in a runner. Physician Sports Med 1990;18(6):76.
57. Hawkins R, Abrams J. Impingement syndrome in the absence of rotator cuff tear (stages 1 and 2). Orthop Clin North Am 1987;18(3):373.
58. Hawkins RJ, Angelo RL. Displaced proximal humeral fractures. Orthop Clin North Am 1987;18(3):421.
59. Hazelman B. Frozen shoulder. In Watson MS, ed. Surgical disorders of the shoulder. New York: Churchill Livingstone, 1991.
60. Hazelman B. Why is a frozen shoulder frozen? Br J Rheumatol 1990;29(2):130.
61. Henry JH, Genung JA. Natural history of glenohumeral dislocation—revisited. Am J Sports Med 1982;10(3):135.
62. Hershman EB, Wilbourn J, Bergfeld JA. Acute brachial neuropathy in athletes. Am J Sports Med 1989;17(5):655.
63. Hooper ACB. Length, diameter and number of ageing skeletal muscle fibres. Gerontology 1981;27:121.
64. Hughes M, Neer CS II. Glenohumeral joint replacement and postoperative rehabilitation. Phys Med 1975;55:850.
65. Jobe FW, Moynes DR, Brewster CE. Rehabilitation of shoulder joint instabilities. Orthop Clin North Am 1987;18(3):473.
66. Keene JS. Ligament and muscle-tendon unit injuries. In Gould JA, ed. Orthopaedic and sports physical therapy. 2nd ed. St. Louis: CV Mosby, 1990.
67. Klawans HL, Topel JL. Neurologic aspects of the shoulder. In Post M, ed. The shoulder: surgical and nonsurgical management. 2nd ed. Philadelphia: Lea & Febiger, 1988.
68. Kline DG, Kott J, Barnes G, et al Exploration of selected brachial plexus lesions by the posterior subscapular approach. J Neurosurg 1978;49:872.
69. Koontz CL, Burkart SL. Thoracic outlet syndrome: diagnosis and management: Pittsburgh AREN Publications/Video Conference, 1986
70. Kozin F. Two unique shoulder disorders: adhesive capsulitis and reflex sympathetic dystrophy syndrome. Postgrad Med 1983; 73(5):207.
71. Kristiansen B, Angermann P, Larsen TK: Functional results following fractures of the proximal humerus. Arch Orthop Trauma Surg 1989;108:339.
72. LeCroy CM, Reedy MK, Seaber AV, et al. Limited sarcomere extensibility and strain injury in rabbit skeletal muscle. Trans Orthop Res Soc 1989;14:316.
73. Leffert RD. Neurological problems. In Rockwood C, Matsen F, eds. The shoulder. Vol. 2. Philadelphia: WB Saunders, 1990.
74. Leffert RD, Rowe CR. Tendon ruptures. In Rowe CR, ed. The shoulder. New York: Churchill Livingstone, 1988.
75. Leslie BM, Harris JM, Driscoll D. Septic arthritis of the shoulder in adults. J Bone Joint Surg 1989;71(10):1516.
76. Lexell J, Henriksson-Larsen K, Winblad B, et al. Distribution of different fiber types in human skeletal muscles: effects of aging studies in whole muscle cross sections. Muscle Nerve 1983; 6:588.
77. Ling SC, Chen CF, Wan RX. A study of the vascular supply of the supraspinatus tendon. Surg Radiol Anat 1990;12:161.
78. Magee DJ. Orthopedic physical assessment. Philadelphia: WB Saunders, 1987.
79. Malone TR, ed. Sports injury management: Muscle injury and rehabilitation. Vol. 1. Baltimore: Williams & Wilkins, 1988.
80. Manske PR, Lesker PA. Flexor tendon nutrition. Hand Clin North Am 1985;1:13.
81. Matsen FA. TUBS, AMBRI—pneumonics to differentiate traumatic instability from multi-directional instability. American Academy of Orthopaedic Surgeons, Summer Institute, San Diego, September 7–11, 1988.
82. Matsen F, Arntz C. Rotator cuff tendon failure. In Rockwood C, Matsen F, eds. The shoulder. Vol. 2. Philadelphia: WB Saunders, 1990.
83. Matsen FA, Arntz CT. Subacromial impingement. In Rockwood C, Matsen F, eds. The shoulder. Vol. 2. Philadelphia: WB Saunders, 1990.
84. Matsen F, Zuckerman J. Anterior glenohumeral instability. Clin Sports Med 1983;2(2):319.
85. May V. Posterior dislocation of the shoulder: habitual, traumatic, and obstetrical. Orthop Clin North Am 1980;11(2):271.
86. McCleery RS, Kesterson JE, Kirtley JA, et al. Subclavius and anterior scalene muscle compression as a cause of intermittent obstruction of the subclavian vein. Ann Surg 1951;133:588.
87. McNab F. Rotator cuff tendinitis. Ann R Coll Surg Engl 1973;53:271.
88. Melvin J, ed. Rheumatic disease in the adult and child: occupational therapy and rehabilitation. 3rd ed. Philadelphia: FA Davis, 1989.
89. Michael R, Matthews L. Lacrosse. In Schneider R, Kennedy JC, Plant NL et al., eds. Sports injuries: mechanism, prevention, and treatment. Baltimore: Williams & Wilkins, 1985.
90. Mohtadi NC. Advances in the understanding of anterior instability of the shoulder. Clin Sports Med 1991;10(4):863.
91. Moran C, Saunders S. Evaluation of the shoulder: a sequential approach. In Donnatelli R, ed. Physical therapy of the shoulder. 2nd ed. New York: Churchill Livingstone, 1991.
92. Moritani T. Training adaptations in the muscles of older men. In Smith EL, Serfass RC, eds. Exercise and aging: the scientific basis. Hillside, N.J.: Enslow Publishers, 1981.
93. Moritani T, DeVries HA. Neural factors versus hypertrophy in the time course of muscle strength gain. Am J Phys Med 1979;58:115.
94. Moseley HF, Goldie I. The arterial pattern of the rotator cuff of the shoulder. J Bone Joint Surg 1963;45B:780.
95. Naffziger HC. Neuritis of the bracial plexus, mechanical in origin: the scalenus syndrome. Surg Gynecol Obstet 1938; 67:722.
96. Neer CS II. Displaced proximal humeral fractures: I. Classification and evaluation. J Bone Joint Surg 1970;52A(6):1077.
97. Neer CS II. Impingement lesions. Clin Orthop 1983;173:70.
98. Neer CS II. Involuntary inferior and multi-directional instability of the shoulder: etiology, recognition, and treatment. Instruct Course Lect 1985;34:232.
99. Neer CS II. Shoulder reconstruction. Philadelphia: WB Saunders, 1990.
100. Neer CS II, McCann PD, MacFarlane EA, et al. Earlier passive motion following shoulder arthroplasty and rotator cuff repair: a prospective study. Orthop Trans 1987;2:231.
101. Neviaser J. Adhesive capsulitis and the stiff and painful shoulder. Orthop Clin North Am 1980;11(2):327.
102. Neviaser J. Adhesive capsulitis of the shoulder: a study of the pathological findings in periarthritis of the shoulder. J Bone Joint Surg 1945;27:211.
103. Neviaser J. Injuries of the clavicle and its articulations. Orthop Clin North Am 1980;11(2):233.
104. Neviaser RJ. Injuries to the clavicle and acromioclavicular joint. Orthop Clin North Am 1987;18(3):433.
105. Neviaser RJ. Lesions of the biceps and tendinitis of the shoulder. Orthop Clin North Am 1980;11(2):343.
106. Neviaser RJ. Ruptures of the rotator cuff. Orthop Clin North Am 1987;18(3):387.
107. Neviaser RJ, Neviaser TJ. Observations on impingement. Clin Orthop 1990;254:60.
108. Neviaser TJ. Adhesive capsulitis. Orthop Clin North Am 1987;18(3):439.
109. Neviaser TJ. The role of the biceps tendon in the impingement syndrome. Orthop Clin North Am 1987;18(3):383.
110. Nicholson GG. Rehabilitation of common shoulder injuries. Clin Sports Med 1989;8(4):633.
111. Nitz A. Physical therapy management of the shoulder. Phys Ther 1986;66(12):1912.
112. Noonan PJ, Garrett WE. Injuries at the myotendinous junction in tendinitis: II. clinical considerations. Clin Sports Med 1992; 2(10):783.
113. Norris TR. History and physical examination of the shoulder. In Nicholas JA, Hershman E, Posner MA, eds. The upper extremity in sports medicine. St. Louis: CV Mosby, 1990.
114. O'Brien M. Functional anatomy and physiology of tendons in tendinitis, part I. Clin Sports Med 1992;11(7):505.
115. O'Brien S, Warren R, Schwartz E. Anterior shoulder instability. Orthop Clin North Am 1987;18(3):395.

116. Osterman AL. The double crush syndrome. Orthop Clin North Am 1988;19(4):147.
117. Pappas AM, Goss TP, Kleinman PK. Symptomatic shoulder instability due to lesions of the glenoid labrum. Am J Sports Med 1983;11(5):279.
118. Payne R. neuropatic pain syndromes with special reference to causalgia and reflex sympathetic dystrophy. Clin J Pain 1986;2:59.
119. Peat M. Functional anatomy of the shoulder complex. Phys Ther 1986;66(12):1855.
120. Perry J. Anatomy and biomechanics of the shoulder in throwing, swimming, gymnastics, and tennis. Clin Sports Med 1983;2(2):247.
121. Peterson TR. Injuries to other parts of the body. In Schneider R, Kennedy JC, Plant NL et al., eds. Sports injuries: mechanism, prevention and treatment. Baltimore: Williams & Wilkins, 1985.
122. Pettrone FA, Nirschl RP. Acromioclavicular dislocation. Am J Sports Med 1978;6(4):160.
123. Post M. Constrained arthroplasty of the shoulder. Orthop Clin North Am 1987;18(3):455.
124. Post M. Fractures of the upper humerus. Orthop Clin North Am 1980;11(2):239.
125. Post M. Orthopaedic management of shoulder infections. In Post M, ed. The shoulder: surgical and nonsurgical management. 2nd ed. Philadelphia: Lea & Febiger, 1988.
126. Post M, Silver R, Singh M. Rotator cuff tear: diagnosis and treatment. Clin Orthop 1983;173:78.
127. Pratt NE. Neurovascular entrapment in the regions of the shoulder and posterior triangle of the neck. Phys Ther 1986; 66(12):1894.
128. Rathbun J, MacNab I. The microvascular pattern of the rotator cuff. J Bone Joint Surg 1970;52B(3):540.
129. Reeves B. The natural history of the frozen shoulder syndrome. Scand J Rheumatol 1975;4:193.
130. Richardson AB. Overuse syndromes in baseball, tennis, gymnastics, and swimming. Clin Sports Med 1983;2(2):379.
131. Rizk T, Pinals R. Frozen shoulder. Semin Arthritis Rheum 1984;11(4):440.
132. Rocobado M. Advanced pathophysiology of the lower cervical spine and shoulder girdle. Course notes, 1990.
133. Roos DB, Owens JC. Thoracic outlet syndrome. Arch Surg 1966;93:71.
134. Roos DB, Wilbourn AJ. Controversies in neurology: thoracic outlet syndrome. Arch Neurol 1990;47:327.
135. Rothman RH, Parke WW. Vasculature anatomy of the rotator cuff. Clin Orthop 1965;41:176.
136. Rowe C. Acromioclavicular and sternoclavicular joints. In Rowe C, ed. The shoulder. New York: Churchill Livingstone, 1988.
137. Rowe C. Acute and recurrent anterior dislocations of the shoulder. Orthop Clin North Am 1980;11(2):253.
138. Rowe C. Dislocations of the shoulder. In Rowe CR, ed. The shoulder. New York: Churchill Livingstone, 1988.
139. Rowe C. Tendinitis, bursitis, impingement, "snapping" scapula, and calcific tendinitis. In Rowe C, ed. The shoulder. New York: Churchill Livingstone, 1988.
140. Rowe CR, Leffert RD. Idiopathic chronic adhesive capsulitis ("frozen shoulder"). In Rowe C, ed. The shoulder. New York: Churchill Livingstone, 1988.
141. Sale DG. Neural adaptation to resistance training. Med Sci Sports Exerc 1988;20:S135.
142. Sallis RE, Jones K, Knopp W. Burners: offensive strategy for an underreported injury. Physician Sports Med 1992;20(11):47.
143. Salter RB. Textbook of disorders and injuries of the musculoskeletal system. 2nd ed. Baltimore: Williams & Wilkins, 1983.
144. Samilson RL, Prieto V. Posterior dislocation of the shoulder in athletes. Clin Sports Med 1983;2(2):369.
145. Schwartz E, Warren RF, O'Brien SJ, et al. Posterior shoulder instability. Orthop Clin North Am 1987;18(3):409.
146. Simkin P. Tendinitis and bursitis of the shoulder: anatomy and therapy. Postgrad Med 1983;73(5):178.
147. Simmonds FA. Shoulder pain: with particular reference to the "frozen shoulder." J Bone Joint Surg 1949;31B(3):426.
148. Skurja M, Monlux JH. Case studies: the suprascapular nerve and shoulder dysfunction. J Orthop Sports Phys Ther 1985;6(4):254.
149. Skyhar MJ, Warren RF, Altchek DW. Instability of the shoulder. In Nicholas JA, Hershman E, Posner MA, eds. The upper extremity in sports medicine. St. Louis: CV Mosby, 1990.
150. Speer KP, Bassett FH. The prolonged burners syndrome. Am J Sports Med 1990;18(6):591.
151. Stanton PE, Nghia MV., Haley P, et al. Thoracic outlet syndrome: a comprehensive evaluation. Am Surg 1988;3:129.
152. Sunderland S. Nerves and nerve injuries. 2nd ed. New York: Churchill Livingston, 1979.
153. Thomas D, Williams R, Smith D. The frozen shoulder: a review of manipulative treatment. Rheumatol Rehabil 1980;19:173.
154. Tibone J, Sellers R, Tonino P. Strength testing after third-degree acromioclavicular dislocations. Am J Sports Med 1992; 20(3):328.
155. Tidball JG. The geometry of actin filament-membrane associations can modify adhesive strength of the myotendinous junction. Cell Motil Cytoskel 1983;3:439.
156. Travell JG. Myofascial pain and dysfunction: the trigger point manual. Baltimore: Williams and Wilkins, 1983.
157. Trotter JA, Hsi K, Samora A, et al. A morphometric analysis of the muscle-tendon junction. Anat Rec 1985;213:26.
158. Turek S. Orthopaedics: principles and their applications. Philadelphia: JB Lippincott, 1967.
159. Tzankoff SP, Norris AH. Effect of muscle mass decrease on age related BMR changes. J Appl Physiol 1977;43:1001.
160. Uhthoff HK, Sarkar K. Calcifying tendinitis. In Rockwood C, Matsen F, eds. The shoulder. Vol. 2. Philadelphia: WB Saunders, 1990.
161. Uhthoff H, Sarkar K. Classification and definition of tendinopathies. Clin Sports Med 1991;10(4):707.
162. Upton ARM, McComas AJ. The double crush in nerve entrapment syndromes. Lancet 1973;2:359.
163. Vandervoort AA, McComa AJ. Contractile changes in opposing muscles of the human ankle joint with aging. J Appl Physiol 1986;61:361.
164. Wadsworth C. Frozen shoulder. Phys Ther 1986;66(12):1878.
165. Warren R. Subluation of the shoulder in athletes. Clin Sports Med 1983;2(2):339.
166. Watson K. Impingement and rotator cuff lesions. In Nicholson JA, Hershman E, Posner MA, eds. The upper extremity in sports medicine. St. Louis: CV Mosby, 1990.
167. Weaver JK, Dunn HK. Treatment of acromioclavicular injuries, especially complete acromioclavicular separation. J Bone Joint Surg 1972;54A(6):1187.
168. White R. The painful shoulder. In Leek J, Gershwin M, Fowler W et al., eds. Principles of physical medicine and rehabilitation in the musculoskeletal diseases. New York: Grune & Stratton, 1986.
169. Wickiewicz TL. Acromioclavicular and sternoclavicular joint injuries. Clin Sports Med 1983;2(2):429.
170. Woo S L-Y, Buckwalter JA. Injury and repair of the musculoskeletal soft tissues. Savannah: American Academy of Orthopaedic Surgeons Symposium, 1987.
171. Woo S L-Y, Tkach LV. The cellular and matrix response of ligaments and tendons to mechanical injury. In Sports induced inflammation. Chicago: American Academy of Orthopaedic Surgeons, 1990:189.
172. Woo S L-Y, Maynard J, Butler D, et al. Ligament, tendon, and joint capsule insertions to bone. In Injury and repair of muscular skeletal soft tissues. Chicago: American Academy of Orthoped Surgeons, 1988.
173. Yamanaka K, Fukuda H. Aging process of the supraspinatus tendon with reference to rotator cuff tears. In Watson M, ed. Surgical disorders of the shoulder. New York: Churchill Livingstone, 1991.
174. Zarins B, Prodromos C. Shoulder injuries in sports. In Rowe CR, ed. The shoulder. New York: Churchill Livingstone, 1985.

Chapter 4

*Gerald R. Williams*
*Joseph P. Iannotti*

# Diagnostic Tests and Surgical Techniques



Martin J. Kelley and William A. Clark: ORTHOPEDIC THERAPY OF THE SHOULDER.

# Rotator Cuff Disease

There are many causative factors, precipitating events, and senescent changes associated with symptomatic syndromes involving the rotator cuff and its surrounding bone and ligamentous structures. Only some of the many factors associated with rotator cuff disease are *intrinsic* to the rotator cuff tendons and its overlying coracoacromial arch. Many other causes of rotator cuff disease are *extrinsic* to these tissues. Extrinsic factors relate to abnormalities of scapulothoracic function secondary to either cervical spondylosis, serratus anterior palsy, scapulofacial muscular dystrophy, or axillary and suprascapular nerve entrapment syndromes. In addition, rotator cuff pathology is often associated with degenerative arthritides of the glenohumeral joint and adhesive capsulitis. When one considers the diverse disorders that affect the rotator cuff either directly or indirectly, it is not difficult to understand why the most important components of the diagnostic evaluation are still, despite all the recent advances in diagnostic imaging, a careful and thorough history and physical examination. The history and physical examination allow the orthopedic surgeon to interpret and place into appropriate clinical perspective both the obvious and subtle anatomic findings of the imaging studies. This section will deal specifically with those disease states which are caused by and related to factors intrinsic to the rotator cuff mechanism and its overlying coracoacromial arch.

## Clinical Presentation

The symptoms associated with primary intrinsic rotator cuff disease include pain, weakness, and limitation of motion. Pain is localized primarily to the anterolateral and superior aspects of the shoulder. It is also commonly seen in the posterior deltoid and periscapular regions, particularly in patients with rotator cuff tears. The pain may be referred to the upper aspect of the arm, often to the level of the deltoid insertion, and rarely is seen distal to the level of the elbow. The shoulder pain is mechanical in nature, in that it is exacerbated by activities requiring use of the arm at and above shoulder level, particularly against resistance, such as with lifting or reaching. The pain may occur at rest but is often less severe than with overhead activities. Pain at night is a common finding and often disturbs the patient's sleep, particularly when the patient lies on the affected shoulder.

The patient may complain of crepitation and weakness of the shoulder, which may be manifested as fatigue symptoms during activities requiring sustained or repetitive elevation of the arm. With severe weakness, the patient often will be unable to elevate the arm above shoulder level. It is sometimes difficult for the patient to discriminate weakness related to pain versus that which is related to true strength deficits.[108,148]

Although loss of passive motion is not a prominent feature of the subjective complaints associated with primary rotator cuff disease, most patients with chronic symptoms will have lost approximately 10 to 15 degrees of forward elevation, cross-body adduction, and rotation.

The onset of symptoms is quite variable. In patients with rotator cuff tears, there is often an episode of minor trauma associated with either the onset or the progression of preexisting symptoms.[148] In older individuals with large, full-thickness rotator cuff tears, the severity of the disease, size of the tear, and chronicity and severity of the symptoms are often inconsistent with the relatively minor trauma associated with the onset of the clinical symptoms. This discrepancy between the severity of the disease and the severity of the initiating traumatic event clearly indicates that in the older age population there are often degenerative and senescent changes associated with the rotator cuff which predate the traumatic event. In some patients these preexisting degenerative changes are associated with more mild chronic symptoms of shoulder pain and limitations of function that are often attributed to recurrent bouts of shoulder "bursitis."

The degree of tenderness about the shoulder in patients with chronic rotator cuff disease is quite variable. Generally, there is only mild and occasionally moderate tenderness about the greater tuberosity, anterior acromion, and region of the bicipital tendon. In patients with acute and severe tenderness, swelling, and erythema, one should consider in the differential diagnosis acute calcific tendinitis or septic subacromial bursitis. In patients with chronic degenerative disease of the rotator cuff, there is occasionally tenderness over the acromioclavicular joint, and this pain may be associated with and exacerbated by passive cross-body adduction. Acute or chronic long head of the biceps tendon rupture, supraspinatus and infraspinatus muscle atrophy, significant weakness of external rotation, accumulation of fluid in the subacromial bursa (i.e., fluid sign), and scapular substitution with attempted elevation of the arm (i.e., shrug sign) are often associated with chronic massive rotator cuff tears. Each of these physical findings has been correlated with a decrease in the functional results following rotator cuff surgery, and each is therefore an important clinical finding that should be assessed and considered in the preoperative evaluation of the patient. Significant pain over the acromioclavicular joint, particularly pain exacerbated by cross-body adduction and associated with significant degenerative changes on imaging studies, is the primary preoperative indication for distal clavicle resection at the time of rotator cuff repair and acromioplasty.

Subacromial crepitance may be elicited with rotation of the humerus, particularly in the abducted position. Significant subacromial crepitance is often associated with significant spur formation and full-thickness rotator cuff tears. Full-thickness rotator cuff tear should be the primary diagnosis in patients with persistent shoulder pain after rupture of the long head of the biceps tendon, since there is a high correlation between rupture of the long head of the biceps, supraspinatus outlet narrowing, and full-thickness rotator cuff tears, particularly in patients over age 50.

Several impingement signs are associated with primary rotator cuff disease, but none is specific for rotator cuff syndrome, and all can be positive because of other causes of shoulder pain. Two impingement signs, that of Neer[133] (Fig. 4-1) and that described by Hawkins and Kennedy[80] (Fig. 4-2), accentuate pain by mechanical irritation of the rotator cuff and biceps tendon beneath the coracoacromial arch. The coracoid impingement sign can be associated with coracoid impingement, although this may be positive in cases of subacromial impingement.[57,73] Of the many diagnostic tests available, the most clinically useful is the selective injec-

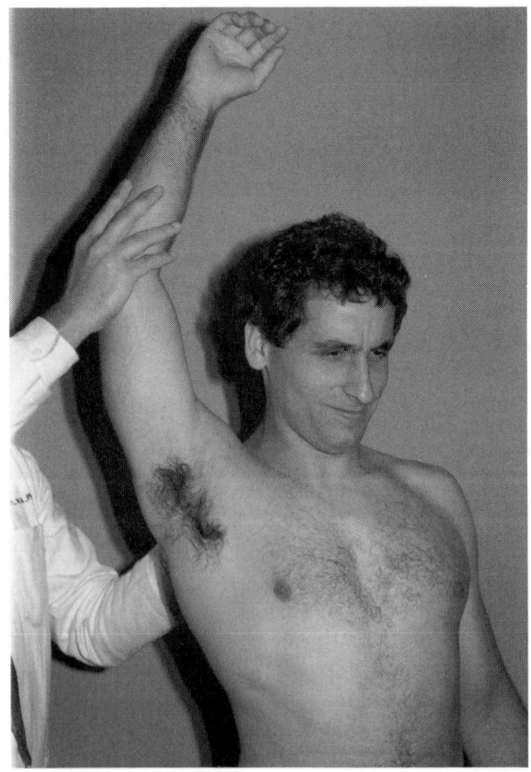

**Figure 4-1.** Neer impingement sign, forced forward flexion in the sagittal plane. (Reproduced with permission from Iannotti JP, ed. Rotator cuff disorders. Park Ridge: American Academy of Orthopedic Surgeons, 1992.)

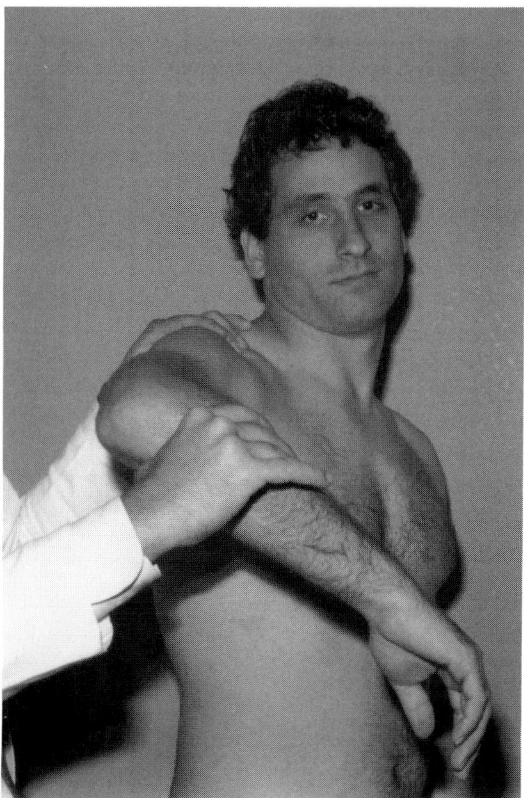

**Figure 4-2.** Hawkin's sign (impingement reinforcement sign, abduction internal rotation impingement sign). The arm is initially placed in neutral rotation and 90 degrees of abduction in the plane of the scapula and internally rotated. (Reproduced with permission from Iannotti JP, ed. Rotator cuff disorders. Park Ridge: American Academy of Orthopedic Surgeons, 1992.)

tion of local anesthetic.[21,80,133] The injection of a local anesthetic is helpful in localizing the pain to a specific anatomic region, thereby adding clinical relevance to the anatomic abnormalities found through imaging studies. The classic impingement test is performed by injecting 8 to 10 cc of local anesthetic into the subacromial space. Then, 5 to 10 minutes after the subacromial injection, the examiner should repeat the physical examination with particular attention to quantifying the pain associated with the impingement signs and the ranges of motion that produce the pain. In general, the pain should decrease at least 50 percent after injection. If it does not, another source of pain should be sought. Alternatively, inaccurate placement of the anesthetic may be responsible. If the pain appears to be associated with the acromioclavicular joint, 2 to 3 cc of local anesthetic injected directly into the acromioclavicular joint may provide an accurate diagnosis. Injection of the subcoracoid space has been described as a means to identify the much less common coracoid impingement syndrome.[28,29]

# Diagnostic Imaging

## PLAIN RADIOGRAPHS

Standard and specialized tilt views are useful in evaluation of symptomatic rotator cuff disease. The standardized views for evaluation of the shape and size of the acromion and acromioclavicular joint include a 30-degree caudad tilt in the anteroposterior plane (Fig. 4-3a), a 10-degree cephalic tilt view in the anteroposterior plane (Fig. 4-4a), and a modified lateral Y view (supraspinatus outlet view) (Fig. 4-5a). These x-rays should be obtained along with the standard anteroposterior view in the plane of the scapula and axillary view (Figs. 4-6 and 4-7). Proliferative degenerative spur formation on the anterior and inferior margins of the acromion and undersurface of the acromioclavicular joint can be assessed with these x-rays. The amount of anterior acromion projecting beyond the anterior border of the clavicle, as seen on the 30-degree caudad tilt view (see Fig. 4-3b), is often associated with significant subacromial impingement.[42,151] Acromial morphology, as described by Morrison and Bigliani,[12,122] is best evaluated on the supraspinatus outlet view (see Fig. 4-5b). Degenerative changes in the acromioclavicular joint are best seen on the 10-degree cephalic tilt anteroposterior view (Zanca view) (see Fig. 4-4b). Degenerative changes in the greater tuberosity, including cyst formation, sclerosis, and occasionally spur formation, are best seen on the anteroposterior view. Unfused acromial apophysis (os acrominale) is best evaluated on the axillary view. Narrowing of the acromiohumeral interval to less than 7 mm is helpful in the diagnosis of chronic large, full-thickness cuff tears.[42,53,75,78,99,102] Cuff arthropathy is demonstrated radiographically as marked cephalad migration of the humeral head, humeral osteopenia, cyst formation, and humeral head collapse[135] (Fig. 4-8). Loss of the articular cartilage of both the glenoid and humeral surfaces results in a nonproliferative glenohumeral narrowing and bone loss. Proliferative degenerative changes of the acromion and acromioclavicular joint are usually associated with cuff arthropathy. These changes are useful in differentiating cuff arthropathy from crystal-induced arthropathy, psoriatic arthropathy, and rheumatoid arthritis. Evaluation of the acromiohumeral interval, calcific deposits, and degenerative changes associated with cuff arthropathy is best demonstrated on anteroposterior scapular plane radiographs.

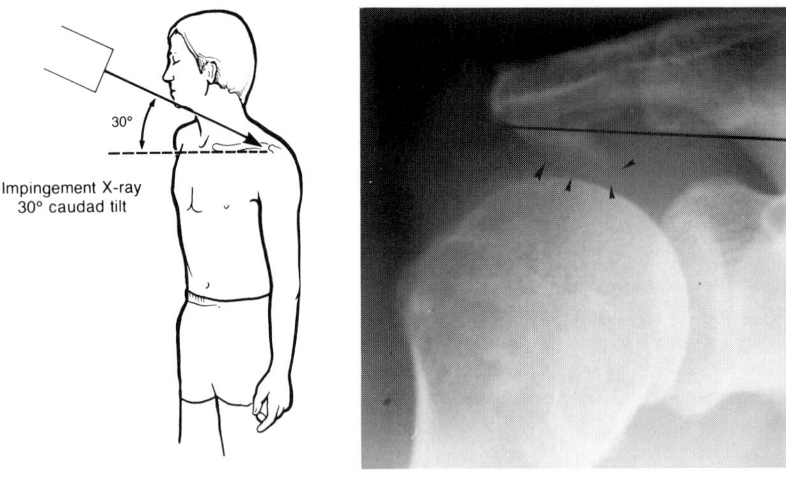


**Figure 4-3.** Rockwood tilt view. (a) This view is anterior/posterior with a 30-degree caudad tilt of the x-ray beam. (b) This x-ray will accentuate anterior projection of an acromial spur (indicated by black arrows). (Reproduced with permission from Rockwood CA, Szalay EA, Curtis RJ, et al. X-ray evaluation of shoulder problems. In: The shoulder. Philadelphia: WB Saunders, 1990.)

## ARTHROGRAPHY

Arthrography is performed by injection of radiopaque contrast material into the glenohumeral joint under sterile conditions (Fig. 4-9a). The arthrogram is the traditional "gold standard" for the imaging diagnosis of full-thickness cuff tears.[68, 75, 98, 107, 159, 181] A full-thickness cuff tear is diagnosed when there is extravasation of contrast material into the subacromial space (see Fig. 4-9b). Extravasation of contrast material into the acromioclavicular joint (Geyser sign) is correlated with massive chronic cuff tears[45] (see Fig. 4-9c).

Although the accuracy of arthrography in determining the size of a full-thickness tear or the presence of partial-thickness tears is not universally accepted, its accuracy in diagnosing full-thickness tears is acknowledged. The specificity and sensitivity of arthrography in full-thickness tears are both better than 90 percent. The positive predictive value of arthrography is higher than 90 percent, and the negative predictive value is approximately 90 percent.

The advantages of shoulder arthrography are that it is easily performed and easily interpreted. It also poses an extremely small incidence of iatrogenic infection. Arthrography is an invasive

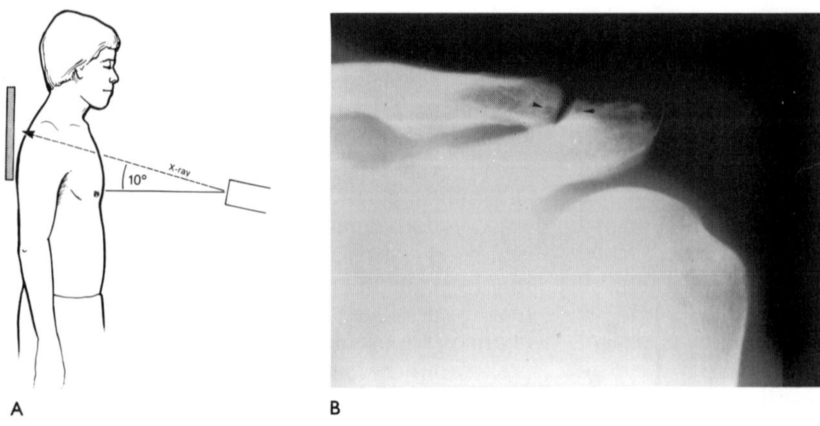


**Figure 4-4.** Zanca view. (a) This view is anterior/posterior with the x-ray beam tilted 10 degrees above the horizontal. (b) This view accentuates the acromioclavicular joint, which allows better visualization of degenerative changes such as cyst formation (black arrows). (Reproduced with permission from Rockwood CA, Szalay EA, Curtis RJ, et al. X-ray evaluation of shoulder problems. In: The shoulder. Philadelphia: WB Saunders, 1990.)

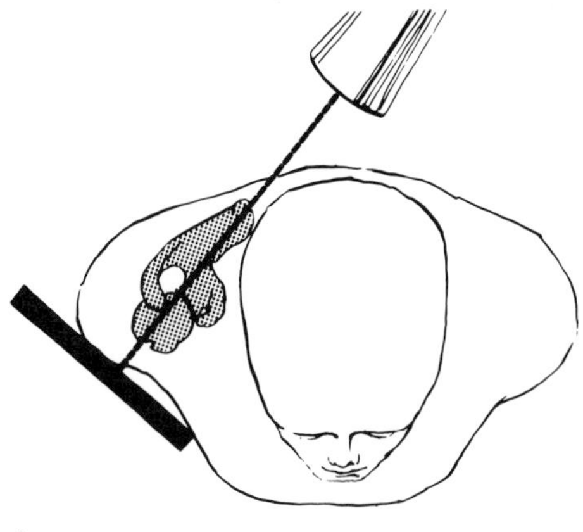

A

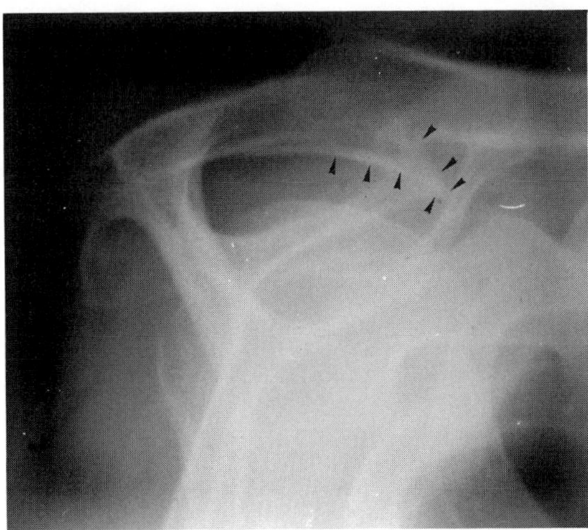

B

**Figure 4-5.** Supraspinatus outlet view. (a) This view is performed in the lateral plane of the scapula with the beam tilted 10 degrees caudad to the horizontal. (b) This view will demonstrate the acromial morphology and inferior and anterior extent of the acromial spur (black arrows). (Reproduced with permission from Rockwood CA Jr, Thomas SC, Matsen FA III. Subluxations and dislocations about the glenohumeral joint. In Rockwood CA, Green DP, Bucholz RW, eds. Fractures. 3rd ed., vol. 1. Philadelphia: JB Lippincott, 1991:1021.)

study and therefore causes discomfort. There is a high incidence of transient increase in shoulder pain that can, on occasion, be significant.[68, 75, 159, 178, 180] The cost is approximately $650. For the purpose of documenting the presence of a full-thickness tear at institutions that do not have a broad experience and documented accuracy using high-resolution ultrasonography or magnetic resonance imaging for cuff disease, arthrography is still the most accurate imaging study, and therefore, it remains the most clinically useful study for surgical decision making.

Arthrography is also reliable for diagnosing a persistent full-thickness tear in a patient who has

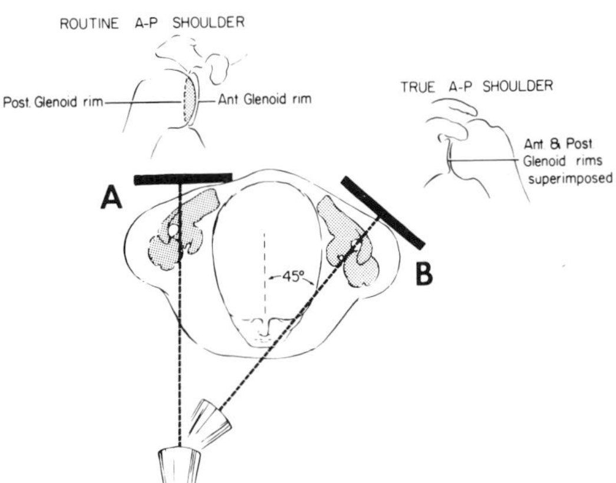


**Figure 4-6.** Anteroposterior radiographs. Anteroposterior radiographs of the shoulder should be taken in the sagital plane (a) and perpendicular to the plane of the scapula (b). Views taken in the sagital plane will show overlap of the glenohumeral articulation, and subtle abnormalities of the glenohumeral articulation may be missed; views taken perpendicular to the plane of the scapula will more clearly demonstrate the glenohumeral articulation. (Reproduced with permission from Neer CS, Rockwood CA, Jr. Fractures and dislocations of the shoulder. In: Rockwood CA, Jr, Green DP (eds.) Fractures. 2nd ed., vol 1. Philadelphia: JB Lippincott, 1984:675.

undergone surgery but whose pain persists. Unfortunately, whether a persistent rotator cuff tear offers an anatomic explanation for persistent pain in this population is subject to question. In a study by Calvert and associates,[27] 17 of 20 patients with clinically satisfactory postoperative results had evidence of contrast material in the

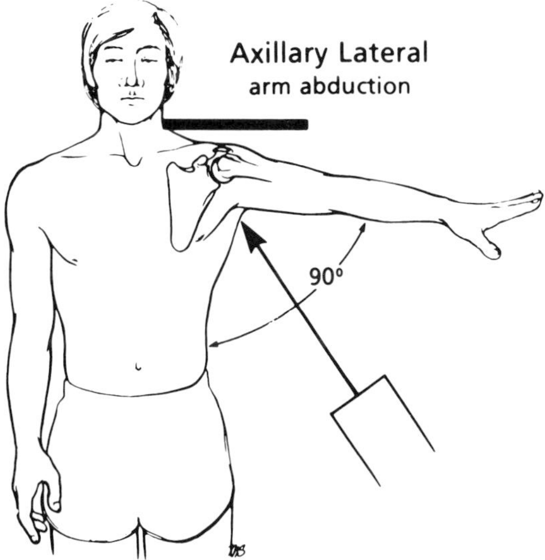


**Figure 4-7.** Axillary lateral view. This view is taken to evaluate the anterior and posterior glenoid margins. (Reproduced with permission from Rockwood CA, Szalay EA, Curtis RJ, et al. X-ray evaluation of shoulder problems. In: The shoulder. Philadelphia: WB Saunders, 1990.)

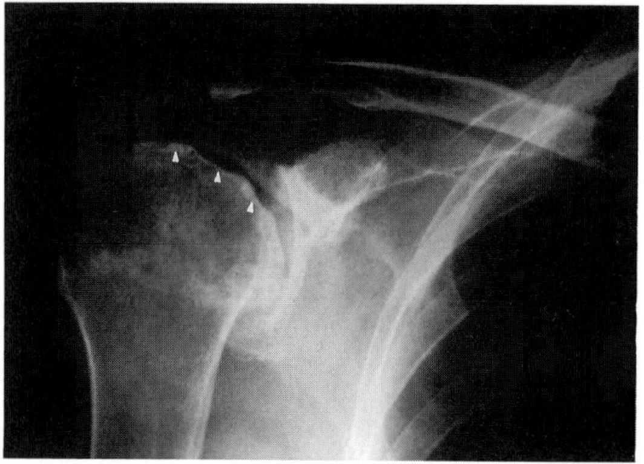

**Figure 4-8.** Anteroposterior radiograph of a patient with rotator cuff tear arthropathy demonstrating humeral head collapse and marked degenerative changes (white arrows).

subacromial space, indicating a persistent full-thickness defect.

## ULTRASONOGRAPHY

Real-time 7-MHz high-resolution ultrasonography of both shoulders has been reported by some investigators to be highly accurate in the diagnosis of full-thickness rotator cuff tears[19,47,49,110,117–119,185] (Fig. 4-10). Most investigators consider high-resolution ultrasonography to be inaccurate in the diagnosis of partial tears. The sensitivity and specificity associated with marked thinning or loss of the normal echogenic signal of the rotator cuff are better than 90 percent. The positive and negative predictive values are 84 and 95 percent, respectively.[119] Other signal abnormalities noted within the rotator cuff by ultrasonography carry an inaccuracy rate of approximately 35 percent. The accuracy of ultrasonography is significantly improved by real-time analysis of the dynamic video images of the cuff as well as experience with the technique.[56,118,119] The entire cuff is difficult to visualize because of the overlying acromion, but this problem can be overcome by arm positioning and with real-time video recording.[48] In studies evaluating the use of ultrasonography after rotator cuff surgery, ultrasonography reported identification of the presence of full-thickness cuff tears.[47,79,110] The criteria for such postoperative diagnoses are different, and such determinations are more difficult to make. A recent study by Harryman et al.[79] using ultrasonography in the postoperative setting following rotator cuff repair has confirmed the findings of Calvert et al.[27] There is a high incidence of recurrent rotator cuff tears, particularly in those patients who preoperatively have two and three tendon tears. The presence of a persistent tear diagnosed by ultrasound

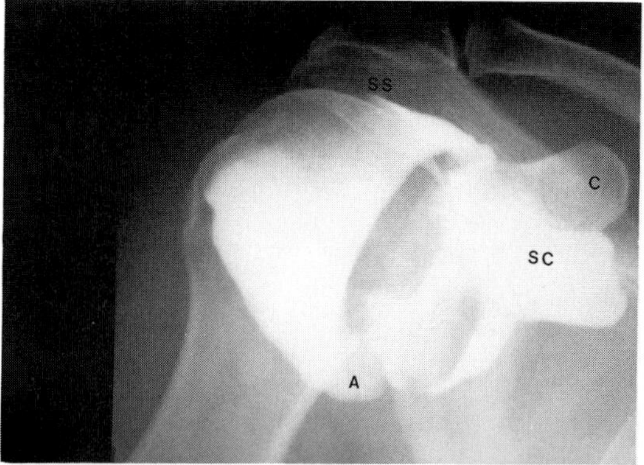


A

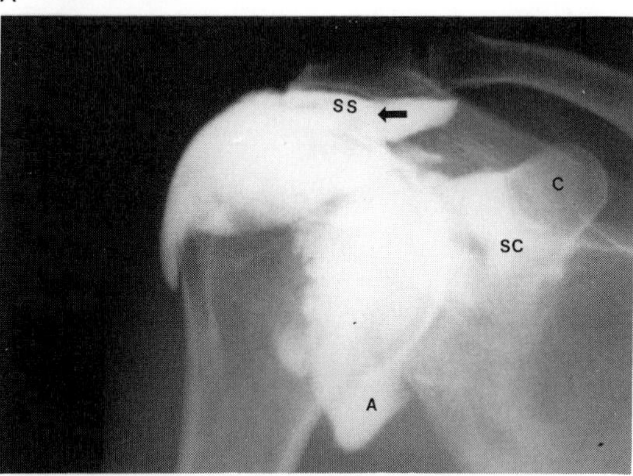


B

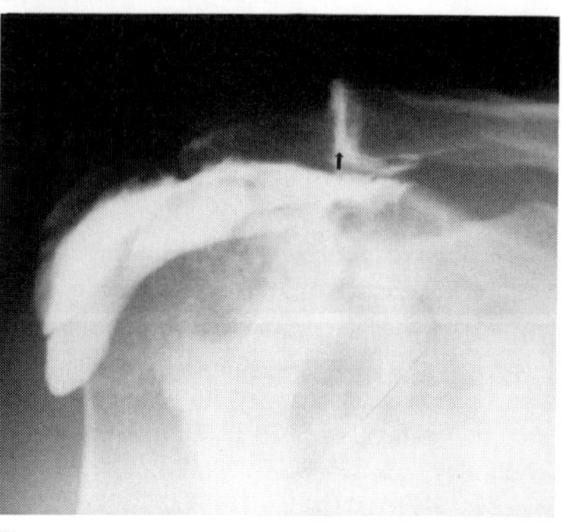

C

**Figure 4-9.** Arthrograms. Anteroposterior radiographs following injection of contrast material. (a) A normal arthrogram demonstrates contrast material which is normally seen below the coracoid (c) in the subcoracoid space (*sc*), as well as in the axillary pouch (*a*). Contrast material is seen around the humeral head but not within the subacromial space. (b) Arthrographic findings for a full-thickness tear of the rotator cuff that demonstrates contrast material within the subacromial space (*ss*) (black arrow). Extravasation of contrast material into the acromioclavicular joint (Geyser sign) (black arrows) is correlated with massive chronic cuff tears. (c) This sign is consistent with large massive chronic cuff tears resulting in erosion of the acromioclavicular joint, thereby allowing contrast material within the acromioclavicular joint space. (Reproduced with permission from Iannotti JP, ed. Rotator cuff disorders. Park Ridge: American Academy of Orthopedic Surgeons, 1992.)

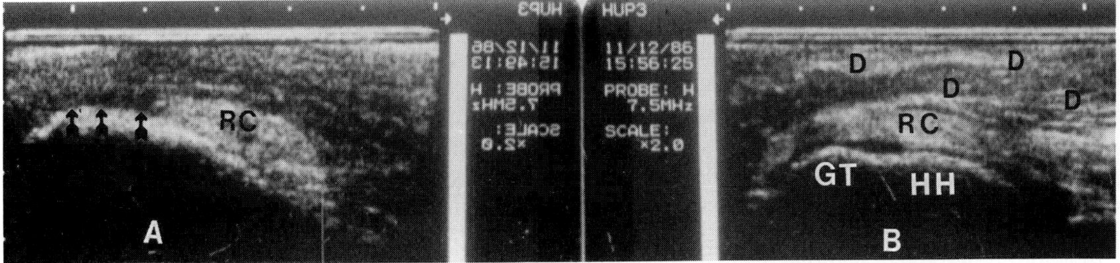


**Figure 4-10.** Ultrasonography. Sagittal plane ultrasonography of the supraspinatus tendon. (a) Right shoulder demonstrating a defect in the rotator cuff (*RC*) indicated by the black arrows. (b) Left shoulder demonstrating a normal signal present in the (*D*) deltoid, a dense normal signal in the (*RC*) rotator cuff, as well as a normal echogenic signal of the (*HH*) humeral head and (*GT*) greater tuberosity.

does not correlate well with the patient's subjective symptoms, since many patients with persistent tears also will have successful outcome of their surgery.

Ultrasonography is noninvasive and costs approximately $450. For these reasons, ultrasonography offers advantages over other diagnostic means, but it has the disadvantage of lacking significant effectiveness in partial-thickness cuff lesions, capsule labral abnormalities, and subacromial impingement.

## MAGNETIC RESONANCE IMAGING

Magnetic resonance imaging (MRI) of the rotator cuff has been wildly studied,[23,61,92,100–103,123,124,181,183] and the criteria for diagnosing full-thickness tears have been fairly well established.[23,92,181,183] The diagnosis is usually based on discontinuity of the tendon on T1-weighted images that is consistent with fluid signal on T2-weighted images (Fig. 4-11). Secondary findings include fluid in the subacromial space (on T2-weighted images), loss of the subacromial fat plane (on T1-weighted images), and proliferative spur formation of the acromion and/or acromioclavicular joint. Large chronic cuff tears often demonstrate spinatus muscle atrophy and show cephalad migration of the humeral head. Full-thickness tears can be reliably diagnosed by MRI if the examiner uses a standardized protocol, off-axis surface coil imaging, and a high-field magnet.[92] The accurate interpretation of MRI requires more training and experience than needed to interpret an arthrogram. The accuracy of MRI depends on the imaging equipment, the technique used, and the experience of the reader. In this last respect, MRI is similar to ultrasonography. The sensitivity and specificity for the diagnosis of full-thickness tears are 100 and 95 percent, respectively. The positive and negative predictive values are 92 and 100 percent, respectively.[92]

Some of the diagnostic advantages of MRI are its ability to evaluate partial-thickness rotator cuff tears, chronic cuff tendinitis, and supra-

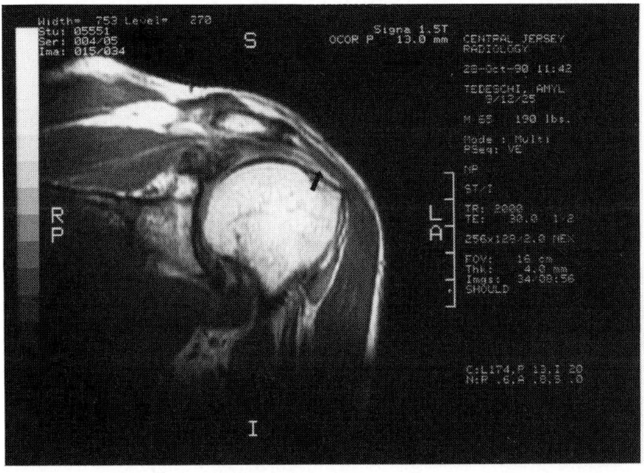


A

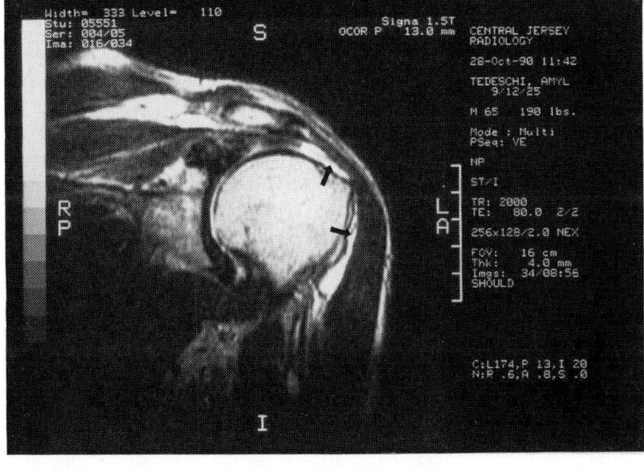


B

**Figure 4-11.** Magnetic resonance imaging. Proton-density no. 15 (a) and T2-weighted no. 15 (b) 30-degree coronal oblique MRI images demonstrating a full-thickness tear (black arrows) with increased signal in both proton-density image and T2-weighted image consistent with fluid within the cuff defect and subacromial space.

spinatus outlet impingement.[150] MRI is able to differentiate cuff degeneration and partial-thickness cuff tears from chronic cuff tendinitis with an intact rotator cuff tendon with a sensitivity and specificity of 82 and 85 percent, respectively. The positive and negative predictive values are 82 and 85 percent, respectively. MRI is very accurate in determining tear size and the presence of spinatus muscle atrophy.[92] MRI in the 30-degree sagittal oblique plane can evaluate the shape of the acromion or the presence of an os acrominale (Fig. 4-12). In addition, if axial imaging of the shoulder is performed, glenoid, labral, and capsular abnormalities can be evaluated.[150] MRI is a noninvasive study that costs approximately $850–$1000. MRI also has been used to evaluate the rotator cuff following rotator cuff surgery. The criterion for diagnosing a full-thickness cuff tear is different in the postoperative shoulder as compared with the unoperated shoulder. In the previously operated shoulder, the diagnosis of a full-thickness cuff tear can be made if there is a distinct discontinuity within the rotator cuff tendon that is filled with fluid, as noted by the marked increase in signal on T2-weighted images. For this specific diagnostic criterion, the accuracy of MRI is reported to be 90 percent. Evaluation of acromion morphology following acromioplasty carries an accuracy of only 75 percent, since there is significant postoperative and metallic artifact that obscures visualization of these structures by MRI.[152]

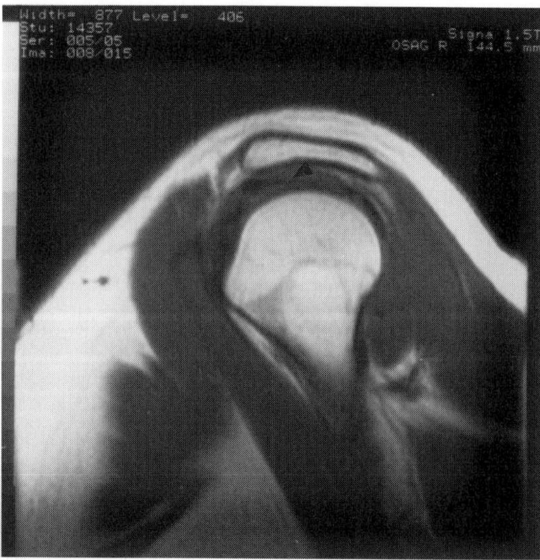


**Figure 4-12.** Magnetic resonance imaging. Proton-density 30-degree sagittal oblique MRI image demonstrating an anteroinferior acromial spur. Type III acromion. (black arrows) (Reproduced with permission from Iannotti JP, ed. Rotator cuff disorders. Park Ridge: American Academy of Orthopedic Surgeons, 1992.)

# Arthroscopy

Arthroscopy of the shoulder for diagnostic evaluation of chronic shoulder pain has been widely used (Fig. 4-13a). In the vast majority of cases, accurate and complete diagnosis often can be made by history, physical examination, and diagnostic imaging studies. In some patients, particularly those having had previous surgery, diagnostic arthroscopy will provide additional information regarding the extent of disease in the osteoarticular and soft tissues of the glenohumeral joint. Most patients with partial-thickness rotator cuff tears will have changes on the articular surface of the rotator cuff (see Fig. 4-13b). The grading system and management protocol for articular surface partial-thickness cuff tears have been proposed by Ellman.[58] The depth and size of the partial-thickness cuff tear are best evaluated by arthroscopy. Arthroscopic evaluation of the rotator cuff followed by arthroscopic surgery for subacromial decompression has been advocated as an effective alternative to open surgery, particularly in patients without full-thickness rotator cuff tears.

# Indications for Surgery

The primary indication for surgical intervention is significant pain that results in disability and functional limitations judged by the patient to be intolerable. In most patients, the indications for surgery include failure of nonoperative management. In selective circumstances, early surgical intervention is recommended. Patients who are active and have moderate or heavy functional demands for recreation or work activities and present with acute traumatic full-thickness rotator cuff tears associated with significant nonantalgic weakness and without a preexisting history of chronic rotator cuff disease are candidates for early surgical repair. This particular subgroup of patients generally constitutes less than 10 percent of most surgical series.[13,76,81,134,157,193] These patients are generally younger, are often less than 40 years of age, and are injured by high-velocity trauma. This group of patients generally does poorly with nonoperative management. With nonoperative management, these patients will often have persistent symptoms, particularly fatigue and weakness associated with their more strenuous activity level. Surgical repair of the rotator cuff is generally easier to perform within the first 6 weeks following injury and is often associated with a more favorable result.[8] In older patients with chronic symptoms and chronic rotator cuff tears, either partial or complete, an

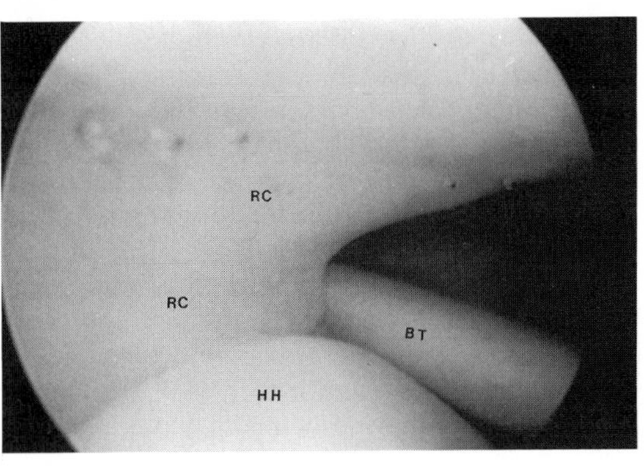


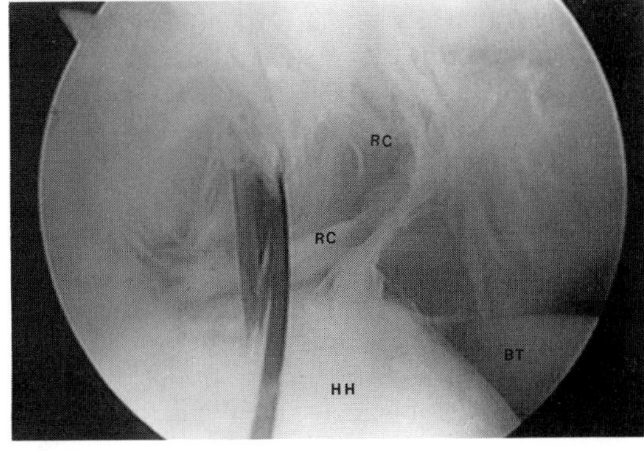


A B

**Figure 4-13.** Arthroscopic views. (a) Normal rotator cuff (*RC*) inserting on the greater tuberosity of the humeral head (*HH*) and a normal intact long head of the biceps (*BT*). (b) Partial-thickness articular surface cuff tear (*RC*) with normal humeral head (*HH*) and intact biceps (*BT*).

initial trial period of nonoperative management is indicated. In this larger group of patients, the adequacy of the nonoperative management program must be assessed prior to a decision to proceed with surgical repair. Nonoperative management would include appropriate rest and avoidance of strenuous activities that precipitate a painful arc and modalities to decrease pain and inflammation, which may include phonophoresis, iontophoresis, ultrasound, local ice and heat, oral anti-inflammatory medication, or corticosteroid injection. A home-based and supervised therapeutic exercise program should include gentle range-of-motion and stretching exercises to maintain or regain passive arcs of motion of the shoulder and gentle strengthening exercises in nonimpingement arcs. In patients with full-thickness rotator cuff tears, this program should be well maintained for approximately a 3-month period. In patients without a full-thickness cuff tear, a nonoperative treatment program of 6 months to 1 year should be considered a prerequisite for surgical intervention. In addition to persistent pain and failure of nonoperative management, the patient should have a positive impingement test, clinical findings that correlate with intrinsic rotator cuff disease, and evidence of mechanical outlet impingement and/or a full-thickness rotator cuff tear by diagnostic imaging studies.

Patients having rotator cuff surgery should be medically fit, cooperative and willing to participate in the rigors of a postoperative rehabilitation program, and ideally should not have other significant causes for shoulder pain (thoracic outlet syndrome, brachial plexus neuropathy, cervical spondylosis).

## Surgical Options

The options for surgical intervention depend on the extent of the disease process. Almost all patients with clinically significant rotator cuff disease show impingement of the rotator cuff by spur formation on the undersurface of the acromion and acromioclavicular joint that results in supraspinatus outlet narrowing. In these cases, therefore, it is important that the surgical management includes adequate decompression of the subacromial space by acromioplasty as well as removal of osteophytes from the undersurface of the acromioclavicular joint and, commonly, resection of the coracoacromial ligament. Regardless of the operative approach, it is important that these specific surgical goals be achieved. In patients who have clinically significant acromioclavicular joint arthropathy, as evidenced by their physical examination, injection test, and imaging studies, partial clavicular resection (Mumford-Gurd procedure) can be performed at the time of acromioplasty.

The management of the rotator cuff lesion is clearly dependent on the extent of the rotator cuff pathology. The articular surface of the rotator cuff is the most common site for partial-thickness rotator cuff tears.[29,39,51,52] The size and depth of the articular surface partial-thickness cuff lesion are best evaluated by arthroscopic means.[58] The management of this lesion is quite controversial, and there is no consensus of opinion in this regard. Surgical options include acromioplasty without specific management of the partial-thickness cuff lesion, acromioplasty plus arthroscopic debridement of the frayed and degenerative portions of the rotator cuff, and lastly, acromioplasty plus excision of the damaged tissue and formal repair of the resulting full-thickness cuff defect. The operative decision is often based on the surgeon's past experience and preference, as well as the extent of the partial-thickness cuff lesion, the age and activity level of the patient, and the presence and extent of outlet impingement.

Several surgical options are available for the management of full-thickness rotator cuff tears. The operative decision in the management of full-thickness cuff tears is again often dependent on the extent and size of the lesion, the quality of the remaining rotator cuff tissue, the age and functional expectations of the patient, and the surgeon's experience and preferences. There is a consensus of opinion that if a full-thickness rotator cuff tear is found and is reparable, then it would be best to repair this by primary means and, in most cases, through reattachment of the torn tendon edge to the greater tuberosity.[39, 57, 76, 79, 145, 193] Successful repair of a full-thickness cuff tear in combination with an adequate subacromial decompression will often lead to improvement of both pain and function. Alternative options for surgical management of a full-thickness rotator cuff tear include use of muscle transfers (subscapularis, latissimus dorsi, and infraspinatus tendons).[38, 74, 146] In patients with irreparable rotator cuff tears, particularly those who are older and have lower functional demands, a satisfactory result may be obtained with adequate decompression alone and limited debridement of frayed and degenerative rotator cuff tissue.[160, 161] There has been limited experience by some surgeons with the use of allograft or prosthetic substitutes in the management of massive rotator cuff tears that could not otherwise be closed by primary repair.[144, 145] The use of these salvage techniques should be limited to those investigators interested in studying the results of these procedures, since their effectiveness has not been adequately defined and requires further evaluation.

## Operative Technique: Authors' Preferred Protocols

### SUBACROMIAL DECOMPRESSION: OPEN ACROMIOPLASTY WITH INTACT ROTATOR CUFF

Anteroinferior acromioplasty, as described by Dr. Charles Neer in 1972,[133] is performed through a 4-cm incision placed within Langer's lines over the anterosuperior aspect of the acromion (Fig. 4-14a). About 2 cm of anterior deltoid origin is removed from the anterior acromion using a Bovie cautery. At the anterolateral corner of the acromion, the deltoid is split within the line of its muscle fibers for a distance of approximately 2 cm (see Fig. 4-14b). The subacromial bursa and coracoacromial ligament are excised from the undersurface of the acromion to the base of the coracoid. Using either an osteotome or an oscillating saw, the acromion, which is projecting anterior to the anterior border of the clavicle, is completely removed (see Fig. 4-14c). The undersurface of the acromion is further decompressed using a high-speed bur (see Fig. 4-14d). The amount of bone removed is judged by palpation of the undersurface of the posterior acromion near the spine of the scapula. Bone along the anteroinferior surface of the acromion is removed so that it is level with the undersurface of the posterior portion of the acromion, thereby creating a flat, or type I, acromial morphology.[12, 122] The amount of bone that can be removed by this two-step acromioplasty can be determined preoperatively by evaluation of the 30-degree caudad tilt view and the supraspinatus outlet view. The undersurface of the acromioclavicular joint is palpated and visualized. Proliferative spur formation at the level of the acromioclavicular joint is removed either with a high-speed burr or a rongeur. The rotator cuff is inspected, and if there is no rotator cuff tear noted either by inspection or palpation, then it is felt that a significant partial-thickness cuff tear is not present. The use of diluted methylene blue placed intraarticularly has been advocated by some as a means to intraoperatively assess undersurface partial-thickness rotator cuff tears.[69] In this technique, the diluted methylene blue stains the degenerative tissues, thereby imparting a discoloration to the damaged area. In these cases, the surgeon may elect to excise the damaged tissue and repair the resulting full-thickness defect. The deltoid is reattached the anterior acromion through drill holes and to the trapezius aponeurosis with heavy nonabsorbable sutures (see Fig. 4-14e). Routine wound closure includes subcuticular closure and Steri-Strips.

### SUBACROMIAL DECOMPRESSION: ARTHROSCOPIC ACROMIOPLASTY WITH INTACT ROTATOR CUFF

Shoulder arthroscopy is performed with the patient in the supine sitting position. A standard-sized 4-mm angled arthroscope is inserted through a posterior portal into the glenohumeral joint. The intraarticular structures are evaluated

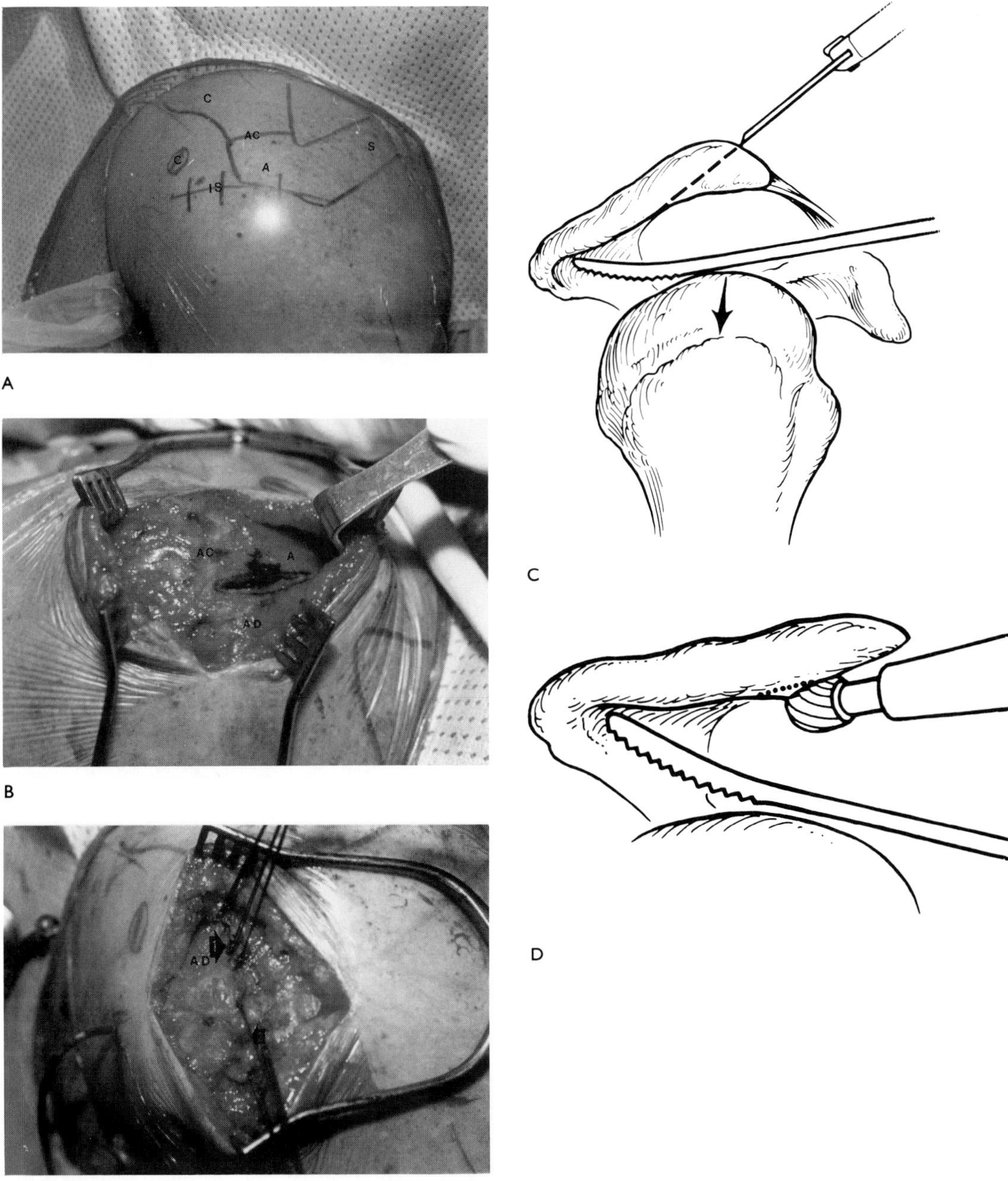


**Figure 4-14.** Open rotator cuff repair and acromioplasty. (a) Incision site for open repair and acromioplasty. The incision is within Langer's lines overlying the acromion (*A*) and lateral to the coracoid (*C*). Landmarks include the acromioclavicular joint (*AC*), clavicle (*C*), and spine of the scapula (*S*). (b) Skin incision is made and subcutaneous flaps prepared. The anterior deltoid origin is incised from the anterior border of the acromion (*A*). The extent of the incision of the deltoid origin is from the acromioclavicular joint (*AC*) to the anterolateral corner of the acromion. (c) Diagrammatic representation of the removal of the anteroinferior acromion for an open Neer acromioplasty. (d) The undersurface of the acromion is further decompressed with a high-speed burr. (e) Closure of the anterior deltoid (*AD*) and middle deltoid (*MD*) back to the acromion with nonabsorbable sutures. For routine rotator cuff repair and open acromioplasty, the anterior deltoid is removed from its bony origin only a distance of approximately 2 cm. (c) and (d) reproduced with permission from Matsen FA, Arntz CT. Subacromial impingement. In: The shoulder. Philadelphia: WB Saunders, 1990.)

for significant articular cartilage disease and labral or capsular abnormalities that may indicate underlying glenohumeral instability. The long head of the biceps tendon is inspected for fraying, and the rotator cuff is evaluated for partial- or full-thickness defects. An anterior surgical portal may be established between the biceps tendon and superior border of the subscapularis, through which is inserted surgical instruments. These instruments may be used for probing, debridement, or repair of the tissues. Articular surface defects in the rotator cuff are often debrided for the purposes of assessing the depth and size of the defect.

Arthroscopic subacromial decompression is accomplished by placing the arthroscope into the subacromial space.[59] This can be achieved either through a posterior portal or a posterolateral portal (Fig. 4-15a). A second anterolateral portal is established, through which a motorized soft-tissue resector is inserted, and the soft tissues on the undersurface of the acromion are removed (see Fig. 4-15b). Care is taken to visualize the entire anterior and anterolateral corner of the acromion as well as the medial aspect of the acromion near the acromioclavicular joint. The undersurface and anterior attachment of the coracoacromial ligament is removed. Soft-tissue resection and resection of the coracoacromial ligament also can be achieved with the use of a cautery. After removal of the acromial attachment of the coracoacromial ligament and the soft tissue on the undersurface of the acromion, the size of the spur is assessed by visual inspection as well as measurement from the preoperative x-rays. Using a high speed burr, all bone anterior to the anterior border of the clavicle is resected (see Fig. 4-15c). The bone remaining on the undersurface of the acromion is tapered posteriorly so that there is a smooth surface that is flat and equal to the level of the undersurface and posterior aspect of the acromion. The acromial surface of the rotator cuff is inspected for partial- or full-thickness cuff defects. Using an end-biting punch, the coracoacromial ligament is further resected. If impingement occurs due to spurs at the level of the acromioclavicular joint, then these are also removed using the burr.

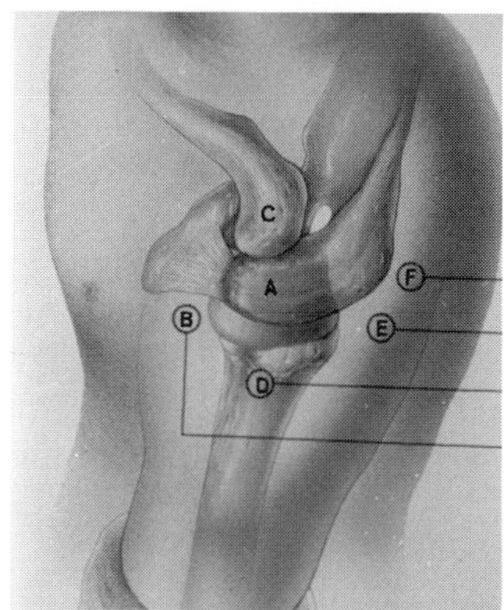


A

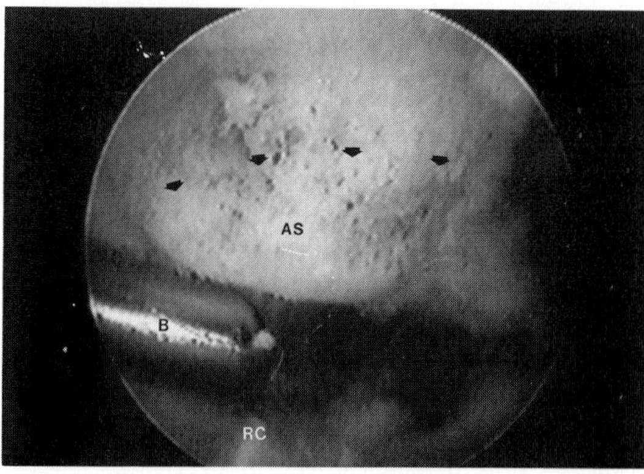


B

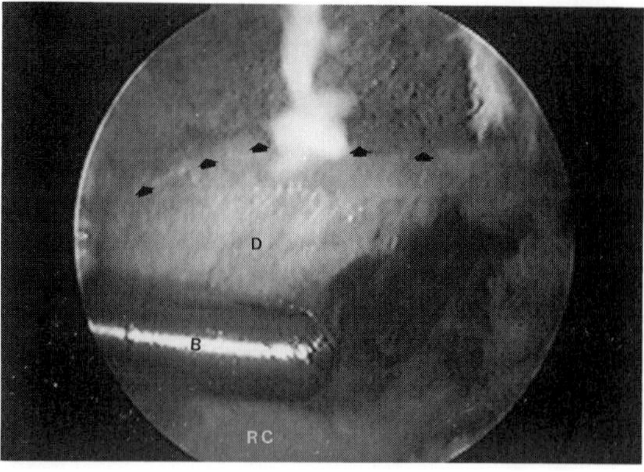


C

**Figure 4-15.** Arthroscopic acromioplasty. (a) Surgical portal sites for arthroscopic evaluation (*CA*, coracoacromial arch; *B*, anterosuperior portals; *D*, lateral portal; *E*, posterolateral portal; *F*, posterior portal). (b) Arthroscopic view demonstrating a large acromial spur (black arrows). The distance between the acromial spur and rotator cuff is approximately 5 mm, as demonstrated by the width of the burr (*B*). (c) Following arthroscopic acromioplasty, the resected margin of the acromion (black arrows) demonstrates the deltoid (*D*) inserting onto the anterior acromion. The distance between the rotator cuff and the anterior acromion is now approximately 1.5 cm. The 5-mm burr (*B*) is demonstrated above the rotator cuff (*RC*). (a) reproduced with permission from Smith-Nephew Dyonics: An illustrated guide to shoulder arthroscopy. Andover, Mass.: 1991.)

## Repair of Full-Thickness Rotator Cuff Tears

Repair of full-thickness rotator cuff tears always includes acromioplasty and coracoacromial ligament resection. In selected cases, distal clavicle resection also may be indicated. Distal clavicle resection is performed in those patients who have significant degenerative changes of the acromioclavicular joint and significant tenderness over this joint that is relieved by selective injection of the joint with local anesthetic. The incision of the deltotrapezius aponeurosis along the anterior and middle deltoid septum is performed (Fig. 4-16a,b). After acromioplasty is achieved (see Fig. 4-16c) and there is no further impingement of the rotator cuff at the level of the acromion or acromioclavicular joint, then rotator cuff repair may be performed. The steps for primary repair of the rotator cuff include finding the margins of the tear, removing mechanically insufficient and frayed rotator cuff tissue at the margins of the tear, and mobilizing the rotator cuff tear, which includes lysis of all adhesions on the acromial and articular surface of the cuff tendons, resection of the coracohumeral ligament (see Fig. 4-16d,e), release of contracted capsule (see Fig. 4-16f), and occasionally placing relaxing incisions in the rotator cuff at the rotator interval. Most tears occur at the bony insertion of the rotator cuff such that the repair requires preparation of a shallow bone trough along the greater tuberosity (see Fig. 4-16g). Drill holes are made through the cortical bone of the greater tuberosity, through which are passed heavy nonabsorbable sutures, and the leading edge of the rotator cuff tear is sewn to the bone trough using a horizontal mattress suture technique (see Fig. 4-16h,i). Some portions of the rotator cuff tear can be repaired with a tendon-to-tendon suturing technique.

Some massive rotator cuff tears cannot be repaired by standard primary repair techniques. In these circumstances, local soft-tissue tendon transfers can be used to augment and close the remaining cuff defect. Soft-tissue transfers that have been used in selected cases include transfer of the subscapularis tendon[38] to substitute for the supraspinatus tendon and transfer of the latissimus dorsi tendon[74] to substitute for the supraspinatus and infraspinatus tendons. These two transfers are active motor transfers and are more complicated and difficult surgical techniques. The long head of the biceps tendon occasionally can be used to reinforce a rotator cuff repair but is considered an inactive transfer and occasionally is used for massive rotator cuff lesions.[146] Other inactive tissue transfers that have been reported sporadically for selected cases of massive rotator cuff tears include the use of allograft or synthetic materials.[144,153] By and large, these inactive biologic and synthetic substitutes have not reached widespread popularity and have only limited follow-up.

Occasionally, patients present with massive rotator cuff tears that are not reparable by primary suturing techniques but are treated by debridement of nonviable rotator cuff tissue and subacromial decompression without rotator cuff repair.[160,161] Patients who have these massive rotator cuff tears and are the best candidates for this operative approach include older patients whose use of the arm excludes heavy recreational or work activities and patients who preoperatively have an intact long head of the biceps tendon and good deltoid function. Preoperatively, these patients have significant pain and weakness of shoulder external rotation but active forward elevation above the shoulder level. Under these clinical circumstances, adequate subacromial decompression without rotator cuff repair often will result in significant improvement of their shoulder pain and, as a result, an improvement in their postoperative function. These patients often will have persistent weakness of the shoulder but will have good functional use for simple overhead activities of daily living. Satisfactory postoperative results require careful strengthening of the anterior and middle deltoid, which is predicated on a well-attached deltoid origin and an innervated deltoid muscle. Patients with rupture of the long head of the biceps tendon often have less favorable results with this procedure.[160,161]

# Operative Technique for Partial-Thickness Rotator Cuff Tears

The operative technique for the management of partial-thickness rotator cuff tears is very controversial. Most partial-thickness rotator cuff tears are found on the undersurface (articular surface) of the rotator cuff. They are often noted near the insertion site of the supraspinatus tendon. These partial-thickness rotator cuff lesions are best evaluated by arthroscopy. The surgical management of such partial-thickness rotator cuff tears is dictated by several factors, including the size of the lesion, the age and activity level of the patient, and the degree of supraspinatus outlet narrowing. In patients who have normal glenohumeral stability and are young and athletically active, particularly with overhead throwing sports, and in whom there is minimal supraspinatus outlet narrowing, arthroscopic debridement of the tear or excision of the remaining tissue and repair of the defect constitute a reasonable surgical option. In patients with small partial-thickness rotator cuff tears who are older and may participate only occasionally in recreational sports or moderate work activities and in whom there is also significant outlet narrowing including subacromial

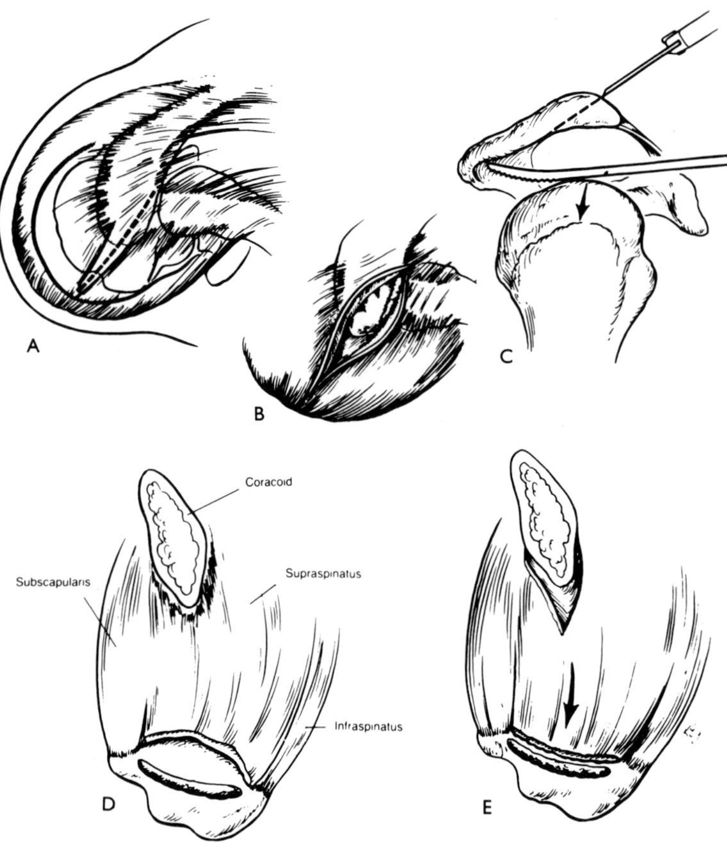


**Figure 4-16.** Repair of full-thickness rotator cuff tear. (a) Incision line. (b) Incision of the deltotrapezius aponeurosis along the anterior and middle deltoid. (c) The line of resection for anterior and inferior acromioplasty. (d,e) Release of the coracohumeral ligament. (f) Release of the contracted capsule in large massive cuff tears for mobilization of capsule and cuff. (g) Preparation of a bony trough in the greater tuberosity. (h,i) Placement of horizontal mattress sutures through tendon and bone. (Reproduced with permission from Matsen FA, Arntz CT. Rotator cuff tendon failure. In: The shoulder. Philadelphia: WB Saunders, 1990.)

spurs, acromioplasty alone will likely provide significant improvement of their pain and adequately minimize progression of the cuff tear. Considering the number of variables in decision making, as well as the wide variability and differing definitions of cuff tear size, youth, and gradations of activity level, it is not difficult to understand the degree of controversy that accompanies the decision making regarding surgical management of partial-thickness cuff tears.

## DISTAL CLAVICLE RESECTION

Distal clavicle resection may be accomplished by both open and arthroscopic techniques. For open procedures, an incision is made as one would for either open acromioplasty or open rotator cuff repair. The deltotrapezius aponeurosis overlying the distal end of the clavicle is incised, and the distal 1.5 to 2.0 cm of clavicle is dissected subperiosteally. Care is taken to avoid injury to the coracoclavicular ligaments. Using an oscillating saw, the distal 1.5 cm of clavicle is removed (Fig. 4-17). The edges of the remaining clavicle are made smooth with either a rasp or a high-speed burr, and the soft tissues of the deltotrapezius aponeurosis are repaired with heavy nonabsorbable sutures. Distal clavicle resection does not significantly alter the coracoclavicular ligaments or vertical stability of the clavicle. The acromioclavicular ligaments are detached, and anteroposterior mobility is increased.

Arthroscopic techniques for distal clavicle resection include visualization of the distal clavicle through a subacromial approach, as described for subacromial decompression, or an acromioclavicular joint approach. In the acromioclavicular approach, a small-diameter arthroscope is inserted directly into the acromioclavicular joint without entering the subacromial space. This technique is used when the only procedure to be performed is distal clavicle resection. In those cases where there is need for both subacromial

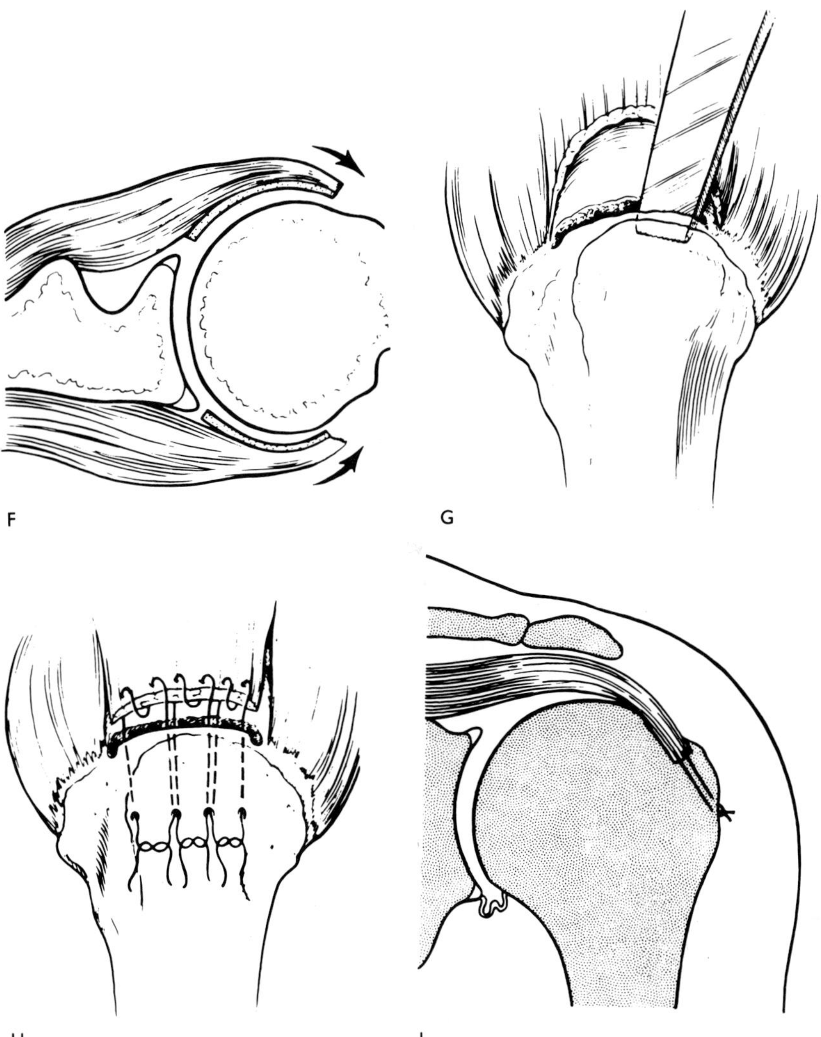


decompression and distal clavicle resection, the subacromial approach is preferred. With either technique, a motorized instrument is used to first define the margins of the distal clavicle and resect the soft tissues within the acromioclavicular joint; thereafter, a high-speed burr is used to resect approximately 1.5 cm of the distal clavicle.

## ARTHROSCOPIC-ASSISTED ROTATOR CUFF REPAIR

Arthroscopically assisted rotator cuff repair is indicated for selected patients with small rotator cuff tears with minimal retraction of the tendon, no significant scarring of the tendon, and healthy rotator cuff tissue. Arthroscopically assisted rotator cuff repair should be in the domain of the experienced shoulder arthroscopist who is familiar with all the principles and techniques of both arthroscopic surgery and standard open rotator cuff repair. Arthroscopically assisted rotator cuff repair includes arthroscopic subacromial decompression, as previously discussed in this chapter, followed by mobilization of the rotator cuff, preparation of a bone trough as one would do for open cuff repair, and placement of sutures at the margin of the cuff tear using arthroscopic suturing instruments. Thereafter, a small arthrotomy is made with a deltoid-splitting incision overlying the greater tuberosity. Sutures are passed through drill holes in the bone trough, and the sutures are tied using a standard technique. The deltoid split is repaired with nonabsorbable suture. Alternative techniques for arthroscopic rotator cuff repair have included use of absorbable tacks and metallic staples. Use of these nonsuture anchoring techniques is easier, but they may have the disadvantages of loss of fixation due to early resorption of the biodegradable material or mechanical loss of fixation due to the soft metaphyseal bone often present at the level of the greater tuberosity.

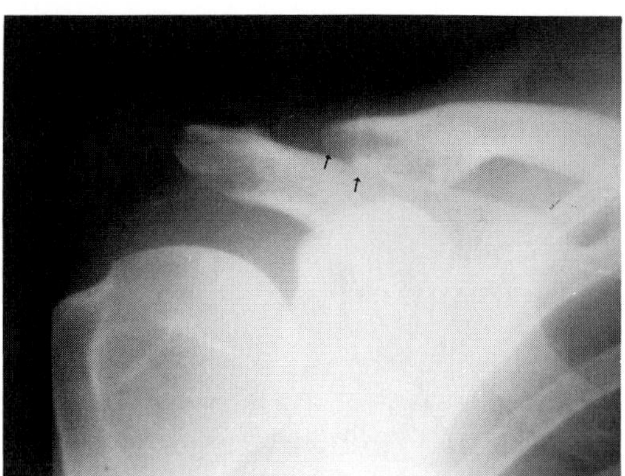

**Figure 4-17.** An anteroposterior radiograph following distal clavicle resection (arrows).

Arthroscopically assisted rotator cuff repair has had relatively limited exposure, and its advantages or benefits over standard open rotator cuff repair have not been defined.

# Rehabilitation

The principles of postoperative rehabilitation are the same regardless of the nature of the operative technique. The rehabilitation program should have clearly defined phases, and the progression of the program should be based on successful completion of the goals defined for each phase of the rehabilitation program. The rehabilitation program must be taught to the patient, understood by the patient, and performed by the patient on a daily basis. With this in mind, the rehabilitation program should be simple and easily performed in a home setting. The rehabilitation program should be directed by the orthopedic surgeon experienced in shoulder surgery and shoulder rehabilitation. The patient should be instructed either by the orthopedic surgeon or by a therapist who has a high level of experience and shares the postoperative goals and philosophy of the operative surgeon.

The goals of the first phase of the rehabilitation are to minimize pain, allow wound healing without risk of disrupting repaired tissues, and begin early joint mobilility to minimize and prevent postoperative stiffness and joint contracture. These goals are accomplished by the immediate postoperative use of cryotherapy and gentle active assisted range of motion of the hand, wrist, elbow, and shoulder. Nonsteroidal anti-inflammatory medication is occasionally useful in minimizing postoperative pain, as is the use of mild narcotic analgesics. Phase I shoulder range-of-motion exercises include pendulums, supine active assisted forward elevation in the plane of the scapula, and external rotation with the shoulder in slight abduction in the plane of the scapula. Standing active assisted extension exercises are also performed in phase I. These phase I exercises are continued until there is only mild pain at the incision site and the exercises are done with ease and have achieved 80 percent of passive arcs of shoulder motion. For arthroscopic acromioplasty, this is usually achieved within 2 weeks; for open acromioplasty, within 2 to 3 weeks; and for rotator cuff repair, within 4 to 6 weeks.

Phase II of the rehabilitation program includes continuation of the phase I stretches with the addition of internal rotation and cross-body adduction and isometric strengthening for the internal and external rotators and anterior, middle, and posterior deltoid. Isometrics should be performed with submaximal effort with the arm in a near-neutral position. Phase II exercises also should include shoulder shrugs, shoulder rolls, and range-of-motion and stretching exercises for the cervical spine. Isometric strengthening for the shoulder should not begin until there is early healing of the rotator cuff tear. For small complete cuff tears with good-quality tissue, this may start as soon as 4 weeks, and for large or massive cuff tears with poor-quality tissue, this may be delayed for up to 8 weeks.

Phase III exercises include progressive resistive exercises with either light weights or elastic materials such as surgical tubing or Theraband®. Phase III exercises should not commence until the patient has regained nearly full passive range of motion of the shoulder and has minimal discomfort. In patients having had arthroscopic acromioplasty, this is usually achieved within 3 to 4 weeks following surgery; for open acromioplasty, 4 to 6 weeks after surgery; for small rotator cuff tears, 6 weeks after surgery; and for larger or massive cuff tears, resistive exercises may be delayed 8 to 10 weeks following surgery. It is our preference that phase III exercises be divided into two steps. The first set of resistive exercises is for internal and external rotation performed in the plane of the scapula with slight abduction of the arm as well as resistive extension strengthening. Resistive exercises are performed with either free weights or elastic bands. The second set of exercises for phase III is not instituted until the patient is able to comfortably perform three sets of 10 repetitions of green Theraband® in external rotation. It is our belief that when the external rotators are strong enough to achieve this level of function, then the rotator cuff is capable of maintaining the humeral head in a depressed position within the glenoid fossa so as to minimize the upward shear stresses of the anterior and middle deltoid when performing forward flexion and abduction strengthening. The second set of glenohumeral strengthening exercises includes the addition of free weights or Theraband® for forward flexion and abduction. Again, these exercises should be done in the plane of the scapula and should be limited initially to below shoulder level. Phase III exercises also include resistive exercises for trapezius, rhomboid, and serratus anterior function. The scapular stabilizers can be strengthened with wall push-ups and shoulder shrugging exercises with light weights. When the patient has full active range of motion of the shoulder, minimal pain with resistive exercises, and forward flexion using up to blue Theraband® or a 10-lb weight, then phase IV of the rehabilitation program may be instituted and should be individualized to the patient's specific goals and future requirements.

Phase IV exercises would include more aggressive resistive exercises. This could employ the use of heavier free weights or isokinetic muscle strengthening, as well as activity-specific strengthening relating either to overhead throwing sport activity or work-related activities.

Phases III and IV of the rehabilitation program must be individualized to the patient's age, expectations, anticipated use of the shoulder, degree of pathology, and response to the rehabilitation program to that date. For example, there are elderly patients with large chronic cuff tears who have significant preoperative atrophy and low functional demands in whom heavy elastic band in phase III exercises and phase IV rehabilitation would be inappropriate and would likely result in a significant increase in their shoulder pain and a poor surgical result. Conversely, young, healthy patients with high expectations should complete a full rehabilitation program including phase IV prior to their full return to sport or heavy work activities. Return to full activity level without complete rehabilitation of the shoulder may precipitate an increase in symptoms or reinjury of the shoulder.

Patients with concomitant cervical spine disease or significant pathology on the contralateral shoulder or other joints of the upper extremity may require further modification of both the technique of rehabilitation and the time course for successful completion of each phase of the rehabilitation. Patients with significant cervical spondylosis should include in their rehabilitation program more specific cervical spine exercises both for range of motion and strengthening of the paracervical musculature.

Complete rehabilitation of shoulder function following rotator cuff surgery varies widely and depends on the type of surgery performed, the age of the patient, and the extent of the pathology. It has been our experience that most patients with full-thickness rotator cuff tears will require a minimum of 6 months for reaching a plateau, and some patients require up to 1 year. Patients having open acromioplasty with an intact rotator cuff will require, on average, 6 months for complete rehabilitation. Patients with arthroscopic acromioplasty usually achieve a functional plateau at 4 months.

# Glenohumeral Arthritis: Total Shoulder Arthroplasty and Glenohumeral Arthrodesis

Diseases that affect the osteoarticular surface of the glenohumeral joint are numerous and varied with respect to etiology, pathology, pathogenesis, progression, and treatment. The most common disorders that affect the osteoarticular surfaces of the glenohumeral joint and can result in the need for surgical intervention include posttraumatic arthritis, degenerative osteoarthritis, osteonecrosis, rheumatoid arthritis, arthritis of glenohumeral instability, rotator cuff arthropathy, and crystal-induced arthritis (hydroxyapatite and urate crystals).[7,34,129] Less common conditions that also result in glenohumeral arthritis include Paget's disease, psoriasis, hemophilic arthropathy, and ochronosis. The common pathology associated with these arthritides that can result in the need for surgical intervention include deformity of the normal articulating surfaces, loss of the articular cartilage, and synovitis associated with generalized joint inflammation. The objectives of diagnosis and treatment of these disorders are to define the nature and the extent of the pathologic condition and to treat this pathology so as to maintain, improve, or restore joint mobility, stability, and strength, as well as diminished pain.

## Diagnosis and Evaluation

Preoperative history and physical examination of the arthritic shoulder should assess the degree to which pain, loss of motion, and loss of strength results in specific limitations of daily, recreational, and work activities. This should include a quantitative assessment of the patient's rest pain, night pain, and pain associated with use of the shoulder. The degree of dysfunction secondary to pain, loss of motion, and loss of strength is the primary criterion for prosthetic joint replacement. The history also should evaluate the patient's goals and expectations such that a clear understanding can be achieved as to the likelihood of achieving these goals following surgical intervention and rehabilitation. Modification of the patient's postoperative activity level may be required due to the nature and severity of the preoperative pathology or secondary to the excessive demands or expectations that a young patient may have that may exceed the functional limitations of any prosthetic replacement. The history also should obtain information regarding the success of nonoperative management, which may include an exercise program, oral anti-inflammatory medication, or cortisone injection. The clinical evaluation of patients with polyarticular inflammatory arthritis also should assess the effectiveness of their systemic arthritis treatment program and the status of the other parts of the musculoskeletal system that may affect the rehabilitation and functional outcome of shoulder replacement surgery. Of particular importance in this regard is the need for ambulatory aids such as crutches and a walker, as well as the function of the hand, wrist, elbow, cervical spine, and opposite shoulder, since these all directly affect the patient's ability to participate in postoperative rehabilitation.

The physical examination should specifically evaluate passive range of motion and external rotation in both neutral and abducted positions. Passive forward elevation, internal rotation, and cross-body adduction also should be measured. Commonly associated with end-stage arthritis of the glenohumeral joint is loss of external rotation, internal rotation, and cross-body adduction. The loss of passive motion due to capsular contracture significantly affects the operative procedure and occasionally adversely affects the postoperative result.[129] In a similar way, significant losses of passive forward elevation also must be addressed by the surgical technique in order to achieve a satisfactory functional outcome. The status of the rotator cuff is one of the most important prognostic factors in determining postoperative function and strength.[7,34,67,129,130] The physical examination may assess the integrity of the rotator cuff by subacromial crepitus, fluid sign, and external rotation strength in the neutral position. Rupture of the long head of the biceps tendon is often associated with large rotator cuff tears. The presence of significant pain over the acromioclavicular joint should be assessed, because distal clavicle resection or acromioplasty is occasionally necessary as part of the operative procedure for joint replacement, particularly in patients with degenerative rotator cuff tears. Patients undergoing prosthetic joint replacement should have an intact deltoid and good periscapular function. As with all patients having shoulder surgery, preoperative evaluation of the shoulder also should include a complete upper extremity neurologic examination and cervical examination to rule out significant concomitant cervical spine disease. This is particularly important in patients with rheumatoid arthritis, who may have instability of the cervical spine.

# Diagnostic Imaging

## PLAIN RADIOGRAPHS

Plain radiographs are the single most important diagnostic test necessary for preoperative evaluation of the arthritic shoulder. The radiographic series should include an anteroposterior view in the plane of the scapula with the arm in 20 degrees of external rotation (Fig. 4-18a). The series also should include an axillary view (see Fig. 4-18b) and a lateral scapular view (Y view). These x-rays should assess the shape of the humeral head, the acromiohumeral interval, the presence of hypertrophic spur formation about the humeral head and glenoid, the presence of acromioclavicular arthritis, subacromial spurring, and glenoid erosion. The size of the humeral canal and the degree of osteopenia should be evaluated. The lateral humeral offset as it relates to humeral head collapse or glenoid erosion should be assessed.[93] Osteoarthritis is characterized by enlargement of the humeral head secondary to peripheral osteophyte formation, subchondral sclerosis, asymmetrical joint space narrowing, subchondral cyst formation, and posterior wear of the glenoid (see Fig. 4-18). When posterior glenoid wear is severe, posterior humeral head subluxation or dislocation may occur. Most patients with osteoarthritis will have an intact rotator cuff, and the acromiohumeral interval is often within normal limits. Patients with rheumatoid arthritis often will have significant osteopenia, symmetrical joint space narrowing, minimal proliferative osteophyte formation (Fig. 4-19), and central or superior glenoid erosion with a decrease in the acromiohumeral interval consistent with marked thinning of the rotator cuff or a rotator cuff tear. Patients with rotator cuff tear arthropathy are characterized by osteopenia, humeral head collapse, superior migration of the humeral head with superior and central erosion of the glenoid, and minimal proliferative osteophyte formation about the glenohumeral joint (Fig. 4-20). Cuff tear arthropathy is often associated with subacromial spurring, acromioclavicular joint arthritis, and erosion of the coracoacromial arch secondary to

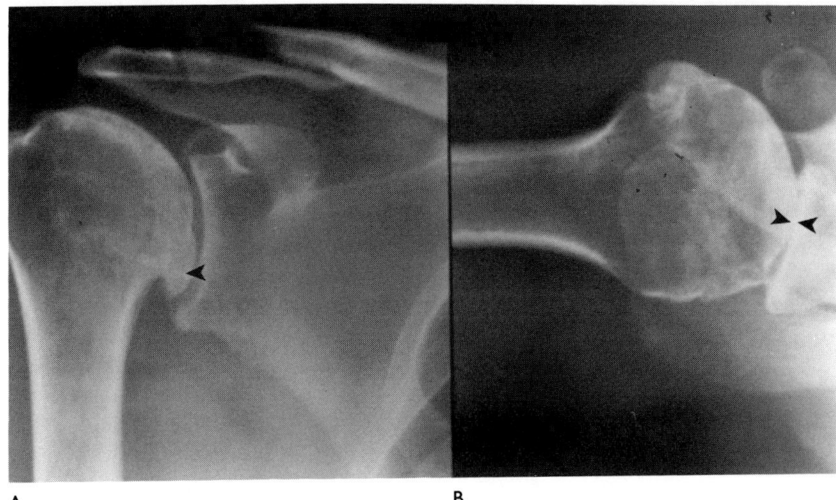


**Figure 4-18.** An anteroposterior (a) and an axillary (b) radiograph demonstrating osteoarthritic changes, including a large osteophyte along the inferior border of the humeral head (a, arrows), subchondral sclerosis, and a loss of articular cartilage with joint space narrowing.

cuff deficiency and cephalad migration of the humeral head. Posttraumatic arthritis may present a varied picture and often is associated with malunion or fibrous union of the greater tuberosities, joint incongruity, and articular cartilage damage that is similar to that noted in osteoarthritis. Osteonecrosis is characterized by severe collapse and fragmentation of the humeral head with less severe changes noted on the glenoid side of the joint (Fig. 4-21). Osteonecrosis is a primary disorder of the humeral head, and therefore, the humeral head demonstrates the most severe pathology, with the glenoid being affected secondarily and late in the disease process. There is often a normal acromiohumeral interval, since the vast majority of these patients have an intact rotator cuff mechanism.

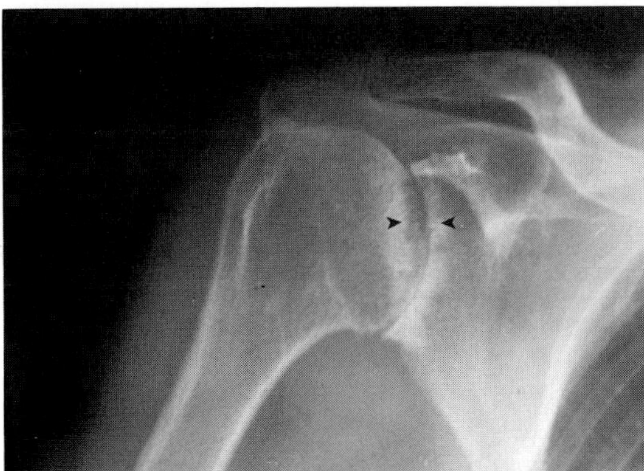

**Figure 4-19.** An anteroposterior radiograph of rheumatoid arthritis demonstrating uniform articular loss of joint space, osteopenia, and osteolysis (arrows).

The diagnosis of the specific arthritic pattern and the status of the rotator cuff are in most cases accurately determined by the patient's past medical history, current history and physical examination, and plain radiographs. In patients with inflammatory arthritides, synovial fluid crystal analysis may be helpful in establishing a specific etiology for the inflammatory process. CT arthrography and MRI are not routine or necessary preoperative studies in evaluating patients with end-stage glenohumeral arthritis.

## CT ARTHROGRAPHY AND MRI

CT arthrography can be used to evaluate both the integrity of the rotator cuff and the degree of glenoid bone loss and glenoid version (Fig. 4-22). This study is particularly useful in patients in whom an adequate axillary view of the shoulder cannot be obtained due to the severity of

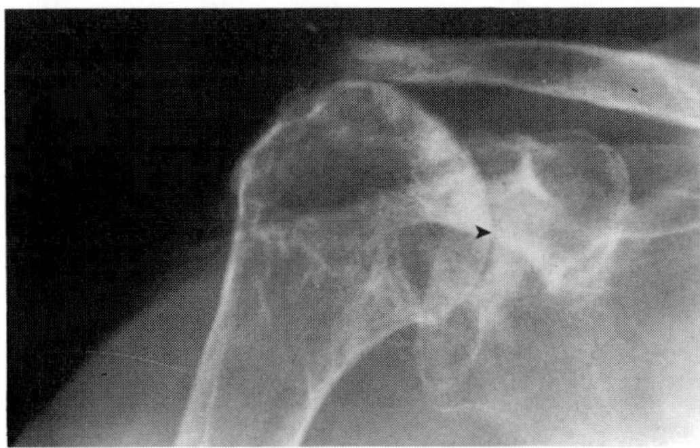

**Figure 4-20.** An anteroposterior radiograph demonstrating rotator cuff tear arthopathy with humeral head collapse, osteopenia, and superior glenoid erosion (arrows).

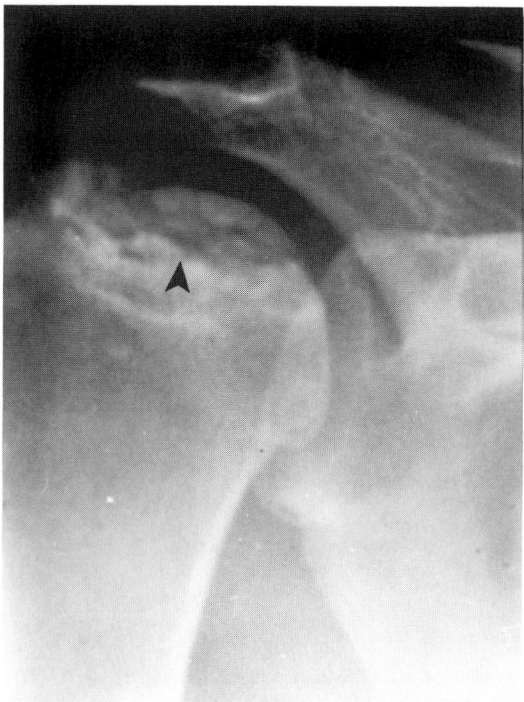

**Figure 4-21.** An anteroposterior radiograph demonstrating osteonecrosis, superior humeral head fragmentation, and collapse (arrows) without significant radiographic evidence of glenoid involvement.

disease and the inability of the patient to be properly positioned for this x-ray view. In these circumstances, a CT scan is quite useful and is recommended for preoperative evaluation. Magnetic resonance imaging (MRI) also can be used for this purpose and may be of value in assessing the status of the rotator cuff, the degree of muscular atrophy, and the degree of glenoid bone erosion (Fig. 4-23). The use of MRI versus CT arthrography is often based on the surgeon's

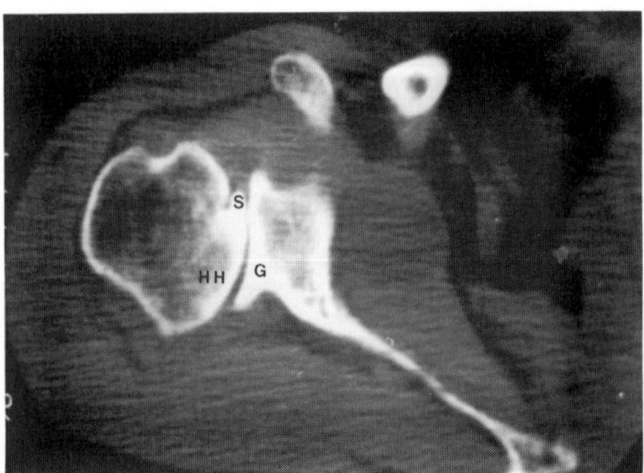


**Figure 4-22.** CT scan. Axial CT radiograph of osteoarthritis with a humeral head (*HH*) spur (*S*) with mild posterior glenoid (*G*) erosion.

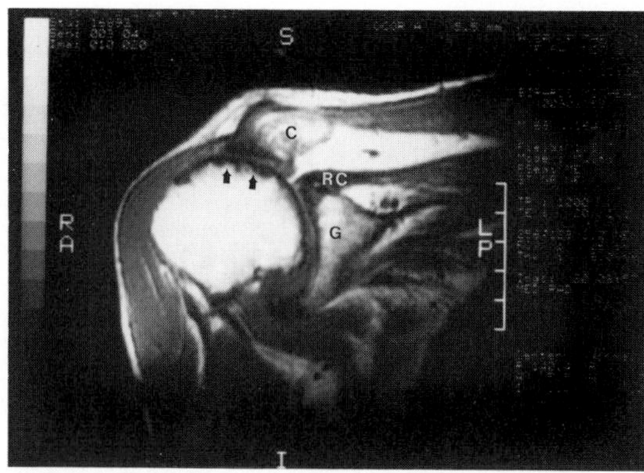


**Figure 4-23.** Magnetic resonance imaging. Proton-density 30-degree coronal oblique image of a patient with rotator cuff tear arthropathy demonstrating subchondral bone collapse (arrows) and retraction of a massive rotator cuff tear (*RC*) to the glenoid margin (*G*) (*C*, clavicle).

preference, experience, and expertise, as well as the availability of the imaging equipment.

# Indications for Surgery

The primary indication for surgical intervention is significant pain that results in limitations of functional activity and is not improved with anti-inflammatory medication, occasional cortisone injections, and a patient- and pathology-specific maintenance exercise program. The degree of pain and disability should be consistent with the degree of pathology noted on the physical examination and x-rays. If there is a significant discrepancy, then an alternative cause of the pain and disability should be considered. For prosthetic joint replacement, the individual should not have a contraindication for surgery. Contraindications for prosthetic joint replacement include a recent history of bacterial infection within the joint or osteomyelitis. The patient should not have a neuropathic arthropathy (syringomyelia or diabetic arthropathy).[31,32,34,129] The patient should have an innervated and intact deltoid and satisfactory periscapular muscular control. The indications for arthrodesis of the glenohumeral joint would include end-stage destructive joint disease with significant pain and patients who have a contraindication for prosthetic replacement, such as septic arthritis, instability of the shoulder, or paralytic shoulder with poor deltoid function.

# Surgical Options

The surgical options for treatment of end-stage glenohumeral arthritis include prosthetic joint replacement, arthrodesis, and resection arthroplasty. In patients who are very young, have maintained near-normal range of motion of the shoulder, and have moderate degenerative changes of the glenohumeral joint, there has been reported limited short-term success with arthroscopic debridement and synovectomy.[154] Arthroscopic surgery is not indicated for the end-stage arthritic joint, particularly in those patients with loss of passive arcs of motion and significant radiographic deformity, since such patients would be better served by the reproducible and predictable results of prosthetic joint replacement. Prosthetic joint replacement could include hemiarthroplasty (proximal humeral replacement) or total shoulder replacement. The indications for hemiarthroplasty include those patients with intact rotator cuff and minimal degenerative changes of the glenoid, particularly patients who are younger in age, or alternatively, those patients who have massive deficiencies of the rotator cuff that are irreparable, as often occurs in rotator cuff tear arthropathy, Milwaukee shoulder (crystal arthropathy), and occasionally rheumatoid arthritis.[63, 67, 131] In patients with massive cuff deficiency, the incidence of glenoid component loosening is significantly greater than in those patients with the same disease process but an intact rotator cuff.[67] As a result of the higher rate of glenoid loosening, hemiarthroplasty is often preferred in this select patient population. In patients with an intact rotator cuff and significant glenoid involvement, the use of a glenoid component will often improve both shoulder mechanics and postoperative pain level.[34, 129] Resection arthroplasty is indicated for those patients with severe bone loss, tumors, failed prior prosthetic replacement with severe bone loss, or sepsis.[106, 113, 184] The functional results after resection arthroplasty are significantly inferior to those after prosthetic replacement, and resection arthroplasty is therefore considered a salvage procedure in patients who have contraindications for prosthetic joint replacement.

## PROSTHETIC JOINT REPLACEMENT

The surgical technique for implanting the prosthetic components of the glenohumeral joint vary considerably depending on the specific design of the prosthesis and the instrumentation available for prosthetic implantation. Despite the specific variations in surgical technique for implanting the prosthesis, many features are common to all prosthetic joint replacements and relate to operative approach and the principles of prosthetic replacement.

The operative approach for prosthetic shoulder replacement maintains an intact deltoid origin and deltoid insertion. The approach involves dissection of the deltopectoral interval along the entire extent of the deltoid muscle (Fig. 4-24a). The upper portion of the pectoralis major insertion site is often incised to allow for easier traction of the humeral head for preparation of the glenoid (see Fig. 4-24b). Often associated with end-stage glenohumeral arthritis is external rotation contracture. This must be corrected at the time of surgery by lengthening of the subscapularis tendon, which can be achieved by removal of the subscapularis from its normal insertion site on the lesser tuberosity (see Fig. 4-24c) and its later reattachment to the surface of the humeral osteotomy, thereby functionally lengthening the subscapularis by approximately 1 cm (see Fig. 4-24d). In patients with more significant external rotation contracture, coronal Z-plasty lengthening of the subscapularis is necessary (see Fig. 4-24e,f). Complete anterior and anteroinferior capsular release and separation of the contracted capsule from the subscapularis are also very important steps in soft-tissue balancing and release of preoperative capsular contracture. Removal of all peripheral osteophytes from the humeral head in a circumferential fashion is also important in achieving appropriate soft-tissue balancing. The humeral head is osteotomized using an oscillating saw and a humeral template that allows for appropriate inclination of the osteotomy cut (see Fig. 4-24g). The normal humeral orientation is 35 degrees of retroversion in relationship to the transverse epicondylar axis of the distal humerus (see Fig. 4-24h). In most cases of glenohumeral arthritis, the prosthesis will be placed in 35 degrees of retroversion. The degree of retroversion of the humeral prosthesis may be altered intentionally to compensate for abnormal version of the humeral component or in selected cases of chronic glenohumeral dislocation or abnormal glenoid version. The need for and degree of alteration of humeral retroversion are often dictated by the preoperative evaluation of the shoulder and radiographs, as well as the preoperative plan to deal with abnormal glenoid version. The rotator cuff and biceps tendon are then inspected, and if a significant rotator cuff tear is present, the cuff tear is mobilized and prepared for later repair as discussed in the preceding section. The coracohumeral ligament is released, and the rotator interval is dissected. The humeral head is then retracted laterally, posterior to the glenoid fossa. The soft tissues around the periphery of the glenoid are removed so as to define the bony contours and borders of the glenoid (Fig. 4-25a). The glenoid is assessed for integrity, volumetric

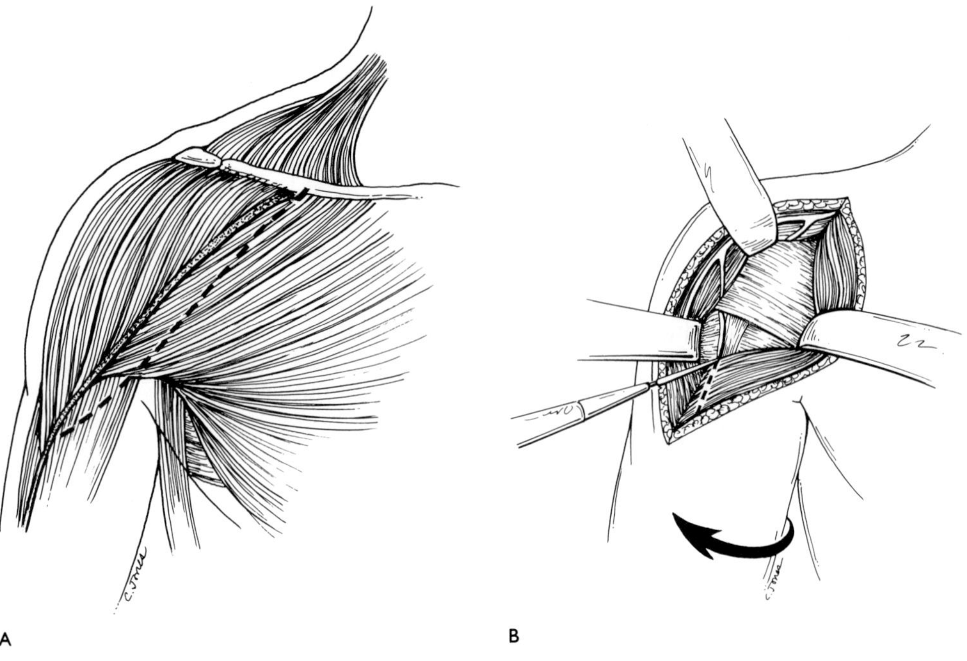


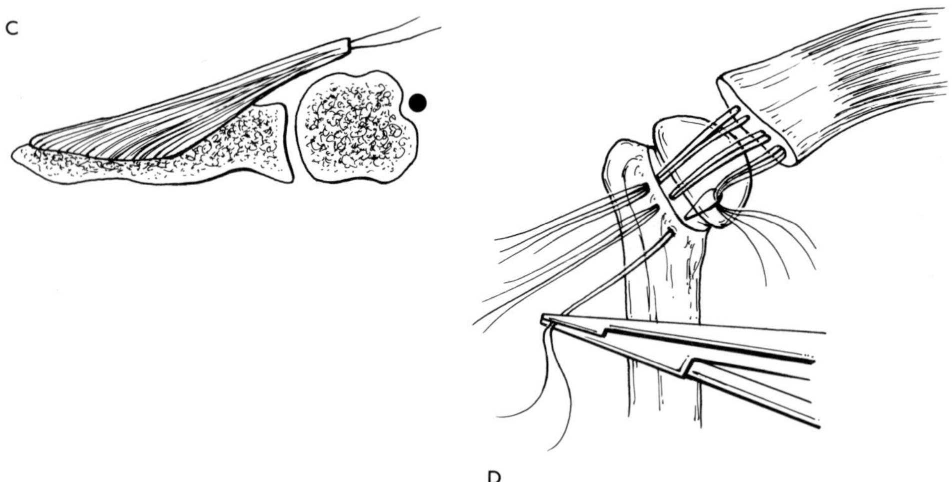


**Figure 4-24.** Total shoulder arthroplasty. (a) Path of incision for total shoulder replacement. (b) Deltopectoral exposure with the deltoid and cephalic vein retracted laterally, the pectoralis major retracted medially, and its upper half incised with a Bovie cautery. (c,d) The subscapularis is released from the lesser tuberosity and, following total shoulder arthroplasty, is reattached to the cut edge of the humeral osteotomy site using heavy nonabsorbable sutures. Removal of the subscapularis from the lesser tuberosity and then repair to the cut edge of the osteotomy functionally lengthen the subscapularis tendon approximately 1.5 cm. (e,f) Coronal Z-plasty lengthening for correction of severe internal rotation contracture. (g) Humeral head osteotomy cut medial to the greater tuberosity and rotator cuff tendons. (h) The humeral head osteotomy is made with the humerus in 35 degrees of external rotation, thereby placing the humeral head prosthesis in an anatomic 35-degree retroverted position.

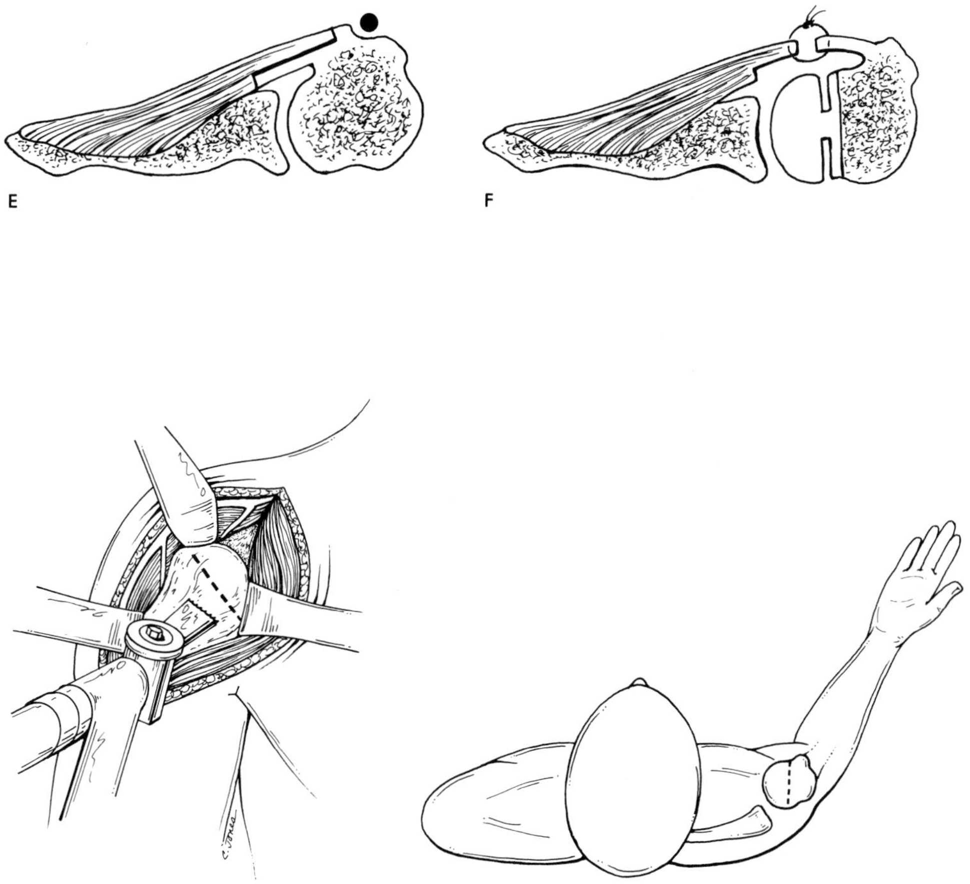


capacity, and degree of bone loss. The glenoid fossa is prepared with reamers as well as handheld instruments so that the fixation pegs of the glenoid component are stable and well seated into the glenoid fossa (see Fig. 4-25b). The principles of glenoid insertion are to maintain a stable and solid bony bed for prosthetic implantation, to minimize loss of subchondral bone, and to avoid perforation of the cortical bone of the glenoid neck. Under ideal circumstances, the glenoid component should be placed in normal version and centered within the metaphyseal bone of the glenoid fossa (see Fig. 4-25c). If there is significant glenoid erosion, then this must be dealt with by either use of a bone graft,[132] asymmetrical reaming of the glenoid, augmentation of the glenoid component[31,37] (see Fig. 4-25d), or a compensatory change in the version of the humeral component. These options are not mutually exclusive, and often, combinations of these options are selected to address glenoid bone loss. The humeral shaft is prepared with successively larger humeral reamers, and a trial humeral component is inserted. All the currently available prosthetic devices have a variety of sizes of glenoid and humeral components so that the optimal size may be selected for the given patient and the pathology that is present. Under ideal circumstances, the size of the prosthesis selected should allow for normal restoration of the glenohumeral relationships and lateral humeral offset and thereby maintain optimal length of the rotator cuff musculature and deltoid moment arm[93] (see Fig. 4-25e). In addition to achieving restoration of the normal lateral humeral offset, it is important to also allow for normal capsular laxity such that there is both a stable prosthesis and satisfactory postoperative passive range of motion.[93] All these factors and goals must be taken into consideration in the selection of a prosthetic implant of the proper size. The patient should have a prosthesis size selected such that at the time of wound closure range of motion is at least 30 degrees of external rotation in adduction, 70 to 80 degrees of external rotation in the abducted position, and at least 150 degrees of forward elevation. Achieving these goals of passive range of motion depends on

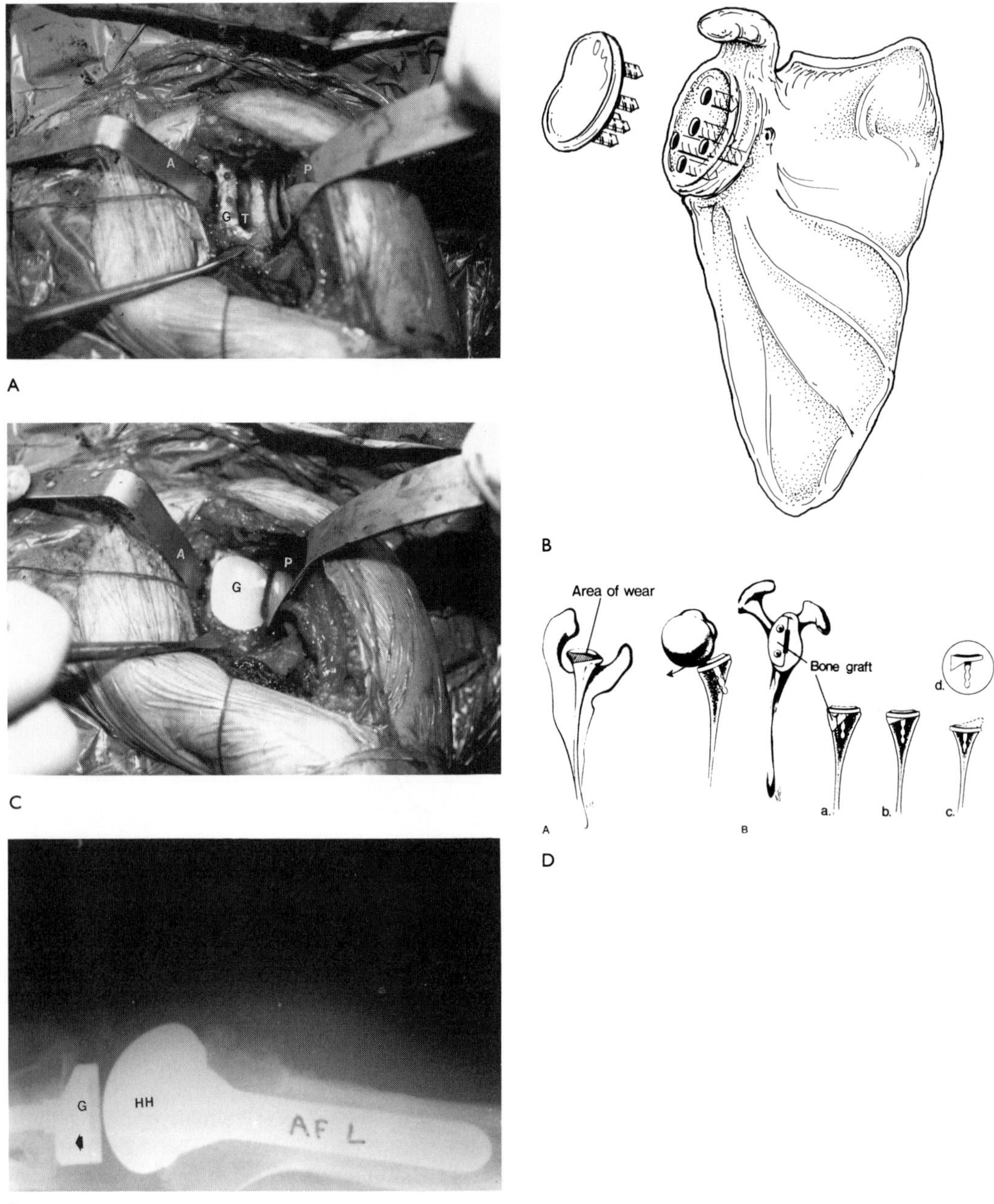


**Figure 4-25.** (a) Operative site for preparation of the glenoid (*G*). A bone trough (T) is made in the central portion of the glenoid for placement of the keel of the polyethylene glenoid component. Anterior (*A*) and posterior (*P*) retractors are placed to adequately expose the glenoid. (b,c) After preparation of the glenoid is complete, the polyethylene glenoid component is inserted. (d) In many patients with osteoarthritis, posterior erosion of the glenoid is present. (*A*) Insertion of the glenoid component in retroversion may lead to posterior dislocation of the humeral head. (*B*) Posterior glenoid wear may be compensated by the use of bone graft (*a*), bone cement (*b*), asymmetrical anterior glenoid reaming (*c*), or a posteriorly augmented glenoid component (*d*). (e) Axillary radiograph following insertion of a Cofield total shoulder arthroplasty with a metal-backed posteriorly augmented component. (d, Reproduced with permission from Neer CS II, Watson KC, Stanton FJ. Recent experience in total shoulder replacement. J Bone Joint Surg 1982;64A:319.)

release of contracted capsule and soft tissues, lengthening of the subscapularis musculotendinous unit, and prosthetic sizing. Occasionally, a smaller prosthesis is used to optimize shoulder motion. Undersizing the humeral component is sometimes helpful in repair of large rotator cuff defects.

After proper selection of prosthetic sizes, the trial implants are removed and the final implants are inserted. On the glenoid side, component insertion and fixation are usually achieved with the use of polymethylmethacrylate (bone cement). There has been limited but successful use of noncemented glenoid components, and the early results are encouraging, but longer follow-up is necessary.[35,36,40] The humeral component is often inserted with press-fit fixation, and in most patients this provides satisfactory stability without the use of bone cement. In those patients with significant bone loss, significant osteoporosis, or tuberosity fractures, the use of bone cement for humeral fixation is necessary. After insertion of the prosthetic components, the subscapularis and rotator interval is closed with heavy nonabsorbable sutures, and if a rotator cuff tear was present, it is repaired to the greater tuberosity. The patient is placed into a sling, and postoperative rehabilitation is started on the day of surgery with passive range of motion of the shoulder.

## ARTHRODESIS

The technique for glenohumeral arthrodesis includes bony fusion between the glenoid and the humerus as well as between the undersurface of the acromion and the humerus. This results in an intraarticular and extraarticular bony union. The principles of glenohumeral arthrodesis include intimate apposition of the cut bony surfaces with healthy viable bone, proper intraoperative positioning of the glenohumeral articulation, and rigid internal fixation. The patient is usually positioned in either the lateral decubitus or sitting position, and the soft tissues overlying the spine of the scapula, acromion, and proximal humerus are dissected, reflecting the deltoid from the spine of the scapula and acromion and splitting the middle deltoid with an attempt to avoid transection of the axillary nerve. If the rotator cuff is still present, it is completely excised from the greater tuberosity, removing the supra- and infraspinatus tendons. This allows for exposure of the glenohumeral joint and subacromial space. All degenerative tissue and articular cartilage are removed from the humeral head and glenoid surface. The arm is positioned in 20 degrees of abduction, 20 to 30 degrees of forward flexion,

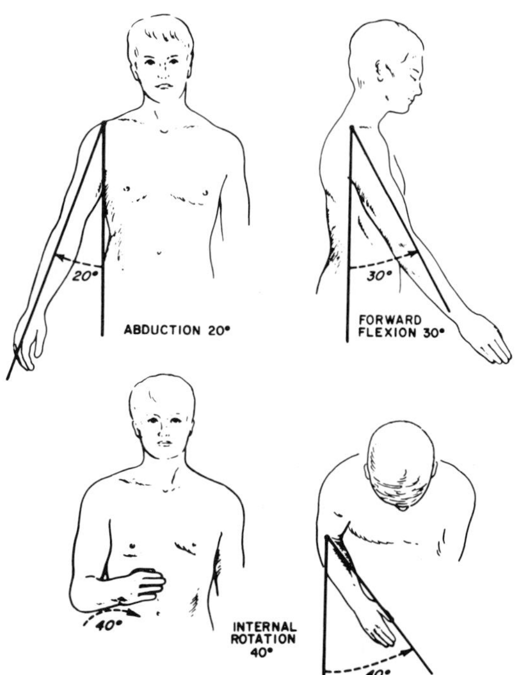


**Figure 4-26.** Arm position for arthrodesis of the shoulder. (Reproduced with permission from Rowe C. Re-evaluation of the arm position in arthrodesis of the shoulder in the adult. J Bone Joint Surg 1974;56A:000.)

and 40 degrees of internal rotation[174] (Fig. 4-26). With the arm held in this position, the glenoid and humeral surfaces are cut so that flat parallel surfaces are achieved. Similarly, the undersurface of the acromion is decorticated, and the superior surface of the humeral head is cut to be parallel with the undersurface of the acromion. The humeral head is shifted superiorly and medially so that there is intimate contact between the surfaces of the humeral head, undersurface of the acromion, and glenoid with the arm held in the proper position. A large 6.5 mm reconstruction plate is shaped to fit over the spine of the scapula, acromion, and lateral portion of the humeral shaft (Fig. 4-27). The plate is fixed to the glenoid through the base of the coracoid with a large screw. Two screws are placed through the plate into the lateral portion of the humeral head and across the glenohumeral articulation. The screws are selected so that there is compression across the cut surfaces of the humeral head and glenoid, thereby achieving rigid internal fixation. In a similar way, two screws are placed through the plate, across the acromion, and into the superior portion of the humeral head. Screws are selected so that again there is compression of the humeral head against the undersurface of the acromion. Screws are then used to complete the

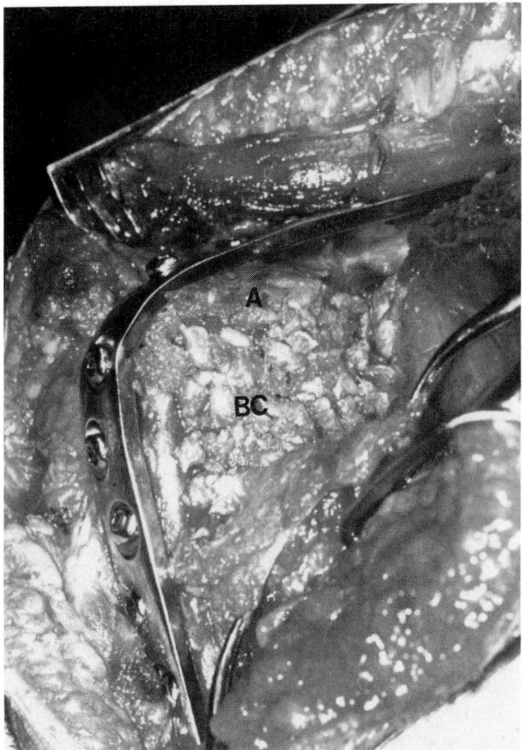


**Figure 4-27.** A large fragment compression plate is placed over the spine of the scapula and acromion (*A*), as well as along the proximal lateral aspect of the humeral head and shaft. Bone graft (*BG*) is placed along the posterior aspect of the humeral head as well as between the humeral head and acromion and humeral head and glenoid.

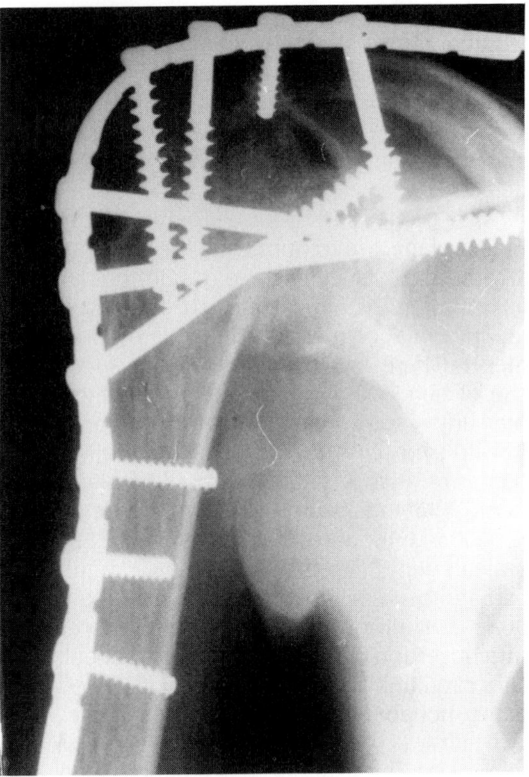

**Figure 4-28.** Postoperative radiograph following glenohumeral arthrodesis demonstrating internal fixation of the glenohumeral joint and acromiohumeral interval using a large fragment decompression plate and multiple bone screws.

fixation of the plate to the humeral shaft and spine of the scapula. Intraoperative x-rays should be obtained if there is any question regarding the proper positioning of the shoulder with respect to the degree of abduction or forward elevation (Fig. 4-28). Bone graft may be obtained locally from the cut surfaces of the humeral head and supplemented with autogenous graft from the iliac crest. Cancellous bone graft should be placed around the fusion site to enhance bony union. The deltoid is closed and reattached to the spine of the scapula, and routine wound closure is achieved. The patient may be placed in a sling, and if rigid internal fixation is achieved and there is good bone quality, rigid external immobilization with use of a brace is usually not necessary.

## RESECTION ARTHROPLASTY

The surgical technique for resection arthroplasty is removal of the humeral head metaphysis to the level of the surgical neck such that the humeral shaft lays below the inferior pole of the glenoid. The goal of this surgery is to minimize bony contact between the humerus and glenoid, and if this achieved, pain is usually improved, although most patients still have some pain.[96,97,104,106,126] Resection arthroplasty results in a shoulder with poor muscle control. Resection arthroplasty may result in either a flail shoulder or functional fibrosis with limited motion at the glenohumeral site.[127] The goal of resection arthroplasty is to improve pain. It is an operation that generally results in only fair functional use of the arm.[33,104,120,184] It is a salvage procedure in patients with severe bone loss secondary to tumor, failed prior arthroplasty, chronic osteomyelitis, or septic arthroplasty.[113,184]

The operative technique may be varied but generally is through a deltopectoral incision. The proximal humerus is identified, dissected subperiosteally, and resected at the level of the surgical neck of the humerus such that the shaft is distal to the inferior pole of the glenoid. Reconstruction of the soft tissues may allow for interposition of the capsule or portions of the rotator cuff between the humeral shaft and glenoid so as to minimize articulation with the cut end of the humerus and glenoid and thereby decrease the chances for postoperative pain.[96,97] Postoperatively, the arm is kept in a sling. Postoperative rehabilitation and exercises are delayed until there is early scarring and fibrosis at the glenohumeral articulation and this affords some stability to the pseudoarticulation.

## Postoperative Rehabilitation

The postoperative rehabilitation for prosthetic joint replacement is, in principle and philosophy, similar to that for rotator cuff surgery. It is similar in that the patient must be directly and primarily involved in the daily exercises for range of motion and strengthening of the shoulder. The exercise program requires a dedicated effort by the patient in performing the exercises several times a day. The exercise program involves the same principles and phases of rehabilitation as outlined in the rotator cuff section.

Phase I of the exercise program begins on the first day of surgery. It involves pendulum and supine active assisted range-of-motion exercises with the use of the opposite hand, exercise wand, or pulley. Forward flexion and external rotation should be achieved within the plane of the scapula, should be done frequently during the course of the day, and should not cause significant pain. External rotation over the first 4 to 5 weeks after surgery should be limited to that which was attained at the time of wound closure. Generally, this should be at least 30 degrees of external rotation with the arm in neutral abduction. Generally, forward flexion should be progressed within the patient's pain tolerance and usually is above 130 degrees prior to discharge from the hospital. The patient is taught submaximal isometric strengthening exercises prior to discharge. Isometrics should be done gently and with approximately 25 percent of the patient's maximum muscular effort. The patients are usually discharged 5 to 7 days following surgery and should be entirely independent in their exercise program prior to discharge. In patients with bilateral shoulder disease or polyarticular rheumatoid arthritis, it is more difficult to achieve these goals, and there is often a need for modification of the exercise program. There is also a greater need for assistance with the exercise program following discharge from the hospital, and occasionally, a limited-goals program is instituted.[128,129] Phase I exercises also should include exercises for the hand, wrist, and elbow to minimize distal hand swelling and stiffness of these joints, as well as gentle shoulder shrugs, shoulder rolls, and range of motion of the cervical spine.

In patients with intact rotator cuff tissues and routine total shoulder arthroplasty, at approximately 6 weeks following surgery, Theraband® strengthening exercises can be instituted. It is our preference that the elastic band exercises be performed in two steps, first achieving good internal and external rotation strengthening and extension strengthening. Once this initial goal is achieve, then abduction and forward elevation isotonic strengthening can be instituted. More aggressive stretches with cross-body adduction, internal rotation, and wall stretches for external rotation and forward elevation can be started 6 weeks after surgery in these uncomplicated patients. In patients with poor-quality soft tissues or a massive rotator cuff tear that was repaired, the rehabilitation program should be altered such that aggressive stretching exercises and resistive isotonic exercises are delayed until there is adequate soft-tissue healing and stability of the glenohumeral components.

The rehabilitation program is continued with progression of the elastic band exercises, use of free weights for strengthening, and stretching exercises on a daily basis for 12 months following arthroplasty. It will often take a patient 12 months to reach a final functional plateau after routine shoulder arthroplasty. Patients are routinely discouraged from participation in heavy recreational or work activities requiring heavy lifting or repetitive activities that result in high forces and loads across the glenohumeral joint. They are discouraged from playing racket sports on a regular basis or any contact sports. Golf, swimming, bicycling, aerobics, and running activities are encouraged as alternative means of exercise fitness in patients with glenohumeral arthroplasty. Most patients who have severe glenohumeral arthritis or poor soft tissues with massive rotator cuff tears fortunately have lower functional demands and are often satisfied with their ability to perform normal daily activities, since it is unlikely that they will do any of the more strenuous activities allowed in patients with less severe tissue damage.

### ARTHRODESIS

Following glenohumeral arthrodesis, the patient is generally placed in a sling, and after initial early wound healing, scapular strengthening exercises and range of motion of the scapulothoracic articulation are started. This usually occurs approximately 1 to 2 weeks after surgery. The patient is encouraged to begin shoulder shrugs, shoulder protraction and retraction exercises, shoulder rolls, and neck range-of-motion exercises. These exercises can be progressed gently with the use of light weights and manual resistive exercises. Bony union usually takes approximately 3 to 5 months from surgery and should be evaluated with anteroposterior tomograms. When there is radiographic evidence of glenohumeral fusion, then the exercise program can be further progressed to more aggressive strengthening, concentrating primarily on serratus anterior, rhomboid, and trapezius function, as well as increasing scapulothoracic mobility. If proper positioning was achieved, the anticipated postoperative active range of motion should allow for 80 to 90 degrees of forward elevation such that the patient should be able to easily touch the top of his or her head and reach to the midline of the ipsilateral buttock, but the arm also should come comfortably to the side without significant scapular winging. The patient should be able to easily perform tasks at waist level and reach to the perineum for daily hygiene.

Following successful fusion and rehabilitation, there are no specific functional limitations that would be placed on the patient other than those which would be anticipated due to the lack of shoulder motion. The patient could participate in strenuous or heavy work activities within his or her limitations of shoulder motion.

# Glenohumeral Instability

Instability of the glenohumeral joint has been recognized for as long as history has been recorded. The Edwin Smith papyrus (3000 to 2500 B.C.) is mankind's oldest book and contains the first report of a shoulder dislocation.[201] Hippocrates,[1] the father of medicine, provided some of the most detailed descriptions of glenohumeral dislocation. Hippocrates described the anatomy of the glenohumeral joint, types of dislocations, methods for closed reduction, and a surgical technique for recurrent dislocations of the shoulder.

Despite its long history, glenohumeral instability remains one of the most difficult and challenging problems encountered by the shoulder surgeon. The management of glenohumeral instability can be quite complex and involves many prognostic factors, including the degree of instability (subluxation versus dislocation), chronicity (acute, recurrent, persistent, and congenital), direction (anterior, posterior, superior, inferior, and multidirectional), and mechanism of injury (traumatic versus atraumatic). Although all these prognostic factors are important, mechanism of injury (traumatic versus atraumatic) is perhaps the most useful in predicting a positive response to surgical intervention.

## Clinical Presentation

Despite the advent of CT arthrography, magnetic resonance imaging (MRI), and arthroscopy, the history and physical examination remain the most important components of a complete diagnostic evaluation for glenohumeral instability. Patient history should be directed toward determining the degree, direction, and mechanism of injury of recurrent glenohumeral instability episodes. Patients with recurrent glenohumeral subluxation fall into two categories: those with a clear-cut history of at least one prior episode of glenohumeral dislocation and those without a history of prior dislocation. In the latter instance, the diagnosis of glenohumeral instability may not be obvious initially. The symptoms of recurrent anterior glenohumeral subluxation can be confused with those of primary subacromial impingement syndrome. A careful history, however, can help distinguish these patients. First, subacromial impingement is unusual before the fifth decade of life (age 40). Second, a history of repetitive overhead athletic activity (i.e., throwing), particularly if it aggravates the patient's symptoms, should raise the possibility of recurrent anterior subluxation. A history of "dead arm syndrome" during throwing or other overhead athletic activities is particularly suggestive of anterior subluxation. Finally, recurrent anterior subluxation episodes are often accompanied by numbness and paresthesias in the arm and hand of the involved extremity.

The direction of recurrent instability episodes is also usually discernible through a good history and physical examination. When eliciting a history, it is extremely important to be as specific as possible with regard to the injury. The position of the arm at the time of the injury can yield significant information. For instance, a football receiver who reports sustaining an anterior blow to his abducted and externally rotated arm while reaching for a pass is likely to have anterior instability. Alternatively, offensive linemen who typically load their shoulders in flexion, adduction, and internal rotation may be more apt to experience posterior instability episodes.

The types of activities associated with recurrent instability episodes also can yield significant information regarding the direction of the instability. Patients with anterior instability frequently will have recurrent instability episodes in the cocking and acceleration phases of throwing. Other overhead athletic activities such as spiking a volleyball or hitting overheads and serves in tennis also can precipitate anterior instability episodes. Occasionally, these recurrent anterior instability episodes may be associated with paresthesias in the involved extremity.

Certain weightlifting exercises which involve bringing the arms behind the plane of the body will precipitate anterior instability episodes. These exercises include benchpresses, incline benchpresses, and military presses with the bar behind the neck. Alternatively, posterior instability is exacerbated by activities that involve flexion, adduction, and internal rotation, particularly when it is associated with an axial load on the glenohumeral joint.

Perhaps the most important information to be gained by the history is whether or not the recurrent instability episodes are traumatic or atraumatic in nature. Historical features associated with traumatic instability include a significant traumatic event, a significant period of disability following the instability episode, dislocation requiring reduction by a physician, and radiographic documentation of the dislocation (Table 4-1). Conversely, an atraumatic dislocation is characterized by insignificant trauma, minimal disability following the dislocation, spontaneous relocation of the dislocation, and lack of radiographic documentation of the dislocation. A particularly troublesome subgroup of patients with atraumatic instability exhibits willful and voluntary dislocations, and the patients frequently are psychologically unstable.[171,173]

Physical examination should be undertaken with the patient unclothed or in a gown that allows visualization of both shoulders. The involved shoulder should be inspected for deltoid, supraspinatus, or infraspinatus atrophy, which could be indicative of chronic axillary nerve injury, suprascapular nerve injury, or significant rotator cuff avulsion in the appropriate age group. In addition, both shoulders should be observed through a complete active range of motion to verify normal scapulothoracic rotation. This helps to verify the integrity of the serratus anterior and trapezius muscles.

Both shoulders as well as all other joints should be examined for the presence of ligamentous laxity. Hyperextension of the elbows, metacarpophalangeal joints, and knees is indicative of generalized ligamentous laxity and should alert the examiner to the possibility of atraumatic instability. Manual stress testing of both shoulders in the anteroposterior and superoinferior planes is performed in order to estimate the amount of translation within the glenohumeral joint. The involved side is compared with the asymptomatic side. Inferior subluxation of the glenohumeral joint with the arm at the side is associated with a dimpling effect just inferior to the acromion that has been termed the *sulcus sign* (Fig. 4-29). This sign has been associated with multidirectional laxity and atraumatic instability, particularly when it is bilateral.

Various apprehension maneuvers have been described as a means of eliciting signs of instability during physical examination. During the anterior apprehension maneuver, the arm is placed in varying degrees of abduction in the coronal plane while a simultaneous external rotation force is applied. The test is positive if the patient becomes anxious that the shoulder will dislocate in this position (Fig. 4-30). Often, patients with recurrent anterior subluxation rather than dislocation will complain of pain rather than true apprehension when the anterior apprehension maneuver is performed. The pain is commonly located in the posterior aspect of the glenohumeral joint and is often relieved by a simultaneously applied posteriorly directed force on the shaft of the humerus. This is typically done in the supine position and is termed the *relocation test*. Although posterior glenohumeral pain is often present during the anterior apprehension maneuver in the presence of anterior subluxation, it is not specific to anterior instability and should be interpreted in conjunction with the remainder of the history and physical examination.

**Table 4-1**

**Characteristics of Traumatic versus Atraumatic Dislocations**

| Traumatic | Atraumatic |
|---|---|
| 1. Significant traumatic event | 1. Insignificant trauma |
| 2. Prolonged disability | 2. Minimal disability |
| 3. Reduction by health professional | 3. Spontaneous reduction |
| 4. Radiographic documentation | 4. No radiographic documentation |

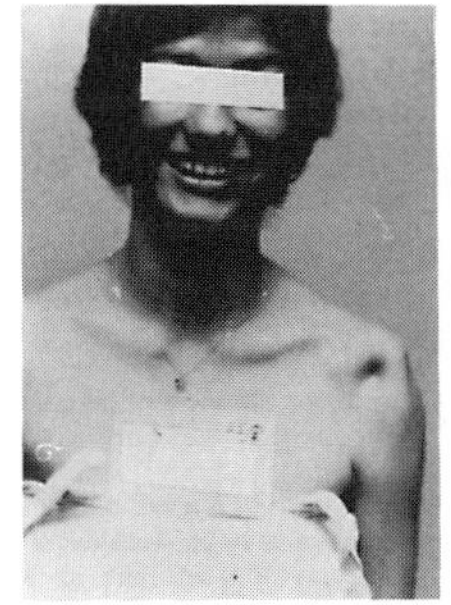

A

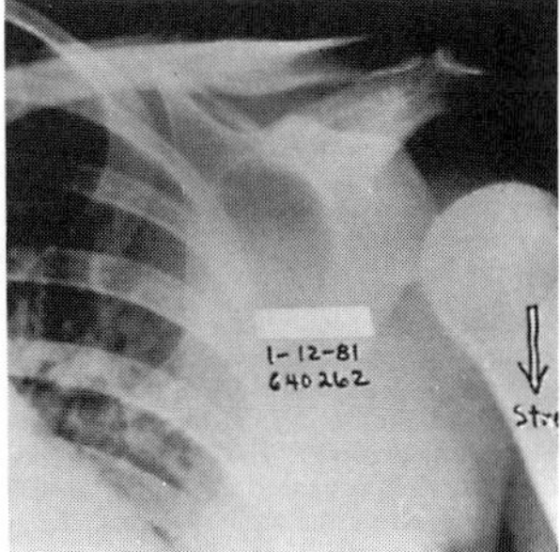


B

**Figure 4-29.** Clinical (a) and radiographic (b) appearance of sulcus sign in a patient with multidirectional laxity. (Reproduced with permission from Neer CS, Rockwood CA Jr. Fractures and dislocations of the shoulder. In: Rockwood CA Jr, Green DP, eds. Fractures. 2nd ed., vol. 1. Philadelphia: JB Lippincott, 1984:675.)

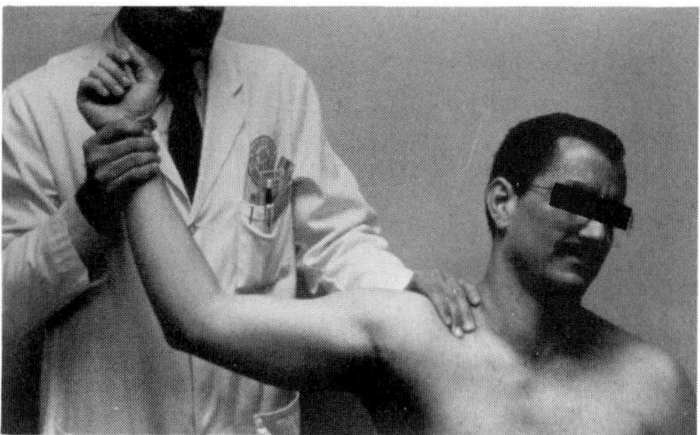

**Figure 4-30.** Positive anterior apprehension maneuver in a patient with recurrent anterior instability.

Posterior instability also may be elicited during physical examination. With the patient in the seated position, the examiner passively abducts the arm to 90 degrees in the plane of the scapula with the arm in neutral rotation. The humerus is placed under axial load, and the shoulder is gradually adducted and internally rotated (Fig. 4-31). Any posterior subluxation or translation should be compared with the opposite side before assuming that it is pathologic. The maneuver can be repeated with the patient in the supine position.

# Diagnostic Imaging

Following completion of the history and physical examination, the examiner should have a strong initial impression regarding the degree, direction, and mechanism of the instability. Although the history and physical examination are the most important components of a complete evaluation, certain diagnostic studies can be of clinical significance with regard to determining whether or not recurrent instability episodes are atraumatic or traumatic in nature. These diagnostic studies include routine radiography, CT scanning, CT arthrography, MRI, and MRI arthrography.

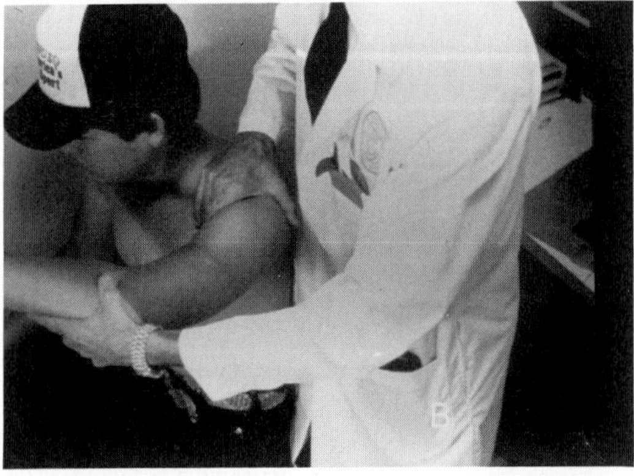

**Figure 4-31.** Simultaneous adduction in internal rotation reproduces posterior instability.

## ROUTINE RADIOGRAPHY

Routine radiographs may not always reveal findings consistent with recurrent instability. Therefore, routine films should be supplemented with certain special views. A complete instability series should include an anteroposterior view of the glenohumeral joint, an axillary lateral view, a West Point view[167] (Fig. 4-32a), a Stryker notch view[77] (Fig. 4-33a), and an apical oblique (Garth) view[71] (Fig. 4-34a). The transcapular or Y view can reveal anterior or posterior dislocation (Fig. 4-35). However, the axillary view is most reliable for posterior dislocation. Radiographic findings associated with traumatic, recurrent anterior instability include calcification along the anteroinferior glenoid rim[24] (see Fig. 4-32b), an indentation fracture in the posterolateral aspect of the humeral head (Hill-Sachs deformity)[89] (see Fig. 4-33b), anterior glenoid rim fracture[14] (see Fig. 4-34b), and flattening of the anterior glenoid rim.[50] Radiographic findings associated with traumatic, recurrent posterior glenohumeral instability include an indentation fracture at the anterolateral aspect of the humeral head (reverse Hill-Sachs deformity)[192] and posterior glenoid rim calcifications and fractures.[149,187,199] Rarely, recurrent posterior instability can be associated with an abnormal posterior inclination (i.e., retroversion) of the glenoid, which may be suggested in the axillary radiograph. Suspected increased glenoid retroversion should be confirmed by CT scan.

## CT SCANNING

History, physical examination, and plain radiography are successful in documenting a diagnosis and formulating a treatment plan in the vast majority of cases. However, CT scanning is helpful in delineating abnormalities of glenoid version, anterior and posterior glenoid deficiencies or fractures (Fig. 4-36), and humeral head defects (Hill-Sachs and reverse Hill-Sachs defects). The CT scan should include both shoulders for comparison. The combination of intraarticular contrast material administration with CT scanning (i.e., CT arthrography) can be useful in demonstrating the presence of anterior capsular and labral abnormalities. Detachment of the anterior glenoid labrum with stripping of the capsule and periosteum from the glenoid neck has become known as the *Bankart lesion*.[4,5] The presence of contrast material extending medial to the anterior glenoid rim on CT arthrography can be indicative of a Bankart lesion. However, this also may represent a false-positive finding and should be

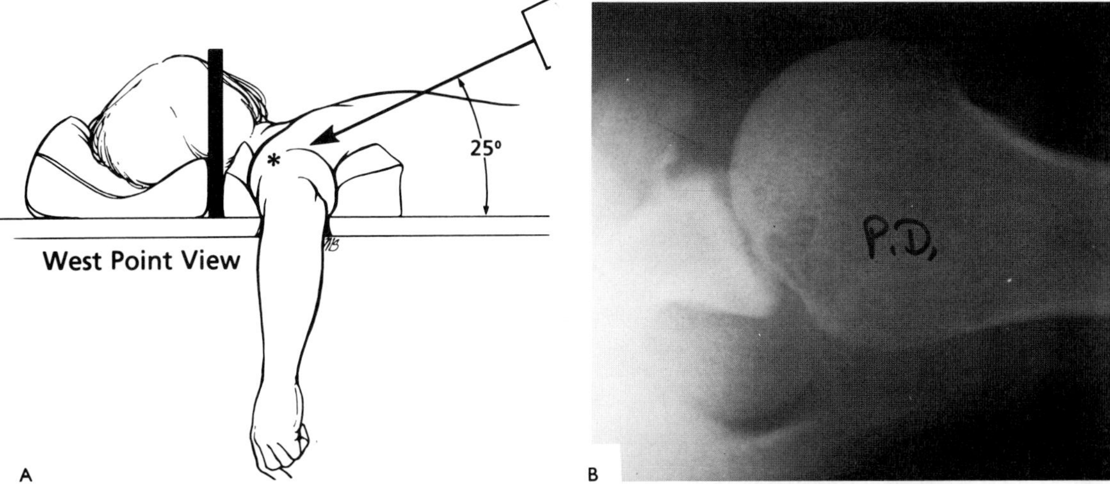


**Figure 4-32.** (a) Radiographic technique for the West Point view (b) Anterior glenoid calcification as demonstrated on the West Point view. (Reproduced with permission from Rockwood CA Jr, Thomas SC, Matsen FA III. Subluxations and dislocations about the glenohumeral joint. In: Rockwood CA, Green DP, Bucholz RW, eds. Fractures. 3rd ed., vol. 1. Philadelphia: JB Lippincott, 1991:1021.)

interpreted in conjunction with history and physical examination.

### MAGNETIC RESONANCE IMAGING

Magnetic resonance imaging (MRI), like CT scanning, should be used only as an adjunct to history, physical examination, and plain radiography. In the vast majority of cases, MRI is not required for adequate diagnosis. In patients over age 40 in whom a significant rotator cuff tear is suspected in conjunction with a dislocation, MRI can provide useful and accurate information regarding the status of the rotator cuff.[92] In difficult diagnostic cases, MRI can provide subtle evidence of a Hill-Sachs defect as well as information regarding the anterior glenoid rim. Abnormalities of the glenoid labrum as well as capsular attachments can be demonstrated using MRI[180] (Fig. 4-37). MRI arthrography using intraarticular gadolinium can enhance the information obtained regarding anterior and posterior capsular attachment as well as glenoid labral abnormalities.[65]

### ELECTROMYOGRAPHY

The most commonly injured nerve in an anterior dislocation of the glenohumeral joint is the axillary nerve.[166] However, injuries to the suprascapular nerve as well as to the entire brachial plexus have been described with anterior dislocation.[155] Although axillary or suprascapular nerve palsy should be strongly suspected on the basis of physical examination, electromyography can provide diagnostic confirmation. Fortunately, the vast majority of neurologic injuries that occur with anterior dislocations recover spontaneously over the course of 6 months to 1 year. Electromyography can be used as an adjunct to physical examination in order to follow the recovery of any neurologic injury.

## Arthroscopy

There has been a recent explosion of interest in arthroscopic procedures related to the glenohumeral joint. Diagnostic arthroscopy as it relates to the evaluation of glenohumeral instability is not required routinely. It should be thought of as an adjunct to and not a substitute for a good history and physical examination. Diagnostic arthroscopy is particularly useful in evaluation of recurrent glenohumeral subluxation in the absence of a previous radiographically documented dislocation or in the evaluation of the symptomatic shoulder after prior surgery. In middle-aged patients, the distinction between primary rotator cuff disease and anterior glenohumeral instability can be extremely difficult to make. In this situation, arthroscopic visualization of an anteroinferior glenoid labral tear or a subtle defect in the posterolateral aspect of the humeral head is suggestive of instability rather than rotator cuff disease.

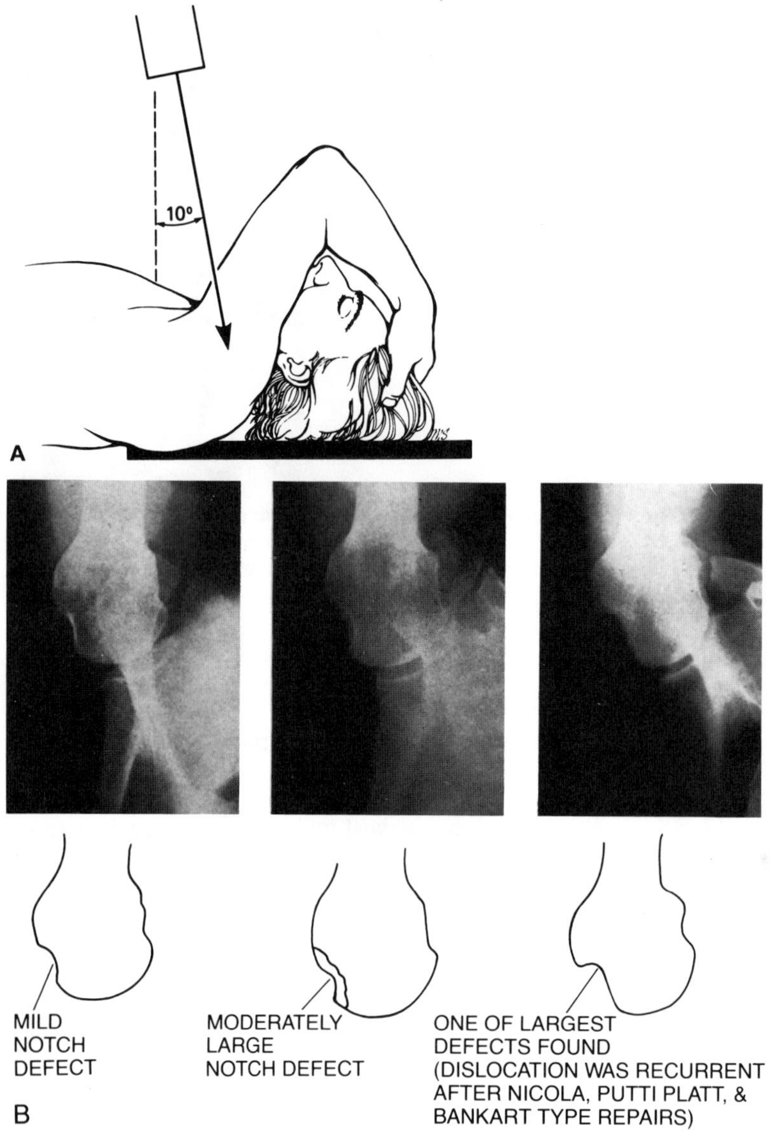


**Figure 4-33.** (a) Radiographic technique for the Stryker notch view. (b) Radiographs demonstrating progressively larger Hill-Sachs defects on the Stryker notch view. (Reproduced with permission from Rockwood CA Jr, Thomas SC, Matsen FA III. Subluxations and dislocations about the glenohumeral joint. In: Rockwood CA, Green DP, Bucholz RW, eds. Fractures. 3rd ed., vol. 1. Philadelphia: JB Lippincott, 1991:1021.)

# Examination under Anesthesia

Examination under anesthesia can provide useful information regarding the direction and degree of instability present in the glenohumeral joint.[41] The amount of translation detected in the affected shoulder should always be compared with the unaffected shoulder to determine the degree of pathologic laxity. However, manual stress testing of the glenohumeral joint under anesthesia can be misleading, particularly in patients with underlying ligamentous laxity. Therefore, the findings should always be interpreted in conjunction with a thorough history and physical examination in the awake patient.

# Indications for Surgery

Surgical stabilization of the glenohumeral joint is reserved primarily for those patients who demonstrate recurrent glenohumeral subluxation or dislocation. The likelihood of a patient undergoing a recurrent episode of glenohumeral

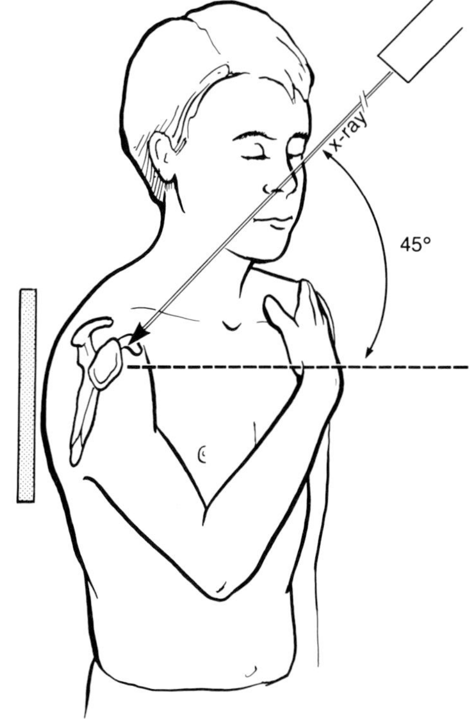


A

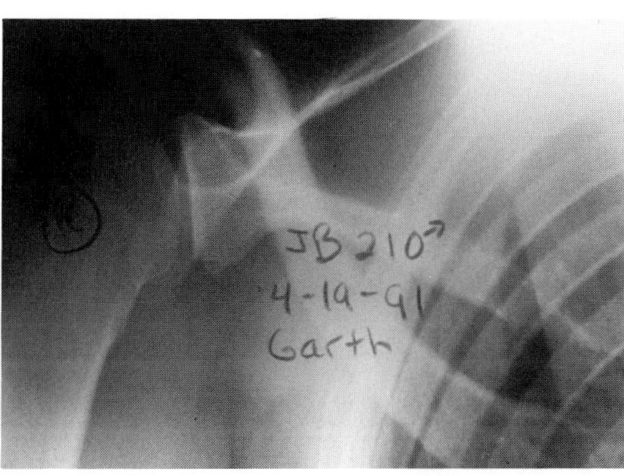

B

**Figure 4-34.** (a) Radiographic technique for the apical oblique (Garth) view. (b) Anterior glenoid rim fracture demonstrated on the Garth view. (a, Reproduced with permission from Rockwood CA Jr, Thomas SC, Matsen FA III. Subluxations and dislocations about the glenohumeral joint. In: Rockwood CA, Green DP, Bucholz RW, eds. Fractures. 3rd ed., vol. 1. Philadelphia: JB Lippincott, 1991:1021.)

instability following an initial glenohumeral dislocation depends on several factors, the most important of which is the patient's age at the time of the initial dislocation.[166] Recurrence rates for anterior dislocation in patients less than 25 years of age have been reported to be as high as 90 percent.[87,116,170] However, the actual rate of recurrence is probably significantly lower than this. Hovelius[91] reported on a 5-year follow-up of 257 shoulders in 254 patients who were between the ages of 12 and 40 years at the time of their initial anterior dislocation. The highest rate of recurrence was 55 percent, and this occurred in the patients who were 22 years of age or less. Patients between the ages of 23 and 29 years had a 37 percent incidence of recurrence, while patients between the ages of 30 and 40 years had a 12 percent incidence of recurrence.

Prior to considering surgical stabilization of the glenohumeral joint in patients with recurrent instability, a well-supervised rehabilitation program directed at the rotator cuff, the three portions of the deltoid, and the scapular stabilizers (serratus anterior and trapezius) should be attempted. The response to exercises is primarily dependent on the etiology of the dislocation. Patients with traumatic recurrent instability respond less favorably than those patients with atraumatic instability.[24]

Posttraumatic recurrent instability responds very predictably to surgical stabilization. Alternatively, operative intervention in patients with atraumatic instability, particularly if the instability is voluntary, is fraught with complications and failure. Consequently, the ideal patient for surgical stabilization is the patient with recurrent instability following a traumatic dislocation who has failed a well-supervised rehabilitation program.

Indications for early surgical stabilization following a primary glenohumeral dislocation are limited. The typical example given is of a high-caliber athlete who sustains a midseason anterior glenohumeral dislocation and would like to avoid missing the next season. If the initial dislocation was traumatic and the patient is a potential scholarship athlete at the college or university level, or if the patient has a legitimate chance to become a professional athlete, it seems reasonable to attempt early stabilization. As mentioned, these circumstances are unusual, and in their absence, surgical stabilization seems best reserved for recurrent episodes of instability following completion of a well-supervised rehabilitation program.

# Surgical Options

## ANTERIOR INSTABILITY

The techniques that have been described for stabilization of anterior glenohumeral instability fall into six general categories. These include muscle sling or tenosuspension operations, muscle

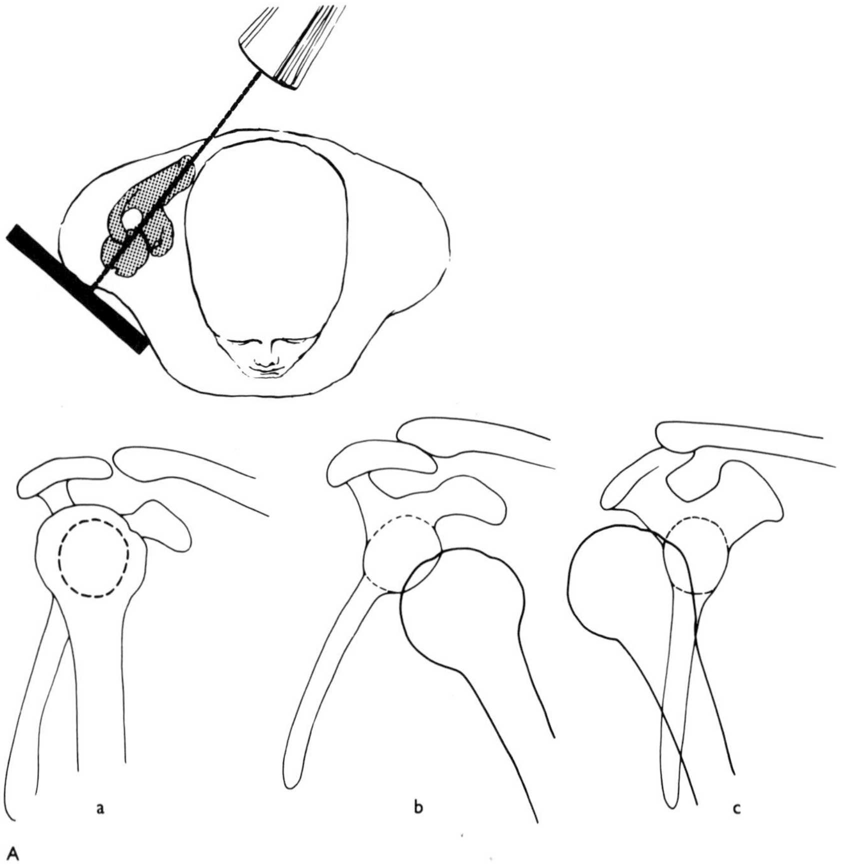


**Figure 4-35.** (A) Radiographic technique for the transcapular (Y) view. Schematic of (*a*) normal alignment, (*b*) anterior dislocation, and (*c*) posterior dislocation of the glenohumeral joint, as demonstrated on a transcapular (Y) view. (B) Radiograph demonstrating posterior dislocation. (Reproduced with permission from Rockwood CA, Szalay EA, Curtis RJ, et al. X-ray evaluation of shoulder problems. In: The shoulder. Philadelphia: WB Saunders, 1990:197.)

transfers, osteotomies (both humeral and glenoid), bone-block procedures, subscapularis procedures, and capsular procedures.

The muscle sling or tenosuspension[64, 86, 147] procedures provide a dynamic muscular sling for inferior support of the anteriorly unstable shoulder. Muscles or tendons used include the posterior deltoid, conjoined tendon, long head of the biceps, and transplanted peroneus longus. In general, these procedures have met with a 30 to 40 percent failure rate and as a result are primarily historical in nature.[163]

Various muscle transfers have been described for stabilization of anterior instability. The Boytchev procedure[18] involves rerouting the pectoralis minor and conjoined tendons deep to the subscapularis. Although this operation is still popular in certain parts of the world, it is of historical interest only in the United States. Saha et al.[176] described transfer of the latissimus dorsi insertion into the insertions of the infrapinatus and teres minor muscles. This was thought to increase the force with which the posterior rotator cuff resisted anterior subluxation in the abducted and externally rotated position. Saha et al. have reported excellent results with this procedure, but it has not met with widespread popularity. Connolly[43] described transfer of the infraspinatus and teres minor into the Hill-Sachs defect on the posterolateral aspect of the humeral head. In general, this is not performed as an isolated procedure. However, in patients with very large Hill-Sachs defects, it can be performed in conjunction with an anterior capsular procedure through an anterior deltopectoral approach.

Both humeral and glenoid osteotomies[175, 196, 197] have been described for anterior instability. Glenoid osteotomies should be reserved for situations in which the glenoid version is abnormal. These are extremely unusual circumstances, and in general, glenoid osteotomies are performed uncommonly for anterior glenohumeral instability. Humeral derotation os-

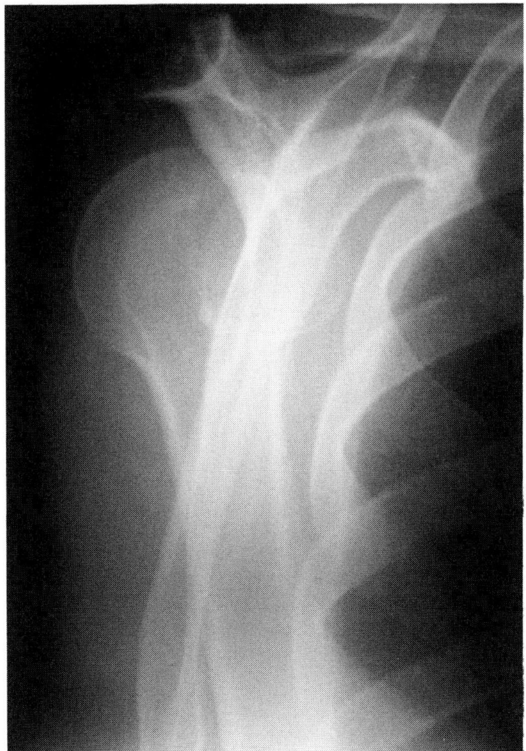

**Figure 4-35B.**

teotomies likewise are reserved for patients whose anterior instability is accompanied by decreased humeral retrotorsion, which is normally 30 to 40 degrees.

The three most common procedures being performed currently for anterior glenohumeral instability are bone-block procedures, subscapularis procedures, and capsular procedures. The prototype of the bone-block procedure is the Bristow-Helfet procedure. This procedure was performed originally by Bristow and reported by his pupil, Helfet[85]—hence the term *Bristow-Helfet procedure*. As originally described, the subscapularis was incised vertically, and the tip of the coracoid process, along with the conjoined tendon, was transferred to the anterior neck of the scapula and sutured into place deep to the subscapularis. Several modifications to the procedure have been described. In its current form, the transplanted coracoid process is stabilized using a screw, and the subscapularis is either split in line with its fibers at the junction of the upper two-thirds and lower one-third or the entire subscapularis is reflected distally from the rotator interval (Fig. 4-38). According to Helfet, the purpose of the procedure was to provide support for the anterior capsular structures as well as to provide a bone block to prevent recurrent anterior dislocation. The procedure is also thought to provide anteroinferior support by preventing the subscapularis from displacing superiorly during abduction and external rotation.

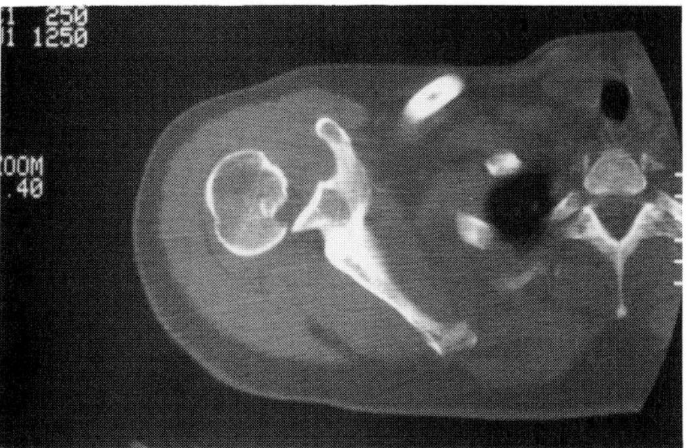

**Figure 4-36.** CT scan demonstrating a moderate-sized reverse Hill-Sachs defect in a patient with traumatic posterior dislocation of the glenohumeral joint.

Subscapularis procedures aim to prevent recurrent anterior dislocation by shortening or transferring the subscapularis. Two main subscapularis procedures have been described: the Putti-Platt procedure and the Magnuson-Stack procedure. The Putti-Platt procedure was reported in 1948 by Osmond-Clarke.[150] The procedure involved dividing the subscapularis tendon and the anterior capsule approximately 2.5 cm medial to the subscapularis insertion on the lesser tuberosity. The lateral flap of subscapularis tendon and capsule was sutured to the soft tissue and/or labrum at the anterior glenoid rim, while the medial flap of subscapularis and capsule was double-breasted over the lateral flap and sutured into place. The major complication associated with this procedure is loss of external rotation and subsequent development of degenerative arthritis or posterior instability.[82] As a result, its popularity is diminishing.

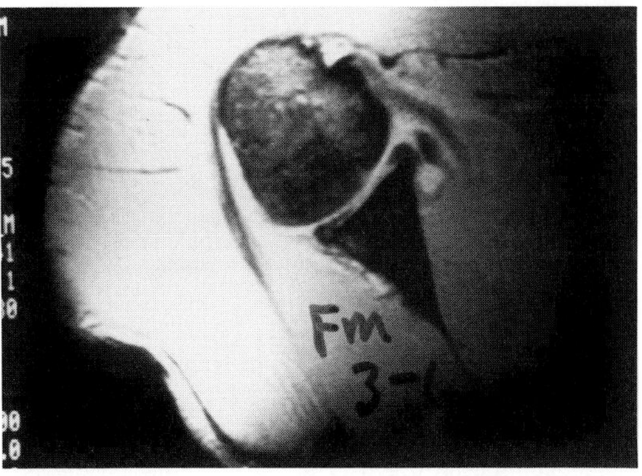

**Figure 4-37.** MRI scan demonstrating anterior labral and capsular detachment (i.e., Bankart lesion).

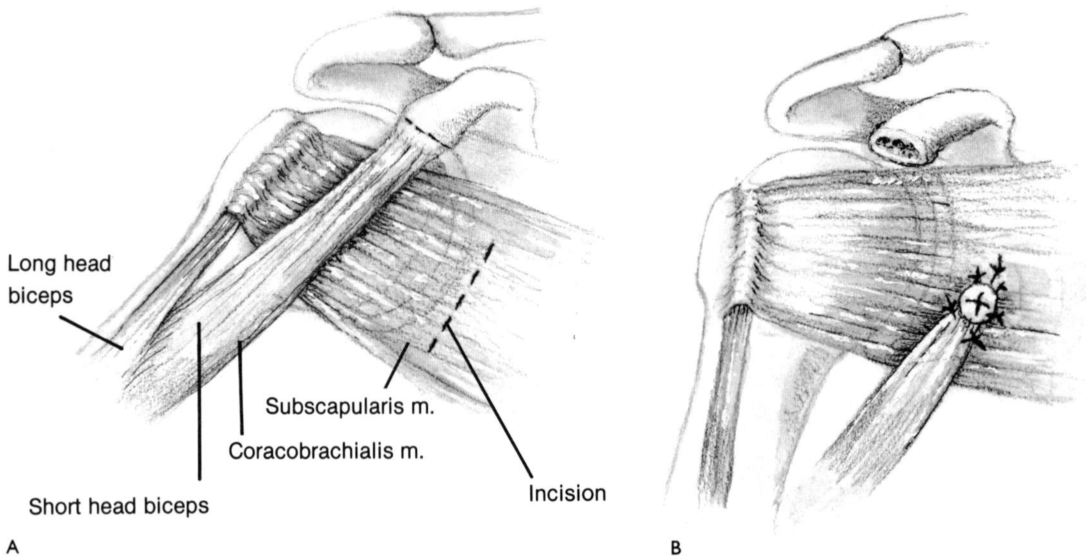


**Figure 4-38.** (a) Schematic drawing representing proposed coracoid osteotomy and subscapularis incision site for Bristow reconstruction. (b) Postoperative drawing with transposed coracoid process fixed with a screw on the neck of the scapula. (Reproduced with permission from DePalma AF. Surgery of the shoulder. 3rd ed. Philadelphia: JB Lippincott, 1983:533.)

Magnuson and Stack described transfer of the subscapularis insertion for treatment of recurrent anterior glenohumeral instability.[111,112] The subscapularis insertion is removed from the lesser tuberosity and transferred laterally and distally on the shaft of the humerus. It is reattached lateral to the bicipital groove to a site on the shaft just below the head of the humerus (Fig. 4-39). The procedure was thought to prevent recurrent anterior dislocation by providing a dynamic sling to support the inferior aspect of the humerus when the arm was placed in abduction and external rotation. This procedure can be associated with loss of external rotation, although to a lesser degree than the Putti-Platt procedure,[158] and as a result also has decreased in popularity.

Capsular procedures are perhaps the most popular procedures currently being performed for recurrent anterior glenohumeral instability. In the case of detachment of the anterior glenoid labrum and capsule from the anterior glenoid rim

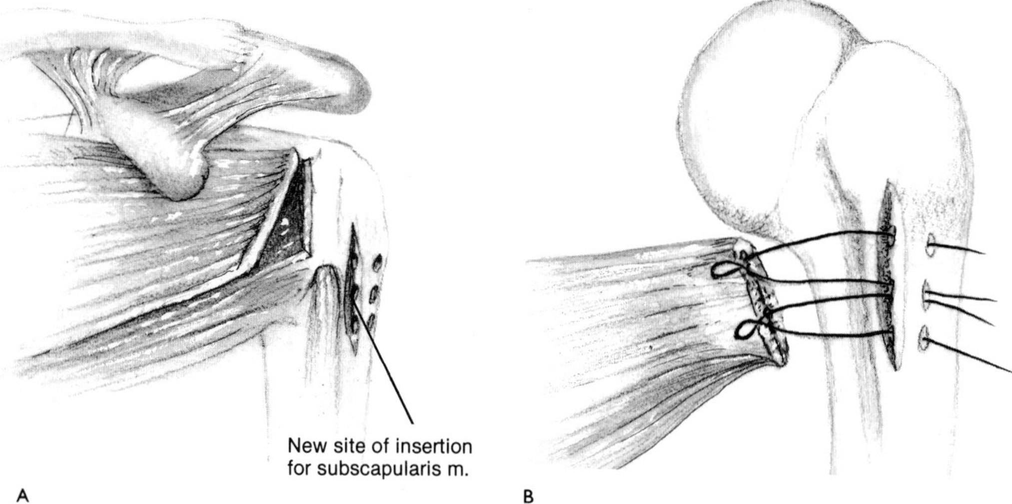


**Figure 4-39.** (a) Schematic depiction of subscapularis reflection and transplant site for the Magnuson-Stack operation. (b) Schematic drawing demonstrating transfer of the subscapularis in a Magnuson-Stack operation. (Reproduced with permission from DePalma AF. Surgery of the shoulder. 3rd ed. Philadelphia: JB Lippincott, 1983:529.)

and neck of the scapula (i.e., the Bankart lesion), the Bankart procedure is performed. If the capsule is not detached from the anterior glenoid rim and instead is redundant, the anterior capsular shift or capsullorhaphy is performed.

The Bankart lesion was described in 1923 by Bankart.[4] This lesion consisted of detachment of the anterior glenoid labrum from the rim of the glenoid with subsequent stripping and avulsion of the capsule and periosteum off the neck of the scapula (Fig. 4-40a). This created a large pouch within which the humeral head could undergo recurrent dislocations. (see Fig. 4-40b). Bankart felt that this was the essential lesion of traumatic recurrent anterior glenohumeral instability. This lesion also was described by Caird[26] (1887), Broca and Hartmann[20] (1890), and Perthes[156] (1906). Perthes described reattachment of the capsule using staples. Bankart described repair of the capsule using sutures placed through drill holes in the rim of the glenoid. Many techniques have been described for reattachment of the capsule, including metallic staples, screws, sutures, metallic ligament anchors, bioabsorbable staples, and ligament "tacks."

In the absence of a Bankart lesion, recurrent dislocation is thought to occur because of capsular redundancy. In this instance, the redundant capsule can be plicated. The concept of capsular plication was introduced by Bardenhauer[6] (1886) and advocated by Thomas[188, 189] (1909).

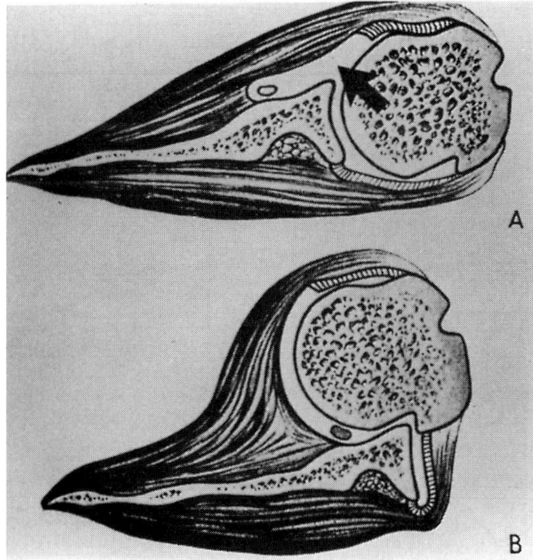


**Figure 4-40.** (a) Superior view of a Perthes or Bankart lesion (arrow). (b) Subsequent dislocation of the humeral head into this lesion. (Reproduced with permission from Rockwood CA Jr, Thomas SC, Matsen FA III. Subluxations and dislocations about the glenohumeral joint. In Rockwood CA, Green DP, Bucholz RW, eds. Fractures. 3rd ed., vol. 1. Philadelphia: JB Lippincott, 1991: 1021.)

However, it was popularized in its current form by Neer and Foster,[142] who described the anteroinferior capsular shift procedure for cases of capsular redundancy.

In general, the capsular procedures have met with a great deal of success. They are approximately 95 percent successful in preventing recurrent anterior dislocations.[166] In addition, they have been associated with a loss of only 5 to 10 degrees of external rotation. However, the Bankart procedure and the capsular shift procedure are both very technically demanding.

There has been a recent trend toward adapting the capsular procedures to arthroscopic techniques. Arthroscopic reattachment of the anterior labrum or capsule is technically straightforward.[28] Methods that have been described for arthroscopic repair of a Bankart lesion include placement of transglenoid sutures, transglenoid screws, metallic or bioabsorbable staples, and bioabsorbable ligament "tacks." Reported results of arthroscopic Bankart repair have been less consistent than open Bankart repair, with a reported recurrence rate in some series as high as 21 percent.[162] However, with proper patient selection and improved arthroscopic techniques, the results may become more consistent and approach those obtained with open techniques.

Arthroscopic capsular shift or capsulorrhaphy is much more difficult than arthroscopic Bankart repair. The technique involves arthroscopic detachment of the anterior labrum and capsule, followed by advancement and reattachment of the capsule and labrum more medially and superiorly. Capsular tension, however, can be very difficult to judge arthroscopically. As a result, the technique has not yet been widely accepted.

## POSTERIOR INSTABILITY

Procedures performed for posterior instability fall into four broad categories: bone-block procedures, glenoid osteotomies, capsular procedures, infraspinatus plicating procedures, and subscapularis transfers. In general, the results of procedures for posterior instability are not nearly as predictable as those of anterior procedures.[83] This may be a function of patient selection as well as of thinner ligaments in the posterior aspect of the shoulder. Care must be taken to select for surgical stabilization primarily those patients with posttraumatic recurrent posterior instability and exclude those patients with atraumatic or voluntary instability.

Posterior bone-block procedures attempt to prevent recurrent posterior instability by providing a bony buttress at the posterior aspect of the glenohumeral joint.[125] The bone graft is most often obtained from the iliac crest and secured into place with an interfragmentary screw. Potential complications include resorption of the graft, degenerative arthritis, and intraarticular screw placement. Currently, these procedures are reserved for cases of posterior glenoid deficiency as well as for revision cases.

The aim of glenoid osteotomies in the treatment of posterior glenohumeral instability is to change the direction of the face of the glenoid to a more anteverted position. This can be performed either by an anterior closing wedge osteotomy or, more commonly, by a posterior opening wedge osteotomy. The posterior opening wedge osteotomy is an extremely demanding procedure and is attended by some significant complications.[83,179] These include intraarticular fracture of the glenoid rim, avascular necrosis of the glenoid, nonunion of the osteotomy, production of anterior instability, and coracoid impingement syndrome. In patients who have normal glenoid version, anteverting the glenoid can lead to stretching out of the anterior capsule subsequent to anterior instability. Therefore, posterior opening wedge glenoid osteotomy is currently reserved for those very few patients who have recurrent posterior instability as a result of an abnormally retroverted glenoid.

The incidence of posterior Bankart lesions in patients with recurrent posterior instability is much less than in those with anterior instability. However, in the presence of a posterior capsular avulsion, the capsule should be repaired to the neck of the glenoid. This is performed most commonly with the use of sutures passed through the glenoid rim. However, other techniques include staples, ligament anchors and "tacks," and screws. Posterior capsulorrhaphy can be performed in conjunction with a posterior Bankart procedure or as an isolated procedure in patients with capsular redundancy rather than capsular avulsion.[190] As mentioned, the posterior capsular procedures are less predictable than anterior capsular procedures. Their predictability is increased when every attempt is made to reserve surgical intervention for those patients with posttraumatic instability rather than atraumatic instability.[9]

Infraspinatus shortening procedures are the posterior counterparts of the subscapularis procedures for anterior instability. The reverse Putti-Platt procedure involves imbrication of the infraspinatus tendon.[165] This procedure is often performed in conjunction with a posterior capsulorrhaphy rather than as an isolated procedure. However, care should be taken not to provide too tight a repair, which will result in an external rotation contracture. In patients with underlying ligamentous laxity, this can cause the patient to begin having recurrent anterior instability. In patients with normal ligamentous laxity, this can cause loss of shoulder motion with decreased elevation, internal rotation, and subsequent development of degenerative arthritis.

Subscapularis transfer is indicated when a reverse Hill-Sachs defect of between 25 and 40 percent of the articular surface is present. McLaughlin[115] described transfer of the subscapularis tendon into the reverse Hill-Sachs defect through an anterior deltopectoral approach. Neer's modification of the McLaughlin procedure involves transfer of the subscapularis along with the lesser tuberosity into the reverse Hill-Sachs defect.[166]

### MULTIDIRECTIONAL INSTABILITY

Patients with underlying ligamentous laxity and generalized laxity of multiple other joints may often present with recurrent episodes of anterior, posterior, as well as inferior glenohumeral instability. The most efficacious form of treatment for these patients is a very prolonged and structured rehabilitation program to strengthen the rotator cuff muscles, the three parts of the deltoid, and the scapular stabilizers. Only after these patients have been compliant but have failed this specific rehabilitation program should surgical stabilization be considered. The procedure that is most likely to diminish the number of instability episodes is the anteroinferior capsular shift procedure, as described by Neer and Foster.[142]

## Authors' Preferred Methods of Treatment

### ANTERIOR INSTABILITY

There is no one surgical procedure that is indicated in all cases of anterior glenohumeral instability. The method chosen should address the pathologic anatomy in an attempt to restore as normal anatomy as possible while maintaining maximum function. In cases of capsular avulsion or Bankart lesion, the Bankart repair is preferred. The skin incision is made at the anterior axillary fold and is extended superiorly to the coracoid process (Fig. 4-41a). The deltopectoral interval is identified, the deltoid and cephalic veins are retracted laterally, and the pectoralis major is retracted medially. In muscular individuals, release of the upper portion of the pectoralis major can aid in exposure. The conjoined tendon of the short head of the biceps and coracobrachialis is retracted medially. Digital palpation is used to identify the axillary nerve, which is protected throughout the procedure (see Fig. 4-41b). The subscapularis is divided approximately 2 to 2½ cm medial to its attachment on the lesser tuberosity. The upper two-thirds is then reflected medially off the anterior capsule. The inferior third is left intact and retracted distally to protect the anterior humeral circumflex vessels and the axillary nerve (see Fig. 4-41c). The capsule is divided from superior to inferior beginning at the rotator interval and extending to the inferior capsular pouch (see Fig. 4-41d). The humeral head is retracted posteriorly through the use of a humeral head retractor. The medial capsule is then reflected anteriorly to expose the underlying Bankart lesion. After the Bankart lesion has been identified, the anterior neck of the scapula is abraded, and the capsule is reattached through drill holes placed in the anterior rim of the glenoid (see Fig. 4-41e–i). The capsule is repaired, and the subscapularis is reattached anatomically (see Fig. 4-41j,k).

Deficiency of the anterior glenoid rim may result from fracture or erosion during repeated dislocation episodes. According to Rowe et al.,[172] loss of as much as 25 percent of the anterior glenoid rim can be tolerated without the need for a bone graft. The capsule is reattached to the remaining anterior glenoid through drill holes. When anterior glenoid deficiency is significant, we prefer the use of a bone graft from the iliac crest. The graft can be placed intraarticularly and secured to the neck of the scapula. The capsule is then reattached to the graft. Alternatively, the graft can be placed extraarticularly on the neck of the scapula so that the anterior capsule is interposed between the humeral head and the graft.

## POSTERIOR INSTABILITY

As in anterior instability, the procedure chosen for recurrent posterior instability should be directed toward restoration of as normal anatomy as possible. In the presence of a posterior Bankart lesion or capsular avulsion, the capsule is reattached to the rim of the glenoid through drill holes. The skin incision begins at the posterior axillary fold and extends toward a point approximately 2 cm medial to the posterior corner of the acromion (Fig. 4-42a). The deltoid is split in line with its fibers beginning at the spine of the scapula and extending 5 or 6 cm distally (see Fig. 4-42b). The raphe separating the upper two-thirds of the infraspinatus from the lower third of the infraspinatus is identified and incised. The upper two-thirds of the infraspinatus is retracted superiorly, while the lower third and the teres minor are retracted inferiorly. The capsule is divided midway between its humeral and glenoid attachments starting superiorly and ending at the inferior capsular pouch (see Fig. 4-42c). The capsule is reflected medially to expose the posterior Bankart lesion. The rim of the glenoid and neck of the scapula are abraded, and the capsule is reattached to the rim of the glenoid through drill holes. The capsule is then imbricated so that neutral rotation is possible with the arm at the side. The split in the infraspinatus is repaired anatomically.

Posterior capsulorrhaphy is performed in the presence of posterior capsular redundancy rather than avulsion. After the infraspinatus has been exposed, it should be examined for redundancy. If the infraspinatus appears redundant, it should be divided approximately 2 cm medial to its attachment on the humerus and reflected off the capsule medially. The capsule is then incised midway between its humeral and glenoid attachments. Sutures are placed in the medial limb, which is then brought laterally and superiorly under the lateral limb of the capsule to create a pants-over-vest effect (see Fig. 4-42d). Care should be taken to perform the capsulorrhaphy so that at least neutral rotation is possible with the arm at the side. The infraspinatus is then imbricated to obliterate its redundancy.

If the infraspinatus is not found to be redundant, it is split along the raphe as mentioned for the posterior Bankart procedure and retracted superiorly and inferiorly. The capsulorrhaphy is performed as noted above, and the infraspinatus is allowed to return to its anatomic position.

On very rare occasions, posterior glenohumeral instability can be associated with increased glenoid retroversion. This is best defined by the CT scan. If it is in fact present, we prefer a posterior glenoid opening wedge osteotomy in conjunction with a posterior capsulorrhaphy. The infraspinatus is again split in line with its fibers and retracted superiorly and inferiorly. The capsule is opened as mentioned above. A flat instrument is placed within the glenoid to estimate the plane of the glenoid articular surface. An extraarticular osteotomy is then made beginning approximately 1 cm medial to the posterior glenoid rim and extending parallel to the plane of the glenoid articular surface (see Fig. 4-42e,f). The osteotomy should be taken up to the anterior cortex, which should be left intact to provide stability to the osteotomy. A wedge of

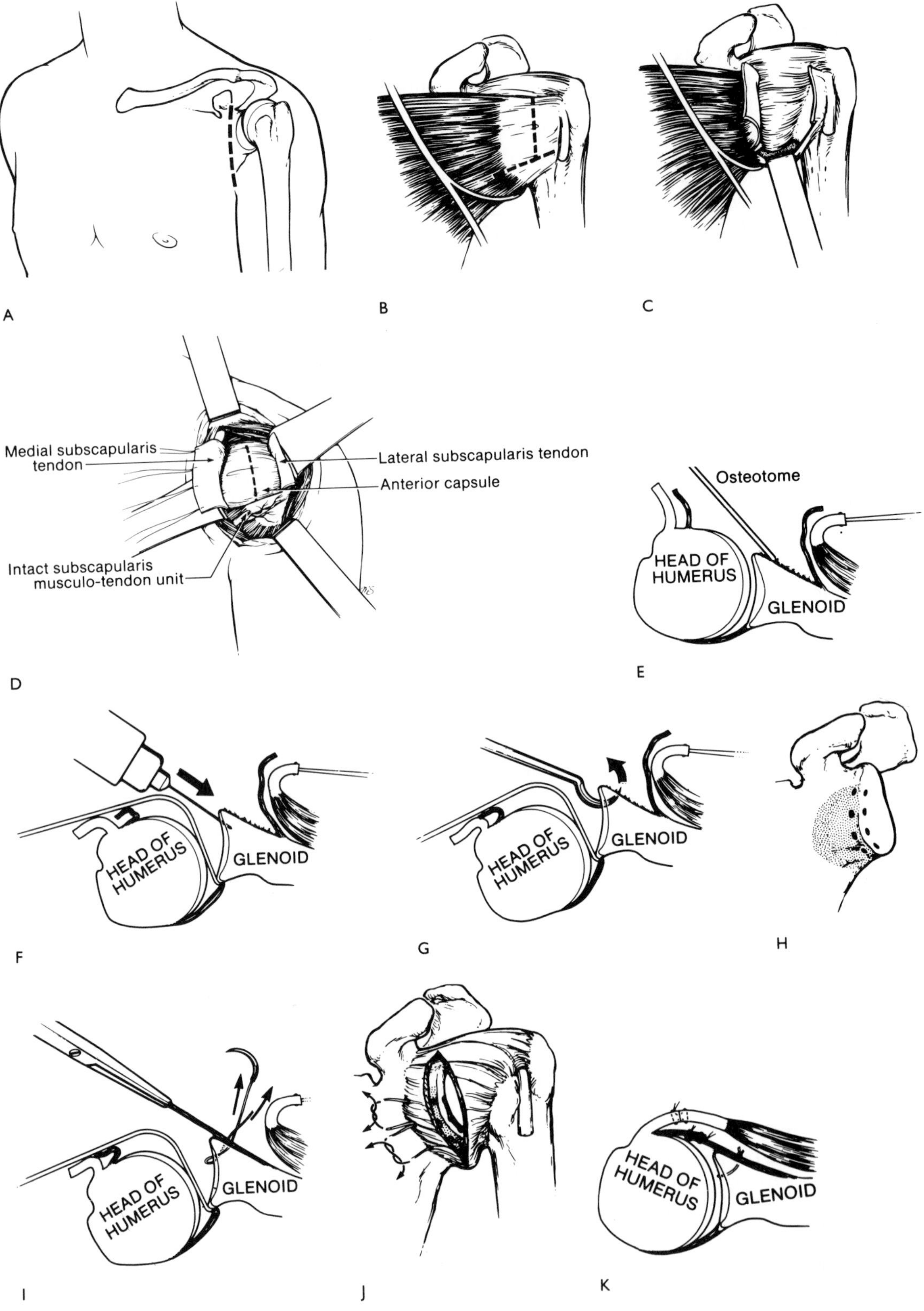
A
B
C
Medial subscapularis tendon
Lateral subscapularis tendon
Anterior capsule
Intact subscapularis musculo-tendon unit
D
Osteotome
HEAD OF HUMERUS
GLENOID
E
HEAD OF HUMERUS
GLENOID
F
HEAD OF HUMERUS
GLENOID
G
H
HEAD OF HUMERUS
GLENOID
I
J
HEAD OF HUMERUS
GLENOID
K

bone taken from the spine of the scapula is placed within the opened osteotomy site (see Fig. 4-42g). If the anterior cortex has been preserved, there is no need for internal fixation. The capsulorrhaphy is performed as mentioned above, and the infraspinatus is allowed to retract to its anatomic position. The final result of the osteotomy is shown in Figure 4-43.

In the presence of posterior glenoid erosion or deficiency, we prefer the use of a bone-graft procedure to bolster the posterior glenoid rim. The graft is taken from the iliac crest and is placed extraarticularly on the posterior glenoid rim and neck of the scapula.

If a reverse Hill-Sachs defect of greater than 25 percent (but less than 40 percent) of the articular surface is present, the McLaughlin procedure is indicated. Through an anterior deltopectoral approach, the subscapularis is subperiosteally removed from the lesser tuberosity and transferred into the reverse Hill-Sachs defect. It is attached through drill holes with heavy nonabsorbable sutures.

### MULTIDIRECTIONAL INSTABILITY

Assuming that the patient has failed the rehabilitation program and is not having voluntary instability, an anteroinferior capsular shift procedure is indicated in order to control multidirectional instability. Multidirectional instability results from a patulous axillary pouch at the inferior aspect of the glenoid. Therefore, obliteration of this pouch will help stabilize the glenohumeral joint. This is done most easily from an anterior approach. The skin incision is the same as described for the Bankart procedure. The subscapularis is reflected medially to expose the anterior capsule. The capsule is then divided from superiorly to inferiorly midway between its humeral and glenoid attachments. The incision is carried all the way around the inferior aspect of the glenoid. Sutures are placed in the medial limb of the capsule, which is then shifted superiorly and laterally under the lateral limb of the capsule to obliterate the axillary pouch. This provides a double breasting of the capsule in its midsubstance (Fig. 4-44a,b). An alternative technique differs from a simple double-breasting procedure and entails incising the capsule at the humeral margin (see Fig. 4-44c). An inferior and superior flap is created by a transverse incision (see Fig. 4-44d). The inferior flap is then pulled superiorly, eliminating posterior and inferior redundancy, followed by inferior advancement of the superior flap (see Fig. 4-44e). The defect in the rotator interval capsule also should be plicated to help prevent inferior subluxation. Care should be taken to perform the capsulorrhaphy with the arm in 30 degrees of external rotation. If the repair is too tight, subsequent posterior instability may result. The subscapularis is repaired anatomically.

## Postoperative Rehabilitation

Although postoperative rehabilitation has been covered in other sections of this text, there are some aspects of postoperative rehabilitation that are unique to the instability patient and therefore deserve special emphasis.

### ANTERIOR INSTABILITY

The goals of postoperative rehabilitation following anterior reconstruction are to maximize return of range of motion, prevent recurrence of instability, strengthen the rotator cuff, deltoid, and scapular stabilizing muscles, and return the patient to premorbid activity level. Rehabilitation begins on postoperative day 1. Pendulum exercises are instituted along with passive external rotation to the extent allowed at the time of surgery. The patient is instructed to perform these exercises six times a day. In addition, the patient is instructed to come out of the sling and use the arm for activities around the house at waist level and within the limits of pain.

The suture is removed at 1 to 2 weeks postoperatively. In addition to maintaining the previ-

**Figure 4-41.** (a) Skin incision for an anterior Bankart repair. (b) Proposed incision site for subscapularis reflection off the anterior capsule. Note the proximity of the axillary nerve. (c) Subscapularis is divided and reflected to expose the capsule. (d) Proposed vertical incision in the anterior capsule midway between the humeral and glenoid attachments. (e) Reflection of the anterior capsule exposes the Bankart lesion to allow for abrasion of the anterior neck of the scapula with an osteotome. (f) Drill holes are placed in the rim of the glenoid. (g,h) Drill holes are connected to anterior glenoid neck. (i,j) Sutures are passed through the drill holes for reattachment of the capsule. (k) Capsule has been repaired to the glenoid. The capsular incision has been closed, and the subscapularis has been reattached anatomically. (Reproduced with permission from Rockwood CA Jr, Thomas SC, Matsen FA III. Subluxations and dislocations about the glenohumeral joint. In: Rockwood CA, Green DP, Bucholz RW, eds. Fractures. 3rd ed., vol. 1. Philadelphia: JB Lippincott, 1991:1021.)

ously instructed exercises, the patient is encouraged to use his or her arm for all daily activities, including overhead function within his or her limits of pain. The patient should refrain from lifting anything heavier than 1 or 2 lb. At 4 weeks, an overhead pulley and supine passive exercises are instituted. In addition, the patient is instructed to begin passively stretching the capsule to increase the range of motion.

At this point, the surgeon should be careful to observe the patient. If the patient appears to be regaining the range of motion more rapidly than desired, the rehabilitation program can be changed accordingly. Likewise, if in spite of this rehabilitation program, the patient appears to be maintaining or increasing stiffness, the passive stretching program can be started before the fourth week.

At approximately the sixth week, the patient will often have regained 80 percent or more of the preoperative range of motion. At this point, strengthening exercises directed at the rotator cuff, deltoid, and scapular stabilizers should be instituted. The patient again should be encouraged to perform these exercises five or six times daily. In an athletic individual, return to sports should be reserved until the patient has 90 percent of the range of motion and strength of the opposite extremity, which usually occurs between 6 months and 1 year from surgery.

## POSTERIOR INSTABILITY

The posterior capsule is much thinner than the anterior capsule. Therefore, rehabilitation is delayed following posterior reconstructive procedures. Postoperatively, the patient is placed in a modified shoulder spica or orthosis that will hold the arm at the side, at or behind the plane of the thorax, in 20 or 30 degrees of external rotation. This relieves pressure on the posterior structures during the early phases of healing.

The brace is maintained for 4 to 6 weeks. Following removal of the brace, the patient is encouraged to use his or her arm for all daily activities within the limits of pain and to avoid lifting weights heavier than 1 to 2 lb. At approximately the eighth week, formal stretching exercises are instituted, with particular emphasis on supine flexion, internal rotation, and cross-body adduction. Once range of motion has approached 80 percent of preoperative values, strengthening exercises directed to the rotator cuff, deltoid, and scapular stabilizers are instituted.

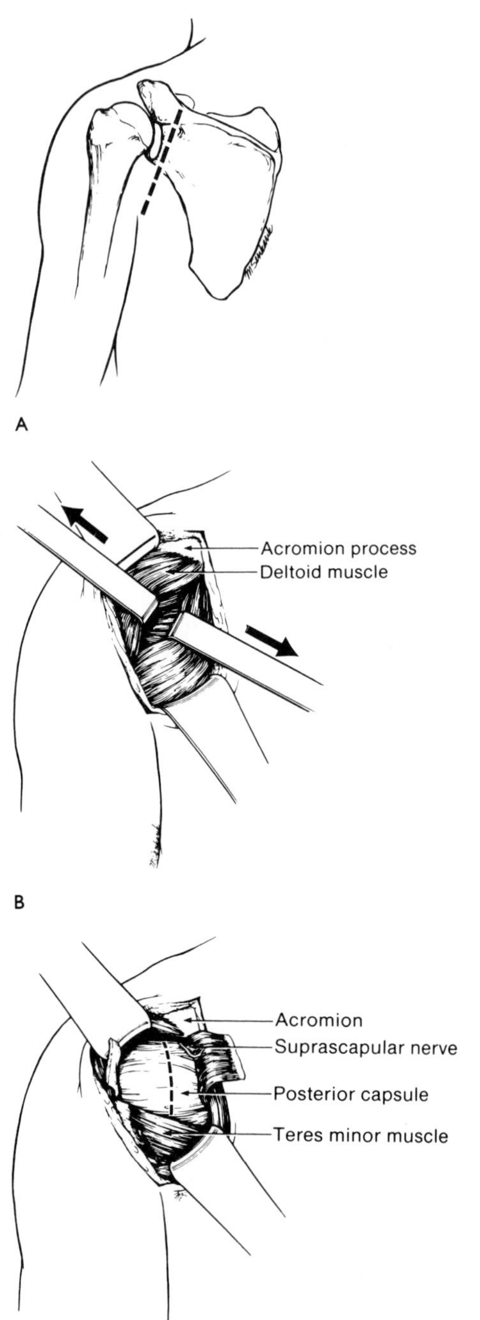


## MULTIDIRECTIONAL INSTABILITY

In general, the rehabilitation program following anterior capsular shift for multidirectional instability is similar to the program used for anterior instability but should proceed more slowly. We have found the use of a brace or cast to be

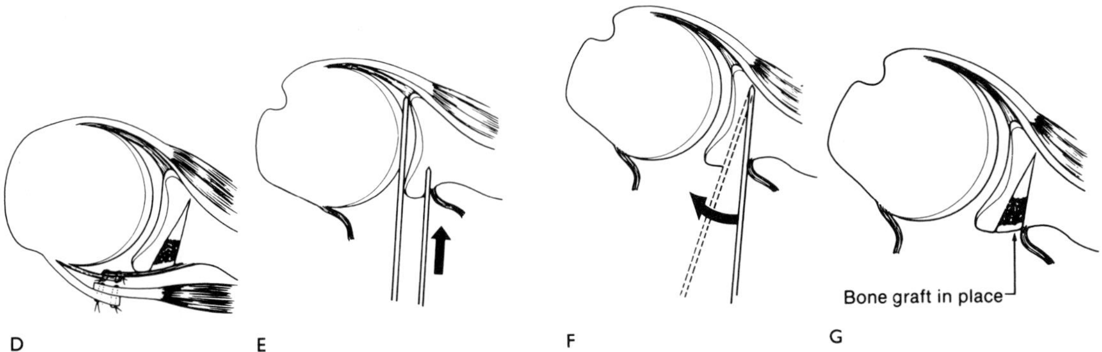


**Figure 4-42.** (a) Utility skin incision for posterior reconstruction of the glenohumeral joint. (b) The deltoid is split in line with its fibers. (c) The infraspinatus is detached from its humeral attachment and reflected medially to expose the underlying capsule, which is incised vertically midway between its humeral and glenoid attachments. Alternately, the infraspinatus insertion can be preserved while the muscle is split and reflected inferiorly and superiorly. (d) The medial capsule is shifted laterally under the lateral capsule. If a posterior Bankart lesion is present, it should be repaired. (e,f) If the glenoid version is required, an opening wedge osteotomy may be performed, the plane of the glenoid articular surface is determined with a flat instrument, and the osteotomy is carried through the neck of the glenoid to the anterior cortex approximately 1 to 1½ cm medial to the articular surface. (g) Bone graft is set in place, followed by closure of the capsule and infraspinatus as seen above. (Reproduced with permission from Rockwood CA Jr, Thomas SC, Matsen FA III. Subluxations and dislocations about the glenohumeral joint. In: Rockwood CA, Green DP, Bucholz RW, eds. Fractures. 3rd ed., vol. 1. Philadelphia: JB Lippincott, 1991:1021.)

counterproductive. These patients are often dependent to a great extent on the tone of the rotator cuff muscles to help maintain stability. Immobilizing the glenohumeral joint for 4 to 6 weeks causes atrophy of the cuff muscles and actually may cause an increase in perceived instability. On the other hand, these patients tend to regain their range of motion extremely rapidly and, as a result, should be observed frequently so that the rehabilitation and stretching program can be tailored appropriately. These patients must maintain a rotator cuff and deltoid strengthening program indefinitely if they wish to remain active and control their instability.

# Fractures of the Proximal Humerus

The age-related incidence of proximal humerus fractures parallels the incidence of proximal femoral fractures. Both these injuries are osteoporosis-related and are seen more commonly in the elderly population.[90, 168] Operative treatment of proximal humeral fractures is therefore complicated by the difficulty in obtaining adequate fixation in osteoporotic metaphyseal bone. Although these fractures often can be comminuted, there are potentially four main fracture fragments.[30, 136] According to Codman,[30] the primary fracture lines tend to follow the epiphyseal scar and may yield a maximum of four major fracture fragments (Fig. 4-45a). These include the articular segment or head, the greater tuberosity, the lesser tuberosity, and the shaft of the humerus. These four components are influenced by the soft-tissue structures that attach to them, resulting in typical displacement (see Fig. 4-45b). Neer[136] subsequently refined Codman's classification and introduced the concepts of displacement of the fragments and avascularity of the head so that the classification system became clinically and prognostically relevant (Fig. 4-46).

According to the Neer classification system, *displacement* is defined as greater than or equal to 1 cm of translation or 45 degrees of angulation as seen on plain radiographs. A nondisplaced or one-part fracture implies that although there may be a comminuted fracture of the proximal humerus, none of the major fragments is displaced. A two-part fracture implies significant displacement of one of the major fracture fragments. The three-part fracture implies displacement of two of the four major segments. A four-part fracture implies significant displacement of all four of the major fragments. Any of these fractures may be associated with an anterior or posterior glenohumeral dislocation.

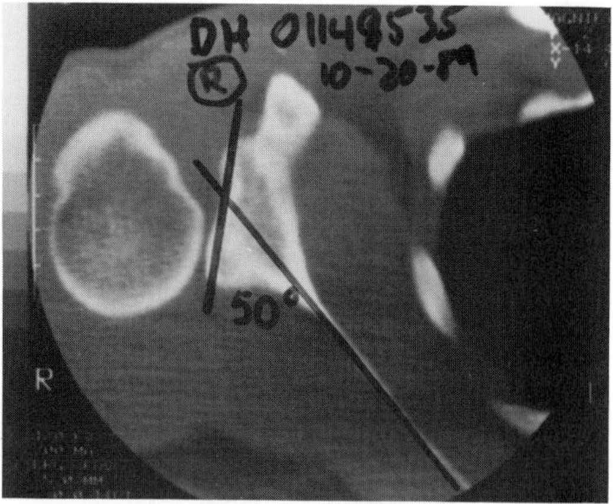


A

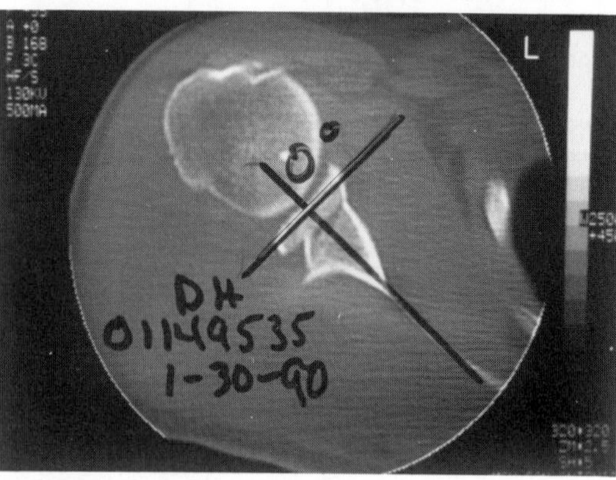


B

**Figure 4-43.** (a) Preoperative CT scan demonstrating 50 degrees of posterior retroversion in a patient with recurrent posterior dislocations. (b) Postoperative radiograph showing correction of the increased retroversion to 0 degrees, following opening wedge osteotomy.

# Clinical Presentation

Methods used for evaluating patients with proximal humerus fractures include history, physical examination, plain radiography, CT scanning, electromyography, and arteriography. The most important of these diagnostic measures are history, physical examination, and plain radiography. A diagnosis and treatment plan can be formulated in over 90 percent of cases with only these three interventional tools.

The patient history should be directed toward determining the mechanism of injury, the presence of any associated injuries, and the medical and functional status of the patient before the injury. The mechanism of injury will often indicate the amount of trauma involved in producing the proximal humerus fracture. In elderly osteoporotic females, the trauma may be as innocuous as a fall from a standing height. Younger patients without osteoporosis who sustain proximal humerus fractures frequently are the victims of severe multisystem trauma. Their other injuries may be life-threatening, and as a result, both the diagnosis and treatment of their proximal humerus fracture may be delayed. It is important to institute treatment of the proximal humerus fracture as soon as is safely possible so that the ultimate end result is not compromised and so that mobilization of the injured patient will be facilitated.

It is important to rule out associated injuries, even in elderly patients who sustain their proximal humerus fractures as a result of apparently minimal trauma. Concommitant injuries that can be seen with proximal humerus fractures include additional fractures at distant sites, hemothorax, pneumothorax, and neurovascular compromise.[11] The patient should be questioned about sources of pain other than the shoulder. If the upper extremity was used to break a fall, there may be fractures of the distal radius and ulna. The presence of hip pain should alert the examiner to the possibility of a concommitant proximal femur fracture. Dyspnea and flank pain may be associated with rib fracture and hemothorax or pneumothorax. Although these concomitant injuries are not seen frequently, their presence should be excluded. The preinjury functional and medical status of the patient is frequently helpful in determining the course of management. Patients with medical problems that make them poor operative risks may be best managed nonoperatively, even in situations that might otherwise be handled by operative means. Conversely, displaced fractures that might be accepted in extremely elderly, inactive patients may be better managed operatively in younger, physically active individuals.

The most common physical finding associated with a proximal humerus fracture is pain. The shoulder girdle often will appear swollen. Ecchymosis is a universal finding but may take 24 to 48 hours to appear. The entire proximal humerus will be tender to palpation, and there may be palpable crepitus with attempted gentle internal and external rotation of the humeral shaft. If the patient complains of pain in areas remote from the injured shoulder, these areas should be examined for the presence of concomitant fractures or injuries.

A complete neurovascular examination of the involved upper extremity is absolutely mandatory in patients with a proximal humerus fracture.[11] Injury to the brachial plexus and axillary

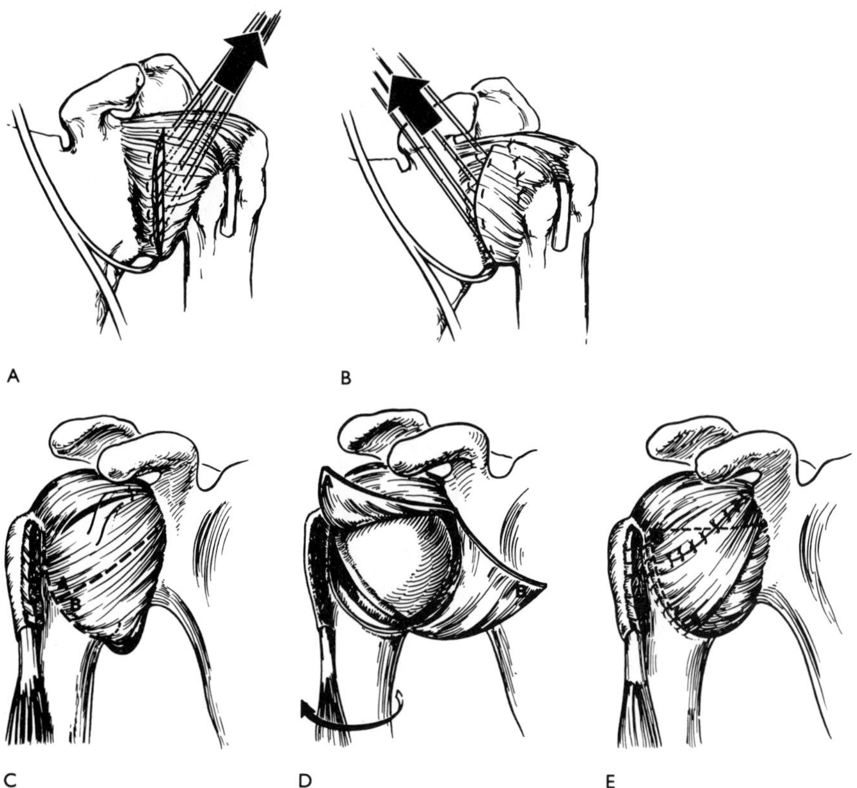


**Figure 4-44.** During a capsular shift procedure, exposure of the capsule is similar to a Bankart procedure. (a) Then the medial limb of the capsule is brought laterally and superiorly under the lateral limb. (b) The lateral limb is double-breasted over the medial limb to form a pants-over-vest arrangement. Note the proximity of the axillary nerve. An alternative surgical technique for the capsular shift involves similar exposure of the capsule as above. (c) Then the capsule is incised at the humeral attachment and transversely. (d) A superior flap and an inferior flap are created by a transverse incision. (e) The inferior flap is advanced superiorly, and the superior flap is brought inferiorly. Closure of the rotator cuff interval is also performed. (Reproduced with permission from Rockwood CA Jr, Thomas SC, Matsen FA III. Subluxations and dislocations about the glenohumeral joint. In: Rockwood CA, Green DP, Bucholz RW, eds. Fractures. 3rd ed., vol. 1. Philadelphia: JB Lippincott, 1991:1021.)

artery have been reported even in undisplaced fractures of the proximal humerus.[94,182] Therefore, it is important that the extremity be tested for the presence of peripheral pulses, good distal capillary refill, and the absence of cyanosis. Sensation is notoriously unreliable for documenting the presence of a neurologic lesion.[15] Therefore, the integrity of all peripheral nerves, including the axillary, musculocutaneous, radial, median, and ulnar nerves, should be verified through motor testing. Even in the acute setting, most patients can contract their deltoid muscle isometrically to verify the integrity of the axillary nerve. Should this not be the case, the patient should be reexamined intermittently until the presence of motor function has been verified. In the absence of motor function to the axillary nerve, an axillary nerve palsy must be suspected. The axillary nerve is the most commonly injured nerve in fractures about the shoulder.[11]

# Diagnostic Imaging

## ROUTINE RADIOGRAPHY

Although history and physical examination are important components of a diagnostic evaluation, proximal humerus fracture is a radiologic diagnosis. Consequently, adequate plain radiographs are mandatory. The trauma series[136] should be obtained and includes a scapular anteroposterior view, a scapular lateral Y view, and an axillary view.

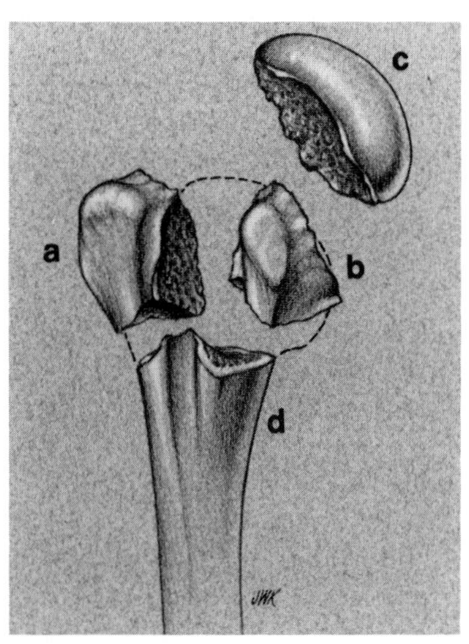


A

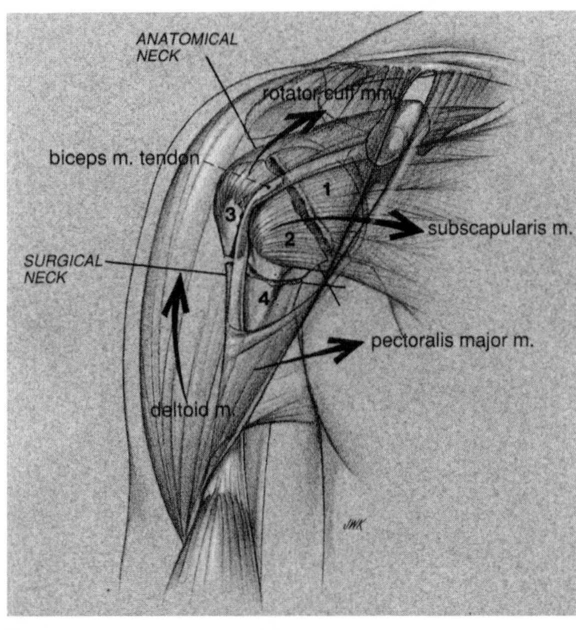


B

**Figure 4-45.** Four distinct fragments of the proximal humerus (a) and their soft-tissue attachments (b) which influence the direction of displacement. (Reproduced with permission from Bigliani LU, Craig EV, Butters KP: Fractures of the shoulder. In: Rockwood CA, Green DP, Bucholz RW, eds. Fractures. 3rd ed., vol. 1. Philadelphia: JB Lippincott, 1991:1021.)

**Displaced Fractures**

| | 2-part | 3-part | 4-part | Articular Surface |
|---|---|---|---|---|
| Anatomical Neck | | | | |
| Surgical Neck | a b c | | | |
| Greater Tuberosity | | | | |
| Lesser Tuberosity | | | | |
| Fracture-Dislocation — Anterior | | | | |
| Fracture-Dislocation — Posterior | | | | |
| Head-Splitting | | | | |

**Figure 4-46.** Neer's classification of proximal humerus fractures. (Reproduced with permission from Bigliani LU, Craig EV, Butters KP. Fractures of the shoulder. In: Rockwood CA, Green DP, Bucholz RW, eds. Fractures. 3rd ed., vol. 1. Philadelphia: JB Lippincott, 1991:871.)

Complete radiographic examination of a proximal humerus fracture requires visualization of both the humerus and the scapula in at least two orthogonal planes.

## CT SCANNING

Although plain radiography is adequate in the vast majority of cases, CT scanning can be useful in certain circumstances. First, CT scanning can help determine whether a fracture has united or has progressed to nonunion. Second, CT scanning can be helpful in evaluating the amount of displacement of greater tuberosity fractures.[121] The amount of articular involvement in head-splitting and humeral head impression fractures also can be quantitated using CT scanning.[11]

## ARTERIOGRAPHY

Arteriography is very rarely required in the evaluation of proximal humerus fractures. Its one indication is a proximal humerus fracture in which arterial injury is suspected on the basis of physical examination. Arteriography in this scenario is useful not only for diagnosis but also for surgical planning.

## ELECTROMYOGRAPHY

Electromyography is not indicated in the acute management of proximal humerus fractures.

However, in a patient whose axillary nerve integrity could not be verified by motor examination, electromyography is useful for documenting the presence of the lesion beginning approximately 21 days from the injury. It can then be used to document reinervation over the ensuing 6 months to 1 year.[15]

# Indications for Surgery

According to Neer,[136, 137] over 80 percent of proximal humerus fractures are minimally displaced and do not require operative intervention. Rose and colleagues[168] and Horak and Nilsson[90] have reported the incidence of nondisplaced fractures to be 78 and 61 percent, respectively. Although the incidence of nondisplaced fracture may be lower than 80 percent, it is clear that the majority of proximal humerus fractures are nondisplaced and do not require operative stabilization (Fig. 4-47).

Depending on the type of fracture, two-, three-, and four-part fractures of the proximal humerus often can require operative intervention in the form of closed reduction, open reduction, and internal fixation or prosthetic replacement. The indications for surgery, as well as the procedure to be performed, depend on the type of fracture present as well as the medical and functional status of the patient.

## TWO-PART FRACTURES

Two-part fractures come in four varieties: anatomic neck, surgical neck, greater tuberosity, and lesser tuberosity.

### ANATOMIC NECK

Displaced fractures through the anatomic neck portend an extremely poor prognosis. Displacement through the anatomic neck causes vascular isolation of the articular segment with a high probability of avascular necrosis.[11] Fortunately, these injuries are extremely rare. Nonoperative management is indicated only in those patients who are extremely poor operative risks or who have little functional use of the involved extremity.

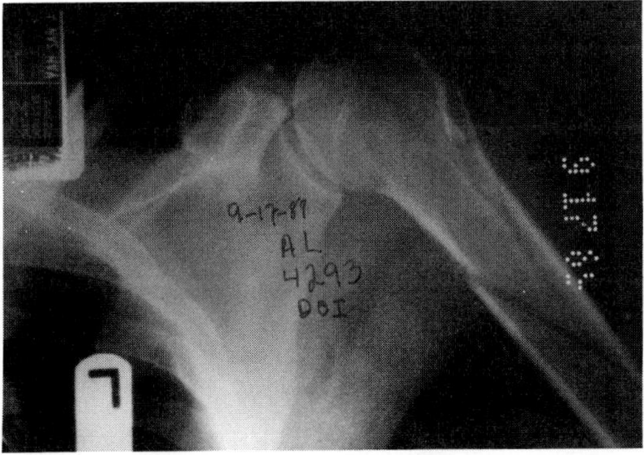

**Figure 4-47.** Radiograph of a nondisplaced proximal humerus fracture.

### SURGICAL NECK

Displacement of a two-part fracture through the surgical neck nearly always involves some component of angulation with the apex anteriorly (Fig. 4-48). In addition, the shaft is usually adducted and internally rotated as a result of the pull of the pectoralis major tendon. Residual angulation of 45 degrees or more is associated with a loss of flexion.[11] Therefore, in active patients who are good operative candidates, reduction of two-part surgical neck fractures is usually indicated.

### GREATER TUBEROSITY

Displaced greater tuberosity fractures occur as an isolated injury as well as with anterior dislocation of the glenohumeral joint. When these fractures occur in combination with anterior dislocation, the likelihood of recurrent dislocation drops to substantially less than 5 percent.[91] This is presumably because the trauma caused fracture of the greater tuberosity rather than an anterior Bankart lesion. Residual displacement of the greater tuberosity is thought to indicate a rotator cuff tear.[138] Healing of the fracture in a displaced position reportedly leads to subacromial impingement syndrome.[138] As a result, displaced greater tuberosity fractures often require operative reduction and stabilization.[11, 138]

### LESSER TUBEROSITY FRACTURES

Two-part fractures of the lesser tuberosity are uncommon and may be isolated or accompanied by posterior dislocation of the glenohumeral joint. Smaller fractures that do not block internal rotation and do not involve a significant portion of the articular surface can be managed nonoperatively. Larger fragments, particularly if they involve the articular surface, should be operatively reduced and stabilized.[11, 138]

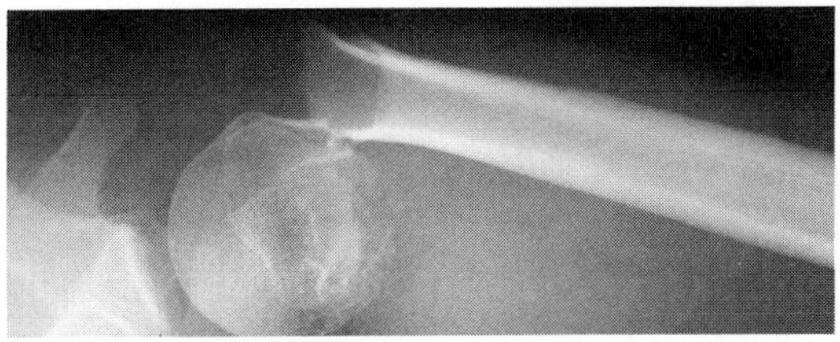

**Figure 4-48.** Two-part fracture of the proximal humerus at the surgical neck revealing typical apex anterior angulation.

## THREE-PART FRACTURES

Three-part fractures are generally unstable injures and are difficult to manage by closed means (Fig. 4-49). They are characterized by a displaced fracture through the surgical neck in combination with either a displaced greater or lesser tuberosity fracture. Depending on which tuberosity remains attached to the head, the articular surface will be facing anteriorly or posteriorly. If the greater tuberosity is intact, the humeral head will be externally rotated and the articular surface will be facing anteriorly. Conversely, in the case of an intact lesser tuberosity, the humeral head will be internally rotated and the articular surface will be facing posteriorly.[11,138] The major deforming force on the humeral shaft is the pectoralis major tendon, which will cause medial displacement of the shaft with respect to the other fragments. In functional patients who are not poor operative candidates, three-part fractures are best managed operatively. Most often, bone quality is sufficient to allow open reduction and internal fixation. However, in the presence of severe comminution or poor bone quality, prosthetic replacement may be preferred.[11,137,138] In older, sedentary patients whose functional demands or underlying medical status mitigate against operative intervention, three-part fractures may be managed nonoperatively.

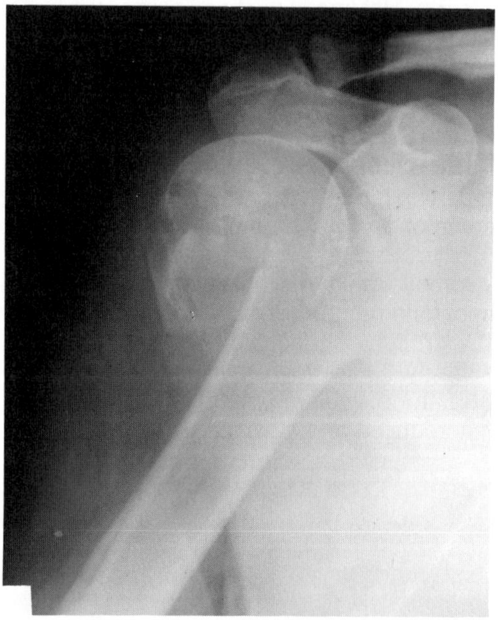

## FOUR-PART FRACTURES

Nonoperative management of four-part fractures is difficult because of gross instability of the fracture fragments as well as vascular isolation of the head fragment (Fig. 4-50). Most series report poor results with nonoperative treatment because of stiffness and avascular necrosis, which has been reported to occur in between 13 and 34 percent of cases.[11] Consequently, four-part fractures are generally treated operatively except in the presence of a medical contraindication to surgery.

## HEAD-SPLITTING AND IMPRESSION FRACTURES

Head-splitting and impression fractures of the proximal humerus do not fit into any set classification of proximal humerus fractures. Head-splitting fractures occur when a coronal fracture line extends intraarticularly through the head, separating the head into two fragments. Impression fractures occur by indentation of the soft cancellous bone of the proximal humerus by the

**Figure 4-49.** Three-part greater tuberosity fracture. (Reproduced with permission from Bigliani LU, Craig EV, Butters KP. Fractures of the shoulder. In: Rockwood CA, Green DP, Bucholz RW, eds. Fractures. 3rd ed., vol. 1. Philadelphia: JB Lippincott, 1991:871.)

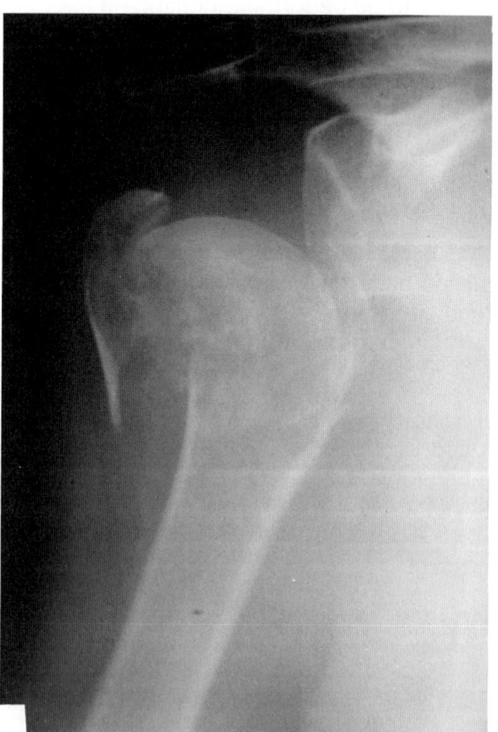

**Figure 4-50.** Four-part fracture. (Reproduced with permission from Bigliani LU, Craig EV, Butters KP. Fractures of the shoulder. In: Rockwood CA, Green DP, Bucholz RW, eds. Fractures. 3rd ed., vol. 1. Philadelphia: JB Lippincott, 1991:871.)

sclerotic margin of the glenoid rim during dislocations. Posterolateral indentation fractures (i.e., Hill-Sachs defects) occur during anterior glenohumeral dislocation, while anterolateral humeral head defects (i.e., reverse Hill-Sachs defects) occur during posterior glenohumeral dislocation.

The need for surgical intervention in displaced head-splitting fractures depends on the degree of displacement, fracture stability, underlying bone quality, and functional status of the patient. In elderly patients with stable, impacted head-splitting fractures, nonoperative management may be indicated. In younger, more active patients, in the presence of significant displacement, operative intervention in the form of open reduction and internal fixation or prosthetic replacement is indicated. The reader is referred to the section on instability for the surgical management of head impression fractures.

# Surgical Options

## TWO-PART FRACTURES

### ANATOMIC NECK

Fortunately, displaced two-part fractures of the anatomic neck are extremely uncommon injuries. The major vascular supply for the humeral head arises from the arcuate artery, which is the terminal branch of the ascending branch of the anterior humeral circumflex artery.[72,105] The arcuate artery is an end artery, and as a result, division of the arcuate artery leads to a very high incidence of avascular necrosis. The artery enters the articular segment just lateral to the articular margin at the superolateral aspect of the bicipital groove.[72] Displacement of a fracture through the anatomic neck disrupts this end artery and leads to a very high incidence of avascular necrosis. As a result, open reduction and internal fixation are indicated only in patients too young to undergo prosthetic replacement. The fracture is best managed in most instances by prosthetic replacement of the proximal humerus. Resurfacing of the glenoid is generally not required.

### SURGICAL NECK

Surgical management of displaced surgical neck fractures includes closed or open reduction combined with internal or external fixation. An initial attempt at closed reduction should be made. The maneuver is most easily performed under general anesthesia. However, an initial attempt in the emergency room under intravenous sedation may be warranted. After achieving a satisfactory closed reduction, the arm is brought to the side, and x-rays are taken. If the reduction is stable, the arm is immobilized in a sling and swath or a shoulder immobilizer, and appropriate postoperative rehabilitation is instituted.

Open reduction is indicated if an adequate closed reduction cannot be obtained. The most common cause for an inability to obtain a closed reduction is soft-tissue interposition (i.e., long head of the biceps or deltoid muscle).[11,138]

In the presence of an unstable closed reduction or an open reduction, several methods of internal fixation have been described. An unstable closed reduction can be handled with percutaneously placed wires from the shaft into the head or with intramedullary devices placed percutaneously through the head and into the shaft of the humerus.[17,95] Open reduction can be combined with intramedullary fixation, extramedullary fixation (i.e., plates and screws, tension band wires, or interfragmentary sutures), or a combination of intramedullary and extramedullary fixation.[11]

### LESSER TUBEROSITY

When operative management of two-part lesser tuberosity fractures is indicated, the preferred approach is open reduction and internal fixation. After open reduction, the lesser tuberosity can be stabilized through the use of interfragmentary screws, interfragmentary wires, or interfragmentary sutures. Any defect in the rotator interval also should be repaired not only to reestablish rotator cuff integrity but also to help maintain the reduction.

### GREATER TUBEROSITY

The goals for surgical management of displaced greater tuberosity fractures are anatomic or near-anatomic reduction of the fracture fragment, stable fixation to allow early motion, and repair of any rotator cuff defects which, when present, typically occur longitudinally at the rotator interval.[11,66,138] Reduction can be performed through either a lateral deltoid splitting approach or a deltopectoral approach. Reduction of the greater tuberosity fracture is facilitated by initially repairing any longitudinal tear in the rotator cuff anatomically. This relieves the displacing forces on the greater tuberosity and allows it to fall into place in its previously anatomic location. Stabilization can be obtained through the use of interfragmentary screws, interfragmentary or tension band wires, or interfragmentary sutures.

## THREE-PART FRACTURES

Surgical management of three-part fractures of the proximal humerus is extremely challenging.

In general, open reduction and internal fixation are the treatments of choice. However, prosthetic replacement may be indicated in a small subgroup of three-part fractures that exhibit extreme comminution and poor bone quality.[11,138]

The underlying principle to be followed in open reduction and internal fixation of three-part fractures, as in all fractures of the proximal humerus, is to obtain adequate fixation in the operating room to allow early postoperative motion so that stiffness can be minimized. Three-part fractures can be thought of as a combination of a two-part fracture of the surgical neck with either a displaced greater or lesser tuberosity fracture. Therefore, operative methods used for open reduction and internal fixation of three-part fractures are combinations of the methods used for two-part surgical neck fractures and displaced tuberosity fractures. The displaced tuberosity is reduced to the remainder of the head and intact tuberosity. It is stabilized with interfragmentary screws, interfragmentary or tension band wires, or interfragmentary sutures. Any longitudinal tear in the rotator cuff is also repaired. The remaining surgical neck fracture is then reduced and stabilized using intramedullary fixation, extramedullary fixation, or a combination of intramedullary and extramedullary fixation. If there is any question regarding the stability of the displaced tuberosity fragment, it should be stabilized to the shaft as well as to the remaining tuberosity and head fragment so as to prevent postoperative tuberosity displacement, which has been associated with poor results.[11,137]

### FOUR-PART FRACTURES

The treatment of choice for nearly all four-part proximal humerus fractures is prosthetic replacement.[11,137,138] Proximal humeral replacement with secure tuberosity reattachment allows for early mobilization and eliminates the possibility of late avascular necrosis. Neer and McIlveen[143] reported 60 of 61 patients with excellent or satisfactory results following proximal humeral replacement for four-part fracture. Although some authors have reported adequate pain relief, others have documented a higher incidence of unsatisfactory results because of postoperative limitation of motion.[11,198]

The role of open reduction and internal fixation in the management of four-part fractures in the young patient is controversial. However, if the goals of satisfactory reduction and rigid enough fixation to allow early mobilization can be achieved, there may be a role for open reduction and internal fixation in patients younger than age 30 who are victims of severe trauma.[11]

### HEAD-SPLITTING AND IMPRESSION FRACTURES

The vast majority of head-splitting fractures occur in elderly patients with osteoporotic bone. Proximal replacement is generally indicated in cases of significant displacement.

## Authors' Preferred Methods of Treatment

### TWO-PART FRACTURES

#### ANATOMIC NECK

In cases of two-part anatomic neck fractures, we prefer proximal humeral replacement. The surgical technique is discussed under management of four-part fractures. However, in brief, the glenohumeral joint is approached through a deltopectoral incision. The subscapularis and capsule are incised 1 to 1½ medial to the subscapularis insertion and reflected medially. The articular segment is excised, an appropriately sized humeral replacement is inserted, and the subscapularis is reattached anatomically.

#### SURGICAL NECK

We prefer an attempt at closed reduction in the operating room under general anesthesia for most cases of two-part surgical neck fractures. If the reduction is stable, no further intervention is required. If the reduction is unstable, however, and there is absence of severe comminution and osteoporosis, we prefer the use of percutaneously placed pins from the lateral shaft into the head (Fig. 4-51a,b). The pins are cut beneath the skin and are removed between the third and sixth week of treatment.

If the fracture cannot be reduced closed, open reduction and internal fixation through an anterior deltopectoral approach are performed. The fracture is approached through a long deltopectoral incision. The fracture site is inspected for interposition of the long head of the biceps or deltoid. After fracture reduction, we prefer stabilization with heavy nonabsorbable sutures. As described by Bigliani,[11] two sutures are placed in figure-of-eight fashion at orthogonal planes to one another. One suture is passed through the rotator cuff and greater tuberosity and through drill holes in the lateral shaft, while the other is placed through the subscapularis and lesser tuberosity into the anterior and lateral shaft. If supplemental fixation is required, we prefer the use of intramedullary fixation.

#### GREATER TUBEROSITY

Although interfragmentary screws may be successful in maintaining a reduction in some

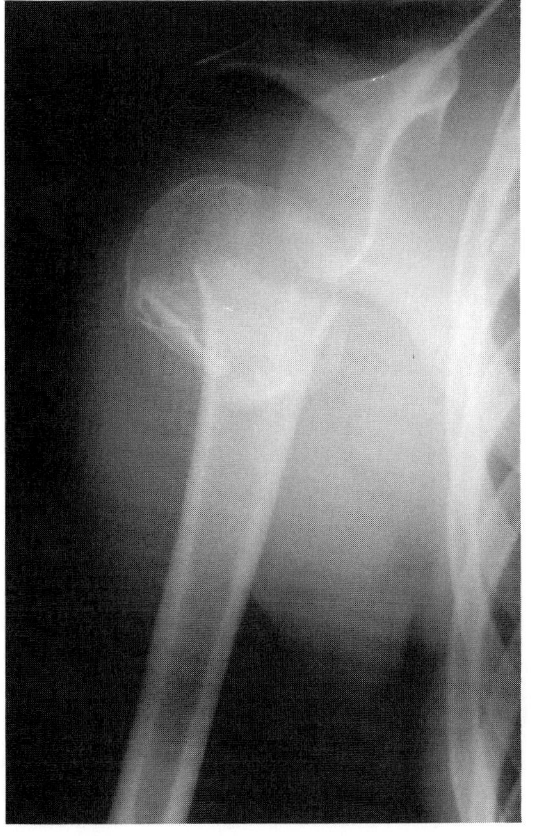

A

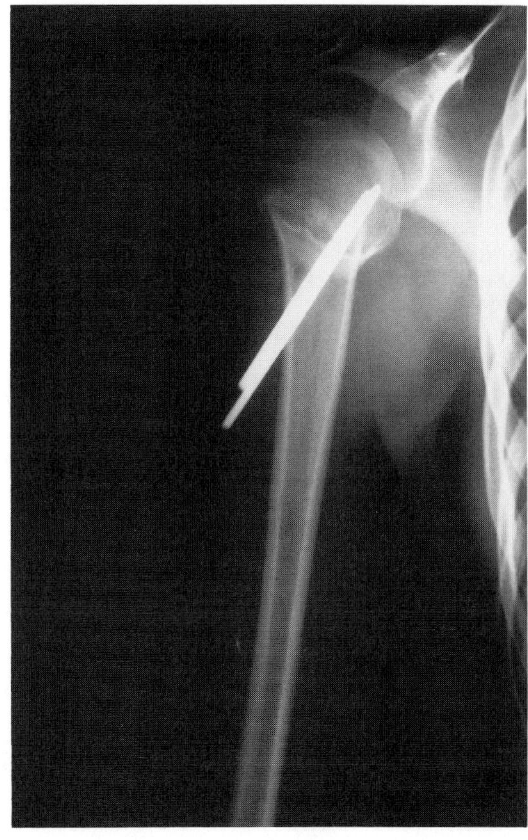

B

**Figure 4-51.** Preoperative radiograph of a two-part surgical neck fracture. (b) Postoperative radiograph following closed reduction and percutaneous pinning.

cases, we prefer the use of interfragmentary suturing using the soft tissues of the rotator cuff to reinforce fixation. Although the fracture can be approached through a superolateral incision using a lateral deltoid split, we prefer an anterior deltopectoral approach. Heavy, nonabsorbable sutures are woven through the rotator cuff, brought through the tuberosity, and fixed to the shaft and lesser tuberosity through drill holes. Repair of the rent in the rotator interval prior to tying the sutures in the tuberosity can aid in achieving and maintaining the reduction.

### LESSER TUBEROSITY

Isolated two-part fractures of the lesser tuberosity that block medial rotation or involve a significant portion of the articular surface are treated with open reduction and internal fixation. Although fixation using interfragmentary screws has been described, the soft cancellous bone of the proximal humerus can lead to loss of fixation and redisplacement of the fracture fragment with ultimate nonunion. Therefore, we prefer interfragmentary fixation using heavy, nonabsorbable sutures through a deltopectoral incision.

## THREE-PART FRACTURES

Open reduction and internal fixation are the treatments of choice for three-part fractures of the proximal humerus. The fracture is approached through a long deltopectoral incision. The deltoid and cephalic vein are retracted laterally, while the pectoralis major is retracted medially. The upper one-third to one-half of the pectoralis major insertion may be incised to aid in visualization of the inferior aspect of the glenohumeral joint. The long head of the biceps is identified and followed to the rotator interval. The displaced tuberosity fracture fragment is identified and reattached to the remaining tuberosity and head fragment through the use of interfragmentary heavy, nonresorbable sutures (Fig. 4-52). Any rent in the rotator cuff is repaired. The shaft is then reduced and stabilized to the proximal fragment in a similar fashion to the

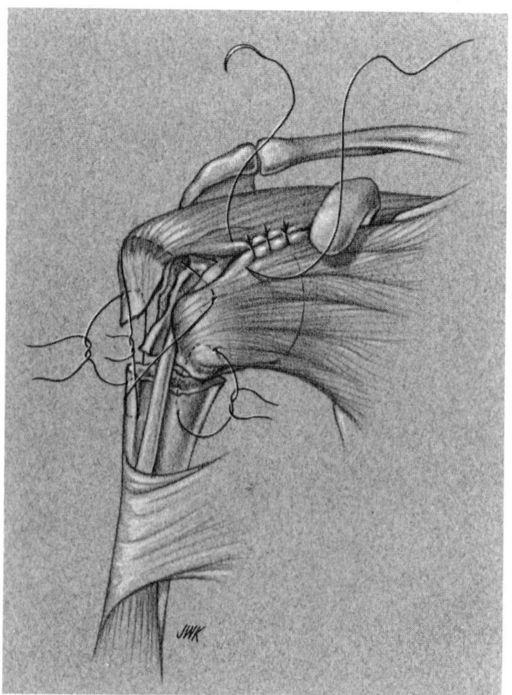

Figure 4-52. Schematic drawing depicting nonabsorbable suture technique for open reduction and internal fixation of three-part proximal humerus fractures. (Reproduced with permission from Bigliani LU, Craig EV, Butters KP. Fractures of the shoulder. In: Rockwood CA, Green DP, Bucholz RW, eds. Fractures. 3rd ed., vol. 1. Philadelphia: JB Lippincott, 1991:871.)

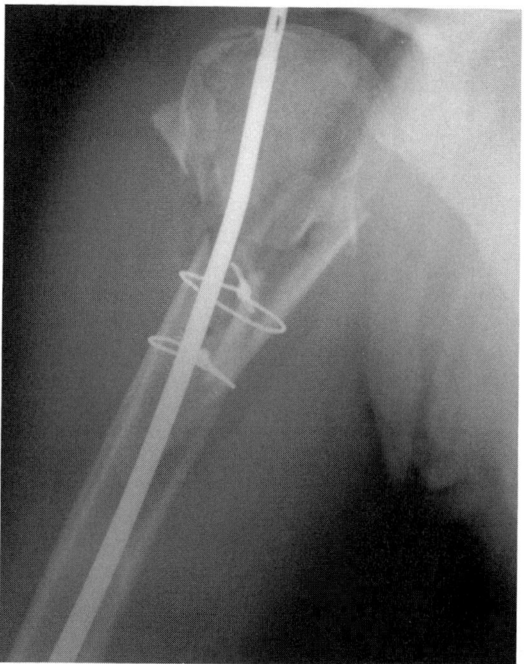

Figure 4-53. Postoperative radiograph of patient with a three-part fracture with communution of the shaft. The greater tuberosity has been sutured to the head, and intramedullary fixation has been used to resist medial displacement. The comminution of the shaft was treated with cerclage wiring.

previously described two-part surgical neck fracture. Care should be taken to reattach the displaced tuberosity to the remaining head and tuberosity fragment as well as to the shaft. And tendency toward medial displacement of the shaft by the pectoralis major can be resisted through the use of supplementary intramedullary fixation (Fig. 4-53).

In selected three-part fractures of the proximal humerus, comminution may be too severe or underlying bone quality may be too poor to allow adequate internal fixation. In these instances, primary humeral head replacement as described in the section on four-part fractures is indicated.

### FOUR-PART FRACTURES

The vast majority of four-part fractures of the proximal humerus are best managed by proximal humeral replacement (Fig. 4-54). The technique is similar to that described for total shoulder replacement.

## Postoperative Rehabilitation

The goal of any surgical procedure in the management of proximal humerus fractures is to achieve adequate enough fixation in the operating room to allow immediate postoperative passive mobilization. However, in cases of less than

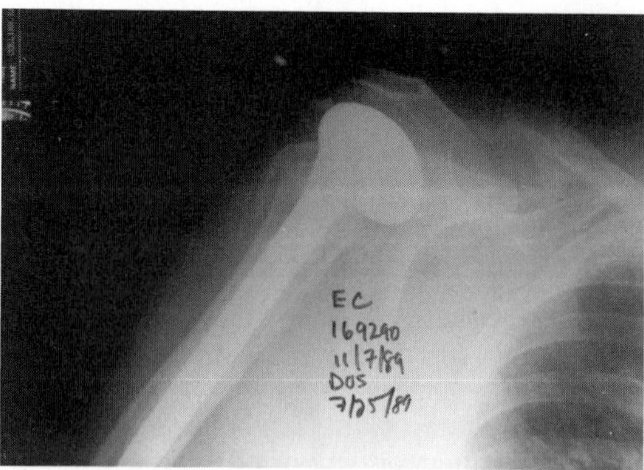

Figure 4-54. Postoperative radiograph of a patient with a four-part fracture of the proximal humerus treated with hemiarthroplasty. Note that the greater tuberosity has been reattached to the shaft.

ideal fixation, the rehabilitation program should be modified so that loss of fixation of the tuberosities or other fracture fragments does not occur. Assuming that adequate fixation has been obtained, pendulum exercises, supine passive flexion exercises, and passive external rotation to the extent allowed on the operating table are initiated on the first postoperative day. An overhead pulley is added in the second postoperative week. In cases of excellent fixation, the pulley can be added slightly earlier. Passive exercises should be performed between four and six times daily using the opposite, unaffected arm to move the operated arm. Once the fracture has healed, passive stretching exercises to increase range of motion along with strengthening exercises for the rotator cuff and deltoid muscles are added. Complete rehabilitation following proximal humeral fractures requires 9 to 18 months.

# Acromioclavicular Joint Injuries

The acromioclavicular joint is a diarthrodial joint located between the lateral end of the clavicle and the medial end of the acromion process. It contains an intraarticular disc and is stabilized by the acromioclavicular ligaments as well as by the coracoclavicular ligament.[165] In general, the acromioclavicular ligaments are capsular structures that provide stability primarily for anterior and posterior (i.e., horizontal) displacement of the lateral end of the clavicle. The coracoclavicular ligament consists of the more medial conoid ligament and the more lateral trapezoid ligament. These ligaments are responsible for superoinferior (i.e., vertical) stability of the lateral end of the clavicle.[70,165,191] Dynamic stability of the acromioclavicular joint is provided by the muscles that cross the joint, namely, the trapezius and deltoid muscles.

Acromioclavicular joint injuries are classified as types I through VI, depending on the integrity of the acromioclavicular and coracoclavicular ligaments and the direction of displacement of the clavicle[165] (Fig.4-55). In a type I injury, the acromioclavicular ligaments are sprained but not torn, and the coracoclavicular ligaments are normal. There is no displacement of the clavicle or acromioclavicular joint. In a type II injury, the acromioclavicular ligaments are completely torn, and the coracoclavicular ligaments are intact but strained. There may be slight widening of the acromioclavicular joint. Type III acromioclavicular dislocation is characterized by complete disruption of the acromioclavicular and coracoclavicular ligaments. There is complete vertical displacement of the acromioclavicular joint. In a type IV dislocation, the acromioclavicular and coracoclavicular ligaments are disrupted, and the clavicle is displaced posteriorly into or through the trapezius muscle. A type V dislocation is characterized by complete disruption of the acromioclavicular and coracoclavicular ligaments and severe vertical displacement of the acromioclavicular joint. The severe displacement associated with a type V injury is presumably a result of complete stripping of the deltoid and trapezius fascia from the distal end of the clavicle, which lies subcutaneously. The type VI dislocation is characterized by inferior displacement of the clavicle with respect to the acromion into either a subacromial or subcoracoid position.

## Clinical Presentation

Patients presenting with acromioclavicular dislocation most often report a direct blow to the lateral aspect of the shoulder in the region of the acromion. This most often occurs as a consequence of a fall on the point of the shoulder. The most common presenting complaint is pain in association with a deformity at the acromioclavicular joint. Patients with severe displacement also may complain of numbness and paresthesias from brachial plexus traction.

Physical findings associated with acromioclavicular dislocation include soft-tissue swelling and deformity at the acromioclavicular joint as well as tenderness. Ecchymosis is also very common but may take 24 to 48 hours to appear. Type II injuries may be associated with significant anteroposterior instability of the acromioclavicular joint, as demonstrated by grasping the shaft of the clavicle and displacing it forward and backward. The vertical instability associated with type III or type V injuries may be reduced most easily by applying a superiorly directed force at the elbow to reduce the arm and shoulder to the clavicle. The function of the coracoclavicular ligaments is to suspend the arm from the clavicle. Rupture of these ligaments causes inferior displacement of the arm and shoulder rather than superior displacement of the clavicle.

In type IV acromioclavicular dislocations, the

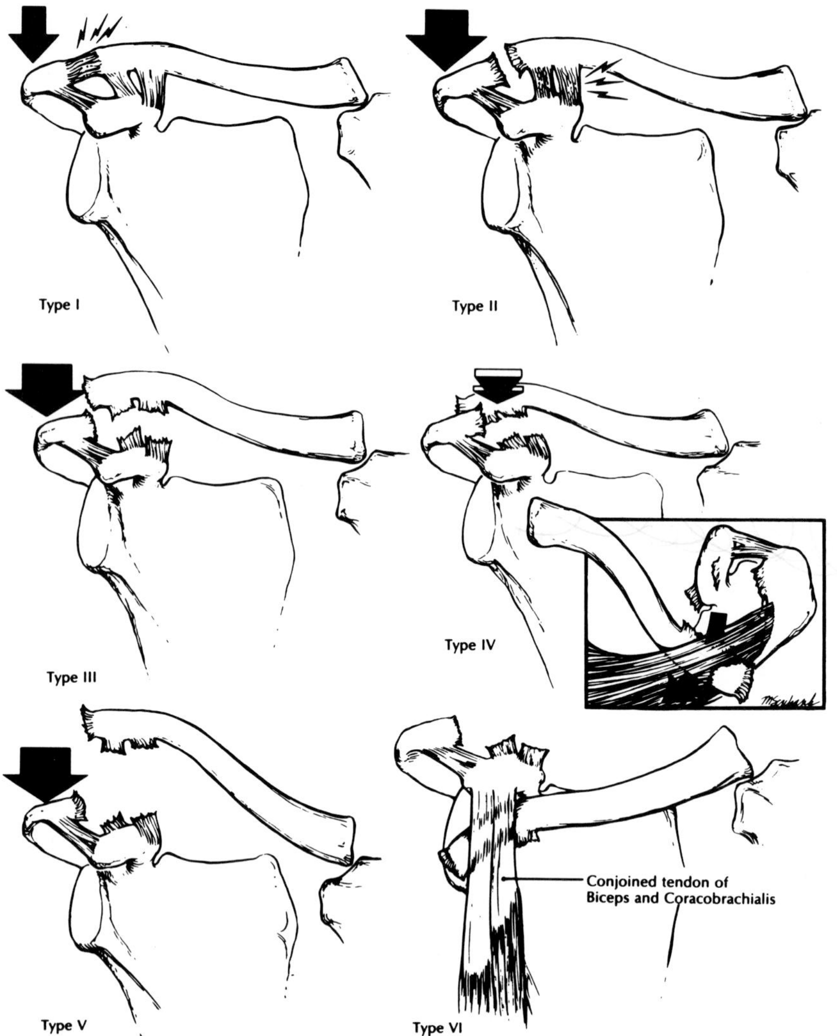


**Figure 4-55.** Classification of acromioclavicular dislocations, types I through VI. (Reproduced with permission from Rockwood CA Jr, Williams GR Jr, Young DC. Injuries to the acromioclavicular joint. In: Rockwood CA, Green DP, Bucholz RW, eds. Fractures. 3rd ed., vol. 1. Philadelphia: JB Lippincott, 1991:1181.)

clavicle is displaced posteriorly into or through the trapezius muscle. This may be observed on physical examination by standing behind the seated patient and looking down on both shoulders from above. The posteriorly dislocated clavicle will be projecting much farther posteriorly than the uninjured clavicle.

Type VI acromioclavicular dislocation, particularly when it is subcoracoid in nature, is frequently the result of severe trauma. As a result, the patient should be questioned and examined for concomitant injuries. Neurovascular examination, which is important in all acromioclavicular dislocations, is particularly important in subcoracoid dislocations, which are frequently accompanied by brachial plexus irritation.

# Diagnostic Imaging

Routine radiography is adequate for diagnosis and treatment of almost all acromioclavicular joint injuries. As with any other musculoskeletal condition, radiographs in at least two orthogonal planes are necessary in order to describe the injury. In addition, stress radiographs have been described in an attempt to classify the acromioclavicular joint dislocation. Certain "special views" also have been described for various unusual situations.

## ROUTINE VIEWS

Routine radiographs of the acromioclavicular joint require approximately one-third to one-half the x-ray penetration required for the glenohumeral joint. Therefore, if the x-ray technique used in imaging the shoulder is not adjusted accordingly, the acromioclavicular joint will be overpenetrated, and small fractures may be overlooked.[165]

Routine anteroposterior views should be standardized so that both arms are hanging unsupported and the same x-ray technique is used for both shoulders. The radiographs should be inspected not only for acromioclavicular displacement but also for the distance between the top of the coracoid and the inferior aspect of the clavicle (Fig. 4-56). The measured coraclavicular interspace is compared with the opposite, uninjured shoulder. An axillary lateral view also should be taken of both shoulders. The axillary view will demonstrate any posterior displacement of the injured clavicle compared with the uninjured side and also will help to delineate fractures of the coracoid process.

### STRESS VIEWS

Acromioclavicular displacement in complete acromioclavicular dislocations can be reduced by contraction of the trapezius aponeurosis as well as by support of the injured extremity with the uninjured arm.[165] Therefore, anteroposterior stress views should be taken in order to quantitate the amount of maximum displacement. Anteroposterior views are taken of both shoulders

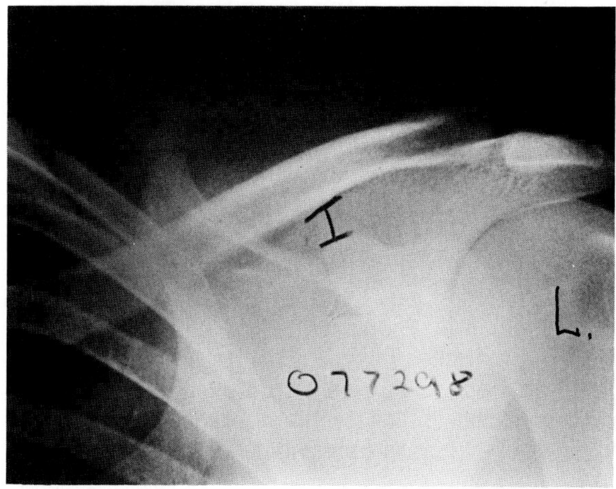


A

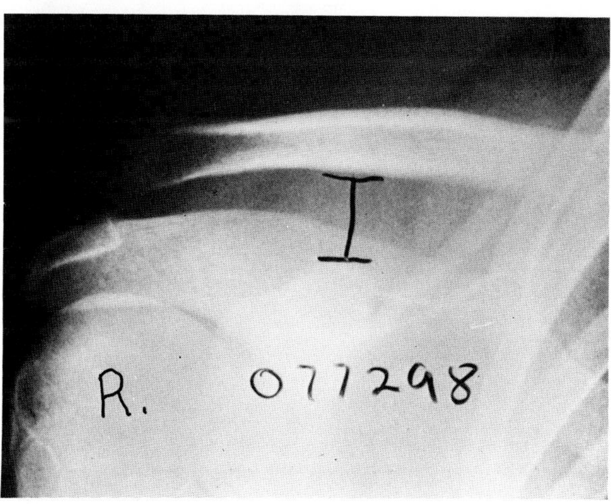


B

**Figure 4-56.** Anteroposterior radiographs should be taken of both acromioclavicular joints with and without weights. Note that the coracoclavicular interspace is greater in part a (the injured side) compared with part b. (Reproduced with permission from Rockwood CA Jr, Williams GR Jr, Young DC. Injuries to the acromioclavicular joint. In: Rockwood CA, Green DP, Bucholz RW, eds. Fractures. 3rd ed., vol. 1. Philadelphia: JB Lippincott, 1991:1181.)

with and without weights suspended from each wrist (Fig.4-57).

Alexander[2] described the "shoulder-forward view." This is a lateral stress view of the acromioclavicular joint. A true transcapular lateral (Y) view is taken with the patient in the relaxed position. The patient is then asked to thrust both shoulders forward. In comparison with the uninjured side, the injured side will reveal that the acromion is displaced anteriorly and inferiorly with respect to the distal clavicle.

### SPECIAL VIEWS

Zanca[200] described a modified anteroposterior view of the acromioclavicular joint (Fig.4-4). He noted that on the true anterior posterior view of the acromioclavicular joint the distal clavicle and acromion were superimposed on the spine of the scapula. Therefore, he recommended both a 10- to 15-degree cephalic tilt and a 30-degree cephalic tilt view in order to project an unobscured image of the joint. The Zanca view is helpful when loose bodies or small fractures of the acromioclavicular joint are suspected in the initial views.

The Stryker notch view[77] is an anteroposterior view with 10 degrees of cephalic tilt with the arm placed on the top of the patient's head see (Fig.4-33). This projects an excellent view of the entire coracoid process. This view is particularly useful when acromioclavicular separation is accompanied by coracoid process fracture. This should be suspected on the routine views when, despite acromioclavicular separation, the coraclavicular interspace is equal to the uninjured side.[165]

## Indications for Surgery

Management of acute acromioclavicular injuries depends on whether or not the injury is a complete or an incomplete dislocation.[25] Type I and II injuries (incomplete dislocations) are most often managed nonoperatively. However, Bergfeld and colleagues[10] and Cox[44] have reported that untreated type I and II injuries may lead to chronic disability.

Type IV, V, and VI injuries require open reduction and internal fixation in the vast majority of cases. Type IV injuries are characterized by extreme posterior displacement of the clavicle into or through the trapezius muscle. This displacement is difficult to reduce closed. Type V injuries are characterized not only by coracoclavicular injury but also by stripping of the deltotrapzeius fascia. This leaves the clavicle in a subcutaneous position and is often best managed by open reduction and internal fixation. Type VI injuries, particularly if they are subcoracoid, cannot be reduced closed and require operative reduction and stabilization.

Treatment of type III acromioclavicular separations is extremely controversial. In the vast majority of cases, nonoperative management will yield good functional results despite resid-

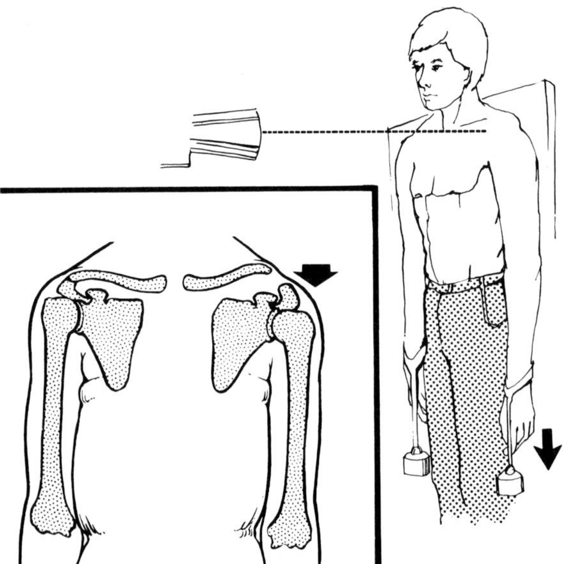

**Figure 4-57.** Technique for obtaining stress views of the acromioclavicular joint. (Reproduced with permission from Rockwood CA Jr, Williams GR Jr, Young DC. Injuries to the acromioclavicular joint. In: Rockwood CA, Green DP, Bucholz RW, eds. Fractures. 3rd ed., vol. 1. Philadelphia: JB Lippincott, 1991:1181.)

ual deformity.[94] Operative repair of type III acromioclavicular dislocations is indicated in patients whose occupation requires heavy manual labor.[165]

## Surgical Options

Three common surgical options are available for treatment of acute, complete acromioclavicular joint injuries. These include intraarticular or acromioclavicular repairs, coracoclavicular repairs, and dynamic muscle transfers. Isolated distal clavicle excision without stabilization in cases of complete acromioclavicular dislocations is generally not indicated.[25,165]

### INTRAARTICULAR ACROMIOCLAVICULAR REPAIRS

Reduction and stabilization of acomioclavicular dislocations using acromioclavicular fixation have been described using both open and percutaneous techniques.[165] Small wires passed from the acromion into the clavicle are prone to breakage and subsequent migration. The use of larger wires or threaded wires or bending the wires outside the skin can help to minimize migration. Acromioclavicular fixation can be associated with an increased incidence of acromioclavicular arthritis, particularly when threaded devices are used.[60]

### EXTRAARTICULAR CORACOCLAVICULAR REPAIRS

Reduction of acromioclavicular dislocation and stabilization using coracoclavicular fixation also have been described by both open and percutaneous techniques.[165] The percutaneous techniques typically involve placement of a screw from the clavicle into the coracoid. In addition to not allowing repair of the coracoclavicular ligaments, this technique is fraught with technical difficulties that have been associated with a 32 percent failure rate in some series.[177] The open technique allows for more accurate placement of the coracoclavicular fixation device as well as for repair of the coracoclavicular ligaments. Various fixation devices have been described, including a coracoclavicular lag screw (i.e., Bosworth or Rockwood screw), loops of steel wire passed around the coracoid and over the clavicle, and loops of coracoclavicular dacron or fascialata.

### DYNAMIC MUSCLE TRANSFERS

Brunelli[22] first reported transfer of the tip of the coracoid process with the attached conjoined tendon to the undersurface of the clavicle for correction of acromioclavicular dislocation. Although some authors have advocated the procedure,[3,54] others have reported a variable success rate,[62] and as a result, the procedure has not enjoyed widespread popularity.

## Authors' Preferred Treatment Protocols

### ACUTE ACROMIOCLAVICULAR DISLOCATION

When operative treatment of acromioclavicular dislocation is indicated, we prefer the use of an extraarticular coracoclavicular repair. The important concepts of surgical treatment include open debridement of the joint, repair of the coracoclavicular ligaments, use of temporary internal fixation to allow ligament healing, and imbrication of the deltotrapezius fascia. The procedure is performed through a straplike incision centered over the clavicle at a point just superior to the base of the coracoid process (Fig. 4-58a). The deltotrapezius fascia is incised longitudinally to expose the clavicle and the acromioclavicular joint. Debris within the joint as well as the intraarticular disc ligament is debrided. The coracoclavicular ligaments (i.e., the trapezoid and conoid ligaments) are identified. Sutures are placed within the ligaments and clamped without tying (see Fig. 4-58b). The acromioclavicular joint is reduced and stabilized through the use of a coracoclavicular lag screw (see Fig. 4-58c). In patients with extremely large, heavy arms or with questionable reliability, this fixation is supplemented with heavy, nonabsorbable sutures passed beneath the coracoid and through drill holes in the clavicle. The sutures in the coracoclavicular ligaments are tied. The screw is then advanced another quarter turn to decrease the tension on the sutures and the repaired ligaments. The deltotrapezius fascia is then imbricated. The screw is removed at 6 to 8 weeks postoperative.

### CHRONIC ACROMIOCLAVICULAR DISLOCATION

In cases of chronic, symptomatic complete acromioclavicular dislocation, isolated excision of the distal clavicle is generally not successful in relieving symptoms. We prefer combining distal clavicle excision with coracoclavicular ligament

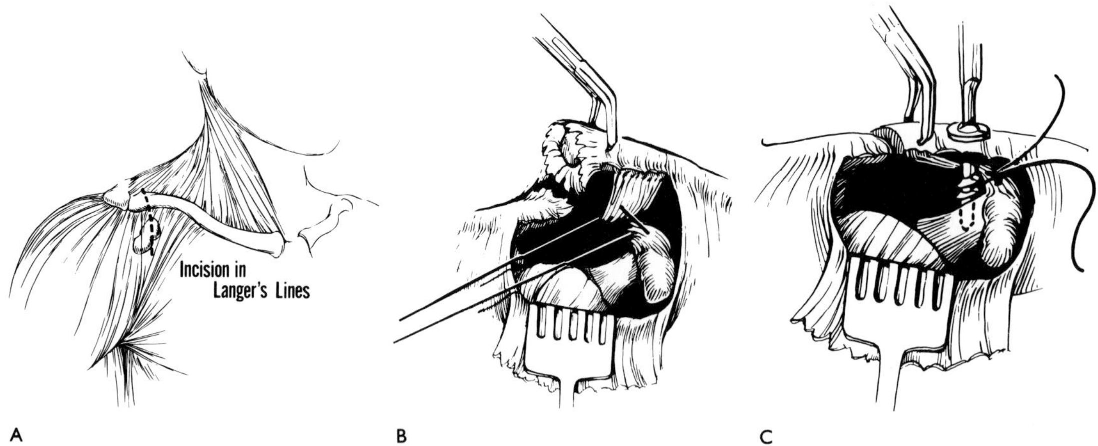


**Figure 4-58.** (a) Skin incision used for open reduction and internal fixation of acromioclavicular dislocation. (b) Sutures are placed within the coracoclavicular ligaments. (c) The clavicle is reduced and held in position with a coracoclavicular lag screw. After placement of the screw and reduction of the joint, the sutures in the coracoclavicular ligaments are tied. (Reproduced with permission from Rockwood CA Jr, Williams GR Jr, Young DC. Injuries to the acromioclavicular joint. In: Rockwood CA, Green DP, Bucholz RW, eds. Fractures. 3rd ed., vol. 1. Philadelphia: JB Lippincott, 1991:1181.)

reconstruction (Fig. 4-59a–h). This technique was originally described by Cadenat[25] and later reported on by Weaver and Dunn.[195] The incision is the same used for acute acromioclavicular dislocation. The distal 2 cm of the clavicle is excised. The acromial attachment of the coracoacromial ligament is removed and transferred into the intramedullary canal of the resected clavicle. The clavicle is stabilized in a fashion similar to that described for the acute acromioclavicular dislocation. The coracoclavicular lag screw is removed 8 to 10 weeks postoperatively.

## Postoperative Rehabilitation

Rehabilitation following surgical management of both acute and chronic acromioclavicular dislocations begins on the day after surgery with pendulum exercises. When not performing pendulum exercises, a sling is worn for the first 2 weeks. Complete overhead elevation of the shoulder is accompanied by 45 degrees of rotation of the clavicle. Therefore, the patient is discouraged from using the arm at or above shoulder height for 6 weeks. The patient is also instructed to avoid lifting anything heavier than 1 lb for 6 weeks. Strengthening exercises for the deltoid and rotator cuff are begun with the arm at the side at approximately 4 to 5 weeks. Trapezius and serratus strengthening exercises are begun at 6 to 8 weeks.

# Fractures of the Clavicle

According to Craig,[46] the subcutaneous location of the clavicle may account for inclusion of fractures of the clavicle in the earliest of mankind's writings. The Edwin Smith papyrus[201] provides some of the earliest descriptions of diagnosis and treatment of clavicle fractures. Craig[46] also has divided fractures of the clavicle into three groups: group I, consisting of fractures of the middle third; group II, consisting of fractures of the distal third; and group III, consisting of fractures of the proximal third.

Fractures of the middle third (group I) are the most common of clavicle fractures, making up 80 percent of clavicle fractures as a whole[46, 88] (Fig. 4-60). This is probably secondary to the fact that the middle third of the clavicle is a junction of the medial and lateral curved ends of the clavicle. In this region, the clavicle's cross section is changing from triangular at the medial side to flattened at the lateral side.

Group II fractures make up 12 to 15 percent of all clavicular fractures[46, 169] (Fig. 4-61). Craig[46] further divides group II fractures into types I through V depending on the location of the fracture fragments and the integrity of the coracoclavicular ligaments. The classic type II distal clavicle fracture is accompanied by vertical instability of the distal fragment secondary to coracoclavicular ligament disruption.[46]

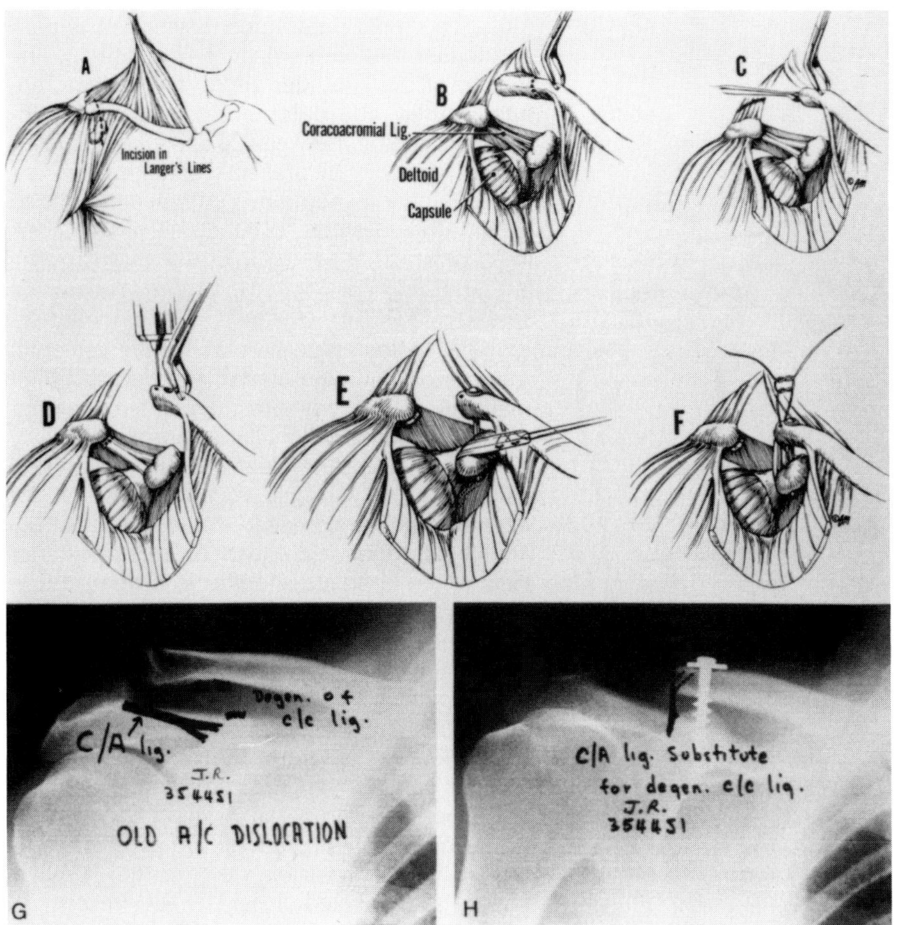


**Figure 4-59.** (a) Skin incision for reconstruction of a chronic acromioclavicular dislocation. (b) Clavicle is displaced superiorly and the coracoacromial ligament is identified. (c) The distal 2 to 2½ cm of the clavicle is excised, and the intramedullary canal is curetted free to accept the coracoacromial ligament. (d) Drill holes are placed within the clavicular shaft. (e) The acromial attachment of the coracoacromial ligament is incised, and sutures are placed within the ligament. The clavicle is stabilized to the coracoid using a coracoclavicular lag screw. (f) The coracoacromial ligament is transferred into the intramedullary canal and brought through drill holes. (g) Preoperative radiograph of a chronic acromioclavicular separation. (h) Postoperative radiographs following acromioclavicular joint reconstruction. (Reproduced with permission from Rockwood CA Jr, Williams GR Jr, Young DC. Injuries to the acromioclavicular joint. In: Rockwood CA, Green DP, Bucholz RW, eds. Fractures. 3rd ed., vol. 1. Philadelphia: JB Lippincott, 1991:1181.)

Group III fractures, fractures of the proximal third of the clavicle, are uncommon and account for 5 to 6 percent of clavicular fractures.[46] It should be remembered that the medial clavicular epiphysis does not fuse with the medial end of the clavicle until the midtwenties. Therefore, injuries to the medial clavicle before this age may well be physeal injuries rather than dislocations of the medial clavicle or fractures through metaphyseal bone.[164]

# Diagnostic Evaluation

Adequate evaluation of clavicle fractures most often involves history, physical examination, and routine radiographs. Occasionally, CT scans or arteriograms may be useful.

## HISTORY AND PHYSICAL EXAMINATION

The subcutaneous location of the clavicle makes inspection and palpation valuable diagnostic

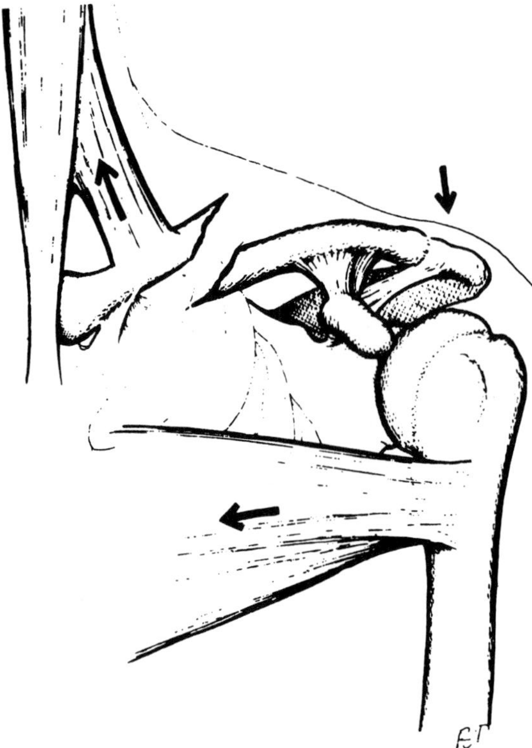

**Figure 4-60.** Group I clavicular fracture demonstrating the superior displacement by the sternocleidomastoid on the proximal segment and gravity on the distal segment. (Reproduced with permission from Bigliani LU, Craig EV, Butters KP. Fractures of the shoulder. In: Rockwood CA, Green DP, Bucholz RW, eds. Fractures. 3rd ed., vol. 1. Philadelphia: JB Lippincott, 1991:871.)

tools. The most predominant symptom is pain and tenderness with palpation. In addition, any motion of the shoulder girdle may cause crepitus. Acutely, the pain is accompanied by localized swelling. Between 24 and 48 hours later, ecchymosis may be present. Distal neurovascular examination should be performed in order to exclude the possibility of subclavian artery laceration or brachial plexus injury.

## ROUTINE RADIOGRAPHY

Routine radiographs should include an anteroposterior view and an axillary view. In minimally displaced fractures, an anteroposterior view with a cephalic tilt of approximately 30 degrees will assist in visualizing the fracture site. In type II distal clavicle fractures in which the fracture is accompanied by coracoclavicular ligament disruption, a comparison anteroposterior view of the opposite shoulder can be useful in order to determine the increase in the coracoclavicular interspace seen on the injured side. Fractures of the medial end of the clavicle, or group III fractures, can be difficult to visualize on routine anteroposterior views. The "serendipity view," or anteroposterior view with 45 degrees of cephalic tilt centered over the sternum, is another plain radiographic view that can assist in the visualization of group III fractures.[164]

The anteroposterior view of the clavicle should be inspected closely for the presence of associated injuries. The presence of a clavicle

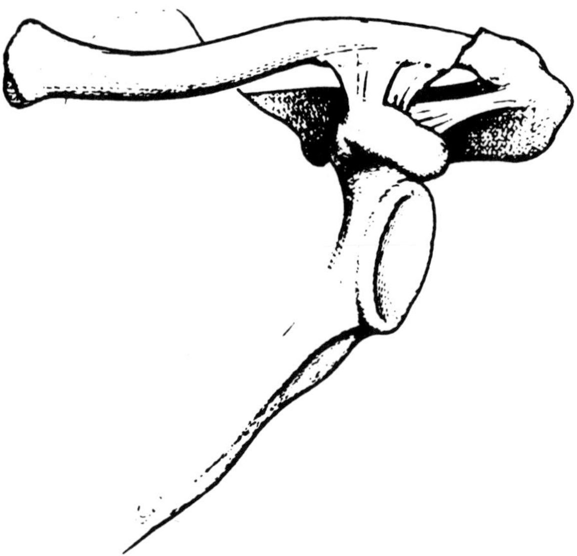

**Figure 4-61.** Group II (type I) fracture of the distal clavicle. (Reproduced with permission from Bigliani LU, Craig EV, Butters KP. Fractures of the shoulder. In: Rockwood CA, Green DP, Bucholz RW, eds. Fractures. 3rd ed., vol. 1. Philadelphia: JB Lippincott, 1991:871.)

fracture in association with fractures of the apical ribs should alert the clinician to the possibility of vascular injury. In addition, the lung field should be examined for the presence of vascular markings all the way to the periphery. If vascular markings cannot be seen all the way to the periphery, a routine chest x-ray should be performed in order to document the presence of pneumothorax.

### ARTERIOGRAPHY

Certain clavicle fractures can be associated with significant vascular injury. As mentioned earlier, a displaced clavicle fracture in association with fracture of the first or second rib should raise the clinician's suspicion for injury to the subclavian artery. In addition, posteriorly displaced fractures of the medial clavicle can be associated with serious neurovascular injury. If a significant vascular injury is suspected on the basis of history, physical examination, and plain radiography, arteriography is indicated.

### CT SCANNING

CT scanning is indicated primarily for group III fractures or fractures of the medial end of the clavicle. Because of the overlap of the underlying ribs, these fractures can be difficult to visualize on routine radiography, even with special views. CT scan is an excellent modality to aid in visualization of the medial end of the clavicle.

## Indications for Surgery

There are very few indications for primary open reduction and internal fixation of any clavicular fracture. Group I, or middle third, fractures routinely result in uneventful union, albeit with some residual deformity, following closed treatment. The reported incidence of nonunion of group I fractures is 0.9 to 4 percent.[46] The one absolute indication for operative treatment of a clavicular shaft fracture is an associated neurovascular injury.[46] Other relative indications include an open fracture requiring operative debridement, a "floating shoulder" (displaced clavicle fracture with a displaced scapular neck fracture), and the presence of multiple trauma.[97]

Operative treatment is indicated in certain types of group II, or distal third, fractures. Nonunion has been reported to be more common in type II distal clavicle fractures than in other clavicle fractures.[46, 139–141] Therefore, open reduction and internal fixation have been advocated for many type II distal clavicle fractures. However, successful union in type II fractures, particularly when the displacement is not severe, is possible with nonoperative means. Furthermore, the presence of nonunion of a type II distal clavicle fracture is not always associated with symptoms disabling enough to require operative intervention.

Closed treatment is routinely indicated for group III fractures unless the injury is associated with serious neurovascular compromise.[46] If operative stabilization of a medial clavicular fracture is indicated, caution should be exercised in stabilization of the fracture with smooth pins. This type of fixation has been associated with severe consequences as a result of pin breakage and migration.[109, 164]

## Surgical Options

Stabilization of group I, or middle third, fractures can be accomplished through the use of intramedullary pins or screws and the use of rigid plates and screws[46] (Fig. 4-62a,b). Each method has its proponents and critics. Both rigid plate fixation and intramedullary fixation have been associated with high rates of union. However, each method has its inherent difficulties and advantages. Plate fixation offers rigid fixation to bending as well as rotational stresses. However, it requires a great deal of subperiosteal stripping of the fragments and produces mechanical stress shielding of the bone. Following healing, refracture at either end of the plate can occur. The plate is usually quite prominent and requires removal. This can be associated with refracture through the previous screw holes. Intramedullary fixation, on the other hand, requires less in the way of soft-tissue stripping. In addition, the devices are load-sharing devices and as a result are not associated with the production of stress shielding and mechanical stress risers. However, they do not provide fixation as rigid as that obtained with plating, particularly in the rotational mode.

Operative stabilization of type II, or distal clavicle, fractures has been performed using fixation techniques similar to those described in the section on acromioclavicular separation. The reported methods have included intramedullary screws or pins and various types of coracoclavicular fixation, including coracoclavicular lag screws and coracoclavicular wires and sutures.

Surgical management of medial clavicular fractures, or group III fractures, is so rarely indicated that experience with any particular fixation technique is lacking. The severe complications associated with pin breakage and migration war-

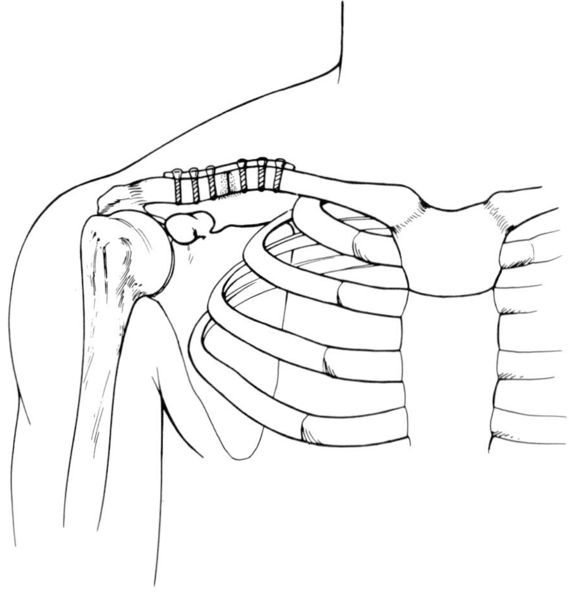


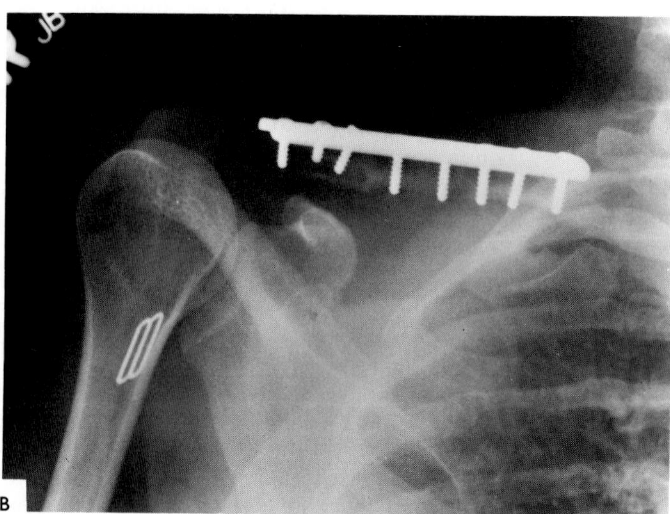


**Figure 4-62.** (a) Illustration of internal fixation for middle third fracture. (b) Radiograph of fixation and use of bone graft. (Reproduced with permission from Bigliani LU, Craig EV, Butters KP. Fractures of the shoulder. In: Rockwood CA, Green DP, Bucholz RW, eds. Fractures. 3rd ed., vol. 1. Philadelphia: JB Lippincott, 1991:871.)

rant extreme caution in the use of these devices in the medial clavicle. If the medial fragment is large enough, plate fixation is perhaps the best option.

## Authors' Preferred Treatment Protocols

We prefer the use of intramedullary fixation for group I, or middle third, fractures of the clavicle that require operative stabilization. The skin incision is made over the fracture site in Langer's skin lines. The deltotrapezius fascia over the fracture site is incised longitudinally. Care should be taken only to incise that portion of fascia which is required to visualize the fracture site. Extraperiosteal stripping should be avoided. A drill is passed retrograde out the distal fragment and is brought through the skin posterior to the shoulder. The drill normally exits slightly posterior and proximal to the acromioclavicular joint. A modified Hagie pin is then passed through the posterior skin wound into the distal fragment and is advanced to the fracture site. The proximal fragment is then drilled, the fracture is reduced, and the modified Hagie pin is passed across the fracture site. The protruding end of the Hagie pin is left slightly prominent in the posterior aspect of the shoulder to allow easier subsequent retrieval. The deltotrapezius fascia is then repaired along with the skin.

In type II, or distal clavicle, fractures, we prefer the use of a coracoclavicular lag screw to reduce the two fracture fragments. The technique for placement of the coracoclavicular lag screw is identical to that described previously for acromioclavicular separation. If the fracture line is oblique and the distal fragment is large enough and not comminuted, the coracoclavicular fixation can be supplemented with interfragmentary fixation.

Fixation of medial clavicular fractures can be extremely difficult. If the medial fragment is large enough, we prefer the use of plate fixation. In the presence of a small medial fragment, we prefer the use of interfragmentary suturing. The skin incision should parallel the medial end of the clavicle and turn distally at the sternoclavicular joint to parallel the border of the manubrium. Care should be taken to avoid injury to neurovascular structures posterior to the clavicle as well as to the costoclavicular and sternoclavicular ligaments. The medial clavicle fracture should be exposed subperiosteally. The fracture is stabilized through the use of plates and screws or sutures passed through drill holes.

## Postoperative Rehabilitation

Stabilization of middle third fractures with an intramedullary device does not provide rigid rotational stability. Therefore, the shoulder should not be brought above shoulder height for 6 to 8 weeks. However, the patient is encouraged to perform pendulum exercises and to use the arm at waist height without lifting anything heavier than 2 lb starting on postoperative day 1. Overhead motion and strengthening exercises are added after fracture healing (usually at 8 to 10 weeks). The pin is removed between 6 months and 1 year postoperatively.

The postoperative rehabilitation for type II, or distal clavicle, fractures is identical to that described for postoperative rehabilitation of acromioclavicular joint injuries.

In fractures of the medial third of the clavicle, the weight of the arm provides significant forces across the fracture site as a result of the lengthy moment arm of the distal fragment. Therefore, sling support should be continued for 3 to 6 weeks. However, the patient is instructed to come out of the sling four to six times daily starting on the first postoperative day in order to perform range-of-motion exercises for the elbow, wrist, and hand and pendulum exercises for the shoulder. Shoulder range-of-motion and strengthening exercises are not instituted for 6 to 8 weeks.

## References


1. Adams FL. The genuine works of Hippocrates. Vols. I and II. New York: William Wood, 1891.
2. Alexander OM. Dislocation of the acromioclavicular joint. Radiography 1949;15:260.
3. Bailey RW. A dynamic repair for complete acromioclavicular joint dislocation. J Bone Joint Surg 1965;47A:858.
4. Bankart ASB. Recurrent or habitual dislocation of the shoulder joint. Br Med J 1923;2:1132.
5. Bankart ASB. The pathology and treatment of recurrent dislocation of the shoulder joint. Br J Surg 1938;26:23.
6. Bardenauer BA. Die verletzungen der oberen extremitaten. Dtsch Chir 1886;63:268.
7. Barrett WP, Franklin JL, Jackins SE, et al. Total shoulder arthroplasty. J Bone Joint Surg 1987;69A:865.
8. Bassett RW, Cofield RH. Acute tears of the rotator cuff: the timing of surgical repair. Clin Orthop 1983;175:18.
9. Bayley IJL, Kessel XX: Posterior dislocation of the shoulder: the clinical spectrum. J Bone Joint Surg 1978;60B:440.
10. Bergfeld JA, Andrish JT, Clancy WG. Evaluation of the acromioclavicular joint following first and second degree sprains. Am J Spors Med 1978;6:153.
11. Bigliani LU. Fractures of the proximal humerus. In: Rockwood CA, Green DP, Bucholz RW, eds. Fractures. 3rd ed. Philadelphia: J B Lippincott, 1991:871.
12. Bigliani LU, Morrison D, April EW. The morphology of the acromion and its relationship to rotator cuff tears. Orthop Trans 1986;10:228.
13. Bigliani LU, McIlveen SJ, Cordasco FA, et al. Operative repair of massive rotator cuff tears: long-term results. Orthop Trans 1990;14:251.
14. Blazina ME, Satzman JS. Recurrent anterior subluxation of the shoulder in athletics: a distinct entity. J Bone Joint Surg 1969; 51A:1037.
15. Blom S, Dahlback LO. Nerve injuries in dislocations of the shoulder joint and fractures of the neck of the humerus: a clinical and electromyographical study. Acta Chir Scand 1970;136:461.
16. Bloom MH, Obata W. Diagnosis of posterior dislocation of the shoulder with the use of Belpeau axillary and angle-up roentgenographjic views. J Bone Joint Surg 1967;49A:943.
17. Bohler J. Perqutane osteosynthese mit dem rontgenbilderstarker. Wiener Klin Wochenschr 1962;74:485.
18. Boytchev B. Treatment of recurrent shoulder instability. Minerva Ortop 1951;2:377.
19. Bretzke CA, Crass JR, Craig EV, et al. Ultrasonography of the rotator cuff: normal and pathologic anatomy. Invest Radiol 1985;20:311.
20. Broca A, Hartmann H. Contribution a l'etude des luxation de l'epaule. Bull Soc Anat Paris 1890;4:312.
21. Brown JT. Early assessment of supraspinatus tears: procaine infiltration as a guide to treatment. J Bone Joint Surg 1949; 31B:423.
22. Brunelli G. Proposta di un nuovo methodo di correzione chirurgia della lussazione acromion clavicolare. Bull Soc Med Chir Bresciana 1956;10:95.
23. Burk DL, Karasick D, Kurtz AB, et al. Rotator cuff tears: prospective comparison of MR imaging with arthrography, sonography and surgery. AJR 1989;153:87.
24. Burkhead WZ, Rockwood CA Jr. Treatment of instability of the shoulder with an exercise program. J Bone Joint Surg 1992; 74A:890.
25. Cadenat FM. The treatment of dislocations and fractures of the outer end of the clavicle. Int Clin 1917;1:145.
26. Caird FM. The shoulder joint in relation to certain dislocations and fractures. Edinburg Med J 1887;32:708.

27. Calvert PT, Packer NP, Stoker DJ, et al. Arthrography of the shoulder after operative repair of the torn rotator cuff. J Bone Joint Surg 1986;68B:147.
28. Caspari RB. Arthroscopic reconstruction for anterior shoulder instability. Techniques Orthop 1988;3:59.
29. Codman EA. The pathology of the subacromial bursa and the supraspinatus tendon. In: Codman EA, ed. The shoulder: rupture of the supraspinatus tendon and other lesions in or about the subacromial bursa. Suppl. Malabar, Fla: Robert E Krieger, 1935:65.
30. Codman EA. The shoulder: rupture of the supraspinatus tendon and other lesions in or about the subacromial bursa. Boston: Thomas Todd, 1934:262.
31. Cofield RH, Briggs BT. Glenohumeral arthritis. J Bone Joint Surg 1979;61A:668.
32. Cofield RH. Unconstrained total shoulder prostheses. Clin Orthop 1983;173:97.
33. Cofield RH. Arthrodesis and resection arthroplasty of the shoulder. In: McCollister Evarts C, ed. Surgery of the musculoskeletal system. New York: Churchill Livingstone, 1983:109.
34. Cofield RH. Total shoulder arthroplasty with the Neer prosthesis. J Bone Joint Surg 1984;66A:899.
35. Cofield RH, Berquist TH. The shoulder. In: Berquist TH, ed. Imaging of orthopaedic trauma and surgery. Philadelphia: WB Saunders, 1986:499.
36. Cofield RH. Preliminary experience with bone ingrowth total shoulder arthroplasty. Orthop Trans 1986;10:217.
37. Cofield RH. Total shoulder arthroplasty with bone ingrowth fixation. In: Kolbel R, Helbig B, Blauth W, eds. Shoulder replacement. Berlin: Springer-Verlag, 1987:209.
38. Cofield RH. Subscapular muscle transposition for repair of chronic rotator cuff tears. Surg Gynecol Obstet 1982;154:672.
39. Cofield RH. Current concepts review: rotator cuff disease of the shoulder. J Bone Joint Surg 1985;67A:974.
40. Cofield RH, Daly PJ. Total shoulder arthroplasty with a tissue ingrowth glenoid component. J Shoulder Elbow Surg 1992;1:77.
41. Cofield RH, Irving JF. Evaluation and classification of shoulder instability: with special reference to examination under anesthesia. Clin Orthop 1987;223:32.
42. Cone RO III, Resnick D, Danzig L. Shoulder impingement syndrome: radiographic evaluation. Radiography 1984;150:29.
43. Connolly JF. Humeral head defects associated with shoulder dislocations: their diagnostic and surgical significance. Instr Course Lect 1972;21:42.
44. Cox JS. The fate of the acromioclavicular joint in athletic injuries. Am J Sports Med 1981;9:50.
45. Craig EV. The geyser sign and torn rotator cuff: clinical significance and pathomechanics. Clin Orthop 1984;191:213.
46. Craig EV. Fractures of the clavicle. In: Rockwood CA Jr, Green DP, Bucholz RW, eds. Fractures. Philadelphia: J B Lippincott, 1991:928.
47. Crass JR, Craig EV, Feinberg SB. Sonography of the postoperative rotator cuff tear. AJR 1986;146:561.
48. Crass JR, Craig EV, Feinberg SB. The hyperextended internal rotation view in rotator cuff ultrasonography. J Clin Ultrasound 1987;15:415.
49. Crass JR, Craig EV, Feinberg SB. Ultrasonography of rotator cuff tears: a review of 500 diagnostic studies. J Clin Ultrasound 1988;16:313.
50. Cyprien JM, Vasey HM, Burdet A, et al. Humeral retrotorsion and glenohumeral relationships in the normal shoulder and in recurrent anterior dislocation. Clin Orthop 1983;175:8.
51. DePalma AF. Surgery of the shoulder. 3rd ed. Philadelphia: JB Lippincott, 1983.
52. DePalma AF, Gallery G, Bennett CA. Variational anatomy and degenerative lesions of the shoulder joint. In: Blount WP, ed. American Academy of Orthopaedic Surgeons Instructional Course Lectures. Vol. VI. Ann Arbor, Mich.: JW Edwards, 1949:255.
53. DeSmet AA, Ting YM. Diagnosis of rotator cuff tears on routine radiographs. J Can Assoc Radiol 1977; 28:54.
54. Dewar FP, Barrington TW. The treatment of chronic acromioclavicular dislocation. J Bone Joint Surg 1965;47B:32.
55. Dines OM, Warren RE, Inglis AE, Pavlov H. The coracoid impingement syndrome. J Bone Joint Surg 1990;72B:314.
56. Drakeford MK, Quinn MJ, Simpson SL, et al. A comparative study of ultrasonography and arthrography in evaluation of the rotator cuff. Clin Orthop 1990;253:118.
57. Ellman H, Hanker G, Bayer M. Repair of the rotator cuff: end-result study of factors influencing reconstruction. J Bone Joint Surg 1986;68A:1136.
58. Ellman H. Diagnosis and treatment of incomplete rotator cuff tears. Clin Orthop 1990;254:64.
59. Ellman H. Arthroscopic subacromial decompression: analysis of one to three year results. J Arthroscopic Rel Surg 1987;3:173.
60. Escola A, Vainionpaa S, Korkala O, Rokkanen P. Acute complete acromioclavicular dislocation: a prospective randomized trial of fixation with smooth or threaded Kirschner wires or cortical screws. Ann Chir Gynecol 1987;76:323.
61. Evancho AM, Stiles RG, Fajmaa WA, et al. MR imaging in the diagnosis of rotator cuff tears. AJR 1988;15:751.
62. Ferris BD, Bhamra M, Paton DF. Coracoid process transfer for acromioclavicular dislcoations: a report of 20 cases. Clin Orthop 1989;242:184.
63. Figgie HE III, Inglis AE, Goldberg VM, et al. An analysis of factors affecting the long-term results of total shoulder arthroplasty in inflammatory arthritis. J Arthroplasty 1988;3:123.
64. Finsterer H. Die operative behandlung der habituellen schulter luxation. Dtsch Z Chir 1917;141:354.
65. Flannigan B, Kursunoglu-Brahme S, Snyder S, et al. MR arthrography of the shoulder: comparison with conventional MR imaging. AJR 1990;155:829.
66. Flatow EL, Cuomo F, Maday MG, et al. Open reduction and internal fixation of two-part displaced fractures of the greater tuberosity of the proximal part of the humerus. J Bone Joint Surg 1991;73A:1213.
67. Franklin JL, Barrett WP, Jackins SE, Matsen FA III. Glenoid loosening in total shoulder arthroplasty. J Arthroplasty 1988;3:39.
68. Freiberger RH, Kaye JJ, Spiller J. Arthrography. New York: Appleton-Century-Crofts, 1979.
69. Fukuda H, Craig EV, Yamanaka K. Surgical treatment of incomplete thickness tears of rotator cuff: long-term follow-up. Orthop Trans 1987;11:237.
70. Fukuda K, Craig EV, An KN, et al. Biomechanical study of the ligamentous system of the acromioclavicular joint. J Bone Joint Surg 1986;68A:434.
71. Garth WP, Slappey CE, Ochs CW. Roentgenographic demonstration of instability of the shoulder: the apical oblique projection: a technical note. J Bone Joint Surg 1984;66A:1450.
72. Gerber C, Schneeberger AG, Tho-Son V. The arterial vascularization of the humeral head: an anatomical study. J Bone Joint Surg 1990;72A:1486.
73. Gerber C, Terrier F, Ganz R. The role of the coracoid process in the chronic impingement syndrome. J Bone Joint Surg 1985; 67B:703.
74. Gerber C, Vinh TS, Hertel R, et al. Latissimus dorsi transfer for the treatment of massive tears of the rotator cuff. Clin Orthop 1988; 232:51.
75. Goldman AB, Dines DM, Warren RF. Shoulder arthrography: technique, diagnosis and clinical correlation. Boston: Little, Brown, 1982:1.
76. Gore DR, Murray MP, Sepic SB, et al. Shoulder muscle strength and range of motion following surgical repair of full-thickness rotator cuff tears. J Bone Joint Surg 1986;68A:266.
77. Hall RH, Isaak F, Booth CR. Dislocations of the shoulder with special reference to accompanying fractures. J Bone Joint Surg 1959;41A:489.
78. Hamada K, Fukuda H, Mikasa M, et al. Roentgenographic findings in massive rotator cuff tears: a long-term observation. Clin Orthop 1990;259:92.
79. Harryman DT, Mack LA, Wang KY, et al. Repairs of the rotator cuff: correlation of functional results with integrity of the cuff. J Bone Joint Surg 1991;73A:982.
80. Hawkins RJ, Kennedy JC. Impingement syndrome in athletes. Am J Sports Med 1980;8:151.
81. Hawkins RJ, Misamore GW, Hobeika PE. Surgery for full-thickness rotator cuff tears. J Bone Joint Surg 1985;67A:1349.
82. Hawkins RJ, Angelo RL. Glenohumeral osteoarthrosis: a late complication of the Putti-Platt repair. J Bone Joint Surg 1990; 72A:1193.
83. Hawkins RJ, Coppert GJ, Johnston G. Recurrent posterior instability (subluxation) of the shoulder. J Bone Joint Surg 1984; 66A:169.
84. Hayes MJ, Van Winkle N. Axillary artery injury with minimally displaced fracture of the neck of the humerus. J Trauma 1983; 23:431.
85. Helfet AJ. Coracoid transplantation for recurrent dislocation of the shoulder. J Bone Joint Surg 1958;40B:198.

86. Henderson MS. Tenosuspension operation for recurrent or habitual dislocation of the shoulder. Surg Clin North Am 1949; 5:997.
87. Henry JH, Genung JA. Natural history of glenohumeral dislocation: revisited. Am J Sports Med 1982;10:135.
88. Heppenstall RB. Fractures and dislocations of the distal clavicle. Orthop Clin North Am 1975;6:447.
89. Hill HA, Sachs MD. The grooved defect of the humeral head: a frequently unrecognized complication of dislocations of the shoulder joint. Radiology 1940;35:690.
90. Horak J, Nilsson B. Epidemiology of fractures of the upper end of the humerus. Clin Orthop 1975;112:250.
91. Hovelius L. Anterior dislocation of the shoulder in teenagers and young adults: five-year prognosis. J Bone Joint Surg 1987; 69A:393.
92. Iannotti JP, Zlatkin MB, Esterhai JL, et al. Magnetic resonance imaging of the shoulder: sensitivity, specificity and predictive value. J Bone Joint Surg 1991;73A:17.
93. Iannotti JP, Gabriel JP, Schneck SL, et al. The normal glenohumeral relationships: an anatomical study of 140 shoulders. J Bone Joint Surg 1991;74A:491.
94. Imatani RJ, Hanlon JJ, Cady GW. Acute complete acromioclavicular separation. J Bone Joint Surg 1975;57A:328.
95. Jaberg H, Warner JJP, Jacob RP. Percutaneous stabilization of unstable fractures of the humerus. J Bone Joint Surg 1992; 74A:508.
96. Jones L. Reconstructive operation for nonreducible fractures of the head of the humerus. Ann Surg 1933;97:217.
97. Jones L. The shoulder joint: observations on the anatomy and physiology: with an analysis of a reconstructive operation following extensive injury. Surg Gynecol Obstet 1942;75:433.
98. Kerwein GA, Rosenburg B, Sneed WR. Arthrographic studies of the shoulder joint. J Bone Joint Surg 1957;39A:1267.
99. Kerwein GA. Roentgenographic diagnosis of shoulder dysfunction. JAMA 1965;194:1081.
100. Kieft GJ, Bloem JL, Oberman WR, et al. Normal shoulder: MRI. Radiology 1986;159:741.
101. Kieft GJ, Bloem JL, Rozing PM, et al. Rotator cuff impingement syndrome: MR imaging. Radiology 1988;166:211.
102. Kneeland JB, Carrera GF, Middleton WD, et al. Rotator cuff tears: preliminary application of high resolution MRI with counter-rotating loop gap resonators. Radiology 1986;160:695.
103. Kneeland JB, Middleton WD, Carrera GF, et al. MR imaging of the shoulder: diagnosis of rotator cuff tears. AJR 1987;149:333.
104. Knight RA, Mayne JA. Comminuted fractures and fracture-dislocations involving the articular surface of the humeral head. J Bone Joint Surg 39A:1343, 1957.
105. Laing PG. The arterial supply of the adult humerus. J Bone Joint Surg 1956;38A:1105.
106. Lettin AWF, Copeland SA, Scales JT. The Stanmore total shoulder replacement. J Bone Joint Surg 1982;64B:47.
107. Lindblom K. Arthrography and roentgenography in ruptures of the tendon of the shoulder joint. Acta Radiol 1939;20:548.
108. Lundberg BJ. The correlation of clinical evaluation with operative findings and prognosis in rotator cuff rupture. In: Bayley I, Kessel L, eds. Shoulder surgery. Berlin: Springer-Verlag, 1982:35.
109. Lyons FA, Rockwood CA Jr. Migration of pins used in operations on the shoulder. J Bone Joint Surg 1990;72A:1262.
110. Mack LA, Matsen FA III, Kilcoyne RF, et al. US evaluation of the rotator cuff. Radiology 1985;157:205.
111. Magnuson PB. Treatment of recurrent dislocation of the shoulder. Surg Clin North Am 1945;25:14.
112. Magnuson PB, Stack JK. Recurrent dislocation of the shoulder. JAMA 1943;123:889.
113. Mason JM. The treatment of dislocation of the shoulder joint complicated by fracture of the upper extremity of the humerus. Ann Surg 1908;47:672.
114. Mc Glynn FJ, El-Khoury G, Albright JP. Arthrotomography of the glenoid labrum in shoulder instability. J Bone Joint Surg 1982; 64A:506.
115. McLaughlin HL. Posterior dislocation of the shoulder. J Bone Joint Surg 1952;34A:584.
116. McLaughlin HL, Cavallaro WU. Primary anterior dislocation of the shoulder. Am J Surg 1950;80:615.
117. Middleton WD, Edelstein G, Reinus WR, et al. Sonographic detection of rotator cuff tears. AJR 1985;144:349.
118. Middleton WD, Reinus WR, Melson GL, et al. Pitfalls of rotator cuff sonography. AJR 1986;146:555.
119. Middleton WD, Reinus WR, Totty WG, et al. Ultrasonographic evaluation of the rotator cuff and biceps tendon. J Bone Joint Surg 1986;68A:440.
120. Mills KL. Severe injuries of the upper end of the humerus. Injury 1974;6:13.
121. Morris MF, Kilcoyne RF, Shuman W. Humeral tuberosity fractures: evaluation by CT scan and management of malunion. Orthop Trans 1987;11:242.
122. Morrison DS, Bigliani LU. The clinical significance of variations in acromial morphology. Orthop Trans 1987;11:234.
123. Morrison DS, Burger P. The use of magnetic resonance imaging in the diagnosis of rotator cuff tears. Presented at the Fourth Open Meeting of the American Shoulder and Elbow Surgeons, Atlanta, Georgia, February 1988.
124. Morrison DS, Otstein R. The use of magnetic resonance imaging in the diagnosis of rotator cuff tears. Orthopedics 1990;13:633.
125. Mowery CA, Garfin SR, Booth RE, Rothman RH. Recurrent posterior dislocation of the shoulder: treatment using a bone block. J Bone Joint Surg 1985;67A:777.
126. Neer CS, Brown TH Jr, McLaughlin HL. Fracture of the neck of the humerus with dislocation of the head fragment. Am J Surg 1953;85:252.
127. Neer CS II. Articular replacement for the humeral head. J Bone Joint Surg 1955;37A:215.
128. Neer CS II. Surgical protocol. Neer II proximal humerus arthroplasty of the shoulder: Neer technique. St. Paul, Minn.: Minnesota Mining and Manufacturing Company, 1982.
129. Neer CS II, Watson KC, Stanton FJ. Recent experience in total shoulder replacement. J Bone Joint Surg 1982;64A:319.
130. Neer CS II, Craig EV, Fukuda H. Cuff-tear arthropathy. J Bone Joint Surg 1983;65A:1232.
131. Neer CS II, McCann PD, Macfarlane EA, Padilla N. Earlier passive motion following shoulder arthroplasty and rotator cuff repair: a prospective study. Orthop Trans 1987;2:231.
132. Neer CS, Morrison DS. Glenoid bone grafting in total shoulder arthroplasty. J Bone Joint Surg 1988;70A:1154.
133. Neer CS II. Anterior acromioplasty for the chronic impingement syndrome in the shoulder: a preliminary report. J Bone Joint Surg 1972;54A:41.
134. Neer CS II. Shoulder reconstruction. Philadelphia: WB Saunders, 1990:495.
135. Neer CS II, Craig EV, Fukuda H. Cuff tear arthropathy. J Bone Joint Surg 1983;65A:1232.
136. Neer CS. Displaced proximal humerus fracture: I. Classification and evaluation. J Bone Joint Surg 1970;52A:1077.
137. Neer CS. Displaced proximal humeral fractures: treatment of three-part and four-part displacement. J Bone Joint Surg 1970; 52A:1090.
138. Neer CS. Shoulder reconstruction. Philadelphia: WB Saunders, 1990:363.
139. Neer CS II. Fractures of the clavicle. In: Rockwood CA Jr, Green DP, eds. Fractures. 2nd ed., Vol. 1. Philadelphia: JB Lippincott, 1984:707.
140. Neer CS II. Fractures of the distal third of the clavicle. Clin Orthop 1968;58:43.
141. Neer CS II. Fractures of the distal clavicle with detachment of the coracoclavicular ligaments in adults. J Trauma 1963;3:99.
142. Neer CS II, Foster CR. Inferior capsular shift for involuntary inferior and multidirectional instability of the shoulder: a preliminary report. J Bone Joint Surg 1980;62A:897.
143. Neer CS, McIlveen SJ. Recent results in technique of prosthetic replacement for four part proximal humeral fractures. Orthop Trans 1986;10:475.
144. Neviaser JS, Neviaser RJ, Neviaser TJ. The repair of chronic massive ruptures of the rotator cuff of the shoulder by use of a freeze-dried rotator cuff. J Bone Joint Surg 1978;60A:681.
145. Neviaser RJ. Ruptures of the rotator cuff. Orthop Clin North Am 1987;18:387.
146. Neviaser TJ, Neviaser RJ. The diagnosis and treatment of incomplete rotator cuff tears. Orthop Trans 1989;15:239.
147. Nicola T. Recurrent anterior dislocation of the shoulder: a new operation. J Bone Joint Surg 1929;11:128.
148. Norwood LA, Barrack R, Jacobson KE. Clinical presentation of complete tears of the rotator cuff. J Bone Joint Surg 1989; 71A:499.
149. O'Connor SJ, Kacknow AJ. Posterior dislocation of the shoulder. Arch Surg 1956;72:479.
150. Osmond-Clarke H. Habitual dislocation of the shoulder: the Putti-Platt operation. J Bone Joint Surg 1948;30B:19.

151. Ono K, Hamamuro T, Rockwood CA. Use of a thirty-degree caudal tilt radiograph in the shoulder impingement syndrome. J Shoulder Elbow Surg 1992;1:246.
152. Owen R, Iannotti JP, Deren J, et al. Magnetic resonance imaging of the rotator cuff after surgery. AJR (in press).
153. Ozaki J, Fujimoto S, Masuhara K. Repair of chronic massive rotator cuff tears with synthetic fabrics. In: Bateman JE, Welsh RP, eds. Surgery of the shoulder. Philadelphia: BC Decker, 1984:185.
154. Pahle JA, Kvarnes L. Shoulder synovectomy. Ann Chir Gynaecol 1985;198 (74 suppl):37.
155. Pasila M, Kiviluoto O, Jaroma H, Sundholm A. Recovery from primary shoulder dislocation and its complications. Acta Orthop Scand 1980;51:257.
156. Perthes G. Uber operationen bei habitueller schulter luxation. Dtsch Z Chir 1906;85:199.
157. Post M, Silver R, Singh M. Rotator cuff tear: diagnosis and treatment. Clin Orthop 1983;173:78.
158. Regan WD, Webster-Bogaart S, Hawkins RJ, Fowler PJ. Comparative functional analysis of the Bristow, Magnuson-Stack, and Putti-Platt procedures for recurrent dislocation of the shoulder. Am J Sports Med 1989;17:42.
159. Resnick D. Shoulder arthrography. Radiol Clin North Am 1981; 19:243.
160. Rockwood CA Jr. Treatment of large tears of the rotator cuff by anterior acromioplasty and debridement of the cuff. Presented at the 53rd Annual Meeting of the American Academy of Orthopaedic Surgeons, New Orleans, February 20–25, 1986.
161. Rockwood CA. The management of patients with massive rotator cuff defects by acromioplasty and rotator cuff debridement. Orthop Trans 1986;10:622.
162. Rockwood CA Jr. Shoulder arthroscopy: a critical review. J Bone Joint Surg 1988;70A;639.
163. Rockwood CA Jr. Dislocations about the shoulder. In: Rockwood CA Jr, Green DP, eds. Fractures. 2nd ed., volume 1. Philadelphia: JB Lippincott, 1984:722.
164. Rockwood CA Jr. Injuries to the sternoclavicular joint. In: Rockwood CA Jr, Green DP, Bucholz RW, eds. Fractures. 3rd ed., vol. 1. Philadelphia: JB Lippincott, 1991:1253.
165. Rockwood CA Jr, Williams GR Jr, Young DC. Injuries to the acromioclavicular joint. In: Rockwood CA Jr, Green DP, Bucholz RW, eds. Fractures. 3rd ed., vol. 1. Philadelphia: JB Lippincott, 1991:1181.
166. Rockwood CA Jr, Thomas SC, Matsen FA III. Subluxations and dislocations about the glenohumeral joint. In: Rockwood, CA Jr, Green DP, Bucholz RW, eds. Fractures. 3rd ed., vol. 1. Philadelphia: JB Lippincott, 1991:1021.
167. Rokous JR, Feagin JA, Abbott HG: Modified axillary roentgenogram: a useful adjunct in the diagnosis of recurrent instability of the shoulder. Clin Orthop 1972;82:84.
168. Rose SH, Melton LJ, Morrey BF, et al. Epidemiologic features of humeral fractures. Clin Orthop 1982;168:24.
169. Rose CR. An atlas of anatomy and treatment of midclavicular fractures. Clin Orthop 1968;58:29.
170. Rowe CR. Prognosis in dislocations of the shoulder. J Bone Joint Surg 1956;38A:957.
171. Rowe CR, Pierce DS. The enigma of voluntary recurrent dislocation of the shoulder. J Bone Joint Surg 1965;47A:1670.
172. Rowe CR, Patel D, Southmayd WW. The Bankart procedure: a long-term end-result study. J Bone Joint Surg 1978;60A:1.
173. Rowe CR, Pierce DS, Clark JG. Voluntary dislocation of the shoulder: a preliminary report on a clinical, electromyographic, and psychiatric study of 26 patients. J Bone Joint Surg 1973;55:445.
174. Rowe CR. Reevaluation of the position of the arm in arthrodesis of the shoulder in the adult. J Bone Joint Surg 1974;56A:913.
175. Saha AK. Theory of shoulder mechanism. Springfield, Ill.: Charles C Thomas, 1961.
176. Saha AK, Bhadra N, Dutta SK. Latissimus dorsi transfer for recurrent dislocation of the shoulder. Acta Orthop Scand 1986;57:539.
177. Saltsou PM. Percutaneous cannulated screw coracoclavicular fixation for acute acromioclavicular dislocations. Clin Orthop 1989;243:112.
178. Samilson RL, Raphael RI, Post L, et al. Arthrography of the shoulder. Clin Orthop 1961;20:21.
179. Scott DJ Jr. Treatment of recurrent posterior dislocation of the shoulder by glenoplasty: report of three cases. J Bone Joint Surg 1967;49A:471.
180. Seeger LL, Gold RH, Bassett LW, et al. Shoulder impingement syndrome: MR findings in 53 shoulders. AJR 1988;150:343.
181. Seeger LL, Ruszkowski JT, Bassett LW, et al. MR imaging of the normal shoulder: anatomic correlation. AJR 1987;148:83.
182. Symth EHJ. Major arterial injury in closed fracture of the neck of the humerus: report of a case. J Bone Joint Surg 1969;51B:508.
183. Soble MG, Kaye AD, Guay RD. Rotator cuff tears: clinical experience with sonographic detection. Radiology 1989;173:319.
184. Steindler A. Orthopaedic operations: indications, technique, and end results. Springfield, Ill.: Charles C Thomas, 1940:302.
185. Stiles RJ, Resnick D, Sartoris DJ, et al. Rotator cuff disruption: diagnosis with digital arthrography. Radiology 1990;154:121.
186. Svend-Hansen H. Displaced proximal humeral fractures: a review of 49 patients. Acta Orthop Scand 1974;45:359.
187. Thomas MA. Posterior subacromial dislocation of the head of the humerus. AJR 1937;37:767.
188. Thomas TT. Habitual or recurrent anterior dislocation of the shoulder: I. Etiology and pathology. Am J Med Sci 1909;137:229.
189. Thomas TT. Habitual or recurrent dislocation of the shoulder: 44 shoulders operated on in 42 patients. Surg Gynecol Obstet 1921;32:291.
190. Tibone JE, Prietto C, Job FW, et al. Staple capsulorrhaphy for recurrent posterior shoulder dislocation. Am J Sports Med 1981;9:135.
191. Urist MR. Complete dislocation of the acromioclavicular joint: the nature of the traumatic lesion and effective methods for treatment with an analysis of 41 cases. J Bone Joint Surg 1946; 28:813.
192. Vichard P, Arnould D. Posterior fracture dislocation of the shoulder: a study of eleven cases. Rev Chir Orthop 1981;67:71.
193. Walker SW, Couch WH, Boester GA, et al. Isokinetic strength of the shoulder after repair of a torn rotator cuff. J Bone Joint Surg 1987;69A:1041.
194. Warner JP, Xianguha D, Warren RF, Torzilli PA. Static capsuloligamentous restraints to superior-inferior translation of the glenohumeral joint. Am J Sports Med 1992;20:675.
195. Weaver JK, Dunn HK. Treatment of acromioclavicular injuries, especially complete acromioclavicular separation. J Bone Joint Surg 1972;54A:1187.
196. Weber BG. Operative treatment for recurrent dislocation of the shoulder: preliminary report. Injury 1969;1:107.
197. Weber BG, Simpson LA, Hardegger F. Rotational humeral osteotomy for recurrent anterior dislocation of the shoulder associated with a large Hill-Sachs lesion. J Bone Joint Surg 1984; 66A:1443.
198. Willems WJ, Lim TEA. Neer arthroplasty for humeral fracture. Acta Orthop Scand 1985;56:394.
199. Wilson JC, McKeever FM. Traumatic posterior (retroglenoid) dislocation of the humerus. J Bone Joint Surg 1949;31A:160.
200. Zanca P. Shoulder pain: involvement of the acromioclavicular joint: analysis of 1000 cases. AJR 1971;112:493.
201. Zimmerman LM, Veith I. Great ideas in the history of surgery: clavicle, shoulder, shoulder amputations. Baltimore: Williams & Wilkins, 1961.
202. Zlatkin MB, Iannotti JP, Roberts MC, et al. Rotator cuff tears: diagnostic performance of MR imaging. Radiology 1989;172:223.

Chapter 5

*Martin J. Kelley*

# Evaluation of the Shoulder



Our thanks to Joel Henry for his contribution on the section entitled Vascular Tests.

Martin J. Kelley and William A. Clark: ORTHOPEDIC THERAPY OF THE SHOULDER.

The arthrokinematic and kinesiologic interdependency of the shoulder complex is complicated and therefore creates a formidable challenge to the clinician's evaluative skills. Clinical evaluation is the keystone to establishing etiology and pathology and to determining a treatment plan; a proper evaluation entails a systematic approach that involves observational skills, the compilation of a detailed and complete history, and the assessment of signs and symptoms. The ability to perform a proficient evaluation rests on the examiner's basic knowledge of anatomy, biomechanics, kinesiology, and pathology. The evaluation process should not be limited to the initial visit. Evaluation should be incorporated into each subsequent treatment visit, either as a formal reexamination or as additional information is gathered through manual and visual feedback. Occasionally, a sign or symptom may not become manifested for several sessions; therefore, constant reassessment is necessary.

To perform a consistent, systematic evaluation of all shoulder patients requires discipline. A thorough evaluation includes the examination and comparison of both the involved and uninvolved extremities. Several important goals are achieved by performing a complete evaluation. It establishes baseline signs and symptoms, thereby allowing the comparison of initial with subsequent findings to determine treatment efficacy. It allows the clinician to identify "normal" abnormalities. For example, many asymptomatic long head of the biceps tendons are tender when they are palpated in the bicipital groove. Without an appreciation of this normality or in the absence of bilateral comparison, erroneous information may be gathered, leading to an incorrect diagnosis and unnecessary treatment.

A systematic evaluation can prevent the exclusion of primary or secondary pathology. For example, a 26-year-old laborer with a history of overhead use presents with signs and symptoms that are consistent with rotator cuff tendinitis. In addition, this patient has primary glenohumeral joint instability. If proper questioning regarding the instability is not done, and if the instability tests are not performed, because the clinician is convinced the problem is an isolated overuse tendinitis, the primary instability may be overlooked, resulting in a partial diagnosis. Although questioning during the history taking often will lead to a diagnosis well before a hand is laid on the patient, the curtailment of a complete examination and "diagnosis prejudicing" must be avoided.

The evaluation visit is the initial contact between patient and clinician and therefore creates a lasting impression for the clinician and the patient. The patient should be made to feel comfortable and trusting. If the clinician conducts a thorough, organized evaluation, and if he or she demonstrates a sound knowledge of current orthopedic concepts and practices by answering the patient's questions regarding incidence, etiology, pathophysiology, and prognosis, the clinician-patient relationship will be strengthened.

# Patient Characteristics

## Age

Patient age provides categorizing information about shoulder pathology. The two most common conditions, rotator cuff disease[4,6,48,49,53] and glenohumeral instability,[26,27,36,61] are both age-dependent. Rotator cuff lesions can occur at any age; they can be initiated by trauma or overuse. However, there is a high incidence of rotator cuff lesions of a degenerative nature in individuals over 40 years of age due to tendon attrition,[47] reduced vascularity,[57] mechanical impingement,[48,49] and decreased tendon tensile strength.[58]

The diagnosis of glenohumeral instability, both primary and recurrent, is found most commonly in patients less than 30 years of age. Traumatic primary glenohumeral dislocations also have a surprisingly similar high rate of occurrence in patients older than 50 years of age.[36,46,61] Differentiating primary from recurrent instability requires clarification. Retrospectic studies[46,61] have demonstrated a high incidence of primary dislocation in patients 50 to 70 years of age, but the recurrence rate is significantly lower (15 percent) compared with the less than 30-year-old population, who demonstrate an 85 percent recurrence rate. Clinicians treat the younger, active patient, and there is therefore a larger body of literature regarding surgery and rehabilitation of the younger, recurrent instability patient population.

## Reactivity

*Reactivity* is a nonspecific term that describes the irritability of the joint and/or its surrounding soft-tissue structures. The categories of reactivity are mild, moderate, and severe. Although a subjective measure, determining a patient's reactivity defines the patients present status and helps to guide the clinician in developing an appropriate therapeutic plan. Determining a patient's reactivity does not establish its source or, necessarily, the extent of the pathology; reactivity does define the generalized degree of inflammation. Patient A, presenting with a mildly reactive shoulder, may have full active and passive range of motion, slight pain at end range, resisted motions that are only painful in abduction, and slight pain elicitation with the impingement sign. Patient B, presenting with a severely reactive shoulder, may have considerably painful restrictions of active and passive range of motion, significant pain and weakness on resisted abduction, external rotation, and flexion, and an exceedingly painful impingement sign. Patient A may have only mild supraspinatus tendinitis, patient B may have a large rotator cuff tear, or both patients may have the same relative tissue involvement yet each appears to be at a different stage of inflammation or healing.

## History

The patient's history often defines pathology prior to clinical examination. Age, occupation, and activities are essential to commence diagnostic categorization. Although rotator cuff pathology is related to degeneration of the tendon and osseous spur formation, there is a correlation between occupations that involve heavy lifting or repetitive or sustained overhead use of the arm and rotator cuff incidence.[23] A patient's general health and other joint involvement may influence symptoms through a systemic or referred mechanism; therefore, details regarding general health and other joint involvement should be outlined. In addition, information on hand dominance, medications, and recreational activities should be obtained. Determining the patient's activity goals will assist in guiding treatment. Table 5-1 lists the subjective information that should be relayed during the history taking.

**Table 5-1**

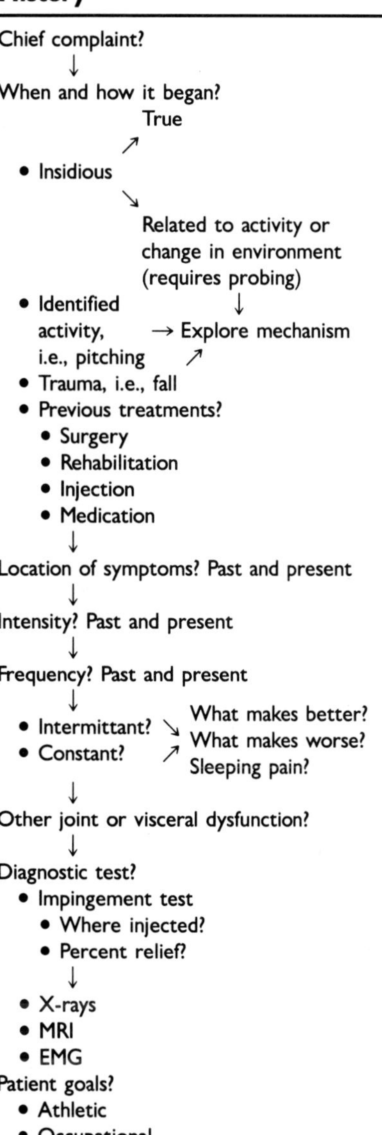

**History**

Chief complaint?
↓
When and how it began?
- Insidious ↗ True
- Insidious ↘ Related to activity or change in environment (requires probing) ↓ → Explore mechanism
- Identified activity, i.e., pitching → Explore mechanism
- Trauma, i.e., fall ↗ Explore mechanism
- Previous treatments?
  - Surgery
  - Rehabilitation
  - Injection
  - Medication

↓
Location of symptoms? Past and present
↓
Intensity? Past and present
↓
Frequency? Past and present
↓
- Intermittant? ↘
- Constant? ↗

What makes better?
What makes worse?
Sleeping pain?

↓
Other joint or visceral dysfunction?
↓
Diagnostic test?
- Impingement test
  - Where injected?
  - Percent relief?

↓
- X-rays
- MRI
- EMG

Patient goals?
- Athletic
- Occupational
- ADLs

## Chief Complaint

Establishing the chief complaint is imperative. What has lead the patient to seek medical attention? Is it pain, instability, weakness, paraesthesia, or difficulty performing activities of daily living? The chief complaint may be isolated or, more typically, a combination of symptoms. Onset and chronology should be investigated and clarified. A specific event, such as a fall, may be easily identified as the precipitating episode.

Insidious onset is characteristic of some conditions, such as adhesive capsulitis. Incidences that initially might seem irrelevant can evade detection by the clinician unless he or she "jogs" the patient's memory by asking specific, activity-related questions. First, a time frame is estimated as to when the symptoms began. Did the patient begin a new job or experience change at work, recreational, or domestic activity, such as moving offices, acquiring a new tennis partner, or painting a bedroom? What the patient considers to be an activity unrelated to his or her present complaint may actually be the cause of it. If a specific event is identified as the potential cause, it requires probing. Was the episode traumatic, such as a high-velocity, uncontrolled fall or a motor vehicle accident? If so, clarify the force and direction affecting the upper extremity. Was the origin of the injury related to a specific sporting event? Replication or breakdown of the specific athletic stroke or technique should be performed. Mechanisms of injuries are similar for specific pathologies, for example, a fall on the superior aspect of the shoulder is consistent with an acromioclavicular joint separation. Frequently, disabling rotator cuff inflammation can result from relatively innocuous activities such as reaching behind the car seat to lift a brief case or simply opening a jammed window. The clinician must elucidate the relationship between pertinent shoulder anatomy and biomechanics, the mechanism of injury, and pathogenesis of common shoulder conditions. During this process, relevant faulty tissue can be identified.

# Characteristics of Pain

## LOCATION

The area of perceived pain helps distinguish the problematic structure. In general, primary pain experienced over the neck, upper shoulder, and/or scapula indicates cervical spine–related tissue, possibly nerve root, dura mater, outer annular disc fibers, or facet joint. Pain can originate from muscles either specific to the cervical spine and/or those sharing shoulder function responsibility. Commonly, the levator scapulae and upper and middle trapezius develop spasm, trigger points, or overuse soreness, primarily or secondarily, in response to primary shoulder or cervical pathology.[65] Knowledge of dermatomal, myotomal, scleratoma (Fig. 5-1), and trigger point reference zones is crucial to the correct interpretation of pain.

Pain around the deltoid, typically laterally, is consistent with dysfunction of the glenohumeral joint and/or associated soft-tissue structures. This region encompasses the C5 dermatome. Escalating inflammation can generate distally into the C5 and C6 dermatomes. A patient with a diagnosis of a supraspinatus tendon tear or tendinitis usually reports achiness over the lateral

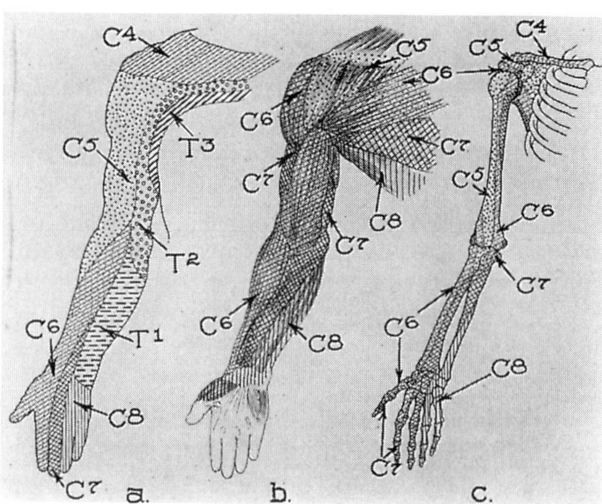


**Figure 5-1.** Upper extremity: (a) dermatomes, (b) myotomes, and (c) scleratomes. (From Inman VT, Saunders JB. Referred pain from skeletal structures. J Nerv Ment Dis 1944;99:660.)

deltoid, not over the tendon. This is *referred pain*. Referred pain can be explained by cerebral and limb bud embryologic development. The supraspinatus tendon is a deep member of the C5 dermatome. A lesion of this structure stimulates the corresponding C5 cerebral cortex, thereby producing a diffuse, often lateral perception of pain. Pain perceived over the acromioclavicular and sternoclavicular joints is characteristic of dysfunction in that corresponding joint, although other portions of the C4 dermatome also can be stimulated.

## INTENSITY AND FREQUENCY

Pain intensity and frequency depict a further sense of tissue reactivity. Considerable inflammation has a high correlation with increased symptoms and tissue reactivity assessment. The foundation of treatment planning is very much dependent on symptom intensity. A visual analog scale can be valuable in providing objective information pertaining to pain intensity.[56] Whether pain is constant or intermittent is important in further deciphering symptom features. Prolonged, constant, unyielding pain is unusual for glenohumeral joint or soft-tissue pathology, except for tumors. Even acute posttraumatic or postoperative patients find relief of constant pain within several days or by appropriate positioning of the arm. Neural irritation or damage can produce uninterrupted pain, but a cervical, brachial plexus, or peripheral nerve examination should identify neural involvement.

Intermittent pain can vary in frequency and intensity. Night pain is quite common with shoulder dysfunctions; most patients with rotator cuff pathology find it difficult to sleep on the involved side. The eventual ability to sleep on the involved shoulder is a sign of recovery and reduced reactivity. The relationship between activity and position requires exploration. For instance, patients with a history of instability may have pain if required to perform activities in a provocative position. Intermittent pain may occur following aggressive activity, overhead use, or the routine performance of the activities of daily living (ADLs). What relieves the pain is also vital information. Patients with a C7 radiculopathy may find relief by placing the arm overhead, yet this position is provocative in those having rotator cuff pathology or instability. Prior utilization and efficacy of the medical intervention, exercise, thermal agents, and medication(s) also should be determined.

## Diagnostic Tests

Diagnostic tests are described in detail in Chapter 4. The physical therapist without special radiographic training typically does not have the ability interprete radiographs and must therefore rely on a radiologist and/or an orthopedic surgeon for interpretation of plain x-rays, MRIs, CT scans, and bone scans. Electromyographs (EMGs) usually are performed and interpreted by a specialist. The clinician should learn and appreciate the appropriate use, limitations, sensitivity, and specificity of diagnostic equipment and results. This knowledge will improve the clinician's evaluative abilities and enable him or her to recommend or suggest further testing when appropriate.

# Postoperative Evaluation

The history reported by the patient should initiate a mental list of differential diagnoses. Regardless of whether a specific diagnosis is provided by the referring physician or if the patient presents following a surgical procedure, the reported history may provide additional information to the therapist that may not have been appreciated previously. The physical examination will then determine the patient's present status.

In order to be able to provide a safe and informative postoperative evaluation, the clinician should understand operative procedures and the associated possible and common complications. Clinicians and surgeons should interact frequently during the management of a postoperative patient. It is a disservice to the patient if the surgeon does not disclose surgical nuances, surgical modifications, or patient tissue idiosyncrasies to the treating therapist. Although surgeons do not always express relevant details to the therapist, therapists are not always ambitious enough to acquaint themselves with surgical procedures. Both scenarios can increase the possibility of patient complications.

When evaluating and treating a patient after rotator cuff repair, particular attention should be paid to the quality of tissue, both rotator cuff and deltoid, its fixation, and if the repair was performed "under tension." The latter refers to repairing the rotator cuff tear by significantly mobilizing the torn tendons toward a bony trough or toward one another to ensure closure. Information regarding chronicity, prior range-of-motion restrictions, strength deficits, and if manipulation was performed at surgery is vital. Tenuous tissue quality and fixation result in slower recovery. If the repair was done under tension because of a chronic retracted cuff tear, discretion regarding adduction and force application is necessary. Significant weakness and unresolved range-of-motion decrements prior to surgery have been shown to depreciate postoperative results.[15]

Patients who are seen following a reconstruction procedure for instability also require special attention. It should be determined if they had characteristics of the traumatic (TUBS) or atraumatic (AMBRI) groups. Information regarding the quality of labral, tendinous, and capsular tissue fixation is essential. Assessment of generalized hypoelasticity and hyperelasticity may be the clinician's greatest guide to evaluation and treatment progression. If a patient with significant hyperelasticity is evaluated at 4 weeks and demonstrates 50 degrees of true glenohumeral joint external rotation with the arm adducted and 150 degrees of elevation, care should be taken to deemphasize range of motion because stability may be sacrificed over time as a result of the pliability of the individual's collagen tissue.

Tissue fixation and healing principles are essential when assessing range of motion and strength. Typically, 4–6 weeks is sufficient for capsular and tendinous tissues to achieve adequate physiologic healing (depending on tissue quality and degree of tension). Controlled, gentle tension can be administered to patients at 2 weeks following a capsular shift or Bankart procedure. Caution is required when stressing tendinous repairs, particularly of the rotator cuff and deltoid. Moderate resistive tension, even at 4 weeks after acromioplasty with good fixation, could detach the deltoid.

Evaluative goals of the postoperative patient are defined by the time period from surgery. Regardless of the procedure, an examination performed on the first day after surgery differs from an examination performed 4 weeks postoperatively. Strength assessment requiring full resistance should be avoided until the relevant tissue can maintain its integrity. The time varies depending on factors previously discussed. Necessary information regarding muscular, structural, and neurovascular intactness usually can be gained with a submaximal contraction within the first 2 weeks. Corroborating evidence to determine if neurovascular integrity is present should be an early goal of all evaluations, but especially following multiple trauma, humeral head fractures, and any surgical procedure. The axillary nerve is vulnerable to injury in all the preceding. Typically, at 6 weeks, a full shoulder evaluation can be performed, although prudence is always required following a rotator cuff repair pertaining to strength assessment.

## Physical Assessment

Skill, experience, and a systematic approach are required in order to gather and interpret signs and symptoms correctly. A consistent evaluation must be done on each patient regardless of history so that the clinician can appreciate "normal" abnormalities, double lesions, and commonly associated lesions (i.e., rotator cuff disease and acromioclavicular joint arthritis). Patient history and physical examination should have correlated findings; if they appear to be unrelated, then further questioning is required. The possibility of a catastrophic etiology should be ruled out early if suspicious signs and symptoms emerge.

The goal of the physical assessment is to determine the source of the chief complaint; to do this, symptoms must be reproduced. Typically, the evaluation process progresses from least to most provocative. As Cyriax[12] discussed, point palpation should be done last, since it can only bias and confuse the clinician and prematurely irritate the patient if it is done early in the examination. The patient should be warned that his or her symptoms may worsen following the evaluation; therefore, the patient should be given appropriate pain relief guidelines to follow.

The patient should be made to understand that the purpose of particular techniques and positions is to reproduce or change the patient's chief complaint, whether it be pain, stiffness, or paresthesia. Clarity is essential in this matter, since patient naiveté can lead to the declaration and interpretation of erroneous and misleading data. If a patient is placed in a particular position and simply asked, "Is that painful?" he or she may respond positively, even though the pain he or she is experiencing is either unrelated to the chief complaint or the chief complaint is unchanged yet the patient is still experiencing it. For example, when assessing resisted shoulder abduction in a patient experiencing constant C5 radicular pain, the patient needs to understand that a "change" in pain related to the resisted motion is being evaluated. If asked, "Is that painful?" while the test is performed, the uninformed patient may give a positive response, misleading the examiner to believe that resisted abduction "increased" the pain, when in fact the pain is unchanged yet still constant.

The order of the physical assessment presented below is based on the authors' preferred performance.

## Observation

An enormous amount of information is gained by general and detailed observations of the patient. General observations regarding upper extremity posturing as well as normal movement patterns, such as taking a shirt off, provide a gauge of reactivity and functional impairment. A patient experiencing pain characteristically protects their upper extremity by maintaining an internally rotated and adducted position. Consistency of motion should always be noted. If a patient can easily place his or her arm overhead while disrobing but then can barely elevate the extremity while active range of motion is being assessed, the clinician notes an inconsistency. A physiologic reason for such a discrepancy must be found; if it cannot be found, then secondary gains or psychosis should be suspected.

Detailed observations to assess soft-tissue and osseous deformity or asymmetry then follow. The patient should be properly exposed; males disrobe from the waist up, and females should wear a gown that allows the appropriate visualization of the complete shoulder girdles and middle to upper thoracic spine. Deformities such as an elevated scapula and short neck found in Sprengel's deformity should be obvious. Bony prominences, particularly of the acromioclavicular and sternoclavicular joints, should be viewed for symmetry. A squared appearance of the lateral shoulder, exposing the lateral acromion, may indicate deltoid wasting or anterior glenohumeral dislocation (Fig. 5-2). Clavicular

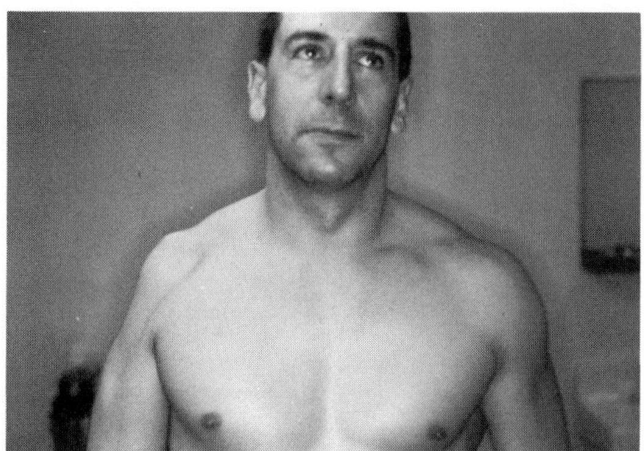

**Figure 5-2.** Significant right deltoid atrophy due to an axillary nerve palsy.

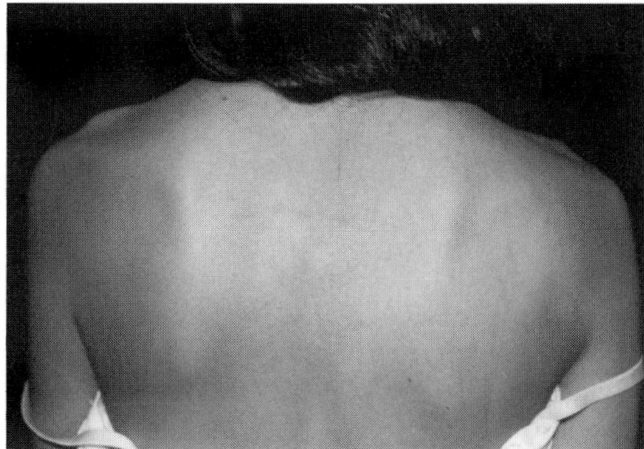

**Figure 5-4.** Atrophy of the supraspinatus and infraspinatus muscles demonstrated by hallowing of the spinati fossa's.

orientation should be appreciated from the anterior view; in the presence of a chronic spinal accessory nerve injury or fascioscapulohumeral muscular dystrophy, the clavicle and associated shoulder girdle may be significantly depressed and protracted due to lost upper trapezius suspensory function (Fig. 5-3).

Muscle contour inspection to determine atrophy or hypertrophy is critical. Complete lesions of the nerve or musculotendinous unit produce conspicuous muscle mass changes; subtle bulk disparity such as in infraspinatus atrophy of a throwing athlete may be more difficult to appreciate. The infraspinatus and supraspinatus fossae and scapular spine should be viewed posteriorly and superiorly (Fig. 5-4). Fossa hollowing indicates pathology of the musculotendinous unit, cervical nerve root, peripheral nerve, or upper plexus. Tendon rupture produces noticeable muscle contour changes, as in the "popeye" muscle that results from long head of the biceps tendon rupture. Detection of muscle bulk changes in unconditioned or obese individuals requires visualization enhanced by active contraction and/or palpation.

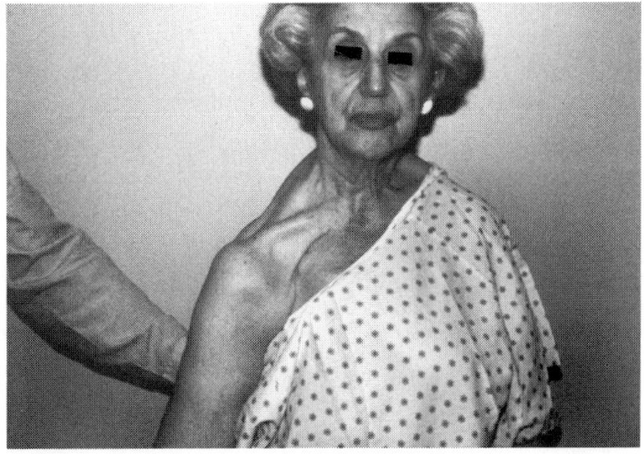

**Figure 5-3.** Patient 11 years after complete and unresolved spinal accessory nerve palsy caused by radiation therapy following a radical mastectomy. Note the inferior clavicular orientation.

## POSTURE

A formal postural assessment is performed to determine scapular and spinal misalignment. Postural alignment should be viewed both sitting and standing and correlated with provoking activities. Spinal alignment directly influences shoulder girdle orientation and function. A sedentary individual sitting or standing in a posterior pelvic tilt, lumbar flexion, increased thoracic flexion, and a forward head position is obliged to anteriorly displace the shoulder girdles. Prolonged chronic placement in this orientation may cause adaptive shortening and stretch weakness of associated spinal, trunk, and shoulder musculature.[37] Attempted arm elevation in this position restricts scapular rotation and retards trunk and rib expansion, thereby causing limited motion (Fig. 5-5.). Repetitive shoulder level or overhead use of the arm while maintaining this posture could predispose the shoulder to soft-tissue trauma, such as trigger point formation or rotator cuff impingement.

Both sitting and standing posture should be viewed posteriorly, laterally, and anteriorly to recognize and correlate postural faults. Particular attention should be directed toward scapular alignment. Posteriorly, the scapular inferior angle should be level with the T7 spinous process; the vertebral border should be 5 to 9 cm, depending on the size of the individual, from the spinous processes.[35,41] Bilateral comparisons should be made. Usually hand dominance affects scapular orientation, although left-handed individuals are inconsistent because they tend to perform many

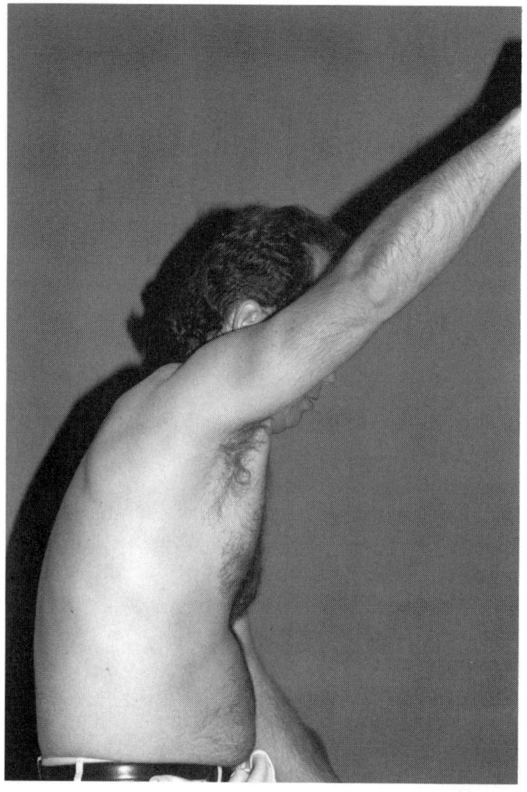

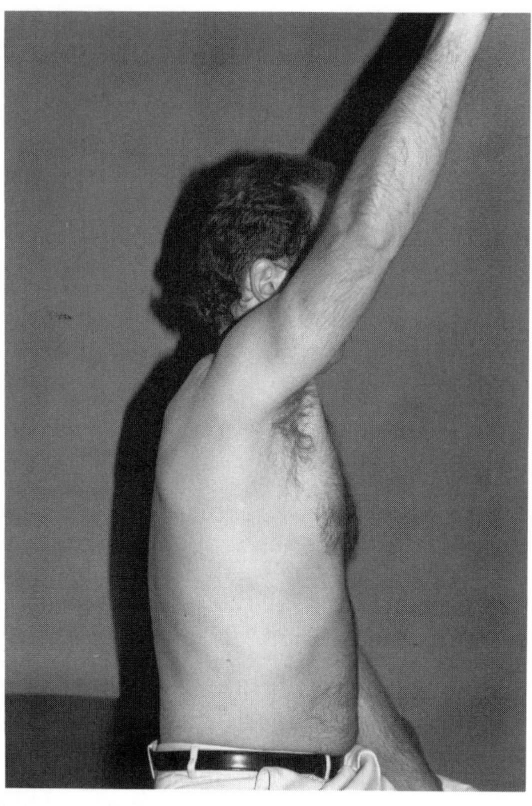

A B

**Figure 5-5.** Restricted arm-trunk elevation with (a) poor posture and appropriate motion with (b) corrected posture.

activities with the right hand. The greater the unilateral activity, the greater is the asymmetry; this is particularly true of pitchers and tennis players.

Scapular orientation has two characteristic presentations: (1) the scapula is abducted and inferiorly displaced relative to the nondominant side, and (2) the scapula is elevated, medially rotated, and forward, yet the acromion is lower compared with the uninvolved side (Fig. 5-6). This occurs because the coracoid is pulled forward, elevating and anteriorly tilting the relatively flat scapula over the curved posterior thoracic wall, thereby displacing the acromion forward

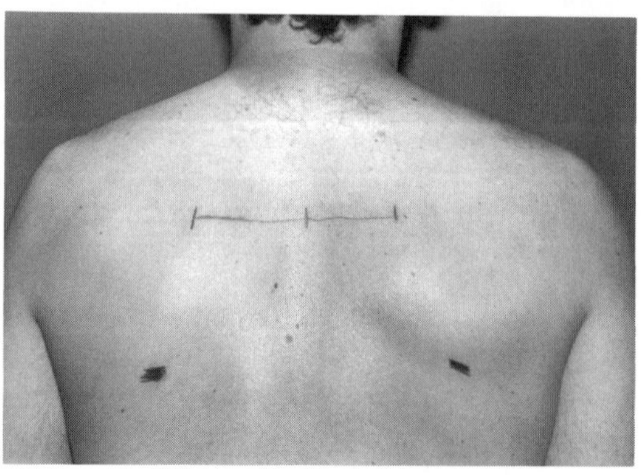

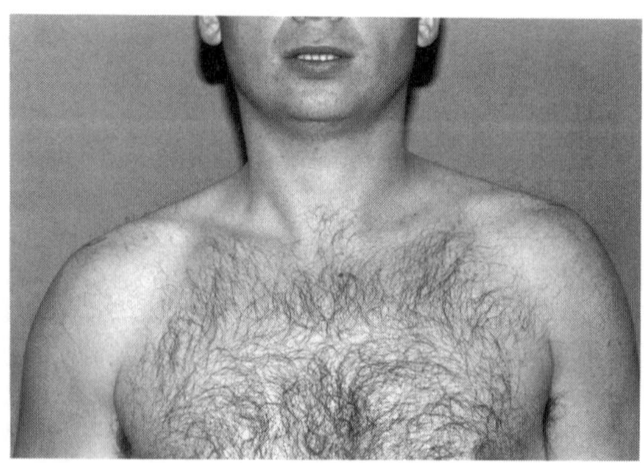

A B

**Figure 5-6.** (a) Posterior view demonstrating typical dominant hand effect (right) on scapular orientation. Note the elevated inferior angle and medial rotation of the scapula. (b) Anterior view, same patient.

and down. The tilting causes the inferior angle to migrate posteriorly away from the thoracic wall; this is often mistaken for scapular "winging." In both the scapular orientations described above, the middle and lower trapezius muscles are elongated, tending to be weak, and the pectoralis minor is tight.

# Cervical Range of Motion

Any time the upper quadrant is involved, the cervical spine requires a screening examination to rule out primary or associated pathology. Active cervical motions are performed in flexion, extension, both side bendings, and rotations. Range of motion and reproduction of symptoms are evaluated and correlated with the chief complaint. Frequently a patient will report upper trapezius or cervical pain or pulling of the stretched side when rotating or laterally flexing away. The patient must distinguish the normal sensation of a stretch from the pain for which they seek medical attention.

A simple technique that helps to determine true, full passive cervical range of motion and also helps distinguish between painful trapezius limitation and restriction from a spinal structure (i.e., disc, facet, ligament, or paravertebral muscle) is to compare cervical range while sitting or standing and while supine. While sitting and standing, the shoulder girdle is depressed by gravity and upper extremity weight, prestretching the upper trapezius muscle, which results in limited contralateral cervical side bending and rotation. Repeating this motion while supine and while manually elevating the shoulder opposite to the head direction allows the upper trapezius to slacken, thus enabling full assessment of true cervical side bending and rotation. To accept cervical side bending and rotation motion as true motion when performed in the sitting or standing position is equivalent to accepting hip flexion motion with the knee extended.

## SPECIAL TESTS

### CERVICAL QUADRANT TEST

The quadrant test is a nonspecific yet excellent test to determine cervical involvement. The head is extended, laterally flexed, and rotated to the ipsilateral side. Overpressure is then applied, which further compresses the posterolateral disc, facet joint, and foraminal space on the side of motion. This test does not always isolate a particular cervical level or structure, but if pain is generated, it is likely there is cervical involvement (Fig. 5-7).

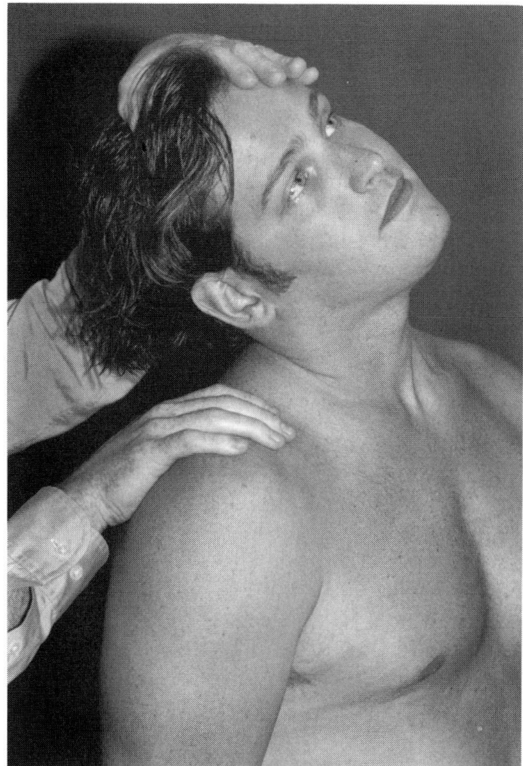

**Figure 5-7.** Quadrant test.

### COMPRESSION AND TRACTION

Compression and traction with the head in a neutral position also assist in determining cervical involvement. Compression is applied by an axial load through the head and neck, which then compresses the disc, nerve root, or facet. Traction is performed to increase foraminal opening and remove cranial weight, thereby arresting compression. Traction can relieve peripheral nerve or dura mater mechanical pressure at the disk level. By expanding the foraminal space, pain due to nerve root compression can be alleviated. A positive compression or traction test indicates a cervical problem due to mechanical compression.

Further cervical evaluation is indicated if there is positive cervical involvement. These techniques will not be described in this text, but a myriad of literature exists regarding in-depth discussion of cervical examination and related pathologies.

# Contractile Versus Noncontractile Tissue

The tissues surrounding the glenohumeral joint are described as either contractile or noncontractile tissue.[12] Before discussing physical examination, further distinction between contractile and noncontractile tissue needs to be reviewed.

Contractile tissue includes muscle belly, tendon, and tendon insertion to bone (tenoperiosteal junction). Noncontractile tissue includes the capsule, ligaments, subchondral bone, labrum, bursa, and nerves.[12] In general, these two groups are evaluatively distinguished by employing static resisted contractions, referred to as *resisted motions*, and by assessing passive range of motion. Contractile element force transmission is a requisite of resisted motions. A lesion within the contractile chain will promote pain when obligated to translate force. Noncontractile tissue is void of any dynamic capacity; it can be assessed grossly by passive range of motion. If passive motion is limited, a correlation is drawn between motion (i.e., external rotation or abduction), tissue stretched during the motion, pain, and the end feel. The clinician also must consider that passive motion can elicit a painful response from a contractile lesion when stretched opposite to its action, for example, supraspinatus elongation during functional internal rotation (reaching up the back) or during external rotation at the side.

When a double lesion exists, one affecting a contractile element and the other affecting a noncontractile element, confusion can arise. A common example of this is a supraspinatus tendinitis coexisting with laxity of the glenohumeral ligaments. Even a full-thickness rotator cuff tear can be considered to involve both contractile (tendon) and noncontractile (capsule and coracohumeral ligament) tissue.

A third mechanism of eliciting pain from either contractile or noncontractile tissue is compression. For instance, the supraspinatus tendon and bursa are both compressed or impinged when forcing the humerus into elevation and stabilizing the scapula. This is the position for the "impingement sign." Full external rotation and horizontal abduction at 90 degrees of abduction or full arm elevation also can result in contractile and noncontractile tissue compromise. In both positions, the supraspinatus tendon can impinge against the posterior glenoid rim.[63,69] Additionally, these positions can stretch or compress the bursa, particularly if it is thickened and fibrotic, while significant stretch of the capsuloligamentous-labral complex results, along with some degree of anterior rotator cuff elongation. If inflammation exists in the stretched or compressed tissue, pain will be elicited.

Visualization and the application of biomechanical and anatomic knowledge are constantly needed during the evaluation. Use of these principles in conjunction with data attained during the examination helps to focus attention on the involved tissue.

# Active Range of Motion

Active range of motion, although nonspecific with respect to distinguishing contractile and noncontractile tissue, does yield valuable information. Active range of motion provides degrees of motion assessment and the ability to complete a fair grade, giving the clinician information regarding reactivity status, symptom location, painful arc presence, and appropriate scapulohumeral rhythm.

Active range of motion is estimated or measured in all cardinal planes and then is compared with the uninvolved side. Elevation, whether flexion, abduction, or scapular plane abduction, is performed to assess range of motion and ability to complete the motion against gravity. External rotation at 90 degrees of abduction and neutral can be assessed quickly in the standing position, as can functional internal rotation (glenohumeral internal rotation, extension, and adduction). Frequently, pain, weakness, or structural restriction produces dysfunctional motion compared with the uninvolved side. Inability or unwillingness to move because of pain helps define tissue reactivity. Location of pain may provide further insight about pathology. The glenohumeral joint and its associated soft tissues usually refer pain laterally over the deltoid, but pain also can be focused more posteriorly or anteriorly. Discomfort associated with biceps tendinitis is commonly felt anteriorly over the groove. The acromioclavicular joint and sternoclavicular joint are implicated when discomfort exists over either joint. Frequently, concomitant pathology of the rotator cuff, biceps tendon, and acromioclavicular joint exists, although the superseding area of pain commonly correlates with the rotator cuff. Active trigger points can further confuse the issue because of characteristic referred pain zones.

Although the Academy of Orthopaedic Surgeons[2] no longer distinguishes flexion from abduction, preferring instead to use the term *elevation*, further information is provided by evaluating elevation in multiple planes. Pain may be present in flexion but not abduction, or vice versa. The correlation between pathology and planar motion cannot always be drawn. However, further insight into the mechanical nature of the subacromial space components and the capsuloligamentous complex (CLC) is elucidated. Mechanical properties can be examined further by changing physiologic motion, for example, by combining flexion while maintaining external rotation, as opposed to allowing the obligatory internal rotation. At times, a patient will experience pain with normal flexion yet be pain-free when external rotation is attempted and elevation is performed in the sagittal plane. During the modified flexion movement, the greater tuberosity and adjoining rotator cuff avoid their journey, and imminent compression, beneath the anterior acromion and coracoacromial ligament. Functional internal rotation is a simple active task that demonstrates the patient's ability to perform glenohumeral internal rotation, extension, and adduction in conjunction with elbow flexion and pronation. A clinician should be aware that the supraspinatus is elongated during this activity and can result in a painful stretch if a tendinous lesion exists. This movement, as well as coronal plane abduction, is almost always limited in a patient presenting with a "frozen shoulder," whether the etiology is idiopathic or traumatic. Both the abducted/externally rotated and the functional internally rotated positions of the shoulder cause a complete twisting of the contracted capsuloligamentous-tendinous complex (CLTC), but in opposite directions.

## PAINFUL ARC

The painful arc has been described by numerous authors.[10, 12, 14, 38, 48, 49] Usually, the painful arc occurs during abduction at between 60 and 120 degrees of elevation (Fig. 5-8). The bursa and rotator cuff are compressed or impinged by some aspect of the overlying coracoacromial arch or inferior acromioclavicular joint. Beyond 120 degrees of elevation, the rotator cuff has traveled past the impinging structures, allowing pain-free motion. Neer[48, 49] describes the painful arc as occurring during flexion when the greater tuberosity passes underneath the anterior acromion. Cyriax[12] believed that the presence of a painful arc is pathognomonic for supraspinatus tendinitis.

A painful arc beginning near the end range and increasing to the end range also has been described.[3, 14, 38, 49] Pathology of the acromioclavicular joint is thought to be responsible for this arc. During end-range elevation, the articular surfaces and disk are significantly compressed, causing pain. Bateman[3] has described subsequent development of acromioclavicular joint arthritis due to attempted range-of-motion compensation in those individuals with restricted glenohumeral motion.

Variations of a painful arc are seen commonly in patients having the same diagnosis. In the presence of reactive tendinitis, bursitis, or a rotator cuff tear, the patient describes pain beginning somewhere between 60 and 90 degrees of elevation that continues *through* the range. This painful arc correlates with compression of inflamed subacromial soft tissues. Frequently, pain due to rotator cuff or bursal compression will only be experienced near end range, mimicking what occurs with acromioclavicular joint arthritis or trauma.

Another painful arc variation occurs during the eccentric phase of the elevating musculature. The patient may experience very little discomfort during elevation, but upon lowering the extremity, a painful arc arises. This may occur because of the eccentric contraction of the rotator cuff and increased load across the intratendinous structures or because of abnormal humeral head translation resulting from poor rotator cuff function and/or joint instability. A third explanation for a painful arc occurring during the arm lowering is based on a reduced contribution of the scapular lateral rotators, particularly of the serratus anterior. Many individuals demonstrate early release of scapular lateral rotation returning from elevation that causes the coracoacromial arch to "clamp down" upon subacromial structures (Fig. 5-9). If the patient is told to "reach forward" while lowering, thereby activating the serratus anterior and associated scapular lateral rotation, the painful arc may disappear. Increased utilization of the serratus anterior during concentric elevation also can negate a painful arc.

The painful arc can be influenced by humeral rotation. As mentioned previously, if the painful arc is present with flexion, the patient is told to elevate the arm with the palm up, which maintains the humerus in a more externally rotated position, preventing the greater tuberosity from passing beneath the anterior acromion. Occasionally, abduction performed in internal rotation is less painful than abduction in neutral or external rotation. Altering the symptoms by modifying humeral head rotation clearly demonstrates the mechanical nature of the condition. This finding can be used to reduce irritation during daily activities and exercise. For example, if external rotation during elevation is found to be less painful the exercise of active assisted flexion can be performed with the forearm supinated or in the neutral position encouraging humeral external rotation and allowing pain-free exercise.

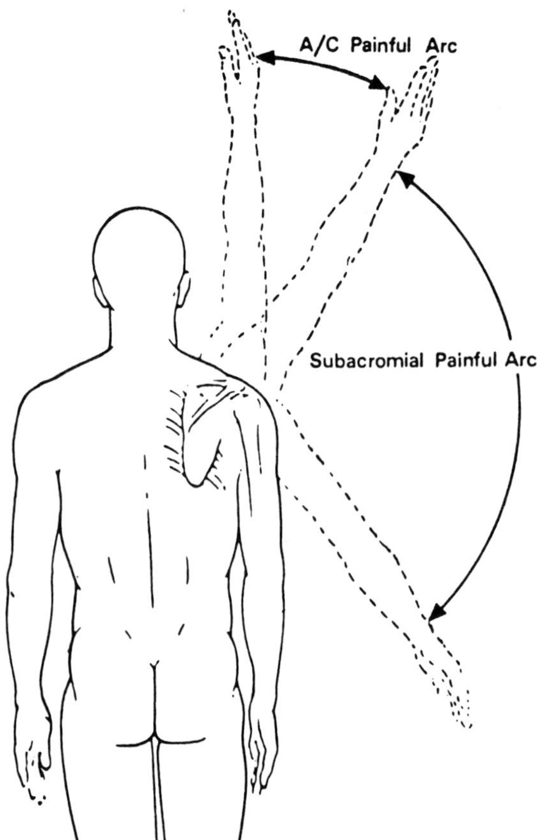


**Figure 5-8.** Painful arcs arising due to subacromial and acromioclavicular pathology. (From Kessell L, Watson M. The painful arc syndrome: clinical classification as a guide to management. J Bone Joint Surg 1977;59B:166.)

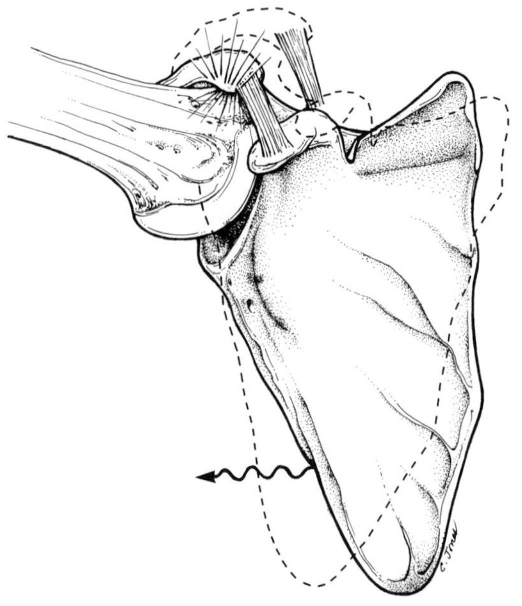

**Figure 5-9.** Subacromial tissue compression caused by weak or dysfunctional scapular rotators.

## SCAPULOHUMERAL RHYTHM

Scapulohumeral rhythm is the smooth and uniform motion of the shoulder girdle joints and muscles allowing full elevation. Proper synchrony is mediated by the healthy state of joints and surrounding soft tissues and proper contraction of muscles. When either pain, pathology, or weakness exists, the rhythm is altered, and further dysfunction is caused. Attempted elevation in the presence of pain, capsular adhesions, or weak musculature commonly will lead to either excessive scapular elevation, lateral rotation, or shrugging; the shrugging can be quite noticeable or subtle (Fig. 5-10). Many times, lumbar hyperextension and contralateral lateral trunk flexion also occur.

A long thoracic nerve palsy will produce obvious "winging" of the scapula during attempted elevation, making the diagnosis simple. The clinician needs to examine the patient closely for subtle scapular "lagging." Inman and Saunders[30] described the setting phase during the initial 30 to 60 degrees of arm abduction or flexion in

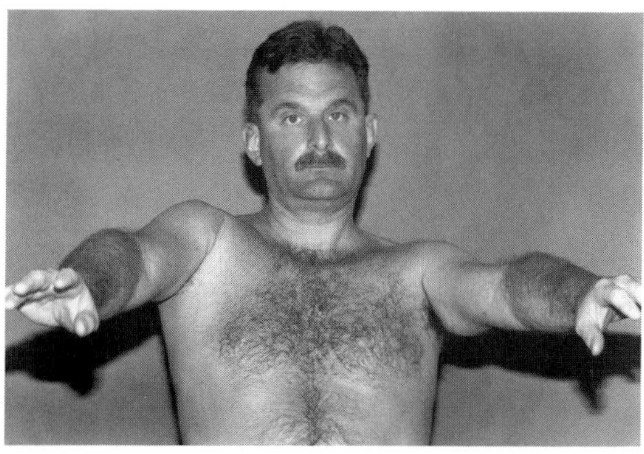

**Figure 5-10.** Patient demonstrating abnormal scapulohumeral rhythm on right by excessive scapular elevation.

which the scapula seeks a position on the thoracic wall. Beyond 60 degrees, the humerus maintains a 2:1 ratio with respect to the scapula. To assess proper scapular rotation, the clinician must palpate the scapular inferior angle. Palpable lateral movement should ensue by at least 70 degrees of arm elevation. If displacement is absent or minimal by 90 degrees, scapular rotator dysfunction exists, probably of the serratus anterior (Fig. 5-11). This is of great clinical significance; the serratus anterior and trapezius need to be strengthened. This is especially important for athletes such as swimmers, who are highly dependent on scapular muscles during endurance and repetitive overhead motions. Once the scapular contribution falters, impingement will soon occur.[50, 52]

# Manual Muscle Testing

The scope of manual muscle testing will not be covered in this text, for there are excellent references describing appropriate techniques. We will discuss the concept of manual muscle testing and how it applies to the shoulder evaluation, in particular to the orthopedic population.

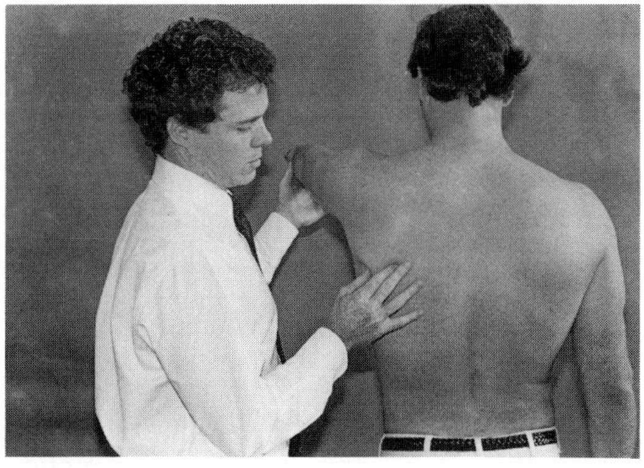

**Figure 5-11.** Assessing proper scapulohumeral rhythm.

Manual muscle testing (MMT) is performed to determine the strength of a particular muscle or group of similar-acting muscles. The grading scheme, based on gravity, was devised by Dr. Robert Lovett during the polio outbreak so that some standardization could be applied to the muscle-testing technique and criteria could be developed for objective grading. This system is still valuable today, particularly for patients with any level of neurologic involvement. Indeed, manual muscle testing can be applied to the orthopedic population, but certain difficulties arise, particularly when evaluating the shoulder. Pain and positioning make strict manual muscle testing difficult to interpret and sometimes impractical to use. We know that pain can invalidate true strength assessment because of reflexive inhibition of the motor units. Consider a patient who presents with a reactive partial tear of the supraspinatus tendon and cannot complete the abduction range against gravity because of pain. Any manual resistance against the abductors causes pain and apparent "weakness." An injection of 10 cc of lidocaine into the subacromial space numbs the involved tendon, rendering associated nerve endings unable to transmit pain. Reexamination of the patient may demonstrate full and painless abduction and the ability of the patient to create significant force when abduction is resisted. Therefore, in fact, this patient does not have true weakness other than that produced by pain.

Positioning also raises problems related to pain. For example, when determining the external rotation strength of an individual presenting 2 weeks after an anterior glenohumeral dislocation, the accepted prone position for MMT requiring the shoulder to be placed in 90 degrees of coronal plane abduction may cause significant pain and apprehension due to recent soft-tissue trauma and an impending sense of dislocating. Testing in this position may indicate a less than fair grade because the individual cannot move through the range of motion against gravity secondary to pain or apprehension. If this individual's external rotators were then tested with the shoulder at the side and in neutral rotation, he or she may in fact demonstrate no weakness of the external rotators at all. Positioning of the glenohumeral joint in elevated ranges also can lead to difficulties when assessing the strength of the scapular muscles, particularly the serratus anterior, rhomboid, middle trapezius, and lower trapezius.

Because of the above-mentioned difficulties, shoulder muscle strength typically is graded using resisted motions and the "break test" at zero elevation and neutral rotation or at some nonprovocative degree of elevation. This will be described shortly under "Resisted Motions."

One element of manual muscle testing that cannot be overlooked is palpation of the primary muscle being tested. It is absolutely essential to palpate during the active and resistive motions. Neurologic involvement following multiple shoulder trauma, contusions, or surgery often can be missed if specific muscle palpation is not performed; this is particularly true of the deltoid. Active elevation in the presence of a partial or even full deltoid palsy may be full, since the rotator cuff and scapulothoracic muscles are quite capable of achieving functional arm elevation. In this case, the deltoid may not be suspected if it is not properly palpated. Clinicians sometimes expect the patient to have pain or be unable to elevate the arm following multiple trauma or postoperatively; thus assessment of the deltoid is deferred. Simple palpation of the deltoid while asking the patient to lift the arm slightly from an elevated position of 45 degrees can determine neurologic intactness.

Although a full description of manual muscle-testing positions will not be presented, Table 5-2 lists the shoulder muscles and gives a brief description of testing technique. Both traditional and alternative muscle-testing positions for the serratus anterior and trapezius will be further discussed. We find that these muscles are frequently overlooked in the evaluation process, as is their contribution to shoulder function. The fact is that weakness or poor endurance of these scapulothoracic muscles results in eventual rotator cuff and capsuloligamentous complex overload and trauma.

## SERRATUS ANTERIOR

When evaluating for scapulothoracic muscle function, the clinician should first assess scapulothoracic rhythm. Significant weakness of the serratus anterior is easy to detect in the presence of a long thoracic nerve palsy. Attempted elevation of the arm, particularly in the sagittal plane, results in scapular winging. The examiner should note less winging when elevation is performed in the coronal plane because of increased trapezius activity, resulting in tethering of the medial scapular border to the thoracic wall. The variation in scapulothoracic muscle activity becomes more important when identifying subtle serratus weakness, which should always be evaluated with the arm in the sagittal plane. Elevation in the sagittal plane requires a greater contribution of the serratus anterior[31,41] and less ability of the trapezius to substitute. If a scapular lag or abnormal rhythm is noted, further selective testing is required.

### WALL PUSH

This is a functional test that requires the patient to place the arms out in front onto a wall and to lean toward the wall by bending the elbows. In the presence of moderate to significant serratus anterior weakness, the scapula's medial border will displace off the thoracic wall (wing), and slight medial rotation will occur (Fig. 5-12).

### QUADRIPED

This position can be used when subtle serratus weakness is suspected. Essentially the patient is asked to assume a hands and knee position and then push up to further displace their trunk toward the ceiling. This significantly challenges the serratus anterior. Weakness will be noted if the scapula displaces off the thoracic wall (Fig. 5-13). A progression of this position is to have the patient perform a push-up from the standard position and then 10 push-ups and reevaluate.

### FUNCTIONAL FLEXION TEST

This is an alternative test for someone who may have difficulty with the quadruped position, yet serratus anterior weakness is suspected. The arm is placed into approximately 120 degrees of sagittal plane elevation. The inferior angle of the scapula is palpated. The examiner pushes the arm toward extension as the patient resists. If the scapula is felt to rotate or wing as resistance is applied, weakness is present in the scapulothoracic muscles, most likely the serratus anterior.[37] If the arm is pushed into extension, yet no motion is felt at the scapulothoracic joint, the glenohumeral joint can be assumed to have moved.

## TRAPEZIUS

The trapezius may be one of the most ignored muscles when a shoulder evaluation is performed. Even in the presence of a complete accessory nerve palsy, patients can be passed from one health care practitioner to another because of an inability to properly evaluate trapezius strength. The primary reason for this ignorance is that many clinicians test trapezius function by shrugging or retracting the shoulders, both of which can be carried out by the levator scapulae and rhomboids.

Atrophy is not always apparent even in extreme cases. By performing a shrugging motion and palpating the upper trapezius fibers, mis-

**Table 5-2**

## Manual Muscle Testing

| Muscle | Nerve Supply | Root Level | Technique |
|---|---|---|---|
| Trapezius<br>Upper | Spinal Accessory n. | CN XI, C3–C4 | Patient upright; place into cervical extension, ipsilateral SB, and contralateral rotation. Pt. elevates scapula while resistance is over distal acromion into depression and at posterior cranium into flexion and contralateral SB. |
| Middle | Same | | Pt. prone; set scapula; arm is brought into 90°; pt. lifts into glenohumeral horizontal abduction and ER, scapular adduction without elevation. Resistance is over the distal scapular spine into scapular abduction. |
| Lower | Same | | Pt. prone; set scapula; arm is brought into 135° of glenohumeral elevation and ER Pt. lifts into scapular depression, and lateral rotation. Resistance is over the distal scapular spine into scapular elevation and abduction. |
| Sternocliedomastoid | Spinal accessory n. | CN XI, C3–C4 | Pt. supine; pt. lifts head into cervical flexion and contralateral rotation. Resistance is over forehead. |
| Serratus anterior | Long thorasic n. | Pretrunk, C5, C6, C7 | Pt. supine; pt. arm at 90° of flexion with elbow flexed. Pt. pushes arm anteriorly. Resistance is over the olecranon pushing posteriorly. |
| Rhomboids/levator scapulae | Dorsal scapular n. | C4–C5 | Pt. prone; set scapula; pt. adducts, elevates, and medially rotates the scapula. Resistance is over the distal scapular spine into abduction and depression. |
| Pectoralis minor | Medial pectoral n. | Medial cord, C8–T1 | Pt. supine; pt. lifts shoulder girdle forward (protract clavicle). Resistance is over the anterior humerus into retraction. |
| Pectoralis major<br>Sternal | Medial and lateral pectoral n. | Lateral and medial cord, C5–T1 | Pt. supine; arm is brought into 135° of coronal abduction; pt. lifts arm into extension and horizontal adduction. Resistance is over the distal humerus opposite the above. |
| Clavicular | Lateral pectoral n. | Lateral cord, C5–C7 | Pt. supine; arm is brought into 60° of coronal abduction; pt. lifts arm into flexion and horizontal adduction. Resistance is over the distal humerus opposite the above. |
| Latissimus dorsi | Thoracodorsal n. | Postior cord, C5–C8 | Pt. prone; pt. lifts arm from neutral into extension and adduction. Resistance is over the distal humerus opposite the above. |
| Teres major | Lower subscapular n. | Posterior cord, C5–C6 | Pt. prone; pt. lifts arm from neutral into extension, adduction and IR. Resistance is over the distal humerus opposite the above. |
| Deltoid<br>Anterior | Axillay n. | Posterior cord, C5–C6 | Pt. upright; pt. lifts arm into elevation 30° posterior to the sagittal plane and some ER. Resistance is over the distal humerus into adduction and extension. |
| Middle | Same | | Pt. upright; pt. lifts arm into coronal plane abduction and neutral rotation. Resistance is over the distal humerus into adduction. |
| Posterior | Same | | Pt. prone; arm is brought into 90° of coronal plane abduction; pt. lifts into horizontal abduction in neutral rotation. Resistance is over the distal humerus into horizontal adduction. |

(*continued*)

**Table 5-2** *(continued)*

**Manual Muscle Testing**

| Muscle | Nerve Supply | Root Level | Technique |
|---|---|---|---|
| Supraspinatus | Suprascapular | Upper trunk, C5–C6 | Pt. upright; pt. lifts arm into scapular plane abduction in IR. Resistance is over the distal humerus into adduction. |
| Infraspinatus | Suprascapular | Upper trunk, C5–C6 | Pt. prone; arm is brought into 90° of adduction with forearm off the table edge; pt. lifts into ER. Resistance is over distal forearm into IR. |
| Subscabularis | Upper and lower subscapular n. | Posterior cord, C5–C8 | Pt. as above; pt. lifts into IR. Resistance is over the distal forearm into ER. |
| Teres minor | Axillary n. | Posterior cord, C5–C6 | Same as for infraspinatus |
| Coracobrachialis | Musculocutaneous n. | C4, C5, C6, C7 | Pt. upright; pt. flexes and horizontally adducts the arm. Resistance is over the distal humerus opposite the above. |
| Biceps brachi | Musculocutaneous n. | C4, C5, C6, C7 | Pt. upright; pt. supinates and flexes elbow. Resistance is over the distal forearm into extension. |
| Triceps | Radial n. | C5, C6, C7, C8 | Pt. prone; arm is brought into 90° of abduction with forearm over the table edge; pt. extends the elbow. Resistance is over the distal forearm into flexion. |

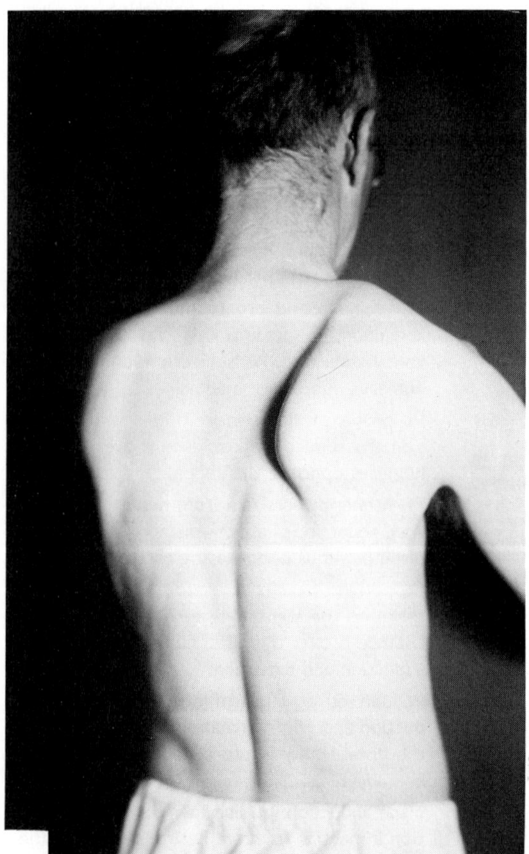

**Figure 5-12.** Medial scapular "winging" in patient with long thoracic nerve palsy.

diagnosis can be avoided. Specific testing of the middle and lower trapezius is essential when positioning allows. A key to trapezius testing is "setting" the scapula into an anatomic position. Normally, when an individual lies prone, the shoulder complex falls forward, thus elevating the shoulder. Testing in this position will only facilitate rhomboid, levator scapulae, and upper trapezius action. To isolate the middle trapezius, the shoulder complex needs to be brought into proper position by pulling the scapula inferiorly and posteriorly so that the inferior angle is somewhat level with the T7 spinous process. The arm is placed into 90 degrees of abduction and full horizontal adduction so that the scapulothoracic

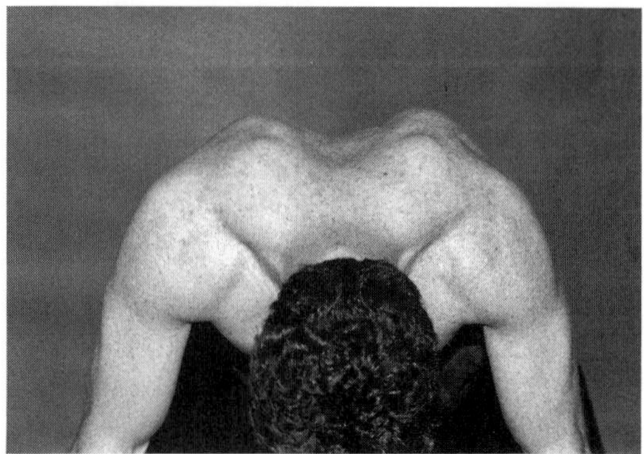

**Figure 5-13.** Slight scapular winging noted on the left in quadraped position.

joint is adducted. The patient is asked to keep the thumb up to encourage external rotation at the glenohumeral joint; this assists in maintaining proper scapular position and in facilitating middle trapezius function. The patient is then asked to hold this position, emphasizing scapular adduction. If the scapula maintains its position on the thoracic wall even if the arm drops due to glenohumeral motion, it is considered a fair grade. If the scapula elevates or abducts, middle trapezius weakness exist. Scapular elevation results from substitution by the rhomboids, levator scapulae and upper trapezius (Fig. 5-14). Resistance can be applied over the posterolateral angle of the acromion toward scapular abduction when performing a break test.

Lower trapezius testing is performed at approximately 135 degrees of elevation while the patient is prone. Again, the patient is asked to maintain the arm in a thumb-up position. The arm is elevated so that the scapula rotates laterally, slightly adducts, and maintains an anatomically normal position with regard to elevation and depression. If the patient can maintain the arm in this position, it is considered a fair grade. To perform the break test, resistance can be placed over the posterolateral acromion toward scapular elevation and abduction. The trapezius muscle testing positions can compromise subacromial tissue and are provocative in a patient with anterior instability. The positions can be modified by keeping the arm in the scapular plane or at the side. Scapular position and direction of resistance should be consistent with those already described.

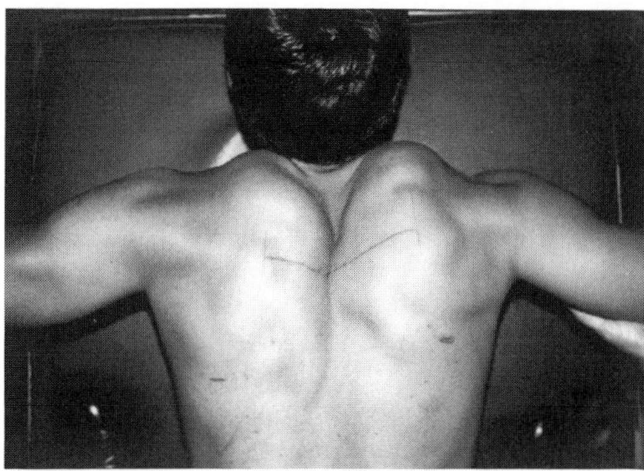

**Figure 5-14.** Manual muscle-testing position for the middle trapezius in a patient with right spinal accessory nerve palsy. Note the correct adducted position of the left scapula. The right scapula is elevated and adducted by substitution of the rhomboids and levator scapulae.

# Resisted Motions

The term *resisted motions* is somewhat confusing because minimal motion occurs; essentially an isometric contraction is performed, followed by an eccentric contraction, as the examiner overcomes the patient's resistance. Resisted motions determine the status of the muscle, tendon, and the tenoperiosteal junction by assessing strength and pain.[12] If a lesion exists within a muscle's contractile chain, pain is caused when resistance is applied in a specific direction that isolates that particular muscle's action. True contractile element isolation is usually ensured by negating any joint motion. There are exceptions to this rule, such as in the presence of arthritic joint changes involving the exposure of subchondral bone. Resisted internal rotation, for example, causes significant joint compression resulting in pain. This is analogous to patellofemoral pain caused with resisted knee extension.

Cyriax[12] emphasized placing the joint near or at midrange when performing resisted motions. He believed that the optimal position is with the arm at the side in neutral rotation. Whenever possible, resistance should be applied over the distal bone to isolate muscle function at a single joint. The exception to this rule is rotation that requires resistance at the distal forearm, thus crossing the elbow. We feel that resisted motions should be performed at various arcs of motion so that reactivity is demonstrated and the mechanical nature of the involved tissue is clearly illustrated. For example, resisted abduction may be moderately painful when performed with the arm at the side, slightly painful when performed at 45 degrees of abduction, and significantly painful when performed at 90 degrees of abduction. The explanation for this scenario is that in the presence of a supraspinatus tendon lesion, the adducted position places a significant degree of tension on the tendon that is further magnified by muscle contraction. At 45 degrees, the tendon is slackened, resulting in less passive tendon tension and pain even though forces are transmitted through the tendon. At 90 degrees, the resisted motion, combined with possible impingement of the tendon against the coracoacromial arch, results in increased discomfort.

## WEAKNESS/PAIN

The presence or absence of pain and/or weakness is of great importance when assessing resisted motions. Five general presentations can occur: strong and painless, strong and painful, weak and painful, weak and painless, and all painful.[12]

If a particular resisted motion elicits no pain even when strong resistance is produced, there is no abnormality of the muscle complex responsible for that motion. Either repetitive resisted motion or an examination after a known aggravating activity is sometimes required for symptom provocation in certain individuals, particularly athletes or those patients with mild reactivity. Frequently, pain may be elicited in an apparently asymptomatic patient by applying an eccentric load. Eccentric loading is known to stress the muscle's passive element, that is, collagen, of which tendons are primarily composed.[11]

A strong and painful presentation upon a resisted motion typically indicates a lesion within a specific muscle, tendon, and/or tenoperiosteal region. Definition of a lesion can range from simple tendinitis, to minimal macro fraying of the tendon, to a partial- or even small full-thickness tear. The problematic musculotendinous unit will be identified by being most painful when tested in its primary direction of action. The degree of reactivity correlates well with associated pain.

A weak and painful response is seen commonly when a reactive or significant tear of the musculotendinous unit exist. This is often seen in patients with large rotator cuff tears, in whom resisted abduction and/or external rotation demonstrates significant weakness and pain. Other pathologies that present in this manner are tubercle fractures or neoplasms. Certainly, following any acute trauma, such as a dislocation, a weak and painful response to resisted motions may be encountered.

If more than one resisted motion is painful or weak, it becomes difficult to determine the primary structure at fault. Lesions involving shoulder musculature other than the rotator cuff are somewhat easier to identify because localized pain is produced during resistance of the muscle's primary motion, and the pain is typically localized away from the rotator cuff reference area. For example, pain associated with a pectoralis major tendon tear is felt along the distal portion of the muscle. It is more confusing to sort out which portion of the rotator cuff harbors a lesion based on resisted motions. The basic anatomy of the rotator cuff provides the answer for the confusion.

The rotator cuff is comprised of the supraspinatus, infraspinatus, teres minor, and subscapularis muscles; each is primarily responsible for a separate motion, yet their tendon fibers overlap, particularly the infraspinatus and supraspinatus, to form a dynamic enclosure posteriorly, superiorly, and anteriorly[8] (Fig. 5-15). The rotator cuff interval is the capsuloligamentous junction between the supraspinatus and subscapularis. Based on this fiber overlap and the rotator cuff interval "bridge," a tear of the supraspinatus is capable of causing pain with resisted abduction, external rotation, and/or internal rotation. Resisted external rotation activates the infraspinatus and teres minor muscles, thereby translating force to the area of overlap with the supraspinatus. Therefore, depending on the size of the supraspinatus tear, pain is elicited during resisted external rotation either by direct fiber association or by indirect involvement of the infraspinatus fibers. The same concept can explain pain with resisted internal rotation in the presence of a supraspinatus tendon tear.

To interpret what portion of the rotator cuff has a lesion, the most painful resisted motion must be identified and related to the muscle responsible for that motion. This becomes more complicated in the presence of moderate to large rotator cuff tears and weakness. Hawkins et al.[22] found that the best indicator of a rotator cuff tear was abduction and external rotation weakness. Even though most of the lesion is of the supraspinatus, the external rotators are found to have a significant strength deficit. This occurs because the external rotators lose their ability to translate force to their bony insertion and supraspinatus tendinous attachment. In the presence of chronic tears, abduction strength may be less

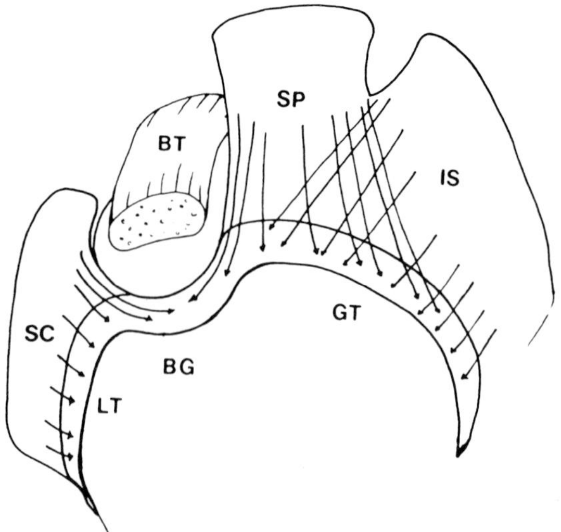


**Figure 5-15.** Rotator cuff fibers interlace and communicate anteriorly and posteriorly. (From Clark JC, Harryman DT. Tendons, ligaments, and capsule of the rotator cuff. J Bone Joint Surg 1992;74A:713.)

affected because of deltoid compensation. Weakness of abduction and external rotation, ruling out neurologic involvement, indicates a tear of the supraspinatus. The size (in centimeters), the completeness of the lesion (partial versus full thickness), the reactivity, and length of time from the last aggravating episode all determine the degree of pain and weakness found in both abduction and external rotation.

If the patient presents with no pain but has weakness, a massive or chronic large rotator cuff tear may be present. Whenever painless weakness is encountered, neurologic involvement also must be investigated to determine if the lesion is located at the cord, cervical root, plexus, or peripheral nerve level; a thorough evaluation by manual muscle, sensation, and reflex testing is essential.

When all resisted motions are painful, an acute inflammatory condition or recent traumatic episode probably exists, as in acute bursitis, the "freezing" phase of adhesive capsulitis (only the very reactive cases) in progressive glenohumeral joint degeneration, or rotator cuff arthropathy. If all clinical and diagnostic tests are negative, a psychogenic disorder or malingering should be considered.

## RESISTED ABDUCTION

Resisted abduction isolates the deltoid and supraspinatus muscles. The deltoid can sometimes be a source of pain in the postoperative patient whose surgery required splitting or elevation of the deltoid from the acromion. Occasionally, poor-quality tissue or too early return to activity results in inadequate fixation or tearing of the deltoid from the acromion. Such a patient is difficult to diagnosis and treat. Many of these patients have undergone rotator cuff surgery or acromioplasty due to impingement; thus the location and type of pain are similar to those associated with the primary problem. Another etiology of deltoid pain is trigger points, either primary or secondary in nature These are frequently seen in patients with a chronically deficient rotator cuff or postoperative rotator cuff repair.

To assess abduction, resistance is applied at the distal humerus at 0, 45, and 90 degrees of coronal plane or plane of the scapula elevation. The effect of position on pain is examined to help determine reactivity and mechanical effect on soft tissue (Fig. 5-16).

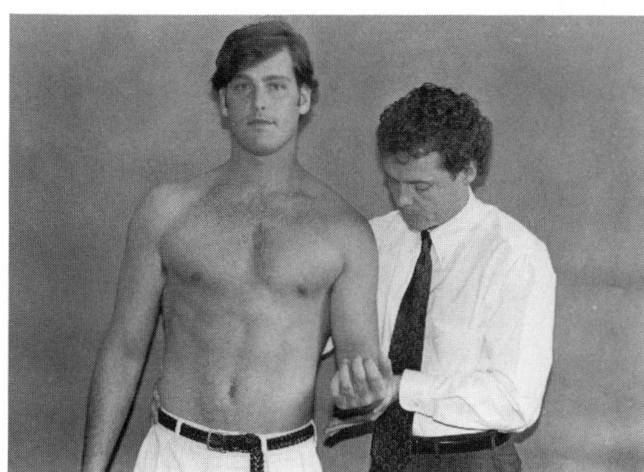

**Figure 5-16.** Resisted abduction at 0 degrees.

Usually when resisted abduction causes pain, a supraspinatus lesion is highly likely. Differentiating between tendinitis, partial-thickness cuff tear, and a small full-thickness cuff tear is very difficult. The degree of pain depends somewhat on the acuteness of the inflammatory state; weakness may or may not be present. A significantly reactive tendinitis may be more painful than a mildly reactive partial- or full-thickness supraspinatus tear. Many individuals have partial-thickness, small full-thickness, and even massive tears and function quite well without significant symptoms.[59] Abduction weakness can be the result of either a moderate (2 to 5 cm) or large (>5 cm) full-thickness rotator cuff tear (supraspinatus tear <2 cm also can cause weakness), C5 nerve root compression, upper plexus lesion, suprascapular nerve palsy, or axillary nerve palsy.

## RESISTED FLEXION

Although the supraspinatus is thought to be a primary abductor, 50 percent of flexion torque output is attributed to the supraspinatus and infraspinatus.[29] Therefore, it is not surprising that a supraspinatus tendon lesion often causes pain during resisted flexion. There appears to be a correlation between tissue reactivity and pain during resisted flexion, since there may be no pain during flexion in a mildly reactive supraspinatus tendonopathy, but there is pain during abduction. The clavicular fibers of the pectoralis major and anterior deltoid are also humeral flexors.

Resistance is applied at the distal humerus to isolate the glenohumeral joint and associated flexor muscles. The test can be performed in the sagittal plane at 0, 45, and 90 degrees. Involvement of clavicular pectoral fiber tears (although rare) is considered if pain is also present during resisted horizontal adduction. Anterior deltoid lesions are uncommon, except in the postoperative case, discussed previously under "Resisted Abduction."

Although the biceps is not considered to be a primary flexor, pain occasionally will be provoked during resisted flexion testing. Location of pain over the biceps groove helps identify the biceps as the culprit.

## RESISTED EXTERNAL ROTATION

The infraspinatus, teres minor, and posterior deltoid all contribute to external rotation, and 80 percent of this force is attributed to the posterior cuff.[55] It is essential to isolate external rotation during the resisted external rotation test. Resistance should be placed at the distal forearm, not the hand. Resistance over the hand, in the presence of lateral epicondylitis, could elicit pain due to wrist extensor activity. As the patient attempts to externally rotate, the clinician should stabilize the distal arm, but not to the point of encouraging abduction. Some patients are natural substituters; they try to either abduct the shoulder or extend or flex the elbow. This substitution allows the external rotators to appear stronger. If elbow flexion or extension substitution is detected, the dorsal aspect of the examiner's second and third middle phalanx is placed against the dorsal wrist. If the patient is employing elbow substitution, the wrist slips off the examiner's fingers (Fig. 5-17).

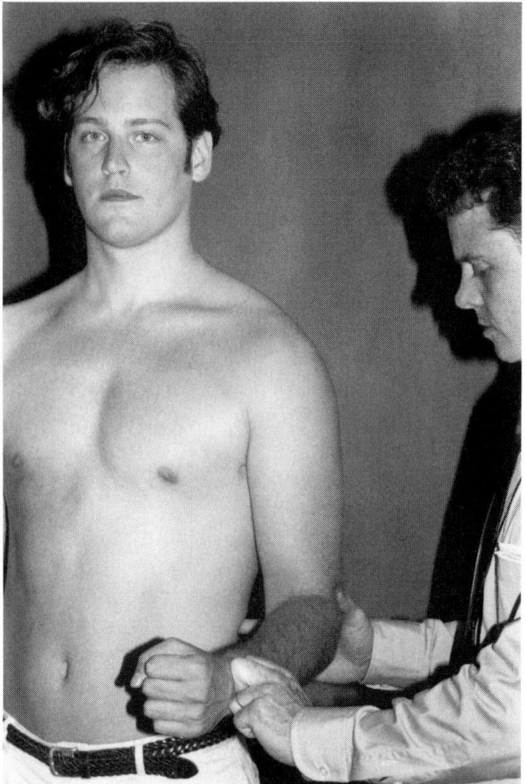

**Figure 5-17.** Resisted external rotation at 0 degrees.

When a supraspinatus lesion is present, pain and/or weakness can be experienced during resisted external rotation. Factors causing the degree of weakness are the same as discussed for resisted abduction.

Frequently, patients are seen who present with pain only during resisted external rotation; further testing then indicates an irritation of the infraspinatus or teres minor tenoperiosteal junction and/or tendon. The infraspinatus may house primary active trigger points that are painful during resisted external rotation and palpation. Commonly, an infraspinatus trigger point refers pain to the anterior shoulder.[65]

## RESISTED INTERNAL ROTATION

The internal rotators are the subscapularis, pectoralis major, teres major, and latissimus dorsi muscles. Pain with resisted internal rotation may indicate subscapularis involvement. Isolated tearing of the subscapularis has been reported to occur during traumatic anterior glenohumeral dislocation.[14] Surprisingly, these tears do not seem to produce chronic pain, although they are thought to contribute to recurrent instability. Trigger points also can cause pain with resisted internal rotation.[65] A supraspinatus tear extending to the rotator cuff interval also may elicit pain with resisted internal rotation due to the pull of the subscapularis on the associated torn fibers.

The clinician must consider the relationship of the capsuloligamentous complex with the rotator cuff when assessing contractile tissue signs in the presence of a capsular pattern (greater restriction of external rotation followed by abduction and less by internal rotation) or capsulitis. We have found a fairly consistent presence of pain during isolated internal rotation, performed with the arm at the side, during the "freezing" phase of adhesive capsulitis. Because the tendon is so intimate with the anterior capsule, tension translates from the subscapularis to the inflamed capsuloligamentous complex, producing pain. This is consistent with the findings of Clark et al.,[9] who mapped out the cohesive areas between the capsuloligamentous complex and the rotator cuff finding that $^2/_3$ of the CLC surface serves as an insertion for the rotator cuff (Fig. 5-18). Pain upon resisted internal rotation also may be present following a Bristow procedure. Because the coracoid is fixed to the scapular neck through the subscapularis or superior to the distal muscle belly, contraction of the subscapularis may be painful.

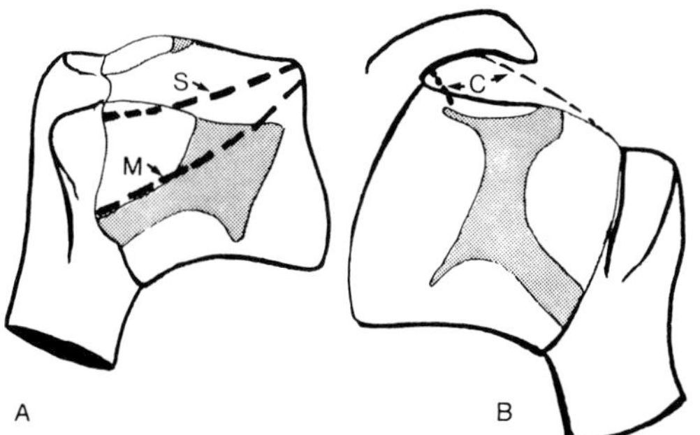


**Figure 5-18.** Zones of rotator cuff adherence to the capsuloligamentous complex. Regions of tendinous attachment are shaded lightly. Areas of muscle fiber attachment are shaded darker. (a) Anterior view. (b) Posterior view. *S*, axes of superior glenohumeral ligament; *M*, axes of middle glenohumeral ligament; and *C*, the margins of the coracohumeral ligament. (From Clark JC, Sidles JR, Matzen FA III. The relationship of the glenohumeral joint capsule to the rotator cuff. Clin Orthop 1990;254:29.)

Assessment of the internal rotators is performed at neutral and with resistance applied over the distal wrist. Strain or tearing of the latissimus dorsi, pectoralis major, and teres major can occur, but because these muscles are multiaction, prestretching them or altering shoulder position to accentuate their activity prior to applying resistance magnifies tension on the involved fibers and assists in identifying the source of pain.

Extensive rotator cuff tears can produce a boutonniere-type lesion through the superior cuff, causing the subscapularis tendon and posterior cuff tendons to slip inferiorly, altering their action from depressors to elevators. Activity of the subscapularis in this case causes superior migration of the humeral head into the coracoacromial arch[45] (Fig. 5-19).

## RESISTED EXTENSION

The shoulder extensors are the posterior deltoid, teres major, latissimus dorsi, and long head of the triceps. Typically, resistance to shoulder extension performed at neutral is painless, even in the presence of significant shoulder pathology. Therefore, information to help identify the source of pain is minimal, although weakness should appreciated if present.

## RESISTED ELBOW FLEXION

Elbow flexion isolates the biceps, brachialis, and brachioradialis; however, only the biceps long and short heads extend to the scapula. Resistance is applied to the distal wrist with the arm adducted, forearm supinated, and elbow flexed to 90 degrees (Fig. 5-20).

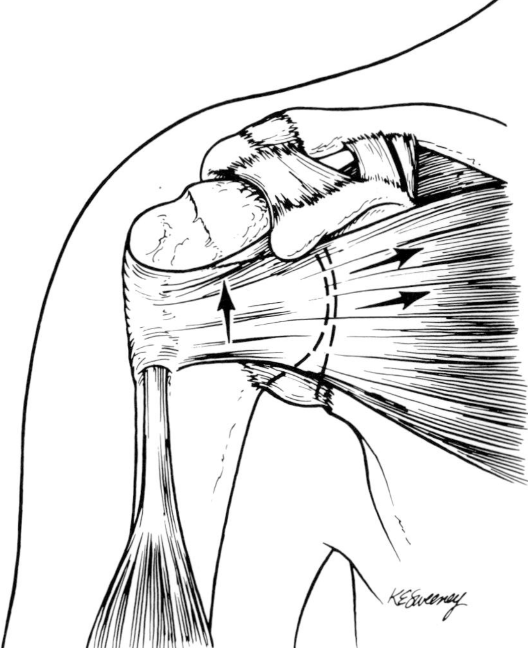

**Figure 5-19.** In the presence of a massive rotator cuff tear with significant cuff retraction, the humeral head can protrude superiorly similar to a "boutonniere" lesion. In this situation, the usual depressive action of the cuff muscles is lost, and the subcapularis causes elevation. (From Matzen FA III, Arntz CT. Rotator cuff tendon failure. In: Rockwood CA, Matzen FA III, eds. The shoulder. Philadelphia: WB Saunders, 1990:647.)

Cyriax[12] reported pain with resisted elbow flexion in the presence of long head of the biceps tendinitis. We have found this to be an unreliable test position in reproducing pain, even in moderately reactive biceps tendon inflammation. Provoking biceps tendon pain sometimes can be accomplished if resistance is applied when the shoulder and elbow are placed in extension in addition to forearm pronation, thereby increasing passive and active tension through the inflamed tendon. Combining humeral external rotation with elbow and shoulder extension further stretches the long head tendon and compresses it against the lesser tuberosity.

## RESISTED ELBOW EXTENSION

The elbow extensors are the triceps, and if pathology exists, commonly of the long head insertion into the infraglenoid rim, pain may be experienced with this test. Tendinitis of the triceps long head can occur in throwing, spiking, or racquet sport athletes. As with elbow flexion, different positions of elevation should be explored to place more tension across the long head and provoke symptoms.

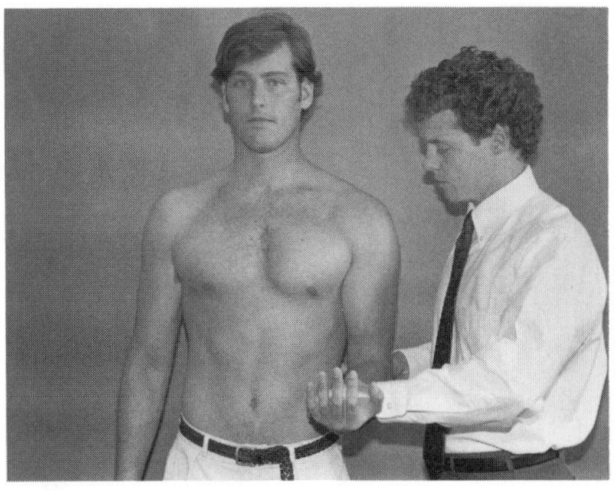
A

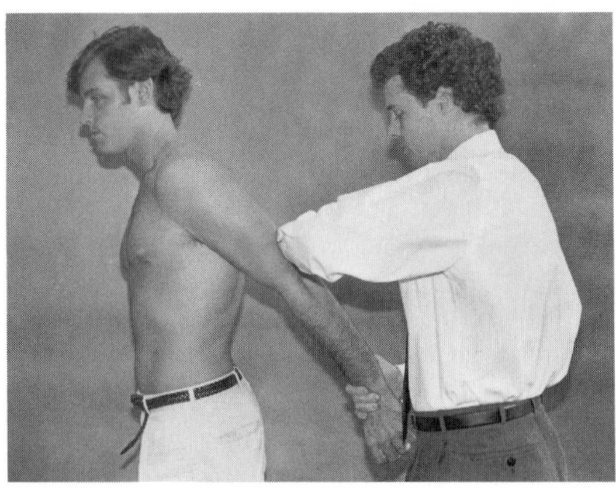
B

**Figure 5-20.** Resisted elbow flexion in (a) neutral shoulder position and (b) more provocative position.

The wrist and finger extensors and flexors as well as the intrinsics of the hand should be evaluated by resisted motions to determine distal muscle weakness either from neurologic or intrinsic myotendinous involvement, thereby completing the upper-quarter screen.

### SUMMARY

Resisted motions are of critical value when differentiating contractile from noncontractile tissue and identifying the involved musculotendinous unit. The examiner must be consistent in positioning, hand placement, and direction of force application yet explore various positions out of the neutral to gain additional information about the mechanical nature of the soft tissue, osseous structures, and their mutual relationship. Resisted-motion testing and the upper-quarter screen flow well together to also determine strength and the involved neurologic level. Completion of the upper-quarter screen by strength testing below the elbow is essential to correlate or confirm neurologic involvement.

## Passive Range of Motion

Assessment of passive range of motion, as opposed to resisted motion, primarily determines the status of noncontractile tissue, particularly the capsuloligamentous complex (CLC). Lesions or adhesions of the capsuloligamentous complex typically lead to restrictions in all planes, although limitations may predominate in one or several planes. Cyriax[12] describes two patterns of general restriction characteristics of all synovial joints: capsular and noncapsular.

The capsular pattern of the shoulder is described as having the greatest restriction in external rotation, followed by abduction and the least in internal rotation. The noncapsular pattern exists if the proportional limitations differ from the capsular pattern. Three pathology categories can result in a noncapsular pattern:

1. Isolated capsuloligamentous lesions
2. Internal derangement
3. Extraarticular limitations

Examples of each at the shoulder include an isolated lesion of the anterior capsule leading to limited external rotation, displaced labral tissue, and acute subdeltoid bursitis causing greater restrictions of abduction.

Four parameters are assessed during passive movement:

1. Range of motion
2. Presence of pain
3. Relationship between pain onset and end-range pain
4. End feel

Normal ranges for active and passive motion were discussed in Chapter 3.

### RANGE OF MOTION

Goniometry is performed to determine passive range of motion. Table 5-3 lists the technique and common substitutions to detect end range. Standardization of technique is absolutely essential in optimizing measurement reliability. Although some clinicians find goniometry unnecessary, we feel that it defines a baseline to gauge progress or regression.

### PAIN

The second parameter important in passive range-of-motion assessment is pain; in particular, when does pain occur? Does pain occur near

**Table 5-3**

**Goniometry**

| Plane of Motion | Excursion (degrees) | Movable Arm | Stationary Arm | Axis | Primary Capsuloligamentous Complex Area Stretch | Subsitution |
|---|---|---|---|---|---|---|
| Flexion | 160–180 | Humeral shaft to lateral epicondyle | Lateral trunk | Halfway between the postero-lateral acromion and axilla | Posterior and inferior | Excessive scapular rotation and/or elevation<br>Lumbar extension<br>Thoracic elevation (rib expansion)<br>Thoracic lateral flexion |
| Abduction (coronal plane) | 160–180 | Humeral shaft to medial epicondyle | In line with sternum | Center of axilla | Anterior and inferior | As above |
| Abduction (POS) | 160–180 | As above | As above | Approx. 1 in lateral to the coracoid process | Inferior | As above |
| Hyperextension | 50–65 | Greater tuberosity to lateral epicondyle | Lateral trunk | Greater tuberosity | Anterior and superior | Scapular anterior tilting and elevation |
| External rotation 90° (coronal plane) | 90–100 | Shaft of forearm to ulnar styloid process | The vertical or horizontal | Olecranon | Anterior and inferior | Scapular posterior tilting and depression |
| External rotation (0°) | 50–76 | As above | As above | As above | Anterior and superior | Scapular adduction |
| Internal rotation 90° (coronal plane) | 40–60 | As above | As above | As above | Posterior and inferior | Scapular anterior tilting and elevation |
| Horizontal adduction | 125–140 | Greater tuberosity to lateral epicondyle | Coronal plane | Superior acromion | Posterior | Scapular adbuction and lateral rotation |
| Horizontal abduction | 40–45 | As above | As above | As above | Anterior | Scapular adduction |

end range, at end range, or when overpressure is applied following end-range arrival? The clinician also needs to determine if a passive painful arc is present. On occasion, pain causing apparent limited motion abates only if further motion is pursued. Varying humeral rotation and plane of elevation can allow further range by mechanically relieving tissue compression.

Pain occurring before true end range, whether full or limited, signifies an inflammatory condition. This is commonly noted in acute bursitis, reactive rotator cuff pathology, and the early stages of reactive adhesive capsulitis. Pain arises from stretching irritated synovial-capsuloligamentous tissue or inflamed or torn tendon or by soft-tissue compression of structures such as the bursa and rotator cuff. The earlier pain is encountered in the range of motion, the greater is the inflammatory intensity or reactivity. Caution is required when evaluating and treating individuals in the early, or "freezing," stage of adhesive capsulitis, since forcing end range by stretching usually intensifies the condition. Pain present as end range is reached indicates less tissue reactivity and is commonly representative of patients in the intermediate, or "frozen," stage of adhesive capsulitis. Stretching should still be approached with caution. Pain sensed after achieving a premature end range demonstrates mild reactivity due to stretching constricted connective tissue. This is noted in the late, or "thawing," stage of adhesive capsulitis, when connective tissue is left thickened and adhesed but may not be inflamed.

## END FEEL

In conjunction with range of motion and pain, the end feel at end range should be scrutinized. *End feel* is the restrictive sensation perceived by the examiner when end range is attained. This tactile impression is valuable in determining the diagnosis and treatment approach. Six end feels have been identified[12]:

1. Soft-tissue approximation
2. Bone to bone
3. Springy
4. Capsular
5. Spasm (muscle guarding)
6. Empty

The former three are uncommon at the shoulder.

Soft-tissue approximation is normally met at several joints, such as the elbow and knee, when full flexion is available and only the soft-tissue mass prevents further motion. A normal bone-to-bone end feel is felt at full terminal elbow extension when a hard, abrupt feel is noted. A springy block end feel results from internal derangement, which is best appreciated at the knee having a displaced meniscal tear. Overpressure at end range engages the derangement between the articular surfaces, producing a "springy" effect.

A capsular end feel is considered normal at all shoulder end ranges. The actual tactile sense has been described as stretching a piece of leather—firm yet pliable.[12] The literature typically incriminates the capsuloligamentous complex as being responsible for normal capsular feel. However, recognizing the intimate relationship between the rotator cuff tendons and the capsuloligamentous complex,[9] tendinous tissue also must participate in the end feel. Turkel et al.[67] found that by incising the subscapularis, external rotation range of motion increased by 18 degrees when performed with the arm at the side. Obviously, this tendon primarily limits external rotation and thus is also responsible for the end feel. A clinical example of this concept is appreciated following a Magnuson-Stack procedure for recurrent anterior instability. The subscapularis tendon is transferred laterally over the bicipital groove, thus limiting external rotation. Examination of these patients postoperatively, regardless of time frame, reveals a "capsular end feel." Although not classically regarded as a component of "capsular" retriction at the shoulder, direct rotator cuff tendon matrix alterations due to inflammation or secondary involvement of the rotator cuff due to functional immobility also can limit range. In essence, it is difficult to rationalize that passive motion is not limited to some degree, whether in the normal or pathologic condition, by the rotator cuff tendons and/or surrounding shoulder musculature.

Cyriax[12] uses the term *spasm* to describe an end feel characterized by involuntary protective muscle activity reflexively initiated by pain. Because spasm has a confusing connotation, we choose the term *muscle guarding*. Two types of muscle guarding have been described, fast and slow.[5] Fast muscle guarding occurs as twinges of protective muscle activity when the arm is moved through the range of motion or at end range. Slow muscle guarding is more controlled yet prevents further motion. The clinician can be fooled by slow muscle guarding because, at some point, undetectable muscle activity limits the motion, mimicking a capsular end feel. This phenomenon was clearly illustrated during personal assessment of individuals with a diagnosis of reactive adhesive capsulitis who were manipulated. Preanesthetization assessment revealed what appeared to be a capsular end feel, yet reevaluation while the patient was unconscious demonstrated up to 30 degrees of increase in range, proving that the pre-anesthetized end feel was due to muscle guarding.

An empty end feel is sometimes encountered in the presence of subdeltoid bursitis; here, pain is so significant that reflexive inhibition of the shoulder muscles occurs. A sense of mechanical limitation is absent at an early end range, with motion limited only by pain. An empty end feel also can be encountered in patients with scapular or acromial fractures or nondisplaced humeral head fractures.

## Accessory Motions (Joint Play)

Passive range of motion can furnish us with a general status of noncontractile tissue regarding hypermobility and hypomobility. Assessment of accessory motion provides specific information concerning joint capsuloligamentous contracture or hyperelasticity. All the joints encompassing the shoulder complex can be evaluated and treated using accessory motions. *Accessory motions* are movements not under voluntary control but essential for normal joint function.[34,43] At the glenohumeral joint, these include anterior, posterior, and inferior humeral head gliding, as well as distraction. All except distraction are considered component motions, defined as and necessary for full active motion.[34,43]

### LOOSE-PACK POSITION

The loose-pack position (LPP) should be used for accessory motion assessment. The glenohumeral joint's loose-pack position falls through the scapular plane and is defined as 55 degrees of abduction and 30 degrees of forward flexion.[34] In the loose-pack position, the capsuloligamentous structures are maximally relaxed, allowing the greatest joint-play excursion. The clinician needs to visually appreciate articular surface orientation so that directional gliding is performed with the articular surfaces parallel to one another. Bilateral comparison is essential to determine mobility asymmetry. As in passive range of motion, reactivity can prevent valid joint-play assessment due to muscle guarding.

The author would like to point out the difficulty in assessing millimeters of motion during glenohumeral accessory motion evaluation. The challenge is attempting to stabilize a relatively free-floating scapula in addition to recognizing soft-tissue (i.e., skin, fat, muscle) "give"; end-feel perception is also influenced. The position for which the author finds greater annecdotal ability to assess joint gliding is with the arm at the side (load and shift test) or in the alternate position for loose-pack position assessment, which will soon be discussed. These positions allow excellent scapular stabilization for assessment in all directions.

### ANTERIOR GLIDE

The loose-pack position is assumed with the patient supine or prone. The proximal humerus is displaced anteriorly and medially, since gliding is considered parallel with the articular surfaces in the scapular plane. When the position is performed supine, the clinician should stabilize across the anterior shoulder to minimize scapulothoracic and sternoclavicular contribution (Fig. 5-21a). The anterior capsuloligamentous complex is isolated primarily during this maneuver. Prone positioning is advantageous because the table stabilizes the scapula, resulting in better glenohumeral isolation. The alternative position to maximize scapular stability and maintain the loose-pack position is sitting (see Fig. 5-21b).

### POSTERIOR GLIDE

The patient is supine, and the arm is in the loose-pack position. The examiner places one hand over the anterior proximal humerus and displaces the humeral head posteriorly and laterally. The posterior capsule is assessed primarily in this position. The clinician must recognize that posterior gliding is normally greater than anterior gliding, with approximately half the humeral head normally translating posteriorly with respect to the glenoid.[19,20]

### INFERIOR GLIDE

The examiner cradles the involved arm between his or her body and arm, securing the patient's proximal arm. The clinician's other hand is placed over the proximal humerus. The slack is taken up in the scapulothorasic joint, and then the humeral head is displaced inferiorly. Inferior glide assessment performed in the loose-pack position evaluates the inferior capsuloligamentous complex (see Fig. 5-21).

A click or clunk may be encountered with directional gliding. This could indicate excessive laxity leading to subluxation or reduction. Clicking itself does not necessarily indicate pathology, but painful clicking can be indicative of a labral tear.

Joint-play assessment of the sternoclavicular, acromioclavicular, and scapulothoracic joint will be addressed in Chapter 7.

## Stability Testing

Stability testing utilizes specific techniques and positions to determine if the glenohumeral joint

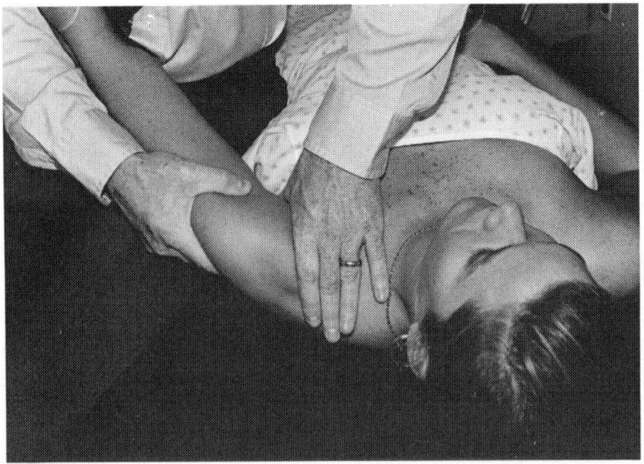

A

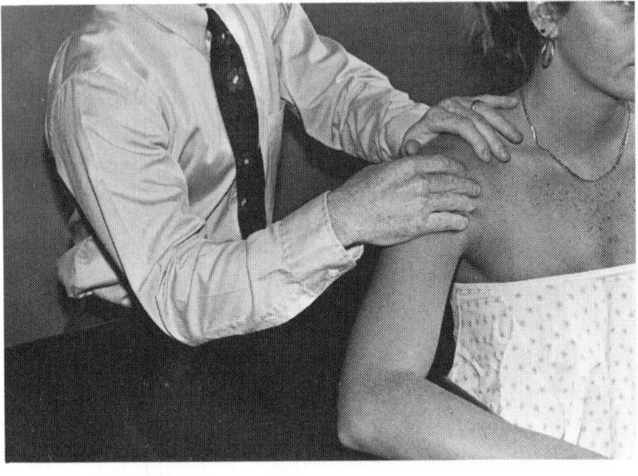

B

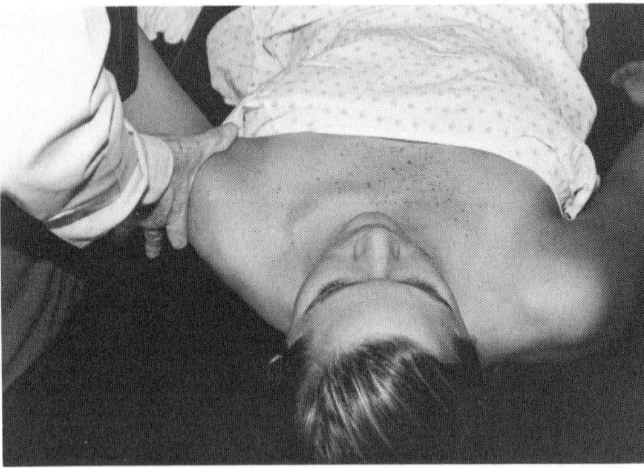

C

**Figure 5-21.** Loose-pack position assessment for (a) anterior glide, (b) alternate position, and (c) inferior glide.

is unstable. Conceptually, these tests are similar to accessory joint motions in their purpose to determine mobility. Some test are similar to joint-play assessment except that they are performed out of the loose-pack position or encompass humeral rotation to further provoke signs and symptoms.

Stability testing should be performed on all patients. Commonly, the history will help determine the presence of instability, but not always. In many instances, the diagnosis of rotator cuff tendinitis or impingement is often applied to a patient when, in fact, symptoms are secondary to a primary instability problem. Bilateral comparison is essential to determine asymmetry. In the multidirectionally unstable patient, capsuloligamentous laxity may be symmetrical, but symptoms may be present on only one side.

A word of caution must be put forth regarding humeral translation assessment. Accessory motions and draw signs are subjective and gain credence when performed in the symptomatic, grossly unstable patient, particularly if excursion findings are asymmetrical. Patient relaxation is absolutely essential. When attempting to quantify excursion in the subtly unstable patient, validity is questionable.[63] Only with standardization of technique and experience does the test attain meaning.

## HYPERELASTICITY/ HYPOELASTICITY

Assessing hyperelasticity or hypoelasticity at other joints is essential. The metacarpophalangeal joints, wrist, elbows, and knees should all be evaluated for mobility (Fig. 5-22). Determining gross connective-tissue hyperelasticity will aide in diagnosis and treatment. Typically, the multidirectional instability (MDI) patient will demonstrate hypermobility of other joints. Determining general connective-tissue elasticity can be a valuable guide in assessing a postoperative patient for recurrent dislocations. Those who are hyperelastic are monitored so that motion does not return too quickly. This contrasts with hastening the rehabilitation in a patient with hypoelastic connective-tissue characteristics who demonstrates early postoperative tightness.

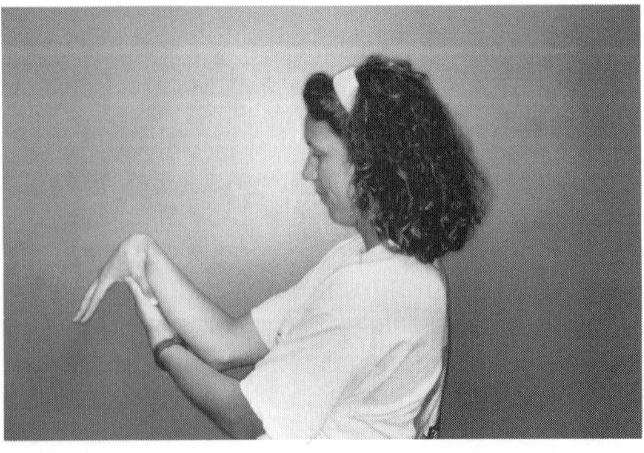

**Figure 5-22.** Patient demonstrating typical hyperelastic feature at the wrist.

## LOAD AND SHIFT TESTS

Hawkins[19,20] described a load and shift test that is a modification of the drawer sign. It is an attempt to quantify directional translation of the humeral head (Fig. 5-23). Before attempting to assess glenohumeral translation, the humeral head is "reduced" or loaded into the glenoid fossa to ensure an appropriate anatomic position. The humeral head is then glided either anteriorly, posteriorly, or inferiorly. "Loading" the joint allows the examiner a better sense of humeral head translation with respect to the glenoid fossa and rim.

The load and shift test is similar to assessing anterior and posterior translation in the loose-pack position, except that it is done with the patient sitting with the arm at the side. Because the glenoid fossa is oriented 30 to 45 degrees to the coronal, the drawer testing should be performed at an oblique angle, perpendicular to the scapular plane. Straight sagittal plane posterior motion would drive the humeral head into the posterior glenoid, while anterior translation would combine lateral distraction, pulling the humeral head away from the glenoid rim.

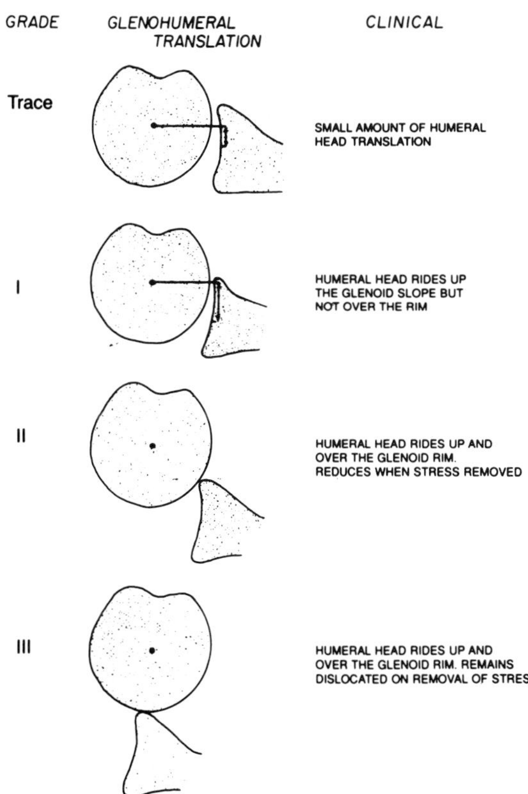


**Figure 5-23.** Representation of load and shift test assessing humeral head glide (translation) relative to the glenoid. (From Hawkins RJ, Bokor DJ. Clinical evaluation of shoulder problems. In: Rockwood CA, Matzen FA III, eds. The shoulder. Vol. 1. Philadelphia: WB Saunders, 1990:67.)

### ANTERIOR DRAWER

The patient is assessed sitting with the arms supported on the thighs. The examiner stabilizes the scapula with one hand and with the other grasp the humeral head between the thumb posteriorly and the fingers anteriorly. The head is loaded and then moved anteriorly and medially so that "true" parallel glide of the joint surfaces is achieved (Fig. 5-24a). Excursion is assessed to determine increased or decreased translation. Painful and painless clicking also should be noted. In some very unstable shoulders, the humeral head can be subluxed manually or even dislocated. Typically, the patient will complain of posterior joint pain.

### POSTERIOR DRAWER

Hand placement is the same as above, but the humeral head is displaced posteriorly and laterally (see Fig. 5-24b). Approximately one-half the humeral head can be normally displaced posteriorly.[20] Thus posterior translation is always considered greater than anterior translation in the normal condition. Care should be taken in "legitimizing" pain with this maneuver. Commonly, the patient reports pain over the biceps groove because of finger compression; this should not be confused with pain associated with increased posterior translation. Both the posterior and anterior drawers can be performed supine.

### MODIFICATIONS

Assessment of the previously described anterior and posterior joint-play techniques can be enhanced by adding humeral rotation. This is very helpful when assessing posterior instability. The arm is examined in the loose-pack position for gliding posterior translation in neutral with respect to humeral rotation. The arm is then internally rotated, tightening the posterior capsule, which should result in very little posterior translation. If increased excursion is still noted compared with the nonsymptomatic side, posterior pathologic instability exists (Fig. 5-25). Humeral external rotation also can be incorporated when assessing anterior gliding and can be compared with the uninvolved side.

### SULCUS SIGN

The sulcus sign is used to determine inferior instability (Fig. 5-26). The arm is kept at the side with the examiner pulling inferiorly at the distal humerus. The examiner's opposite hand palpates the space between the anterolateral acro-

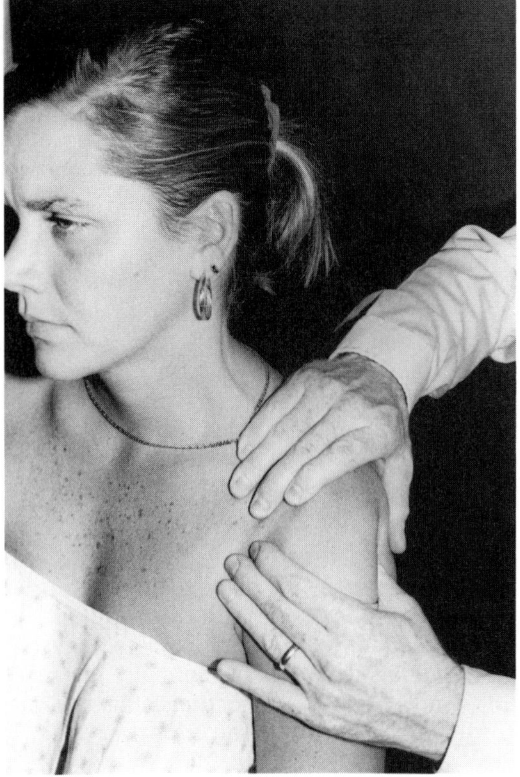

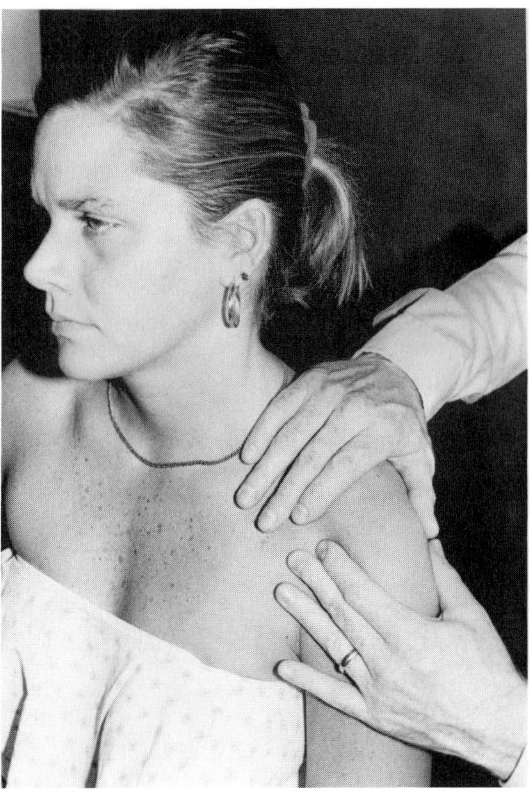

A B

**Figure 5-24.** Position for load shift testing for (a) anterior and (b) posterior draw assessment.

mion and the humeral head. Minimal separation should occur. Increased or asymmetrical gapping will cause a depression or "sulcus" of the skin inferior to the acromion, indicating laxity. As with all tests assessing translation, the patient needs to be relaxed when performing the sulcus sign; if not, increased activity of the deltoid or rotator cuff results in a false-negative result.

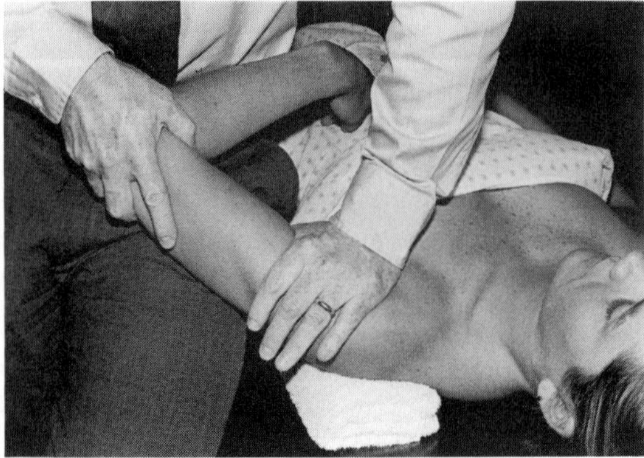

**Figure 5-25.** Modification of loose-pack position for assessing posterior instability.

## APPREHENSION SIGN (CRANK TEST)

The apprehension sign is used to reproduce the symptoms associated with anterior instability by using the provocative position (Fig. 5-27). The patient can be sitting or supine, and the arm is placed in 90 degrees of coronal plane abduction, followed by external rotation of the humerus. The patient having anterior glenohumeral instability will muscle guard because of *posterior* joint pain or react with apprehension, sensing imminent subluxation. This reaction is considered positive and is called a *positive apprehension sign*. The report of pain by itself does not indicate instability.

## FULCRUM TEST

The fulcrum test uses the provocative position of 90 degrees of abduction and external rotation while attempting to lever the humeral head anteriorly with the examiner's opposite hand. This further challenges the anterior capsuloligamentous-labral complex, and if a deficit exist, pain, apprehension, and possibly subluxation result (Fig. 5-28).

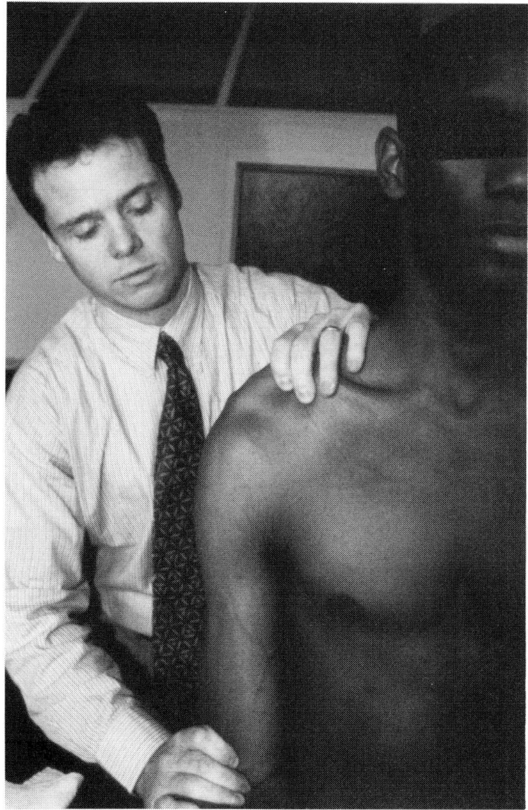

**Figure 5-26.** Sulcus sign.

## RELOCATION TEST

This test was described initially by Jobe and Moynes[32] to assist in identifying patients with subtle anterior subluxation. The test position is similar to that of the apprehension sign. The arm is placed in 90 degrees of coronal abduction, followed by humeral external rotation. If pain or apprehension is demonstrated, the examiner repeats the test but manually displaces the humeral head posteriorly (Fig. 5-29). By doing so,

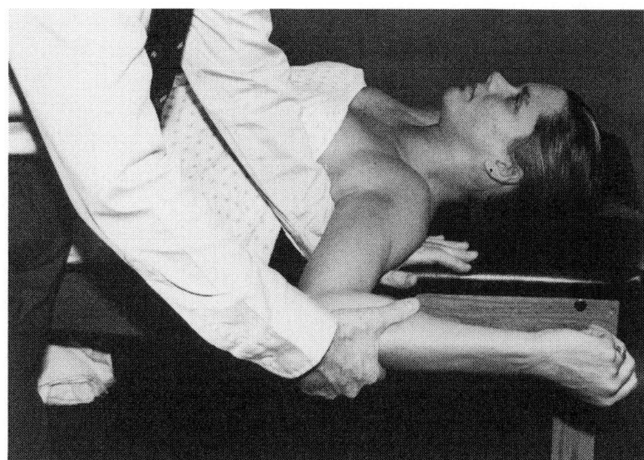

**Figure 5-28.** Fulcrum test.

theoretically, the anterior subluxation is reduced or "relocated"; if pain or apprehension lessens, the test is considered positive.

We have found this test to be helpful in identifying patients with subtle anterior instability as well but also have found it positive (for pain) in older patients with rotator cuff pathology and no instability. There appears to be two mechanisms through which the relocation test is positive in those patients with only rotator cuff pathology. In a patient with pain at full external rotation end range at 90 degrees of abduction, the greater tuberosity and associated rotator cuff tendon (particularly the supraspinatus) contact the posterior glenoid rim and labrum. This recently has been confirmed arthroscopically and by CT scan.[69] By manually displacing the humeral head posteriorly, the supraspinatus is lifted from the glenoid rim, relieving "impingement" and thus decreasing symptoms (Fig. 5-30). Rotator cuff impingement on the posterior glenoid rim also has been demonstrated in the fully elevated position by magnetic resonance imaging.[63] The second mechanism is related to the coracoacromial arch and appears in patients who have limited

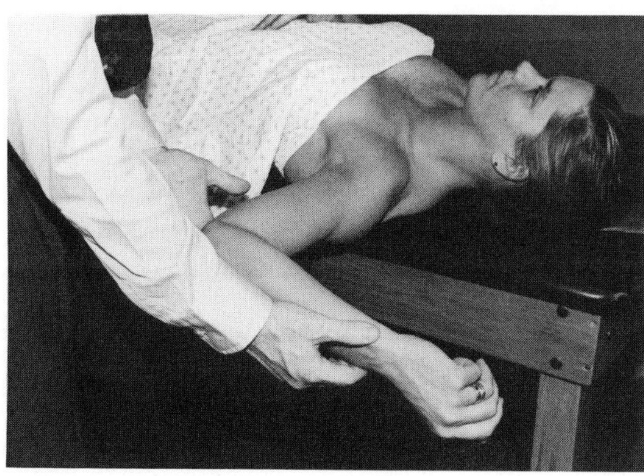

**Figure 5-27.** Apprehension sign.

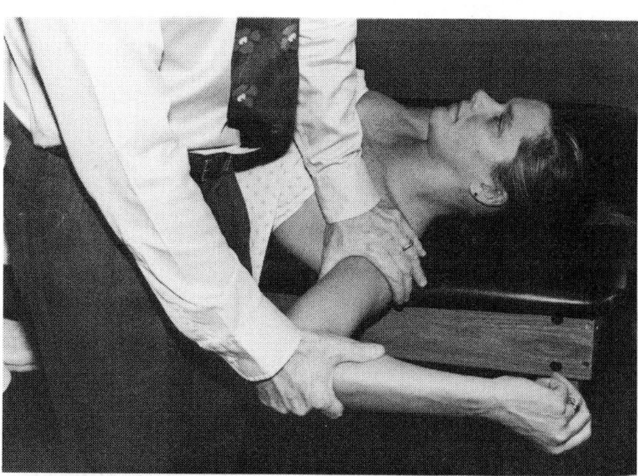

**Figure 5-29.** Relocation test.

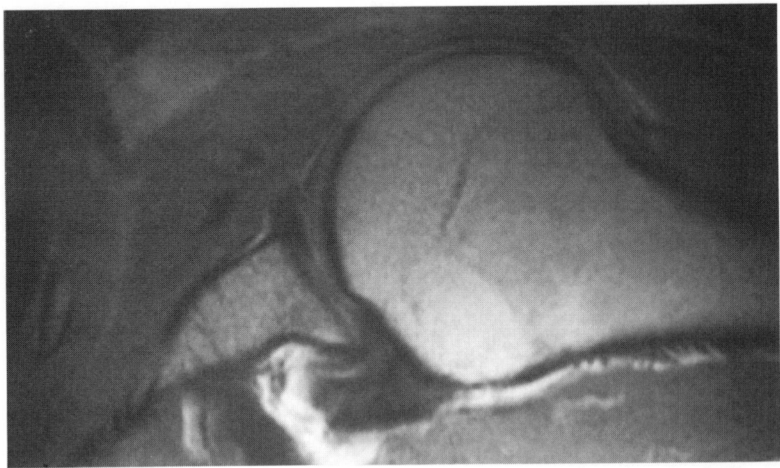

A

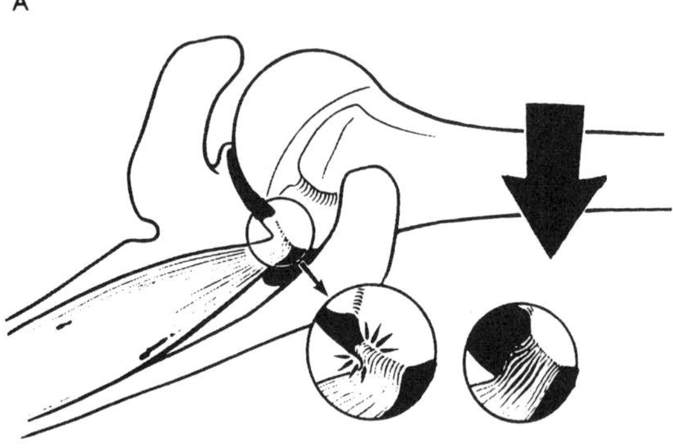

B

**Figure 5-30.** (a) CT scan demonstrating supraspinatus impingement against the poste.ior glenoid rim in 90 degrees of abduction, full external rotation, and horizontal abduction. (b) Schematic of impingement and mechanism of pain relief due to posterior glenoid impingement during relocation test. (From Walch G, Boileau P, Noel E, Donell T. Impingement of the deep surface of the supraspinatus tendon on the posterior glenoid rim: an arthroscopic study. J Shoulder Elbow Surg 1992;1:239.)

and painful external rotation of 30 to 60 degrees and muscle guarding or a soft end feel at end range. Posterior displacement of the humeral head changes the orientation of the rotator cuff tendons and bursa to the coracoacromial arch, which relieves painful impingement and allows further motion.

## POSTERIOR APPREHENSION TEST

Patients with posterior instability typically experience subluxation as opposed to frank dislocation; therefore, it is sometimes more difficult to provoke symptoms or subluxation when performing the posterior apprehension test.

The arm is placed in 90 degrees of elevation and horizontal adduction while applying a posterior axial load to the humerus (Fig. 5-31). Subluxation may be felt with application of the posterior force, or reduction may be imparted to the examiner's hand as the arm is moved toward the coronal plane; either is considered a positive test. Posterior pain due to stretching of the posterior cuff and capsule without posterior mechanical displacement occurs and helps determine posterior instability. This test is typically found painful soon after a dislocation or painful subluxation episode.

## SUMMARY

Accessory motion and stability testing assess the restrictive status and capabilities of the capsuloligamentous soft tissue surrounding the

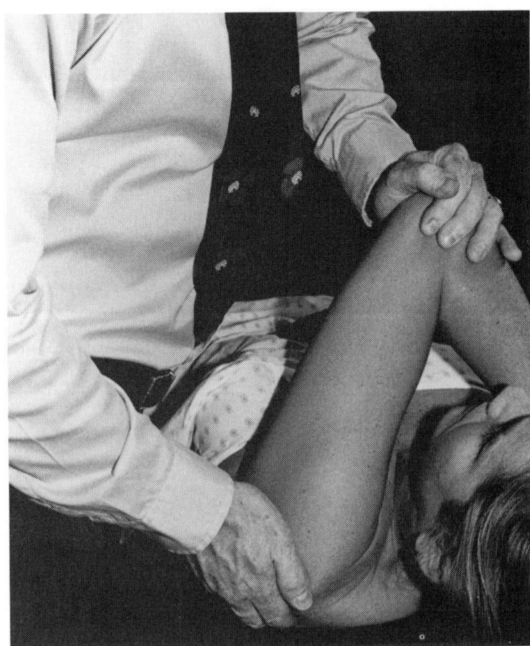

**Figure 5-31.** Posterior apprehension test.

shoulder joint by determining if excessive or reduced motion is allowed. To gain valid information from this portion of the evaluation, the clinician must (1) posses knowledge of positional influence on the static restraints, (2) stabilize the proximal segment when able to, and (3) compare findings with the uninvolved side. Experience and correlation with the history and diagnostic tests are absolutely vital.

# Special Tests

Numerous special tests and signs have been reported in the literature over the years. These help to further elucidate the involved structures and are helpful in determining diagnosis.

## IMPINGEMENT SIGN

This maneuver was popularized by Charles Neer[48] in the early 1970s. He overwhelmingly felt that the anterior acromion was the sight of impingement of the rotator cuff. To perform the test, the patient's arm is passively elevated while the scapula is stabilized (Fig. 5-32a). This maneuver reduces scapular rotation and thus causes the inflamed supraspinatus tendon and bursa to impinge against the anterior acromion. If the patient reacts painfully, the test is considered positive. Hawkins modification of this maneuver has been described by the placing the arm into elevation and then forcibly internally rotating the humerus. This is felt to impinge the supraspinatus tendon against the coracoacromial ligament[21] (see Fig. 5-32b).

We feel that performing this test at 20-degree intervals from the sagittal plane to posterior of the coronal plane helps determine the mechanical influence of position on the rotator cuff–bursa complex, as well as the reactivity status. Although not demonstrated by a controlled study, we feel that there is a change in the rotator cuff–bursa orientation to the overlying arch depending on the plane of elevation (Fig. 5-33). The author's anecdotal sense is that pain in one plane of elevation as opposed to another indicates the lesion size and general location on the rotator cuff or degree of inflammation. For example, a positive impingement sign when performed in the sagittal plane and negative in all other plane tested indicates a smaller lesion and less reactivity. This contrasts with pain felt when the impingement sign is performed at 20-degree intervals from the sagittal plane to posterior of the coronal plane, indicating a large cuff lesion or significant inflammation of the rotator cuff–bursa complex. If pain is felt only when the arm is placed posterior to the coronal plane, one can speculate that a posterior cuff lesion is present. In this position, the supraspinatus is no longer under the coracoacromial arch; instead, the infraspinatus and teres minor fill the subacromial space (see Fig. 5-33c).

The clinician should be careful not to spontaneously deduce that the presence of a positive impingement sign resulted from true mechanical impingement; one does not necessarily indicate the other. For example, a baseball pitcher completes a nine-inning game and has significant discomfort the following day. If an impingement sign is performed, it is positive not because of mechanical impingement, but because his rotator cuff tendons are inflamed and swollen from overuse due to tensile loading and the "position" of the impingement sign compresses the inflamed tissue. After a number of days, the inflammation resolves, the impingement sign is negative, and the pitcher is ready to throw again.

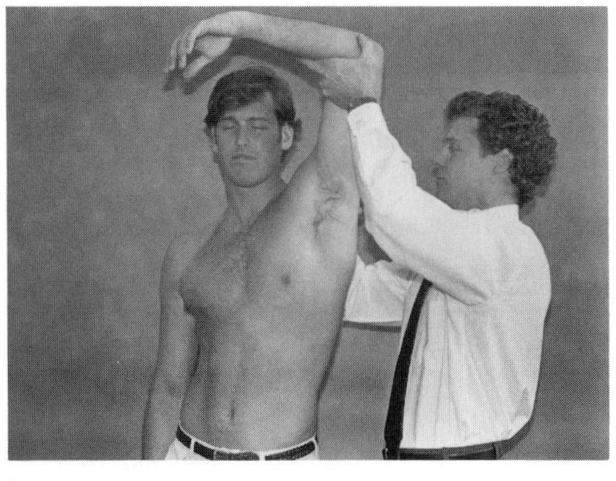

A B

**Figure 5-32.** Impingement sign: (a) Neer and (b) Hawkins.

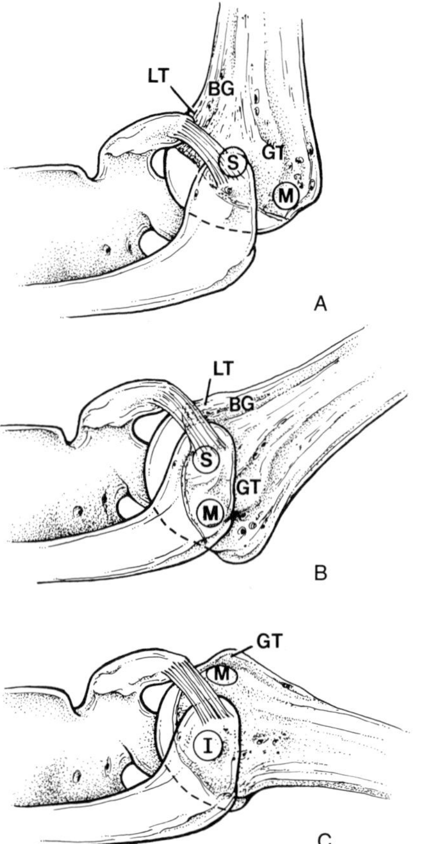


**Figure 5-33.** Multiangle impingement sign showing change in orientation of the rotator cuff insertions to the coracacromial arch. LT: lesser tubercle; BG: biceps groove; GT: greater tubercle; S: superior facet; M: middle facet; I: inferior facet.

The impingement test can follow a positive impingement sign. Here, 10 cc of lidocaine or marcaine is injected into the subacromial space, which numbs the inflamed bursa and rotator cuff tendons. After approximately 5–10 minutes, the impingement sign is repeated. If the patient demonstrates a significant reduction in pain, the test is considered positive. A positive test indicates rotator cuff and/or bursal involvement. The subacromial space may then be injected with cortisone to reduce tissue inflammation. If the patient has no change in pain or only partial relief, occasionally the biceps tendon and/or the acromioclavicular joint is then injected and the impingement sign is performed again. This demonstrates how both the impingement sign and the impingement test are used diagnostically to isolate the involved tissue. If no relief of symptoms is noted after the impingement test, a different etiology should be suspected.

## SUPRASPINATUS ISOLATION TEST (ABDUCTION/INTERNAL ROTATION)

The supraspinatus isolation test differs from the impingement sign in that it is performed actively and is followed by resistance. This position has been demonstrated to isolate the supraspinatus by EMG testing.[32]

The patient is asked to elevate the arm to 90 degrees in the scapular plane and then internally rotate the humerus by pointing the thumb down. (Fig. 5-34). This may be painful, since it replicates an impingement sign position. The examiner then applies resistance into adduction. If a tendinous supraspinatus lesion exists, a painful and/or weak response is evoked. Contralateral comparison is essential in determining weakness, since most individuals can easily be "broken" from the test position.

The test also should be performed at 45 degrees of abduction, which is below the impingement zone. In this position, subacromial tissue compression or impingement is avoided, yet the musculotendinous unit is still isolated due to the manual resistance applied. If pain significantly reduces and/or strength improves compared with the 90-degree position, impingement of the bursa without significant tendon involvement should be suspected.

The examiner must consider the effect this test has on the biceps tendon. Many patients presenting with biceps tendinitis also will report pain with this test. The examiner needs to further differentiate between the biceps tendon and the rotator cuff if both conditions exist simultaneously.

## REVERSE IMPINGEMENT SIGN

This sign, to the authors knowledge, has not been described previously in the literature. It is

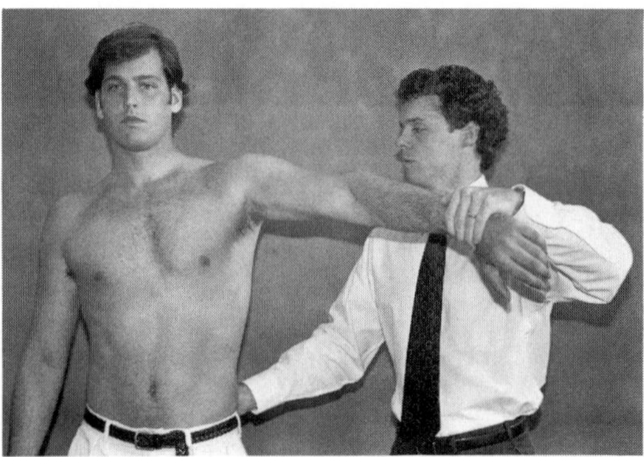

**Figure 5-34.** Supraspinatus isolation test (abduction/internal rotation).

occasionally present when a positive impingement sign exists and frequently when a painful arc and/or pain is present during passive external rotation at 90 degrees of coronal plane abduction. If pain is present during external rotation, the arm is brought back to neutral rotation. The examiner manually glides the humeral head inferiorly by applying a proximal force; external rotation is again attempted. If external rotation range of motion significantly improves because pain is alleviated, the sign is considered positive. This maneuver also can be performed during active or passive abduction. The patient is placed supine, and the test is performed with either active or passive abduction, depending on which is painful. Again, the humeral head is moved inferiorly while abducting, and change in pain noted. If symptoms reduce significantly during the performance of the reverse impingement sign, it is an indication that the subacromial tissue is the source of pain because of mechanical impingement. By manually displacing the humeral head, the subacromial space is widened, and its contents are allowed to move unencumbered, thus relieving pain and increasing range. The reverse impingement sign appears more consistently in patients having small cuff lesions or low reactivity.

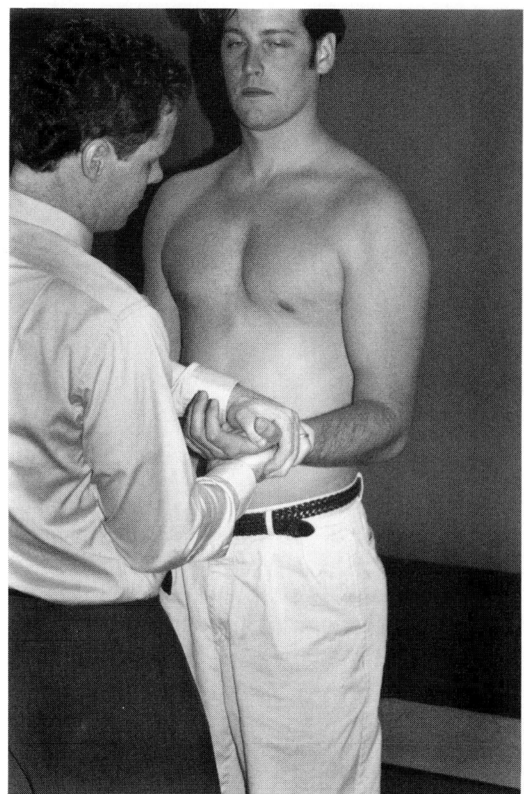

**Figure 5-35.** Yergason's sign (supination sign).

## YERGASON OR SUPINATION SIGN

Yergason first published the following test in 1931, crediting Dr. F. J. Caulter with its origin.[70] He described the test as having the patient's elbow flexed to 90 degrees with the forearm pronated. The patient actively supinate's while the examiner resists at the distal forearm (Fig. 5-35). The sign is consider positive when pain is reproduced over the bicipital groove. During this test, the inflamed long head of the biceps and sheath are pulled against the lesser tuberosity causing pain. When biceps tendinitis is present, we have found pain reproduction with resisted supination more consistently than pain with resisted elbow flexion. The examiner should be cautious about concomitantly resisting external rotation during the Yergason test. Patients unconsciously attempt to externally rotate while they supinate. If rotator cuff pathology exists in the presence of an ill-performed Yergason maneuver, a misleading positive Yergason sign will be interpreted. Supine placement of the patient can assist in better stabilization and isolation of supination.

## SPEED'S TEST

This test is performed to provoke pain associated with biceps inflammation. The patient is asked to elevate the arm to 60 degrees in the sagittal plane with the forearm supinated. Resistance is applied at the wrist, thus activating the biceps (Fig. 5-36). The location of pain over the biceps groove is important to note, since Speed's test also can produce symptoms in the presence of rotator cuff pathology.

## LUDINGTON'S TEST

This test is directed primarily toward provoking pain from the long head of the biceps tendon. The patient places the hands to the top of the head. The patient then contracts the biceps; if pain is increased, the biceps tendon may have a lesion. If the muscle belly is palpated and felt to contract weakly or lack any contraction, a rupture to the long head may be present.[42]

## PASSIVE HORIZONTAL ADDUCTION

A painful response when placing the upper extremity into horizontal adduction can indicate several pathologies or dysfunctional structures: (1) the acromioclavicular joint, (2) coracoid impingement, (3) posterior instability, (4) posterior

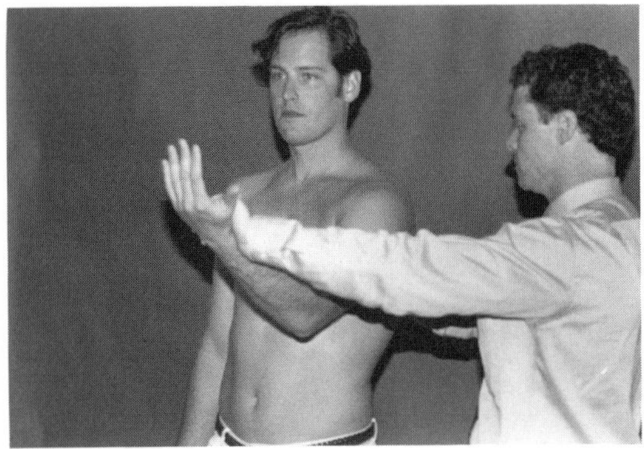

**Figure 5-36.** Speed's test.

capsular tightness, or (5) a rotator cuff lesion. In part, the location of pain will help distinguish the structure at fault. The examiner should keep in mind the presence of double lesions. Commonly, rotator cuff pathology exists in conjunction with acromioclavicular joint arthritis (Fig. 5-37).

### ACROMIOCLAVICULAR PATHOLOGY

A grade II or grade III separation of the acromioclavicular joint may be easily identified by history, palpation, and x-ray. A grade I separation or joint arthritis can be difficult to detect by history or palpation. Horizontal adduction results in tension of the superior acromioclavicular joint ligament and also causes joint compression. Pain is localized over the joint when positive.

### CORACOID IMPINGEMENT

Although the same maneuver is performed, the location of pain differs in the presence of coracoid impingement, being medial to the biceps tendon and lesser tuberosity, over the coracoid. During horizontal adduction, the coracoid bursa can be compressed by the lesser tuberosity, producing pain.

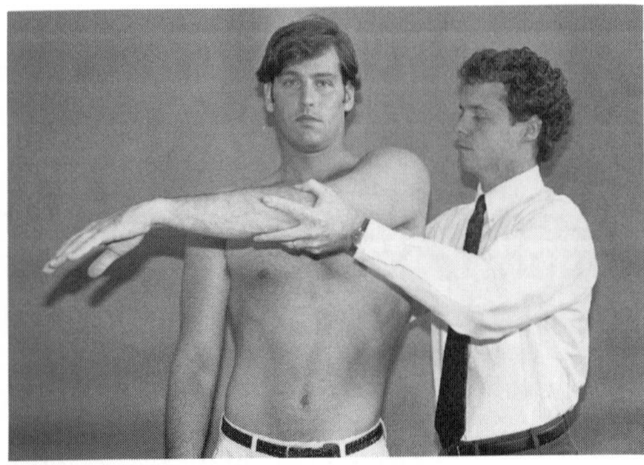

**Figure 5-37.** Passive horizontal adduction.

### POSTERIOR INSTABILITY (REFER TO POSTERIOR APPREHENSION TEST

### POSTERIOR CAPSULAR TIGHTNESS

Restriction of the posterior joint soft tissues can lead to mechanical subacromial impingement during elevation and flexion.[44] Horizontal adduction can identify tightness by stretching the posterior capsule and rotator cuff; pain may or may not be produced.

To assess posterior capsular/cuff tightness accurately, the examiner should stabilize the lateral scapula, preventing scapular abduction and lateral rotation and thus isolating glenohumeral motion (Fig. 5-38). The degree of restriction is then estimated by measuring, in inches, the olecranon's relationship to the nose or by goniometric measurement. The opposite arm is then assessed and asymmetry noted. Commonly, the dominant hand side is found to be restricted.

### ROTATOR CUFF PATHOLOGY

Placing the arm into horizontal adduction can painfully compress the subacromial soft tissue, causing pain. Differentiating acromioclavicular pain from rotator cuff pain depends on the location of the pain. Rotator cuff pain is commonly felt laterally or superiorly yet diffusely or is localized anterior to the acromion, as opposed to localized acromioclavicular joint discomfort.

# Neural Tests

## SENSATION/REFLEXES

Sensation testing is imperative to determine neurologic involvement demonstrated by cutaneous disruption. Light touch, pin prick, and thermal descrimination should be determined in all dermatomes.

Reflexes need to be examined bilaterally at the biceps (C5), brachioradialis (C5–C6), and triceps (C7). Reflex absence or sluggishness is recorded and correlated with other findings.

## ELVEY TEST

This test is analogous to the straight-leg raise in the lower extremity. Tension is placed throughout the upper extremity's peripheral neurologic network with primary focus on the median nerve and the C5–C7 nerve roots. This test is very useful in determining the presence of a subtle brachial plexopathy.

The test is performed with the patient supine and the involved extremity positioned at 90 de-

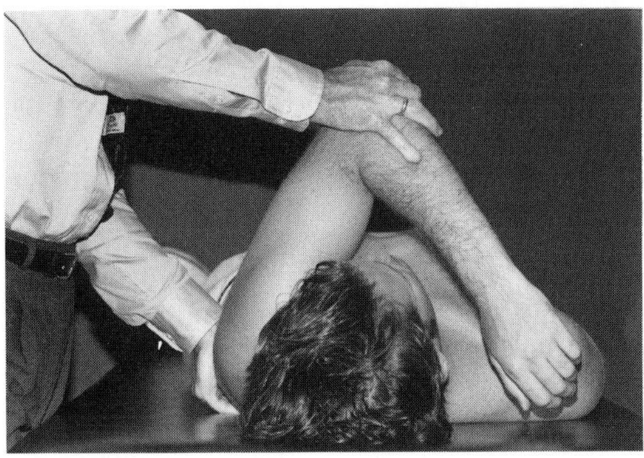

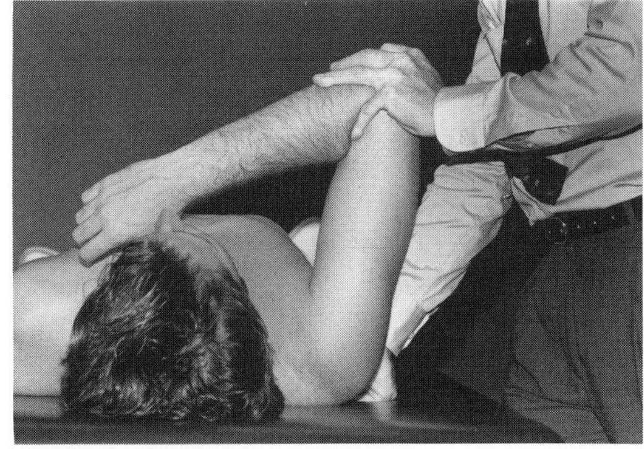

A B

**Figure 5-38.** Passive horizontal adduction with scapular stabilization to assess glenohumeral motion. (a) Normal. (b) Restricted.

grees of abduction and external rotation, keeping the elbow flexed. The examiner determines symptom changes as the shoulder girdle is depressed while moving the arm into horizontal abduction. The elbow is then extended, keeping the forearm supinated and the wrist extended (Fig. 5-39). The patient may experience radicular pain, a stretch or ache in the shoulder or cubital fossa, or paresthesia. To accentuate the stretch, cervical contralateral side bending can be performed. Comparison must be made with the asymptomatic side using the degree of elbow extension and symptoms as a reference.

## TINEL SIGN

This test has been described as eliciting tenderness from a neuroma.[25] In fact, paresthesia caused by compression of neural tissue will be augmented when assessing this sign's presence. The test can be performed anywhere along the nerve path, but the sign is best elicited over the more superficial areas of neural tissue. Areas the sign is best assessed are Erb's point, the medial arm, the ulnar groove, medial to the common flexor tendon origin, the middle of the volar aspect of the wrist, and over the pisiform. The test is performed by tapping over the choosen area; if paresthesia or pain is produced at the region or more typically within the involved nerve sensory distribution, the sign is considered positive. This indicates involvement of the nerve at that level and/or somewhere proximal along the neural track. For example, a positive Tinel sign is commonly elicted at the ulnar groove, yet the lesion may be in the brachial plexus.

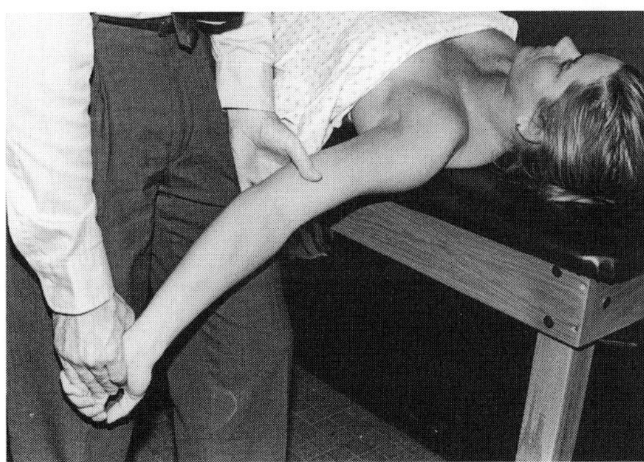

**Figure 5-39.** Elvey sign.

# Vascular Tests

The clinical diagnosis of vascular compromise is suggested by provocation or relief of signs and symptoms by selective anatomic positioning and alteration of tissue tensions.

The examiner must attempt to evaluate changes induced in the arterial, venous, and nervous systems during each diagnostic maneuver. Three or more distinct anatomic sites in the shoulder girdle region can be involved in the production of thoracic outlet syndrome. The classic diagnostic maneuvers attempt to provoke neurovascular disturbances by introducing mechanical forces at these specific sites.

Test maneuvers and general examination for vascular compromise are performed with the patient seated and well stabilized. All tests are performed bilaterally and compared. The examiner should begin with observation of the hands, resting palms up on the thighs. Notation of color is made in the dependent position and observed for change when in the test position. Skin temperature and moisture are noted. With the palms down and forearms pronated and resting on the thighs, the radial pulse is monitored at the wrist. The pulse volume or strength is assessed bilaterally in the rest position. Bilateral brachial blood pressures can be taken and compared. A difference of more than 30 mmHg is significant.[39]

Symptom reproduction or intensification is one objective of the following tests. The patient is asked to report the location, nature, and intensity of symptoms before each diagnostic maneuver while in the rest position and provide commentary on perceived changes during and immediately following each test.

## ADSON MANEUVER

This test position was designed by Alfred Adson to produce compression on the subclavian artery within the interscalene space. His original description is as follows:

> The test consists of having the patient take a long breath, elevate his chin and turn it to the affected side. This is done as the patient is seated upright, with his arms resting on his knees. An alteration or obliteration of the radial pulse or change in blood pressure is a pathognomonic sign of the presence of a cervical rib or the scalenus anticus syndrome.[1]

Primarily a vascular test, there is also strong probability that the brachial plexus becomes partially compressed when the artery is displaced posteriorly against trunks of the plexus.[1,19] The venous system is not influenced directly because the subclavian vein is not normally located in the interscalene space. A variation in the test includes turning the chin to the opposite side, which exerts greater compression in certain individuals.[1,7,19]

A common error is removing the arm from its supported position on the thigh or placing traction on the limb. Once this occurs, the examiner has introduced stretch on the course of the neurovascular bundle, losing localization of forces exerted only in the interscalene region. The author's preferred method of testing is performed in three stages, as shown in Figure 5-40.

Halstead's test extends the neck and turns the head to the opposite shoulder; then downward traction is given to the ipsilateral limb.[19]

If the test is found to be positive when performed in this manner, it can only be interpreted as a general indicator of neurovascular disturbance. This becomes an important consideration when planning corrective exercises or surgical intervention.

## COSTOCLAVICULAR MANEUVER

The exaggerated military posture is used to produce compression on the retroclavicular portion of the neurovascular bundle in the costoclavicular space. With the patient seated, forearms resting on the thighs, palms down, the radial pulse is monitored at the wrist. The patient is instructed to sit upright, protrude the chest, and pull both shoulder blades down and back together. This position is held for a minimum of 10 seconds while the radial pulse is monitored resting on the lap. Bilateral comparisons of pulse volume are made.[7,19,39]

An alternate position places the patient supine on the examining table with the hands resting on the abdomen. Using the thenar pad of one

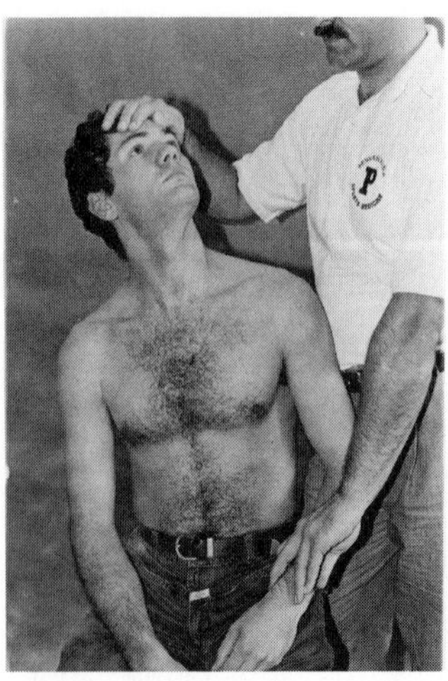

A

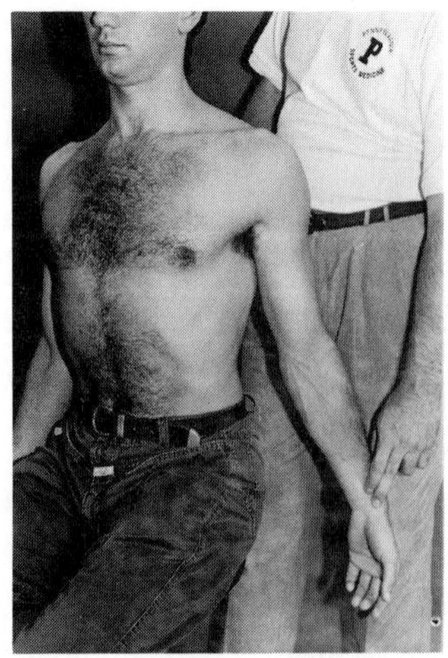

B

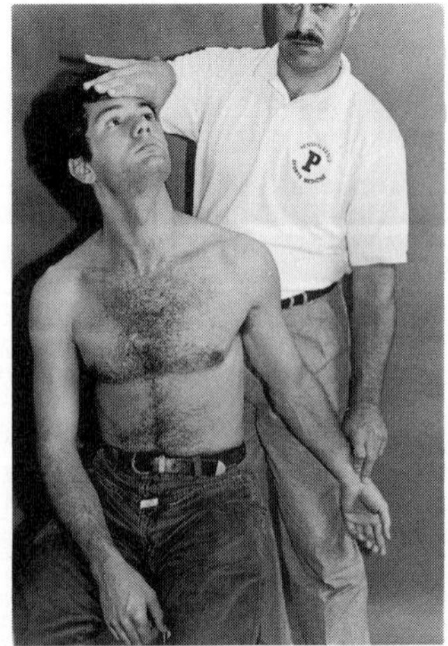

C

**Figure 5-40.** Adson test. (a) Isolated cervical motion. (b) Isolated upper extremity motion. (c) Completed test position.

hand, the examiner applies manual pressure directed down and back on the medial clavicle, while the other hand monitors the pulse.

## SHOULDER GIRDLE RELIEF POSITION

This test can be used when signs or symptoms are already present before performing the costoclavicular diagnostic maneuver or after symptoms have been provoked by the latter test. The patient is seated or standing. The examiner grasps the patient's arms and passively elevates the shoulder girdle up and forward, thereby increasing the dimensions of the costoclavicular spaces. It is important that the shoulder girdle be elevated passively by the therapist to eliminate adverse influences of muscle tension. (Fig. 5-41) With some patients who find it difficult to relax, the test works better sidelying with the side to be tested placed upward. This position should be maintained for a minimum of 30 seconds, and the patient is queried about changes in symptoms. Prolonged neurogenic compression is typically described as "numbness" in the forearm and hand, frequently in the ulnar distribution. When pressure is relieved from the nerve trunk, this perceived numbness changes to "pins and needles" or tingling. As ischemia is relieved and circulation increases in the nerve, some pain may occur at that location, but distal symptoms continue to abate. This progression of symptoms is sometimes referred to as the *release phenomenon*. Arterial relief is evidenced by increased pulse volume, increased hand temperature, and color changes from white or mottled to pink. Venous relief is detected by reduction in venous engorgement and cyanotic appearance of the hands.

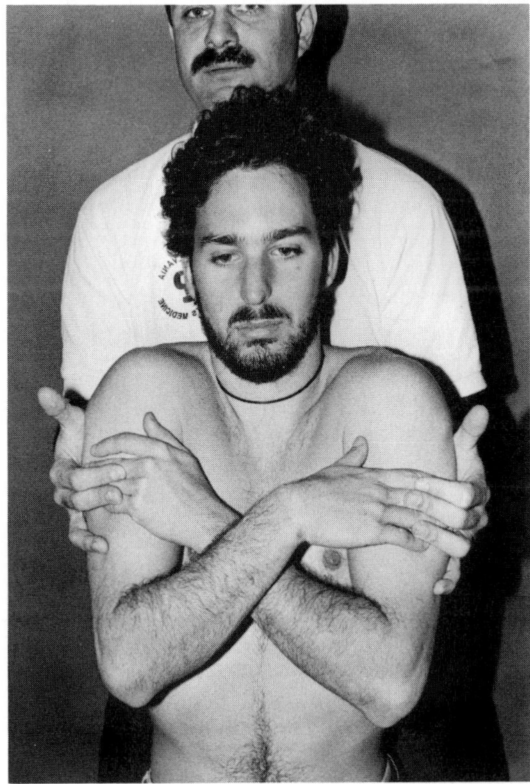

**Figure 5-41.** Shoulder girdle relief test.

## HYPERABDUCTION TEST MANEUVER

Wright identified two additional anatomic sites of potential neurovascular irritation: the subclavius muscle, costocoracoid ligament, and clavipectoral fascia in the infraclavicular region and the insertion of the pectoralis minor tendon at the coracoid process. The hyperabduction, or Wright's, test produces both compression and strong stretch on the neurovascular bundle.[7,19,39]

The radial pulse is monitored in the rest position with the patient seated. The upper extremity is passively positioned with the elbow in approximately 45 degrees of flexion and elevated to the level of the patient's eyes. The limb is drawn posterior to the coronal plane, and effort is made to draw the pectoralis minor and clavipectoral fascia taut. This results in increased soft-tissue compression and strong stretch around the coracoid, which functions now as a pulley to intensify the stretch. This stretch probably is distributed to some extent along the nerve pathway distal and proximal to site, decreasing the specificity of the test to the pectoral region.[7,19,60]

## ELEVATED ARM STRESS TEST

The elevated arm stress test (EAST), also referred to as the *Roos test*,[60] attempts to provoke symptoms by combining exercise to increase metabolic demand with positioning to reduce vascular supply. The patient is seated, and the arms are elevated to 90 degrees of abduction and external rotation and then brought posterior to approximate the scapulae. The patient closes and opens the grip repeatedly at a rate of approximately one repetition per second. The test is continued for up to 3 minutes. The examiner should coach the patient to maintain the correct position throughout the duration. The test is timed, and the point of fatigue or quitting is recorded. The patient is then examined for vascular signs such as pallor, venous engorgement, and skin temperature and is queried on the occurrence, location, and nature of symptoms produced.

The elevated arm stress test is useful to detect thoracic outlet syndrome in less pronounced cases, but because it stresses the entire upper extremity, neck, and shoulder girdle simultaneously, it is not specific to the location or mechanism involved.

### DIFFICULTIES IN TESTING

Diagnostic accuracy can prove difficult for several reasons. The list of signs and symptoms attributed to thoracic outlet syndrome is extensive, but the signs and symptoms are typically intermittent in nature. Changes in the radial pulse volume occur in many asymptomatic individuals; the absence of change in the radial pulse suggests the lack of significant arterial compression but does not rule out venous or neurologic involvement. Inflamed nerves will be sensitized to stretch or compression distal to the site of the lesion, and more than one lesion can coexist.

### SUMMARY

Special tests are extremely reliable in identifying the structure at fault, but the clinician should not solely rely on a specific test to determine the diagnosis. For example, a positive impingement sign is typically thought to indicate primary mechanical impingement; however, the clinician must correlate the history and information compiled about muscle strength, restricted soft tissues, and stability testing to determine if the positive impingement sign is just identifying *symptoms* (subacromial tissue inflammation), whereas the *primary* problem is muscle weakness, tight or lax static restraints *causing* rotator cuff overuse, or mechanical compression of the cuff tendon and bursa. Table 5-4 correlates some physical assessment signs and tests with commonly seen pathologies.

## Palpation

Palpation is performed to detect temperature changes, atrophy, and swelling and to identify bony landmarks and structures such as muscle bellies and tendons. Temperature change can give an indication of inflammation or reduced circulation. Warmth commonly exists following surgery as the healing process continues. In severe to moderate reactive rotator cuff irritation, warmth may be noticed about the greater tuberosity.

Subtle swelling or atrophy may be palpated by symmetrically "smoothing" with the fingers the areas around the deltoid and scapular fossae for contour asymmetry. Occasionally, a defect can be palpated at the supraspinatus/infraspinatus insertion in patients with large rotator cuff tears. Crepitus and clicking are palpated for during both active and passive range of motion. Crepitus can indicated articular or rotator cuff deficits, while clicking about the shoulder can be quite normal. Tracing clicking to soft-tissue, labral, or articular origin can be challenging because of the ability of bones to transmit vibration. Symptomatic clicking should be noted and entered into evaluation data. Painless clicking, such as that which occurs at the biceps tendon when throwing, can become painful with repetitive mechanical irritation.

The examiner needs to gain appreciation for normal tender areas responding to deep palpation. These include the biceps groove, coracoid process, inferior posterior deltoid fibers, and lesser tubercle. Without prior knowledge of vulnerable tenderness or if palpated without contralateral comparison, significant erroneous information can be gathered. Knowledge of referred pain zones and trigger points is invaluable in establishing a diagnosis and treatment plan. The clinician may become frustrated when palpation is performed over the reference pain area, since the lesion lies elsewhere.

Lastly, accurate palpation can only be performed if the clinician has appropriate knowledge of anatomy and biomechanics. Anatomic visualization is essential to strip away the overlying tissue, and biomechanical principles are required to fully expose the underlying structures. For example, although the supraspinatus insertion to the greater tuberosity lies anterior to the acromion in the resting position, full exposure is gained through humeral internal rotation, extension, and adduction.[13,68]

### STERNOCLAVICULAR JOINT

The sternoclavicular joint can be found easily just lateral to the sternal notch. (Fig 5-42) Movement is felt as the shoulder girdle is elevated, depressed, protracted, or retracted. Abrupt joint motion occurring as the arm is elevated could indicate subluxation.

### ACROMIOCLAVICULAR JOINT

The acromioclavicular joint is found at the distal lateral clavicle junction with the acromion. Point tenderness could indicate pathology, and contralateral comparison is required. Following a grade II or grade III separation, the scapula depresses as a consequence of coracoclavicular and acromioclavicular ligament tearing. This results in a noticeable prominence of the distal

Table 5-4

**Correlation of Some Physical Findings with Common Shoulder Pathologies**

| | Supraspinatus Tendinitis | Supraspinatus Partial Tear | Rotator Cuff Full-Thickness Tear (1–5 cm) | Rotator Cuff Full-Thickness Tear (>75 cm) | Infraspinatus Tendinitis | Subscapularis Tendinitis | Biceps Tendinitis | Adhesive Capsulitis Stage I | Stage II | Stage III | Anterior Instability[x] | Posterior Instability[x] | Multidirectional Instability[x] | Acute Bursitis | Chronic Fibriotic Bursitis | Acromioclavicular Joint Sprain/Arthritis | Glenohumeral Joint Arthritis |
|---|---|---|---|---|---|---|---|---|---|---|---|---|---|---|---|---|---|
| *Passive:* | | | | | | | | | | | | | | | | | |
| G-h abduction | f− | f+/− | f+/− | f/sl +/− | f− | f− | f− | sl/ml + | ml+ | sgl +/− | f− | f− | f− | sgl + | f+ | f+ | sl/ml +/− |
| Elevation | f− | f+/− | f+/− | f/sl +/− | f− | f− | f+/− | sl/ml + | ml+ | sgl +/− | f− | f− | f− | sgl + | f+ | f+ | sl/ml +/− |
| ER at 90° | f− | f+/− | f+/− | f/sl +/− | f− | f+/− | f+/− | sl/ml + | ml+ | sgl +/− | f/sl + | f− | f/sl + | sgl + | f+ | f+/− | ml/sgl +/− |
| ER at 0° | f− | f+/− | f+/− | f/sl +/− | f− | f+/− | f+/− | sl/ml + | ml+ | sgl +/− | f+ | f− | f− | sgl + | f+/− | f+ | ml/sgl +/− |
| IR at 90° | f− | f+/− | f+/− | f/sl +/− | f+/− | f− | f− | sl/ml + | ml+ | sgl +/− | f− | f− | f− | sgl + | f+ | f+ | ml/sgl +/− |
| Functional IR | f+/− | f/sl + | sl/ml + | sl/ml + | f+/− | f− | f+/− | sl/ml + | ml+ | sgl +/− | f− | f− | f− | sgl + | f+/− | f+ | ml/sgl +/− |
| Horizontal add | f+/− | f+/− | f+/− | f+/− | f+/− | f+/− | f+/− | sl/ml + | ml+ | sgl +/− | − | f+/− | f+/− | sgl + | f+/− | f+ | sl/ml +/− |
| Painful arc (80–120°) | + | +/− | +/− | +/− | +/− | +/− | +/− | − | − | − | − | − | − | − | +/− | − | − |
| *Resisted* | | | | | | | | | | | | | | | | | |
| Abduction | +/− | + | + | + | +/− | +/− | +/− | +/− | +/− | − | − | − | − | + | − | − | +/− |
| Flexion | +/− | + | + | + | +/− | +/− | +/− | +/− | +/− | − | − | − | − | + | − | − | +/− |
| ER | +/− | + | + | + | + | − | − | +/− | +/− | − | − | − | − | + | − | − | +/− |
| IR | +/− | +/− | +/− | +/− | − | +/− | +/− | +/− | +/− | − | − | − | − | + | − | − | +/− |
| Elbow flexion | − | − | − | − | − | − | +/− | +/− | − | − | − | − | − | + | − | − | − |
| Elbow extension | − | − | − | − | − | − | − | +/− | − | − | − | − | − | +/− | − | − | − |
| Abd/IR 90° | + | + | + | + | + | +/− | +/− | + | +/− | − | − | − | − | + | +/− | − | +/− |
| Abd/AR 45° | + | + | + | + | + | +/− | +/− | + | +/− | − | − | − | − | + | − | − | +/− |
| Impingement sign | + | + | + | + | + | − | +/− | + | + | − | − | − | − | + | + | +/− | +/− |
| *Apprehension sign | − | − | − | − | − | − | − | − | − | − | + | − | + | − | − | − | − |
| IRelocation test | +/− | +/− | +/− | +/− | +/− | − | +/− | − | − | − | + | − | + | − | +/− | − | − |

*Codes:* **f** = full motion; **sl** = slight limitation (<25%); **ml** = moderate limitation (25–75%); **sgl** = significant limitation (>75%); + = painful; − = painless; * = apprehension not pain; I = pain or apprehension; and x = resisted motions are painful if tendons inflamed.

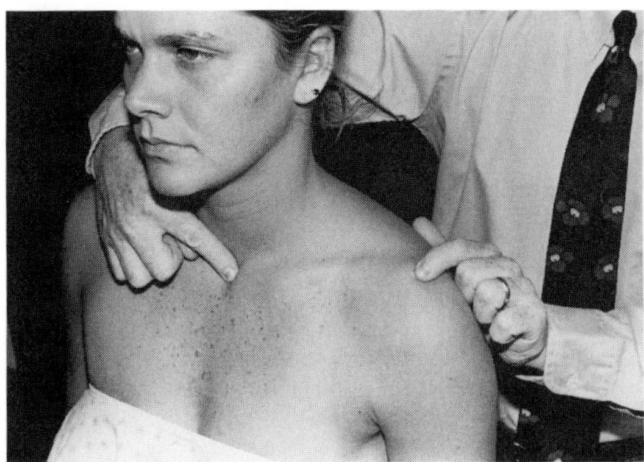

**Figure 5-42.** Palpation of the sternoclavicular and acromioclavicular joints.

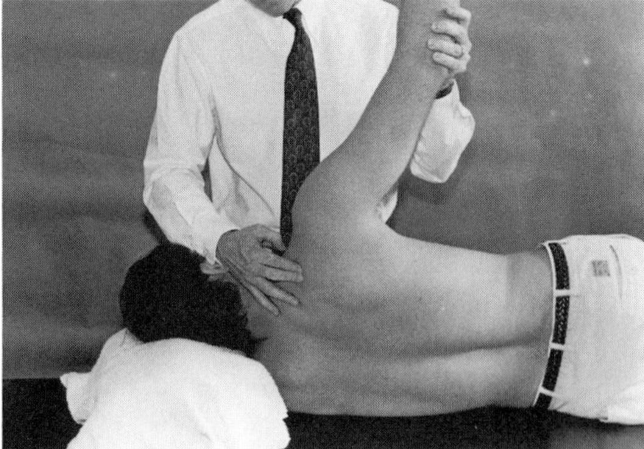

**Figure 5-43.** Isolated palpation of the supraspinatus muscle belly.

clavicle compared with the uninvolved side (see Fig. 5-42).

## SUPRASPINATUS

### BELLY

The supraspinatus muscle belly can be difficult to isolated because the upper trapezius blankets it superiorly. Commonly, in a chronic condition such as a large rotator cuff tear or a suprascapular nerve injury, atrophy is appreciated by hollowing of the fossa. Atrophy may not be present in a recent injury, and palpation to determine supraspinatus contraction during active elevation is frustrating because of the trapezius obligatory activity. To better palpate the supraspinatus muscle belly, the patient is placed side lying on the uninvolved side; this places the trapezius in a relatively gravity-eliminated position for arm elevation. The examiner then passively places the patient's involved upper extremity into abduction to approximately 60 degrees, and then, while palpating over the supraspinatus belly, the patient is asked to maintain this position. The supraspinatus belly can be felt to contract through the relatively inactive trapezius. If no contraction is felt, interruption of the muscle tendon unit or innervation is suspected (Fig. 5-43).

### MUSCULOTENDINOUS JUNCTION

Cyriax[13] describes palpation of the supraspinatus musculotendinous junction just posterior to the distal clavicle and anterior to the suprascapular spine. Pain at this location could indicate the lesion location.

### TENDON

Full exposure of the supraspinatus tendon insertion should be gained by placing the patient's arm into functional internal rotation (Fig. 5-44). This position completely exposes the tenoperiosteal junction and tendon.[13,67] Using the anterolateral acromion as a reference, move approximately 2 cm inferiorly; this is where the tendon and tenoperiosteal junction are palpated. The subacromial bursa also can be palpated in this position.

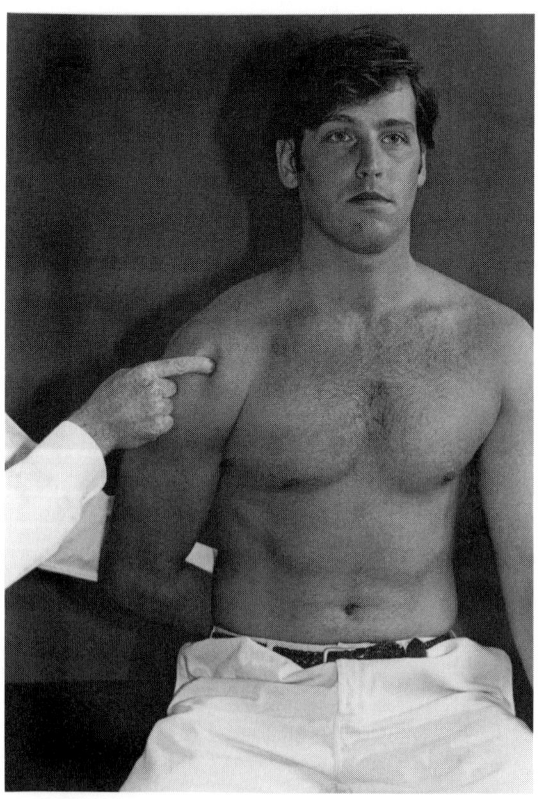

**Figure 5-44.** Supraspinatus tenoperiosteal junction and tendon.

## INFRASPINATUS

### BELLY

The infraspinatus muscle belly is readily palpated in the infraspinatus fossa, since no overlying musculature is present (Fig. 5-45).

### TENDON

The patient can be placed prone or seated with the arm at 90 degrees of flexion, slight horizontal adduction, and in external rotation. This displaces the infraspinatus insertion posteriorly and inferiorly to the acromion. Identify the posterior lateral acromion, and palpate inferiorly approximately 1 cm. The tendon can be found distal to the muscle belly (see Fig. 5-45).

## SUBSCAPULARIS

### BELLY

The subscapularis muscle belly is difficult to palpate because its origin is on the ventral surface of the scapula. A position has been described for trigger point assessment in which the patient is placed supine with the arm abducted to 90 degrees, causing lateral rotation of the scapula[64] (Fig. 5-46). The examiner identifies the anterior latissimus dorsi border and palpates deep into the exposed subscapularis muscle belly. Trigger points of the subscapularis are believed to be a source of pain and potentially restrict shoulder range of motion.

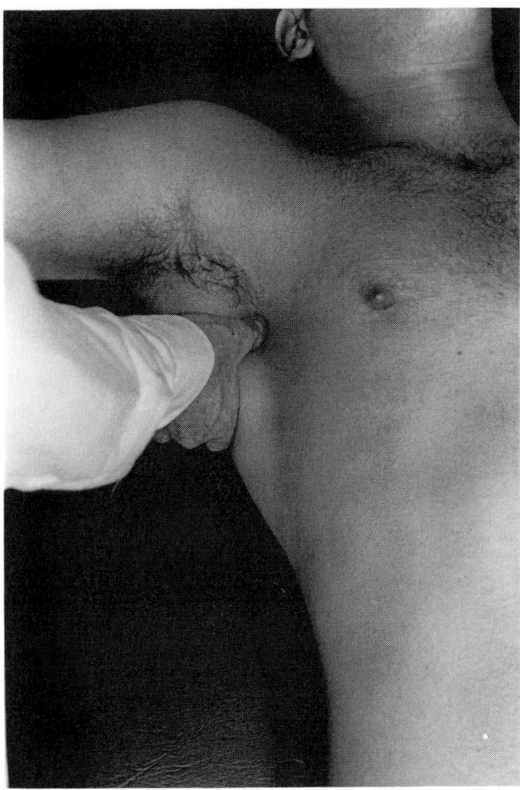

**Figure 5-46.** Subscapularis muscle belly.

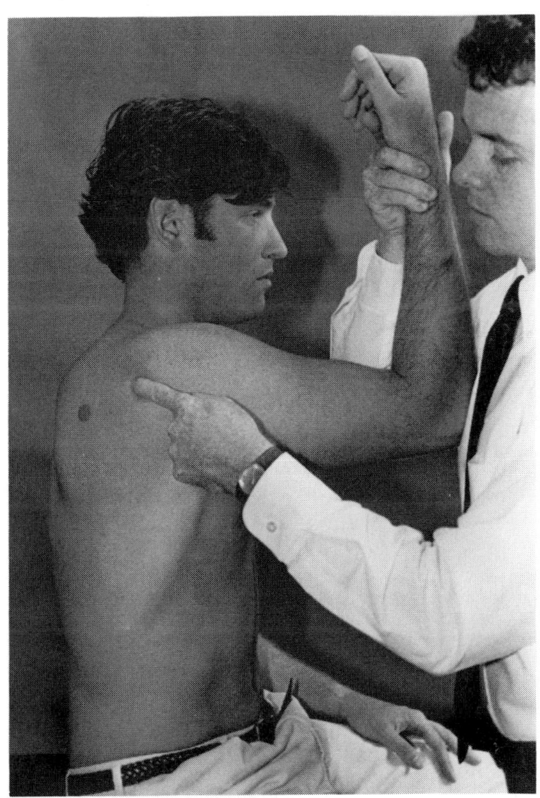

**Figure 5-45.** Infraspinatus tendon and muscle belly (dot).

### TENDON

The subscapularis tendon and insertion into the lesser tubercle can be a source of pain. To palpate, the patient is placed upright or supine, and the lesser tubercle is located by using the anterolateral acromion as a landmark. The examiner palpates inferiorly approximately 2 cm, and the arm is rotated internally and externally beneath the thumb. Movement of the tuberosities and groove is appreciated underneath the thumb. In external rotation, the lesser tuberosity is palpated; as the arm is internally rotated, the finger falls into the groove and then onto the anterior greater tuberosity (Fig. 5-47). To gain greater exposure of the insertion and tendon, the humerus should be externally rotated approximately 50 degrees.

## BICEPS

### TENDON

This structure is intraarticular and extraarticular. Trauma to the tendon has been described as commonly occurring as it wraps laterally around

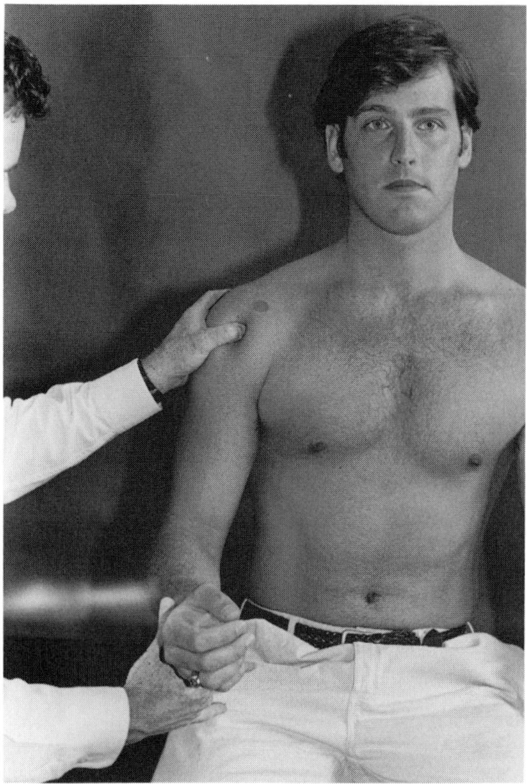

**Figure 5-47.** Long head of biceps in the groove and intraarticular (dot). Subcabularis tendon is found with external rotation of the humerus, medial to the lesser tuberosity prominence.

the lesser tuberosity. This is an area of friction which, over time, can cause fraying and eventual rupture.[25] The intraarticular component also can be traumatized by impingement against the over lying coracoacromial arch.

### GROOVE

This is a normally tender area even in the asymptomatic shoulder, and bilateral comparison is essential. The patient's arm is placed at approximately 10 degrees of internal rotation, placing the groove anteriorly. Find the groove position relative to the tuberosities, as discussed under subscapularis tendon palpation (see Fig. 5-47). The actual tendon cannot be appreciated because it lies tight in the groove and is covered by the anterior deltoid. Many clinicians mistakenly "palpate" the biceps tendon in the groove, but further discrimination reveals the septum between the anterior and middle deltoid heads. The intraarticular component can be identified over the humeral head as it runs an oblique course to the supraglenoid tubercle. This is best palpated in a very thin individual or in the presence of marked deltoid atrophy.

## DELTOID

The deltoid can harbor trigger points, particularly in a patient with a chronically painful shoulder. The deltoid heads require palpation for tenderness and comparison with the uninvolved side. Commonly, the symptomatic trigger point is found in the distal anterior portion of the middle deltoid (Fig. 5-48). We have found the inferior fiber of the posterior deltoid to be normally tender, possibly due to the axillary nerve superficial location.

## EVALUATIVE FRICTION MASSAGE OR ACUPRESSURE

Once a tender region of the contractile element has been identified friction massage can be performed to determine the effect on signs and symptoms. The patient is initially examined and painful ranges and resisted motions determined. Friction massage or acupressure is then performed for 3 to 5 minutes to the suspected soft-tissue element. The patient is then reassessed, and the percentage reduction of pain reported. In essence, this is a noninvasive equivalent to the impingement test. This is more appropriate in the less reactive patient. If an area is exquisitely tender, particularly if the examination determines a high degree of reactivity, evaluative friction massage or acupressure should be deferred.

As discussed previously, palpation should be performed last to prevent premature irritation of the involved structures as well as avoiding "diagnosis prejudging." Palpation assessment, quite literally places the "finishing touches" on the evaluation process. Results should confirm the history and previously gathered information regarding symptom etiology and diagnosis.

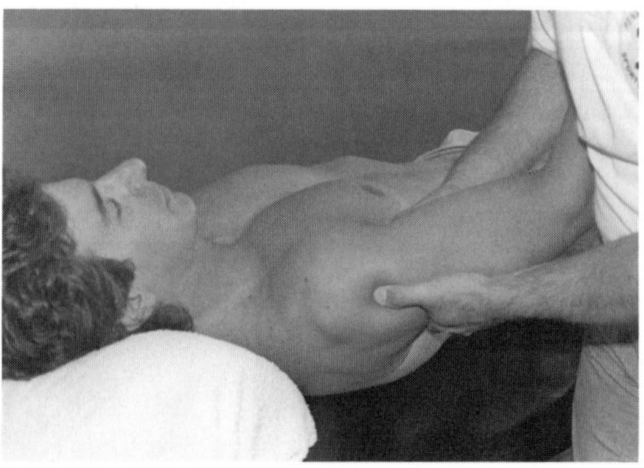

**Figure 5-48.** Middle deltoid.

# Summary

The goal of this chapter was to integrate knowledge of anatomy, biomechanics, and pathogenesis into an effective, scientifically based evaluation process. As much as we attempt to achieve this goal, the clinician must realize that experience and "art" play a major role in assessing a patient.

The evaluation process is more than a search for the source of pain. It provides a "current status" and a gateway to the treatment approach. For example, three patients may present with a similar diagnosis of rotator cuff impingement, yet all three may manifest a different level of reactivity and have a myriad of findings that individualize their specific treatment. In closing, take nothing for granted, prove it to yourself!

# References


1. Adson AW. Cervical ribs: symptoms, differential diagnosis of section of the insertion of the scalenus anticus muscle. J Int Coll Surg 1951;16:546.
2. American Academy of Orthopaedic Surgeons. Joint motion: method of measuring and recording. Chicago: American Academy of Orthopaedic Surgeons, 1965.
3. Bateman JE. The shoulder and neck. Philadelphia: WB Saunders, 1971.
4. Booth RE, Marvel JP. Differential diagnosis of shoulder pain. Orthop Clin North Am 1975;6:353.
5. Bowling RW, Rockar PA, Erhard R. Examination of the shoulder complex. Phys Ther 1986;66:1866.
6. Brewer BJ. Aging of the rotator cuff. Am J Sports Med 1979; 7(2):102.
7. CIBA Publication. Thoracic outlet syndrome. Summit, NJ:CIBA, 1971.
8. Clark JC, Harryman DT. Tendons, ligaments, and capsule of the rotator cuff. J Bone Joint Surg. 1992;74A:713.
9. Clark JC, Sidles JR, Matzen FA III. The relationship of the glenohumeral joint capsule to the rotator cuff. Clin Orthop 1990;254:29.
10. Codman EA. The shoulder. Boston: Thomas Todd, 1934.
11. Curwin S, Standish WD. Tendinitis: its etiology and treatment. Lexington, Ky.: Collamore Press, 1984.
12. Cyriax J. Diagnosis of soft tissue lesions. In: Textbook of orthopaedic medicine. 8th ed., vol. 1. Baltimore: Williams & Wilkins, 1970.
13. Cyriax J, Cyriax P. Illustrated manual of orthopaedic medicine. London: Butterworth, 1983.
14. DePalma AF. Surgery of the shoulder. Philadelphia: JB Lippincott, 1973.
15. Ellman H, Hanker G, Bayer M. Repair of the rotator cuff: end-result study of factors influencing reconstruction. J Bone Joint Surg 1986;68A:1136.
16. Elvey RL. The investigation of arm pain. In: Grieve GP, ed. Modern manual of therapy of the vertebral column. Edinburgh: Churchill Livingstone, 1986.
17. Harryman DT, Sidles JA, Clark JM, et al. Translation of the humeral head on the glenoid with passive glenohumeral motion. J Bone Joint Surg 1990;72A:1334.
18. Harryman DT, Sidles JA, Harris SL, Matzen FA III. The role of the rotator interval capsule in passive motion and stability of the shoulder. J Bone Joint Surg 1992;74A:53.
19. Hawkins RJ, Bokor DJ. Clinical evaluation of shoulder problems. In: Rockwood CA, Matzen FA III, eds. The shoulder. Vol. 1. Philadelphia: WB Saunders, 1990:167.
20. Hawkins RJ, Hoebeika P. Physical examination of the shoulder. Orthopedics 1983;6:1270.
21. Hawkins RJ, Kennedy JC. Impingement syndrome in athletes. Am J Sports Med 1980;8:151.
22. Hawkins RJ, Misamore GW, Hobeika PE. Surgery of full-thickness rotator cuff tears. J Bone Joint Surg 1985;67A:1349.
23. Herberts D, Kadefors R, Anderson G, Petersen I. Shoulder pain in industry: an epidemiological study in welders. Acta Orthop Scand 1981;52:299.
24. Hitchcock HH, Bechtol CO. Painful shoulder: observations on the role of the tendon of the long head of the biceps brachii in its causation. J Bone Joint Surg 1948;30A:263.
25. Hoppenfeld S. Physical examination of the spine and extremities. New York: Appleton-Century-Crofts, 1976.
26. Hovelius L. Recurrences after initial dislocation of the shoulder. J Bone Joint Surg 1983;65A:343.
27. Hovelius L. Anterior dislocation of the shoulder in teenagers and young adults: five-year prognosis. J Bone Joint Surg 1987;69A:393.
28. Howell SM, Galinat BJ, Renzi AJ, Marone PJ. Normal and abnormal mechanics of the glenohumeral joint in the horizontal plane. J Bone Joint Surg 1988;70A:227.
29. Howell SM, Imobersteg AM, Seger DE, Marone PJ. Clarification of the role of the supraspinatus muscle in shoulder function. J Bone Joint Surg 1986;68A:398.
30. Inman VT, Saunders JB. Referred pain from skeletal structures. J Nerv Ment Dis 1944;99:660.
31. Inman VT, Saunders JR, Abbott LC. Observations on the function of the shoulder joint. J Bone Joint Surg. 1944;26:1.
32. Jobe FW, Moynes DR. Delineation of diagnostic criteria and a rehabilitation program for rotator cuff injures. Am J Sports Med 1982;10:336.
33. Jobe FW, Moynes DR, Brewster CF. Rehabilitation of shoulder joint instabilities. Orthop Clin North Am 1987;18:473.
34. Kaltenborn FM. Mobilization of the extremity joints: examination and basic treatment techniques. Oslo: Olaf Bokhandel, 1980.
35. Kapandji I. The physiology of joints. Vol. 1. Baltimore: Williams & Wilkins, 1970.
36. Kazar B, Relovsky E. Prognosis of primary dislocation of the shoulder. Acta Orthop Scand 1969;40:216.
37. Kendall FP, McCreary EK. Muscle testing and function. 3rd ed. Baltimore: Williams & Wilkins, 1982.
38. Kessell L, Watson M. The painful arc syndrome: clinical classification as a guide to management. J Bone Joint Surg 1977;59B:166.
39. Koontz CL, Burkart SL. AREN Publications/Video Conference: Thoracic outlet syndrome: diagnosis and management. 1986; Pittsburgh.
40. Kuhlman JR, Iannotti JP, Kelley MJ, et al. Isokinetic and isometric evaluation of the shoulder: implications for clinical assessment of rotator cuff strength. J. Bone Joint Surg 1992; 74A:1320.
41. Laumann U. Kinesiology of the shoulder joint. In: Kolbel R, Helbig, Blauth eds. Shoulder replacement. Berlin: Springer-Verlag, 1987.
42. Ludington NA. Rupture of the long head of the biceps flexor cubiti muscle. Ann Surg 1923;77:358.
43. Maitland GD. Peripheral manipulation. 3rd ed. London: Butterworth, 1991.
44. Matzen FA III, Arntz CT. Subacromial impingement. In Rockwood CA, Matzen FA III, eds. The shoulder. Philadelphia: WB Saunders, 1990:623.
45. Matzen FA III, Arntz CT. Rotator cuff tendon failure. In: Rockwood CA, Matzen FA III, eds. The shoulder. Philadelphia: WB Saunders, 1990:647.
46. McLaughlin HL, Cavallaro WU. Primary anterior dislocation of the shoulder. Am J Surg 1950;80:615.
47. Moseley HF. Ruptures to the rotator cuff. Springfield, Ill.: Charles C Thomas, 1952.
48. Neer CS II. Anterior acromioplasty for the chronic impingement syndrome in the shoulder: a preliminary report. J Bone Joint Surg 1972;54A:41.
49. Neer CS II. Impingement lesions. Clin Orthop 1983;173:70.
50. Nuber GW, Jobe FW, Perry JP, et al. Fine wire EMG analysis of the shoulder during swimming. Am J Sports Med 1986;14:7.
51. Pappas AM, Zawacki RM, Sullivan TJ. Biomechanics of baseball pitching. Am J Sports Med 1985;13:216.
52. Perry J. Anatomy and biomechanics of the shoulder in throwing, swimming, gymnastics and tennis. Clin Sports Med 1983;2:247.
53. Pettersson G. Rupture of the tendon aponeurosis of the shoulder joint in anterior inferior dislocation. Acta Chir Scand Suppl 1942;77:1.

54. Poppen NK, Walker PS. Normal and abnormal motion of the shoulder. J Bone Joint Surg 1976;58A:195.
55. Poppen NK, Walker PS. Forces at the glenohumeral joint in abduction. Clin Orthop 1978;135:165.
56. Price DD, McGrath PA, Rafii A, Buckingham B. The validation of visual analogue scales a ratio scale measures for chronic and experimental pain. Pain 1982;17:45.
57. Rathbun JB, Macnab I. The microvascular pattern of the rotator cuff. J Bone Joint Surg 1970;52B:540.
58. Reeves B. Experiments on the tensile strength of the anterior capsular structures of the shoulder region. J Bone Joint Surg 1968;50B:858.
59. Rockwood CA, Williams GR, Birkhead WZ. The long results of acromioplasty and debriedment of irreparable degenerative lesions of the rotator cuff. J. Bone Joint Surg 1994.
60. Roos DB, Owens JC. Thoracic outlet syndrome. Arch Surg 1966; 93:71.
61. Rowe CR. Prognosis in dislocations of the shoulder. J Bone Joint Surg 1956;8A:957.
62. Rowe CR, Sakellarides HT. Factors related to recurrences of anterior dislocations of the shoulder. Clin Orthop 1961;20:40.
63. Sidles J. Shoulder Biomechanics. Presentation at the American Society of Shoulder and Elbow Therapist Meeting, Vail, Colorado, 1992.
64. Terry GC, Hammon D, France P, Norwood LA. The stabilizing function of the passive shoulder restraints. Am J Sports Med 1991;19:26.
65. Travell JG, Simon DG. Myofascial pain and dysfunction: the trigger point manual. Baltimore: Williams & Wilkins, 1983.
66. Turek S. Orthopaedics: principles and their applications. Philadelphia: JB Lippincott, 1967.
67. Turkel SJ, Panio MW, Marshal JL. Stabilizing mechanism preventing anterior dislocation of the glenohumeral joint. J Bone Joint Surg 1981;63A:1208.
68. Vaes PH, Annaert JM, Clarys P, Opdecam P. Shoulder position and access for palpation to the rotator cuff tendons: an anatomical and kinesiological study. Presented at the IFRAMT Meeting, June 1992; Vail (CO).
69. Walch G, Boileau P, Noel E, Donell T. Impingement of the deep surface of the supraspinatus tendon on the posterior glenoid rim: an arthroscopic study. J Shoulder Elbow Surg 1992;1:239.
70. Yergason RM. Supination sign. J Bone Joint Surg 1931;13A:160.

# Chapter 6

G. Kelley Fitzgerald
Susan L. Michlovitz

# Modality Therapy



Physical agents, including heat, cold, pulsed ultrasound, and electrical stimulation, are used commonly as adjunctive treatment in shoulder rehabilitation programs for reducing inflammation, pain control, or muscle activation/reeducation. The efficacy of treatment with physical agents is determined in part by the physical therapist's clinical decision-making ability. Several factors require consideration when deciding how and when to use physical agents in a shoulder rehabilitation program.

Perhaps the most important factor to consider when making decisions to incorporate physical agents in rehabilitation programs is the nature of the clinical problem, that is, the type and stage of dysfunction. For example, the treatment approach to an inflammatory process will vary in acute versus chronic inflammatory conditions. Limitations in joint mobility that result from joint capsule and ligament restrictions versus limitations due primarily to pain and protective muscle guarding may be approached differently with physical agents. The approach to managing instability differs from that for hypomobility. A thorough understanding of the problem by evaluation and reevaluation of each patient will allow the therapist to determine the most appropriate and potentially effective treatment. Table 6-1 offers a clinical decision-making scheme.

Knowledge of the biophysical effect(s) of physical agents also will help the therapist determine an appropriate treatment approach for a particular clinical problem. Depending on treatment parameter settings, some physical agents may have thermal or nonthermal effects on tissues. If the desired biophysical effect for altering the clinical problem involves a nonthermal effect, the therapist should select the type of physical agent and treatment parameters that are most appropriate.

The anatomic structures associated with the clinical problem must be considered. The type and depth of the affected tissues may dictate the type of physical agent and the parameters used in treatment. Patient positioning also may be determined by the anatomic location of the af-

Martin J. Kelley and William A. Clark: ORTHOPEDIC THERAPY OF THE SHOULDER.

**Table 6-1**

**Clinical Decision-Making Scheme**

| Stages of Injury | Clinical Problems | Solutions |
|---|---|---|
| Acute | Reduce inflammation | Cryotherapy<br>Pulsed ultrasound<br>Phonophoresis*<br>Iontophoresis |
| | Maintain mobility | PROM, gentle AROM |
| | Control pain | Cryotherapy<br>TENS |
| | Muscle guarding | Cryotherapy<br>TENS |
| Subacute | Control pain and muscle guarding | TENS<br>Superficial heat<br>Ultrasound |
| | Improve mobility | ES with AROM,<br>Heat with prolonged stretching<br>Cryokinetics |
| Chronic | Muscle atrophy | Motor level ES (isometric or with AROM) |
| | Residual loss of motion | ES with AROM<br>Heat with prolonged stretching |

* Low-intensity ultrasound is recommended for phonophoresis treatment of acute inflammatory conditions.

fected tissues in relation to therapeutic application. For example, if the therapist wants to apply ultrasound over the rotator cuff tendons, the arm should be positioned in a manner that would expose that tendon from under the acromion. However, if electrical stimulation is being used to cause contraction of the infraspinatus muscle, positioning should optimize the length/tension relationship of that muscle, for example, avoiding the extremes of ranges of internal or external shoulder rotation.

Criteria for evaluating patient response to treatment and treatment effectiveness should be considered at the onset of treatment. Adverse reactions to physical agent treatment modalities should be understood and monitored by the therapist. Clinical signs and symptoms such as pain at rest, during movement, and during functional activities; skin temperature; joint mobility; and muscle performance should be identified and used as measures of treatment effectiveness. The therapist should include periodic reevaluation as part of the overall treatment plan. If improvement in the clinical problem with respect to identified criteria is not observed in a reasonable amount of time, the treatment should be changed or terminated.

There are probably few, if any, instances in which physical agents alone will be sufficient to resolve the clinical problem. Therefore, the therapist must consider the role of the selected physical agent in conjunction with other treatment interventions. The therapist should understand how physical agents may enhance or inhibit the effectiveness of other treatments being utilized in the rehabilitation program. For example, cold applications may increase the stiffness of connective tissues, such as joint capsules.[1,44] If the therapist is treating a patient with limited joint mobility secondary to capsular restrictions, applying cold modalities prior to the mobility exercises may reduce the effectiveness of the exercise program. Conversely, heating connective tissues may enhance connective-tissue extensibility.[27] Applying a heat modality prior to exercise in this patient may enhance the effectiveness of the exercise program.

Physical agents can be used to treat a variety of shoulder dysfunctions. Categorizing shoulder dysfunctions into groups of clinical problems can be helpful in facilitating appropriate clinical decision making. For the purpose of this chapter, shoulder dysfunctions are categorized into three groups: (1) inflammation, (2) pain and muscle guarding, and (3) limitations in joint mobility. Treatment alternatives with physical agents will be identified for each of these groups. Mechanisms for altering the clinical problems, suggested patient setups, treatment parameter selection, and precautions for each treatment alternative will be discussed. The use of physical agents in conjunction with other treatment interventions and criteria for altering or discontinuing treatment also will be discussed. Case studies will be presented to illustrate examples of treatment intervention with physical agents for each of the shoulder dysfunction categories.

# Inflammation

Physical therapists may encounter a variety of inflammatory conditions when treating patients with shoulder dysfunction. Rotator cuff injuries, tendinitis, bursitis, and capsulitis are generally the most common types of inflammatory processes related to shoulder dysfunction. Thermal agents, pulsed ultrasound, and electrical stimulation can be used to treat these conditions.

## Thermal Agents

### BIOPHYSICAL MECHANISMS

Heat and cold modalities are used commonly to treat inflammation. An understanding of the biophysical effects of these modalities on body tissues is necessary for selecting an appropriate treatment for a given inflammatory condition. Modalities used in cryotherapy (treatment with cold modalities) may have several biophysical effects on tissues that may alter an inflammatory process. Rippe and Grega[37] reported that cooling of tissues reduces the effect of histamine on capillary permeability. A reduction in capillary permeability can alter the inflammatory process by impeding leukocyte infiltration into the affected tissues and assisting to control edema. Schaubel[38] and Farry et al.[15] reported that decreases in leukocyte counts were associated with cooling of tissues.

A reduction in metabolic rate secondary to cold application also may alter the inflammatory process. Phagocytic activity of leukocytes has been shown to be limited by reducing tissue temperatures,[13] which may imply that metabolic activity is reduced. Knight[26] hypothesized that reducing metabolic activity of inflamed tissues using cold treatments may decrease secondary hypoxic injury to these tissues. The beneficial effects of cryotherapy are considered to be most effective in the early stages of inflammation.

Continuous-wave ultrasound at 0.1 to 0.2 W/cm$^2$ or pulsed ultrasound at 0.5 to 1.0 W/cm$^2$, 20 percent duty cycle, may be effective in treating soft-tissue injuries during the inflammatory stage of wound healing through nonthermal effects on tissues. According to Dyson and Luke,[14] low-intensity ultrasound stimulates mast cell degranulation, which results in the release of chemotaxic agents. These chemotaxic agents attract fibroblasts and endothelial cells to the injured area, enhancing the healing and tissue repair process. Dyson and Luke[14] hypothesize that low-intensity ultrasound does not suppress inflammation but rather accelerates the inflammatory stage of wound healing so that tissue repair occurs faster than under conditions when ultrasound is not used.

Ultrasound has been used in an attempt to administer anti-inflammatory medications through the skin, for example, phonophoresis. Phonophoresis is proposed to have its effects by a thermal mechanism and possibly by an increase in cell permeability associated with nonthermal doses of ultrasound. Acoustic streaming, the movement of fluids along cell membranes as a result of a mechanical pressure wave, may contribute to changes in ion fluxes. This streaming has been associated with changes in ion fluxes and subsequent changes in cellular activity found with ultrasound application. As of this writing, the authors are unaware of any well-controlled clinical trials to support the use of phonophoresis for reducing inflammation.

Pulsed shortwave diathermy administered at nonthermal dosages has been proposed to promote healing of soft tissues. Depolarization of cell membranes has been associated with cellular injury.[4] Theoretically, it is believed that pulsed shortwave diathermy may play a role in repolarizing the damaged cell membrane, which, in turn, may enhance the healing process. Therefore, pulsed shortwave diathermy may be useful in treating acute inflammatory conditions. To date, though, these claims are still speculative at best.

Modalities that deliver heat to body tissues, such as moist hot packs, continuous-wave ultrasound at intensities of 1.0 W/cm$^2$ or greater, and continuous shortwave and microwave diathermy, may exacerbate acute inflammatory conditions. Application of heat results in increased metabolism of vasoactive chemicals and increased local blood flow, which, in turn, increases capillary hydrostatic pressure. The increase in vasoactive amines and capillary hydrostatic pressure may increase edema formation. Because of these physiologic responses of tissues to heat, heat modalities are not desirable for treatment of acute inflammatory conditions.

Heat modalities may be beneficial in subacute and chronic inflammatory conditions. During this phase of inflammation, the goal of treatment is to promote tissue healing. The increased blood flow associated with heating of tissues may bring nutrients necessary for healing to the affected area and assist in the removal of inflammatory exudates and debris from the affected area. Heating may increase the metabolic rate in tissues. An increase in metabolic rate may expedite the processes necessary for tissue repair.

Physiologic responses to thermal agent application depend on the type and intensity of thermal agent used in treatment. The physical therapist must consider the stage of inflammation and the desired physiologic response to treatment when selecting a thermal agent for treatment.

## TREATMENT TECHNIQUES WITH THERMAL AGENTS

Cryotherapy is usually the treatment of choice in acute inflammatory conditions. Acute rotator cuff tendinitis, biceps tendinitis, and subacromial bursitis can be treated with a variety of cryotherapy modalities. The most practical cold modalities for application to the shoulder are ice massage, ice packs, and commercial cold packs.

When preparing for ice massage, the patient should be positioned to best expose the anatomic structure(s) to be treated and to allow comfort throughout the treatment session. If the rotator cuff tendons or subacromial bursae are to be targeted, the patient should be seated with the affected arm supported by pillows. If tolerated, the humerus should be in slight extension and internal rotation to expose these structures from under the acromion process.

When the patient is positioned appropriately, the ice massage is performed by moving the ice cup over the anterior and superior shoulder in a steady, circular manner. Treatment duration is approximately 5 minutes. This time period should allow for effective cooling of tissues in a well-defined area. Longer periods are probably not necessary because the ice is applied directly to a small area of the patient's skin. The therapist should monitor the skin for signs of potential tissue injury. Wheals, which are erythematous raised borders with blanched centers on the skin, are a sign that the treatment dosage may be too intense or the patient is hypersensitive to cold. If this occurs, ice should be discontinued. The patient should be instructed to perform the ice massage as often as needed, usually three to four times per day, during the acute stage of inflammation. A period of 45 to 60 minutes between treatments is recommended to avoid undesired effects of prolonged cold application. The patient also may be advised to use ice massage before and/or after exercise or physical activity.

When preparing the patient for ice massage to the biceps tendon, the patient can be seated with the arm supported on pillows and the humerus externally rotated so that the epicondyles are in the coronal plane. The biceps tendon can be located anteriorly in this position. The ice is then applied to the anterosuperior aspect of the shoulder as described above. The frequency and duration of treatment, as well as skin monitoring, are all performed as described above.

The methods for applying ice packs or commercial cold packs are similar. The ice pack is prepared by wrapping crushed ice or ice cubes in a wet terry cloth towel. The commercial cold pack is prepared by wrapping the pack in a wet towel. Wrapping the ice or the commercial cold pack in a wet towel reduces the amount of airspace between the modality and the skin, which allows for more efficient heat exchange between the two surfaces, that is, more efficient cooling.[31] Some clinicians use crushed ice in a plastic bag applied directly to the patient's skin for ice pack treatment. This treatment alternative is also acceptable, and our experience is that there is no increased risk for thermal tissue damage using this method.

Patient positioning for treatment of rotator cuff tendinitis, subacromial bursitis, and biceps tendinitis with ice and commercial cold packs can be the same as described for ice massage treatment. The packs can be applied for 15 to 20 minutes to the affected area. A longer duration of treatment is used for ice pack application compared with ice massage because the ice or cold pack is not in direct contact with the skin and more time is needed for cold penetration. The skin should be monitored periodically to ensure safety from tissue injury. The patient also can be instructed to perform these treatments three to four times per day.

When larger muscle masses about the shoulder, such as the deltoid, upper trapezius, and infraspinatus muscle bellies, have been contused, strained, or exhibit protective muscle guarding, ice packs and commercial cold packs can be an effective way of applying cold treatment to these structures. The arm should be supported to ensure patient comfort and allow easy access to the target tissues. Positioning the arm in the scapular plane is usually good for patient comfort. The frequency and duration of treatment are the same as described above.

The therapist should be aware of adverse systemic reactions to cold therapy. Patients who are hypersensitive to cold treatment may experience flushing of the face, a sharp reduction in blood pressure, increased pulse rate, and syncope.[31] Patients with systemic disorders such as multiple myeloma, leukemia, systemic lupus erythematosus, and rheumatoid arthritis may be prone to cryoglobinemia (where an abnormal blood protein precipitates and can result in ischemia or gangrene). Cold therapy for inflammation in patients with these diseases should be used with caution.

Low-intensity continuous-wave or pulsed ultrasound can be used to treat acute inflammatory conditions of the shoulder. The patient should be positioned appropriately to expose the target anatomic structure (Fig. 6-1). If the rotator cuff tendons and/or subacromial bursa are treated, ultrasound at 3 MHz may be most appropriate. At this frequency, ultrasound is attenuated (absorbed) by structures within 1 to 2 cm of the skin surface.[45] Ultrasound at 1 MHz may be more appropriate in treating deeper structures, such as capsular tissue and deep muscles.

The skin over the treatment area should be covered with an aqueous-based ultrasound gel. The therapist can begin treatment by applying a firm contact of the applicator to the skin of the treatment area and slowly moving the applicator in a rhythmic pattern of longitudinal stroking or overlapping circular movements. Movement of the applicator at a rate of approximately 4 cm/s has been recommended.[36] The applicator should always be moved to distribute energy evenly.

The size of the treatment area should be considered when determining treatment duration. The total area covered is usually two to three times the size of the effective radiating area (ERA) of the crystal for every 5 minutes of exposure.[36] Because the treatment area for rotator cuff tendons is small, the duration of treatment probably does not need to exceed 5 minutes. If larger surface areas such as the anterior and inferior capsule are to be treated, the duration of treatment should be increased accordingly.

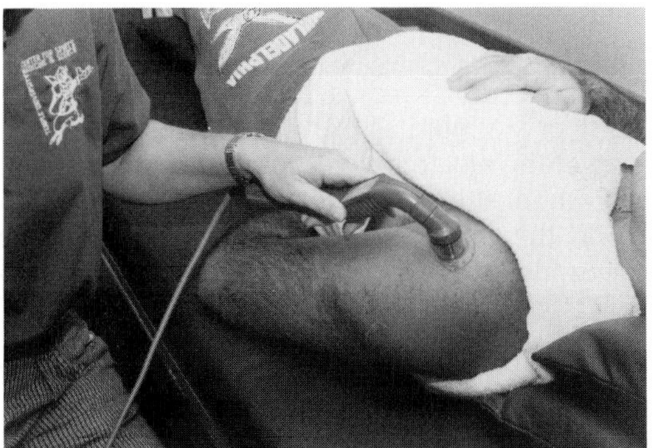

**Figure 6-1.** Positioning of the shoulder during ultrasound treatment of the rotator cuff.

Phonophoresis is another treatment alternative suggested for acute inflammatory conditions of the shoulder. A number of media (e.g. couplants with medication) are used for phonophoresis. The type of medium used may influence the effectiveness of treatment. Davick et al.[11] found greater penetration of 10% cortisol than 5% cortisol in dog skin. There may be a trend toward greater efficacy of phonophoresis with 10% versus 1% hydrocortisone cream for treating epicondylitis and subacromial bursitis.[24] This finding, however, needs further substantiation under a well-controlled study. Benson and McElnay[5] reported that most media typically used in phonophoresis treatment do not transmit ultrasound energy effectively and could therefore result in less effective treatment. A number of media have been found to transmit ultrasound energy adequately (0.05% betamethasone with ultrasound gel, Lidex gel, Thera-Gesic cream).[6] However, ultrasound transmission *through* a medium has not yet been equated with tissue penetration of the substance.

The medium used for phonophoresis should be rubbed into the skin overlying the treatment area, reducing air bubbles and thus improving ultrasound transmission. Patient positioning and duration of treatment are generally determined in the same manner as for ultrasound treatment. The literature is unclear with regard to optimal ultrasound parameter settings for this procedure. Pulsed ultrasound has been used for phonophoresis, but to date, the authors are unaware of any supporting evidence for the efficacy of this mode. Generally, it is recommended that ultrasound intensity be set within the patient's tolerance. A recent study by Ciccone et al.[9] suggests that ultrasound at intensities sufficient to cause tissue heating may exacerbate acute conditions and offset beneficial effects of anti-inflammatory medications. The intensity probably should not exceed a level beyond which the patient reports the sensation of minimal warmth in the treatment area.

Pulsed shortwave diathermy also may be a treatment consideration for acute inflammatory conditions of the shoulder. This modality may be particularly effective when larger surface areas are treated, such as multiple muscular strains about the shoulder girdle. For the interested reader, Kloth et al.[25] have recently written a literature review on the applications of shortwave diathermy.

Once the inflammatory process has progressed beyond the acute stage, the therapist may select physical agents that deliver heat to the tissues. Continuous-wave ultrasound at 1.0 to 1.5 W/cm$^2$ and continuous shortwave diathermy are common modalities used to treat chronic inflammatory conditions.

The intensity of the ultrasound may be set at a level that allows the patient to experience a mild sensation of warmth. Sensations of intense warmth, burning, or aching pain may indicate that the ultrasound is too intense. The use of preselected intensity dosages, such as 1.5 W/cm$^2$, is not logical because absorption of ultrasound energy by nonhomogeneous tissues and target tissue depth are variable from patient to patient.

## Electrical Stimulation

Electrical stimulation may be useful in treating inflammatory conditions of the shoulder by motor level electrical stimulation (electrical stimulation that induces muscle contraction) for edema control or iontophoresis for delivery of medication secondary to an ongoing inflammatory process. Motor-level stimulation via neuromuscular electrical stimulation (NMES) can be used after acute trauma or surgery, when the patient is having difficulty or is unable to contract the muscles of the shoulder. The stimulation should be applied in a manner that induces a tetanic contraction of muscles. These muscle contractions should simulate the muscle-pumping action of voluntary muscle contraction, improving local circulation and venous return, which may in turn reduce edema. This technique should be used prudently and should be avoided when muscle contraction is contraindicated. The therapist should consult with the surgeon regarding motor-level stimulation treatment in postoperative patients to ensure that this method is not contraindicated.

Pulsed or burst modulated alternating current (ac) can be used for neuromuscular electrical stimulation for edema control.[40] The pulse-rate range may be from 10 to 15 pulses per second. The pulse duration of the waveform should be greater than 100 μs. The amplitude should be great enough to elicit a tetanic muscle contraction. A 1:1 on/off time ratio, or 50 percent duty cycle, may be desirable. Electrode placement should be determined by identifying appropriate shoulder muscles for stimulation and then using the motor point of these muscles as sites for electrodes.

Some clinicians use sensory-level stimulation for edema control using high-voltage monophasic pulsed current (HVPC). Although there is some evidence based on data from animal models to suggest that this may be effective in reducing the rate of edema formation,[16] sensory-level stimulation has not been found to be effective in reducing edema in studies using human subjects.[32] Therefore, motor-level stimulation is recommended when the purpose of electrical stimulation treatment is to reduce edema. Further research regarding the efficacy of sensory-level electrical stimulation for edema control in humans is needed before it should be considered a reasonable clinical technique.

Electrical stimulation can be used for iontophoresis to manage inflammatory conditions of the shoulder. The charge of the free ions in the solution of medication used for iontophoresis will determine the electrode placement. Positively charged ions will be repelled by the anode; therefore, the anode would be the treatment electrode if the medication of choice is positively charged, and vice versa if the medication is negatively charged. Direct current (dc) is necessary for iontophoresis so that unidirectional flow of ions is maintained.

Dexamethasone and dexamethasone mixed with lidocaine have been found to effectively penetrate tissues during iontophoresis.[19] Corticosteroids have not been found to penetrate tissues sufficiently during iontophoresis procedures.[8] Logically, a drug that penetrates through skin is chosen for treatment.

Prior to iontophoresis, the patient should be screened for drug allergies. The patient should be positioned comfortably but in a manner that will best expose the structure targeted for treatment with iontophoresis (Fig. 6-2). The skin over the area to be treated should be cleaned with rubbing alcohol, and any excess hair should be shaved.

The therapist may select copper, tin, aluminum, or platinum as the electrode material. The size of the electrode will affect the current density under the electrode. The smaller the electrode, the greater is the current density. Smaller electrodes are recommended when treating specific structures (i.e., a tendon), and larger electrodes are recommended when treating a less localized treatment area (i.e., a muscle group).[20] A sponge or gauze soaked in the desired medication is placed between the patient's skin and the treatment electrode. Commercially available disposable electrodes that provide a well into which

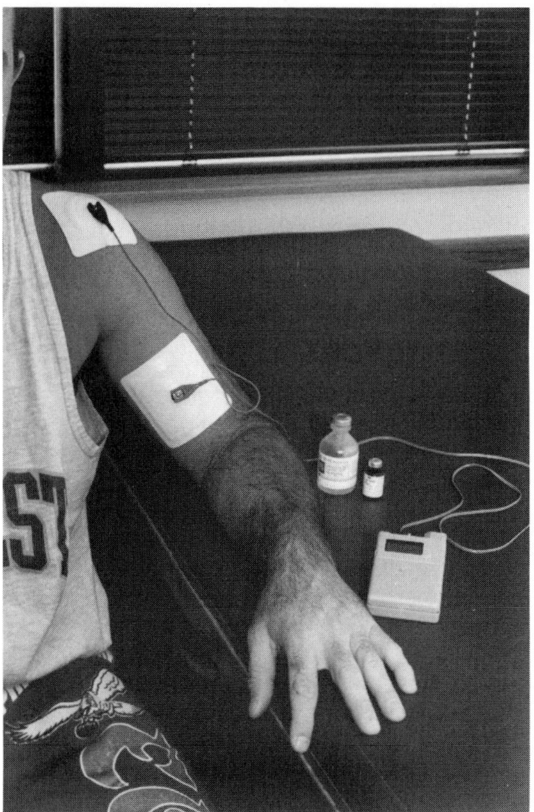

Figure 6-2. Iontophoresis treatment of the anterosuperior shoulder.

the medication is injected also can be used; however, these electrodes are expensive. These electrodes eliminate the need for sponges in the treatment setup. The nontreatment electrode is placed on the skin adjacent to the treatment area. The optimal distance between electrodes has not been determined. Electrodes should be placed so that they do not overlap with each other. The therapist should remember that current density will decrease as electrodes are moved further apart. According to Glick and Snyder-Mackler,[20] most recent studies have reported a current intensity of 3 to 5 mA for durations of 10 to 20 minutes.

Because direct current is used in iontophoresis procedures, the therapist and patient need to monitor the patient's skin for adverse reactions to the stimulation, that is, galvanic burns. This is more likely to occur under the cathode because alkaline chemical changes associated with the cathode are more irritating to the skin. Using a cathode that is larger than the anode will help reduce the current density under the cathode and thus reduce the occurrence of galvanic skin burns. The therapist also should be aware of adverse reactions to the medication being used during treatment and what the appropriate actions are should any of these reactions occur. The patient's physician should be notified when the patient has an adverse reaction to treatment.

## Other Considerations

The use of physical agents in any rehabilitation program must be considered in context with other therapeutic interventions. When to use a physical agent to enhance overall treatment is as important as selecting the most appropriate type of agent. Considering the phase of inflammation and the immediate goals of rehabilitation may assist the therapist in determining when to use a specific physical agent. For example, if the patient is experiencing an acute inflammation of the shoulder, the immediate goals of rehabilitation are to reduce the inflammation and maintain joint mobility. The therapist would probably administer the physical agent of choice at the beginning of treatment, followed by a mild joint mobility program. During the chronic phase of inflammation, improving joint mobility and function becomes more emphasized. Heat modalities may be used prior to exercise, and then cold modalities may be used following the exercise to minimize exacerbations of inflammation resulting from increased activity. Decisions regarding when to use physical agents with other treatments should be guided by the immediate goals of treatment and a knowledge of the effects the physical agent will have on other treatments.

When to stop treatment also should be guided by the goals of rehabilitation. Patients with inflammatory conditions typically have pain during some functional activity, pain on palpation of the involved structures, elevated skin temperatures over the involved structures, and sometimes pain at rest. Goals of rehabilitation usually will be directed at resolving these signs and symptoms. Therefore, treatment with physical agents should be continued, altered, or terminated depending on the effects they have on signs and symptoms. If signs and symptoms improve with treatment, continue the treatment. If signs and symptoms plateau or become worse, change the treatment approach. If the goals for a particular treatment intervention have been met, terminate the treatment. Our clinical experience suggests that changes in signs and symptoms from treatment with physical agents should be observable within 3 to 5 treatments. Decisions to continue, change, or terminate treatment should be made within this time period.

## CASE REPORT 1

S.P. is a 29-year-old female who works on an assembly line moving 5-lb containers from waist to above-shoulder level. She complained of left hand pain and tingling. Her primary care physician diagnosed her as having carpal tunnel syndrome. She began physical therapy at the local hospital and was placed on a program of progressive resisted exercies including overhead presses. She reports that she was "no better" from therapy and went to see an orthopedic surgeon with her complaints now of right shoulder pain. The primary source of her pain is the long head of the biceps. S.P. was referred to physical therapy for resolution of the right shoulder pain and instruction in proper work posturing and movements. The area over the long head of the biceps was tender and warm to palpation and swollen. Pain symptoms were reproduced during resisted isometric muscle testing of shoulder elevation, elbow flexion, and supination. The initial session of physical therapy included ice massage (and instruction for home use) to the area over the long head of the biceps (Fig. 6-3). The shoulder was positioned into slight external rotation of the arm to expose the biceps tendon. Ice massage was applied for approximately 5 minutes. This was followed by instruction in proper posture during functional activities to avoid further aggravation by mechanical irritations. S.P. also was told to avoid elevation over 90 degrees. Ice massage was continued at subsequent visits while S.P. was instructed in pendulum exercises and pain-free isometric strengthening for the rotator cuff muscles. Subsequent plans include a work-site visit.

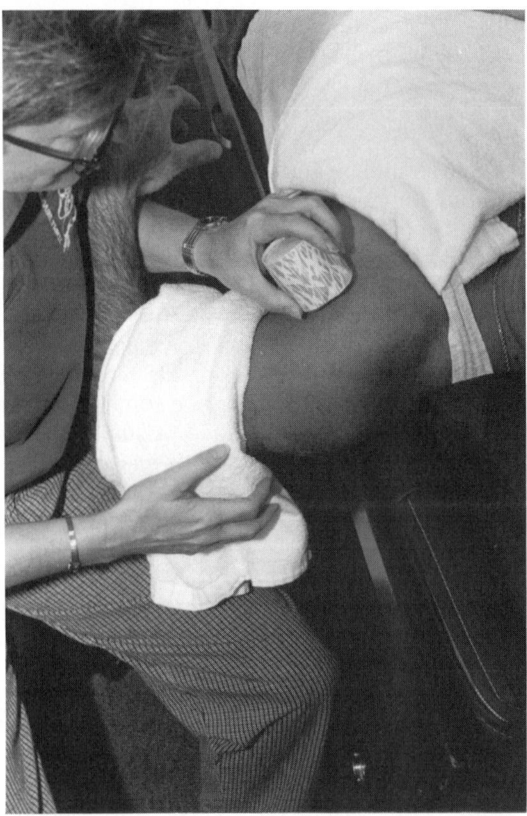

**Figure 6-3.** Ice massage treatment to the long head of the biceps brachii tendon.

## CASE REPORT 2

J.M. is a 45-year-old female with rheumatoid arthritis. She has had a flare-up of her right shoulder and has as primary findings a tendinitis of the supraspinatus tendon. The initial physical therapy plan is based on the goals of controlling pain and reducing inflammation. Dexamethasone iontophoresis was selected for its anti-inflammatory properties.[19,22] The arm was positioned in extension to clear the supraspinatus tendon from under the acromion. The arm was not adducted due to pain complaints. The dexamethasone was placed under the positive electrode, and the negative electrode of the circuit was placed over the middle deltoid. The electrodes used were commercially available. Stimulation was provided at 4 mA for 10 minutes.

# Pain and Muscle Relaxation

# Thermal Agents

## BIOPHYSICAL MECHANISMS

The mechanisms by which thermal agents relieve pain and induce muscle relaxation are based on the physiologic responses to the application of heat and cold on vascular and neurologic systems. These vascular and neurologic effects and their implications for reducing pain will be described for heat and cold modalities.

Heat increases local blood flow, which may help remove accumulated chemical mediators, such as prostaglandins, bradykinin, and histamine, from injured tissue. These mediators are thought to sensitize nociceptors, making them more reactive to stimuli. When cold is applied to tissues, the metabolic rate is decreased, which may result in a reduction in the amount of vasodilator substances released into tissues that are responsible for sensitizing nociceptors.

Heat and cold may reduce pain through a

counterirritation mechanism.[17] The application of heat or cold to the skin will increase the amount of sensory input from thermoreceptors to the central nervous system, overriding input from nociceptors and resulting in a reduced sensation of pain. The mechanism that Melzack and Wall[30] called a *spinal gate*, blocking pain perception, may be synonymous with counterirritation.

The application of heat to the body seems to have a general relaxation effect. There may be some influence of heating on descending pain inhibitory systems, but this has not yet been substantiated with scientific data.[34] This general relaxation effect may help to reduce protective muscle guarding associated with pain and injury.

## TREATMENT TECHNIQUES

Pain and muscle guarding often can reduce the willingness and ability of patients to move their shoulder after injury or surgery. This may result in joint stiffness or capsular adhesions and interfere with the normal healing of tissues. Heat and cold modalities can be used to minimize pain and promote muscle relaxation, facilitating the ease with which exercise can be performed and thus optimizing recovery.

Cold modalities are often used to reduce pain so that joint motion is more tolerable for the patient. Hayden[23] and Grant[21] have described a treatment approach using cold prior to exercise to reduce pain, which they have termed *cryokinetics*. This approach can be applied to patients with shoulder pain. The therapist performs an ice massage to the painful area of the shoulder until the sensation of pain is diminished (approximately 5 minutes). The patient then performs the shoulder mobility program. If the pain begins to return, the ice may be reapplied, followed by resumption of exercise. This cycling of ice massage with exercise may continue for three to four cycles, depending on patient tolerance. The obvious concern with this technique is that because pain has been masked temporarily due to cold treatment, there may be potential for reinjury if the exercise is too intense. Therapists must therefore use caution when prescribing exercise in conjunction with cold treatment.

Ice packs and commercial cold packs also can be used to reduce pain and protective muscle guarding of the shoulder complex. The patient should be positioned in a manner that exposes the involved structure yet allows for sufficient relaxation. For example, if ice packs were to be applied over the upper trapezius, rotator cuff, and deltoid muscles, the patient may be in the sitting position to allow easy access to these structures, but pillows also should be used to support the weight of the upper extremity so that these muscles can relax. The duration of treatment is usually 15 to 20 minutes.

Some patients are hypersensitive to cold treatment and respond more favorably to heat modalities. Positioning concerns for treatment with heat modalities are the same as for cold modalities. When using hot packs, selecting the proper size hot pack will ensure better contact between the hot pack and the treatment area, which may allow for more effective heating. For example, if the patient is sitting, a cervical hot pack may be appropriate because it can be draped over the shoulder to cover anterior, posterior, and superior aspects of the shoulder. The duration of treatment with the hot pack is usually 20 minutes. This time period should be enough for adequate heating, and most hot packs will not maintain enough heat to induce a therapeutic temperature for longer periods.

Ultrasound and shortwave diathermy can be used for deep heating of the shoulder complex to decrease pain and relax protective muscle guarding. Ultrasound and shortwave diathermy intensities should be consistent with those needed for thermal effects. The patient should experience a mild warmth in the treatment area during application. The duration of ultrasound treatment should be determined by the size of the surface area to be treated. The size of the treated area probably should not exceed two to three times the size of the effective radiating area. If larger areas require treatment, these areas should be divided into treatment fields, each field being treated separately. The duration of diathermy treatment is usually 15 to 20 minutes to obtain a heating effect.

Myofascial trigger points (hyperirritable spots within muscle or fascia that are painful on compression and give rise to characteristic referred pain, tenderness, and autonomic phenomena[42]) are commonly found in the shoulder complex. When present, pain and muscle spasm from these trigger points may limit shoulder mobility. Ice massage, vapocoolant sprays, or ultrasound can be used to desensitize these trigger points so that pain is reduced and mobility can be restored.

Treatment of trigger points with thermal agents is initiated by positioning the patient in a manner that places the involved muscle in a lengthened position. For example, the infraspinatus muscle is a common site for myofascial trigger points in the shoulder region. Before applying the thermal agent, the patient should be positioned so that the arm is internally rotated with some flexion and horizontal adduction to increase the length

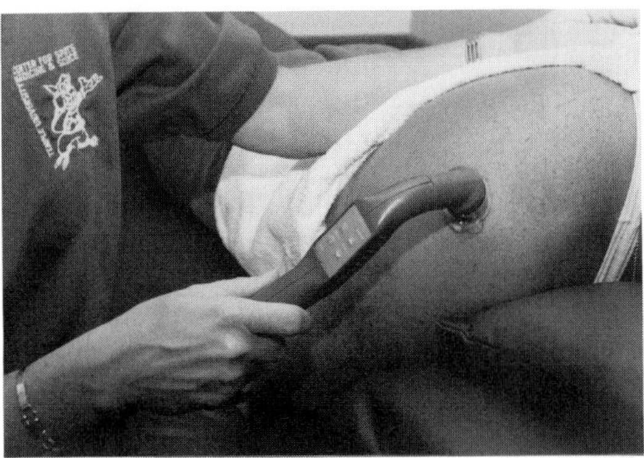

**Figure 6-4.** Ultrasound treatment over the distal infraspinatus muscle. The patient's upper extremity is positioned in slight flexion and internal rotation to increase the length of the muscle.

of the infraspinatus muscle (Fig 6-4). The upper trapezius and levator scapulae muscles are also common sites for trigger points in the shoulder complex. Patients should be positioned accordingly to lengthen these muscles prior to treatment.

When the patient has been positioned appropriately, the selected treatment modality can be applied directly over the area of the trigger point. Because the goal is to achieve greater movement without triggering pain symptoms, treatment should include lengthening of the involved muscle after application of the physical agent used to desensitize the trigger point. Depending on patient tolerance, therapists sometimes repeat two to three bouts of thermal agent application followed by increasing the length of the muscle in a single treatment session.

# Electrical Stimulation

A large number of electrical stimulation devices for the treatment of pain are available. There are two basic premises to keep in mind that may help physical therapists from becoming overwhelmed by the vast numbers of stimulators on the market. The first is that all electrical stimulation devices used by physical therapists for pain control are transcutaneous electrical nerve stimulators (TENS). Although stimulators may vary in waveform, pulse rates and durations, amplitude range, and the modulations offered, they are technically TENS units.

The second premise is that therapists should decide what parameters (i.e., pulse rate, pulse duration, amplitude) are needed to achieve the desired clinical affect and then select a device that provides these parameters. Therapists need not memorize the uses for high-voltage versus interferential versus electrical muscle stimulators. Many of these units can be used for the same purposes. If the therapist knows what parameter settings are needed to induce a desired affect, the therapist can use any device that allows for control of the necessary parameters.

## BIOPHYSICAL EFFECTS AND MODES OF STIMULATION

According to Snyder-Mackler,[39] there are three basic types of stimulation used for pain control: sensory-level, motor-level, and noxious-level stimulation. The proposed biophysical effects of electrical stimulation for pain control will be described in terms of these levels of stimulation.

*Sensory-level stimulation* is defined as stimulation at or above the sensory threshold but below the motor threshold.[39] The pulse rate is approximately 50 to 100 pulses per second (pps) and pulse duration is 2 to 50 μs. The amplitude is set within patient tolerance levels, making this type of stimulation relatively comfortable. The proposed mechanism of pain control for this level of stimulation is by direct peripheral block of transmission or by a central inhibitory mechanism secondary to stimulation of large-diameter fibers (gate control mechanism). There is a fairly quick response to treatment, but this response is not long lasting when the stimulation is discontinued. Sensory-level stimulation is recommended for acute pain but may not be the best alternative for chronic pain conditions.

*Motor-level stimulation* refers to a level of stimulation that results in a visible muscle contraction. The pulse rate is 2 to 4 pulses per second with a pulse duration of approximately 150 μs or greater. Depending on the desired affect, the amplitude may be set to within patient tolerance or to a level that results in painful muscle contraction. The mechanism of pain control for nonpainful motor-level stimulation is probably similar to that for sensory-level stimulation.[39] Painful motor-level stimulation may work via release of endogenous opiates that act to increase an individual's pain threshold.[39] This level of stimulation may be more suited for patients with chronic pain. The response to treatment may be delayed, but this level of stimulation seems to have longer-lasting effects than sensory-level stimulation.

*Noxious-level stimulation* implies that pain and discomfort are induced at this level of electrical stimulation. Noxious-level stimulation may occur with and without muscle contraction. The pulse rate may be either 1 to 5 pulses per second or greater than 100 pulses per second. Pulse duration can be as great as 1 s. Amplitude settings are high enough to induce discomfort. The mechanism for pain control with noxious stimulation is believed to involve the systemic release of endogenous opiates that reduce the patient's pain threshold.[39] Noxious-level stimulation should be considered as an approach to pain control when less uncomfortable levels of stimulation have been unsuccessful.

## TREATMENT TECHNIQUES

When planning electrical stimulation treatment for pain control, stimulation characteristics (pulse rate, pulse duration, and peak amplitude) and sites for electrode placement must be determined. Sensory-level stimulation is usually the first approach for acute painful conditions of the shoulder. Patients accept this stimulation level well, and if pain relief will occur, it will begin during the treatment. Motor-level stimulation may be used when the therapist wishes to relax muscle or when muscle contraction is not contraindicated. Some therapists will use a combination of sensory-level and motor-level stimulation in the same treatment. The therapist may first begin with sensory-level stimulation to obtain quick pain relief and then switch to motor-level stimulation after 10 to 15 minutes of treatment to potentially induce longer-lasting treatment effects. The initial use of sensory-level stimulation may make motor-level stimulation more acceptable to the patient.

The type of stimulator used for treatment can be selected once the therapist has identified the necessary stimulus parameters for treatment. Electrical stimulators may be portable or clinical stimulators (portable = battery operated; clinical = power cord to wall socket). Table 6-2 provides a brief description of the common types of electrical stimulators used by physical therapists for pain control. Table 6-3 is a listing of the available parameter settings for devices listed in Table 6-2. Information from the instrument manual regarding pulse rate, pulse duration, and amplitude should allow the therapist to determine if the device is capable of administering the desired level of electrical stimulation. Many devices now have the capability of multiple modes of electrical stimulation for pain control.

Electrode placement sites are determined based on patient evaluation findings. If pain is localized and superficial, electrodes can be placed so that the current crosses over the area of pain. Electrodes also may be placed along the complete distribution of referred or projected pain. Dermatomes, myotomes, sclerotomes, acupuncture points, and myofascial trigger points are all possible alternatives for electrode placement sites.[29] When motor-level stimulation is desired, the motor points of the target muscle(s) is(are) selected.

The distance between electrodes needs to be considered. Current density increases as the distance between electrodes decreases. Electrodes can be positioned relatively close to focus the current in a small area, such as a myofascial trigger point. Electrodes should be placed farther apart if a larger area is to be treated. The size of the electrodes also will affect the concentration of current in an area. Smaller electrodes focus current in a localized manner, and large electrodes distribute current over larger areas.

**Table 6-2**

**Common Electrical Stimulators Used for Pain Control**

| Type of Stimulator | Current | Time-Dependent Factors | Amplitude-Dependent Factors | Electrode Systems |
|---|---|---|---|---|
| HVPC | Twin pulsed monophasic | On/off time | Ramp | One or two channels* |
| TENS | Pulsed monophasic | Modulation of pps and bursts | Modulation of amplitude | One or two channels, parallel or crisscross for sensory-level stimulation |
| Interferential current | ac, two independnt channels | Beats | | two-circuit crisscross |
| Low volt† | Pulsed or bursted ac, dc | On/off time | Ramp | Probe, pads |
| Microcurrent devices | Pulsed monophasic | Pulses per second (pps) | Ramp | Probe, pads |

* *Caution:* Make sure circuit is completed by adding a dispersive electrode.
† NMES devices are low-voltage devices and can be used for motor-level stimulation to control pain.

**Table 6-3**

**Pain-Control Stimulus Characteristics**

| Level of Stimulation | Stimulus Characteristics | Units Available |
|---|---|---|
| Sensory-level stimulation | Pulse rate: 50–100 pps or bps<br>Pulse duration: 2–50 μs<br>Amplitude: To sensory level | HVPC<br>TENS<br>Interf'l<br>Low volt |
| Motor-level stimulation | Pulse rate: 2–4 pps<br>Pulse duration: ≥150 μs<br>Amplitude: To motor level | TENS<br>Low volt |
| Noxious-level Stimulation | Pulse rate: 1–5 pps or ≥100 pps<br>Pulse duration: Up to 1 s<br>Amplitude: To noxious sensory level | Low volt (Neuroprobe) |

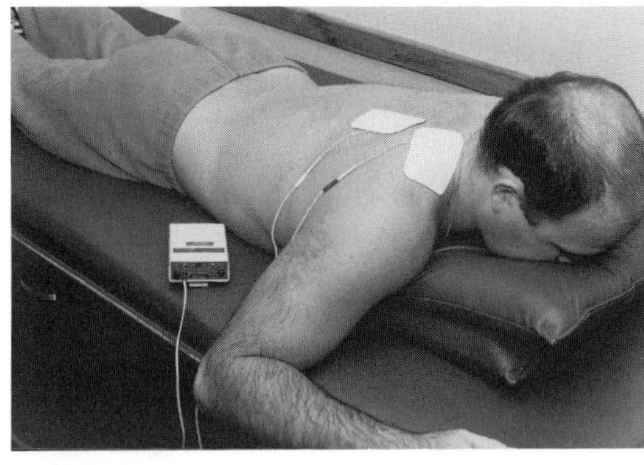

**Figure 6-5.** Neuromuscular electrical stimulation to the trapezius muscles.

Neuromuscular electrical stimulation (NMES) has been recommended for relaxing protective muscle guarding.[35] The goal of treatment is to fatigue the muscle, which, in turn may promote relaxation. High pulse rates (80 to 100 pulses per second) and low on/off time ratios (1:1) may expedite muscle fatigue. Consider a patient with complaints of muscle pain and guarding in the trapezius muscle (Fig. 6-5). Electrodes can be placed over the belly of this muscle, the pulse rate can be set at 80 to 100 pulses per second, on/off time can each be set at 10 s each, and the duration of treatment may be 15 to 30 minutes.[41]

Electrical stimulation treatment for pain control should be coordinated with therapeutic exercise and functional activities. Electrical stimulation can be administered before, during, and after these activities. The ultimate goal is to achieve performance of activity without the need for electrical stimulation. Therefore, therapists should frequently reevaluate and adjust treatment so that the least time of electrical stimulation necessary for adequate pain reduction is used during activity. A gradual reduction in treatment time with electrical stimulation should be considered as the patient's condition improves.

## CASE REPORT 3

M.M., a 48-year-old male, fell down the stairs and landed on outstretched hand. He sustained an impacted fracture of the proximal humerus. His arm was immobilized for 3 weeks in a shoulder immobilizer, after which an order was received to begin therapy for gentle range-of-motion exercises. Initially, the patient was apprehensive about moving. There was generalized protective muscle guarding about the shoulder girdle, as evidenced by painful attempts at active shoulder motion and palpation of shoulder girdle muscles.

Hot packs were used to provide surface heat and reduce muscle guarding through reflex mechanisms. The patient was positioned in a semirecline posture with a wedged pillow behind him. An 8 × 10 in hot pack was sufficiently covered with towels and placed behind the shoulder. Another pack of the same size was placed over the superior and anterior shoulder to cover as much total surface area around the shoulder as possible (Fig. 6-6). Hot packs were left in place for 20 minutes. The patient was instructed in gentle pendulum exercises after removal of the heat.

Therapy progressed well over the next 3 weeks, but M.M. developed a dull ache around the shoulder that was limiting his ability to perform range-of-motion exercises. Prior to joint mobilization and active assisted exercises in forward elevation, 15 to 20 minutes of motor-level electrical stimulation was applied for pain control. Two channels were utilized, one over the middle deltoid and upper trapezius and the other over the infraspinatus and anterior deltoid. Electrical stimulation was followed by grade II joint mobilization of the glenohumeral joint followed by elevation in a scapular plane using overhead pulleys for an assist. Electrical stimulation and instruction in self-mobilization and overhead pulleys were provided for home use.

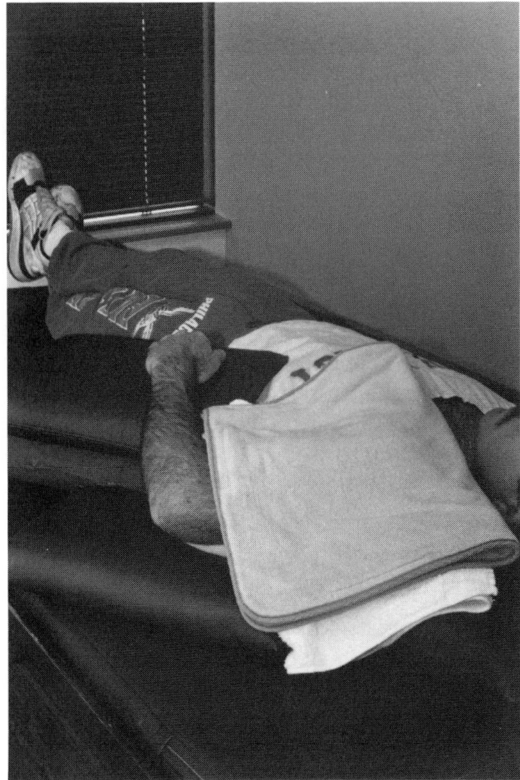

**Figure 6-6.** Hydrocollator pad application to the anterior and posterior shoulder with the patient in a reclined position.

# Limitations in Joint Mobility and Stability

Pain, adaptive shortening of tissues, and compromised muscle performance after shoulder injury or surgery can limit shoulder mobility and stability. This section will describe the use of physical agents in treating limitations in shoulder mobility and instability due to shortening of tissues and poor muscle performance.

## Thermal Agents

### BIOPHYSICAL EFFECTS

Increasing the temperature of connective tissues tends to increase the extensibility of these tissues[18,27,37] and reduce joint stiffness.[1,44] The increased temperature alters the viscoelastic properties of connective tissue so that less force is required to lengthen the tissue. Decreasing the temperature of tissues apparently has the opposite effect. *Joint stiffness*, defined as the amount of torque required to passively move a limb segment through a range of motion, was found to decrease following heat application and increase with the application of cold treatment.[1,44] Therefore, if the purpose of using physical agents is to enhance joint mobility programs, it would seem logical to use modalities that can elevate tissue temperatures.

### TREATMENT TECHNIQUES

Physical agents that provide heat to tissues are combined with stretching techniques to improve the mobility of the shoulder. Data from animal studies investigating the effectiveness of heat combined with stretching in lengthening tissues support this practice. Few controlled clinical studies, however, have been done to examine this treatment approach on contracted human tissues. Based on the data available, supplementing shoulder mobility programs with heat modalities would seem to be a logical treatment approach.

The glenohumeral joint–capsuloligamentous complex is probably the structure of most concern when significant restrictions in motion occur at the shoulder; however, adaptive shortening of muscles and tendons also may contribute to this problem. A deep-heating modality such as ultrasound seems most appropriate to target these deeper tissues. Ultrasound treatment parameters should be consistent with those necessary to produce a thermal effect (continuous-wave ultrasound from 1.0 to 1.2 W/cm$^2$ over the shoulder). The duration of treatment should be determined by the size of the treatment area (refer to the section on inflammation).

Determining the location of the tissue restriction is important for deciding which area of the shoulder is to be treated with ultrasound. This can be done by identifying the motions that are limited. For example, limitations in abduction and external rotation may indicate that the tissue restrictions are anterior and inferior to the glenohumeral joint. Therefore, ultrasound should be applied to the anterior and inferior aspects of the glenohumeral joint. The patient's arm should be positioned at or near the end of the pain-free range of abduction and external rotation while the ultrasound is applied to these areas (Fig. 6-7). This would place the target tissues in a lengthened position during heat application. Maintaining the patient in this position

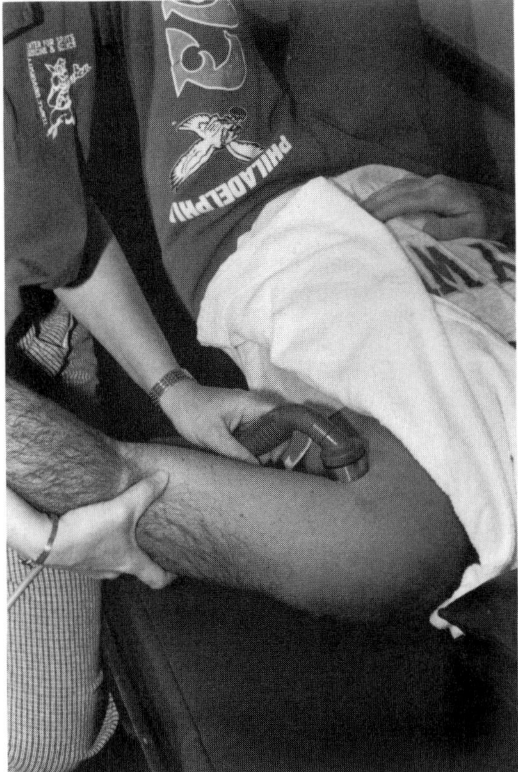

**Figure 6-7.** Ultrasound treatment directed at the anterior and inferior tissues of the shoulder.

for several minutes after ultrasound treatment may enhance the effectiveness of the mobility program.[27]

# Electrical Stimulation

## Biophysical Effects

When muscles that normally produce movement at a joint are compromised by disuse or guarding due to pain, joint mobility may be reduced due to the lack of movement. Neuromuscular electrical stimulation (NMES) can induce muscle contraction to cause movement of limb segments so that the mobility of the joint can be maintained. NMES programs have been described in the literature for the wrist and hand, knee, and ankle joints.[3,7,33,43] Producing shoulder motion through NMES is probably not practical due to the complexity and interaction of muscles acting about the shoulder.

If the patient is able to actively elevate the arm through a partial range of motion, NMES may be used to assist in increasing the amount of active motion at the shoulder. Volitional movement has been shown to improve by combining NMES with exercise programs.[7,28,43] Although these reports have not included the shoulder joint, it seems logical that the same principles may apply to the shoulder. Further research investigating the use of NMES for improving shoulder mobility and strength is needed.

After shoulder injury or surgery, patients may sometimes be unable to voluntarily contract the muscles around the shoulder. If this condition continues, the muscles may become atrophied and weakened. NMES may be used to reduce the rate of atrophy and strength loss until voluntary muscle contraction has been restored.

### TREATMENT TECHNIQUES

Before initiating an NMES program for shoulder rehabilitation, the therapist must consider the parameters that are necessary to induce a smooth muscular contraction. Delitto and Robinson[12] have outlined the essential parameters needed for NMES. The instrument used for treatment should have controls for pulse rate and amplitude, ramp modulation, and on/off time duty cycles.

Table 6-4 outlines stimulus parameters for NMES. The pulse rate control should include a range from at least 40 to 50 pulses per second. Pulse rates greater than this will cause more rapid fatigue of muscle. The amplitude should be great enough to allow for smooth muscle contraction yet remain tolerable to the patient. Ramp modulation allows for a gradual increase up to the treatment amplitude, providing greater comfort to the patient during treatment. A ramp up of 2 to 4 s is commonly used in treatment. Although most instruments provide a ramp-down control,

**Table 6-4**

**Available Units and Stimulus Characteristics for NMES**

| Treatment Purpose | Stimulus Characteristics | Units Available |
|---|---|---|
| Muscle relaxation | Pulse rate: 80–100 pps<br>Pulse duration: 20 μs<br>On/off time ratio: 1:1<br>Ramp: 0 to 2 s | Low volt<br>HVPC |
| Muscle reeducation | Pulse rate: 35–50 pps<br>Pulse duration: 20–1000 μs<br>On/off time ratio: 1:3, 1:5<br>Ramp: 2–4 s | Low volt |

this is usually not necessary for patients with musculoskeletal conditions. The on/off duty cycle allows the therapist to select the amount of time that stimulation will be on and the amount of rest from stimulation. This control is important in preventing fatigue of the muscle during treatment. An on/off time ratio of 1:3 (e.g., 10 s on, 30 s off) to 1:5 is usually recommended to prevent muscle fatigue. Some instruments allow for control of pulse duration, but many do not. The instrument should provide a range of pulse duration from 200 to 300μs for adequate muscle contraction.

A number of electrical stimulators can be used for NMES treatment. Most portable stimulators provide sufficient amplitude for NMES treatment in shoulder rehabilitation. If an adequate muscle contraction is not achieved due to limitations in power output with a portable unit, therapists may try a clinical unit as an alternative, when available.

Electrodes are usually placed over the motor point or the muscle belly of the muscle being stimulated. The size of the electrodes varies depending on the size of the muscles to be activated and their proximity to muscles that the therapist does not wish to activate. Caution should be taken to avoid electrodes that are too large, thus dispersing current to ineffectual levels or recruiting unwanted muscles. Conversely, with very small electrodes, the increased current density may be uncomfortable.

NMES is typically used to retard muscular atrophy and/or promote joint stability after shoulder injury or surgery. Isometric cocontraction of multiple muscles surrounding the shoulder joint may be induced with NMES for this purpose. Therefore, instruments used in treatment should allow for simultaneous stimulation on both channels of the instrument.

When using NMES to assist in increasing the available active motion of the shoulder, therapists must identify the muscles involved in producing the desired motion. For example, if forward shoulder elevation is to be improved with NMES, the infraspinatus muscle (joint stability) and the anterior deltoid (prime mover) should be identified as electrode placement sites for NMES treatment. The patient is asked to perform forward shoulder elevation actively using maximum effort while the stimulator is on. NMES treatment may be continued as a supplement to active range-of-motion exercise until the therapist determines that the patient can elevate the arm to the desired range of motion without stimulation.

There is some controversy as to whether NMES treatment is useful in conditions in which muscle is denervated. Some experts believe that the minimal and temporary benefits of NMES under these conditions are not worth the time and effort.[10,12] Baker[2] suggests that if therapists believe there may be potential for improvement, a trial of NMES treatment may be appropriate. If, however, improvement is not observed within a few weeks, it is probably not worth continuing this approach.

NMES can be incorporated into the patient's home rehabilitation program. Once the treatment parameters have been determined, most patients and their family members can be instructed in the use of NMES devices for home use. There is usually adequate third-party payer reimbursement for rental or purchase of these devices. If the therapist believes that the cognitive state of the patient or family is not conducive to safe operation of NMES devices for home use, then this treatment application should be avoided.

### CASE REPORT 4

K.S., a 48-year-old computer salesman, had an acromioplasty 1 year ago for a chronic impingement syndrome. Two months ago he slipped on the stairs and sustained a bad bruise of the soft tissues around the shoulder. Unfortunately, he developed a "frozen" shoulder. He was referred to physical therapy, and after an evaluation, the therapist chose to use ultrasound combined with stretching to improve motion. K.S. was positioned with the affected limb at end-range flexion. Ultrasound was applied at 1.2 W/cm$^2$, continuous mode, 1 MHz, for 5 minutes to the inferior glenohumeral capsule and 5 minutes to the anterior capsule. Joint and soft-tissue mobilization techniques were performed in an attempt to increase external rotation and elevation following the ultrasound application.

## Summary

The use of physical agents as a treatment supplement for inflammation, pain, and joint mobility and stability in shoulder rehabilitation programs has been discussed. Case reports have been provided to illustrate the use of various physical agents for these clinical problems. Therapists are encouraged to identify the clinical problem and the biophysical effects needed to alleviate the problem before selecting a physical agent for treatment. The treatment parameters should be consistent with the biophysical effect that is to be achieved with the physical agent. The effectiveness of physical agents as a supplement to a shoulder rehabilitation program is dependent on sound clinical decision making on the part of the physical therapist.

# References


1. Bäcklund L, Tiselius P. Objective measurement of joint stiffness in rheumatoid arthritis. Acta Rheum Scand. 1967;13:275.
2. Baker LL. Neuromuscular electrical stimulation in the restoration of purposeful limb movements. In: Wolf SL, ed. Electrotherapy. New York: Churchill Livingstone, 1981:25.
3. Baker LL, Yeh C, Wilson D, Waters RL. Electrical stimulation of wrist and fingers for hemiplegic patients. Phys Ther 1979;59:1495.
4. Becker RO, Murray DG. Method for producing cellular dedifferentiation by means of very small electric currents. Ann NY Acad Sci 1967;29:606.
5. Benson HAE, McElnay JC. Transmission of ultrasound energy through topical pharmaceutical products. Physiotherapy 1988; 74:587.
6. Cameron MH, Monroe LG. Relative transmission of ultrasound by media customarily used for phonophoresis. Phys Ther 1992; 72:142.
7. Carnstam B, Larson L, Prevec T. Improvement of gait following electrical stimulation: I. Investigations on changes in voluntary strength and proprioceptive reflexes. Scand J Rehabil Med 1977: 9:7.
8. Chantraine A, Lundy JP, Berger D. Is cortisone iontophoresis possible? Arch Phys Med Rehabil 1986;67:38.
9. Ciccone CD, Leggin BG, Callamaro JJ. Effects of ultrasound and trolamine salicylate phonophoresis on delayed-onset muscle soreness. Phys Ther 1991;71:666.
10. Cummings J. Electrical stimulation of healthy muscle. In: Nelson RM, Currier DP, eds, Clinical electrotherapy. East Norwalk, Conn.: Appleton-Century-Crofts, 1987:81.
11. Davick JP, Martin RK, Albright JP. Distribution and deposition of tritiated cortisol using phonophoresis. Phys Ther 1988;68:1672.
12. Delitto A, Robinson AJ. Electrical stimulation of muscle: techniques and applications. In: Snyder-Mackler L, Robinson AJ, eds. Clinical electrophysiology, electrotherapy, and electrophysiologic testing. Baltimore: Williams & Wilkins, 1989:95.
13. Dorwart BB, et al. Effects of heat, cold, and agitation on crystal-induced arthritis in the dog. Arthritis Rheum 1973;16:540.
14. Dyson M, Luke DA. Induction of mast cell degranulation in skin by ultrasound. IEEE Trans Ultrason Ferroelec Frequency Control UFFC 1986;33:194.
15. Farry PJ, et al. Ice treatment of injured ligaments: an experimental model. NZ Med J 1980;12:12.
16. Fish DR, Mendel FC, Schultz AM, Gottstein-Yerke LM. Effect of anodal high-voltage pulsed current on edema formation in frog hind limbs. Phys Ther 1991;71:724.
17. Gammon GD, Starr I. Studies on the relief of pain by counterirritation. J Clin Invest 1941;20:13.
18. Gersten JW. Effect of ultrasound on tendon extensibility. Am J Phys Med 1955;34:362.
19. Glass JM, Stephen RL, Jacobsen SC. The quantity and distribution of radiolabeled dexamethasone delivered to tissue by iontophoresis. Int J Dermatol 1980;19:519.
20. Glick E, Snyder-Mackler L. Iontophoresis. In: Snyder-Mackler L, Robinson AJ, eds. Clinical electrophysiology, electrotherapy and electrophysiologic testing. Baltimore: Williams & Wilkins, 1989: 247.
21. Grant AE. Massage with ice (cryokinetics) in the treatment of painful conditions of the musculoskeletal system. Arch Phys Med Rehabil 1964;45:233.
22. Hasson S. Exercise training and dexamethasone iontophoresis in RA: a case study. Physiother Can 1991;3:11.
23. Hayden CA. Cryokinetics in an early treatment program. Am Phys Ther Assoc 1964;44:990.
24. Kleinkort JA, Wood F. Phonophoresis with 1 percent versus 10 percent hydrocortisone. Phys Ther 1975;55:1320.
25. Kloth LC, Morrison M, Ferguson B. Therapeutic microwave and shortwave diathermy: a review of thermal effectiveness, safe use, and state-of-the-art. Washington: Center for Devices on Radiological Health, DHHS, FDA 85-8237, 1984.
26. Knight KL. Cryotherapy: theory, technique and physiology. Chattanooga, Tenn.: Chattanooga Corp, 1985:154.
27. Lehmann JF, Masock AJ, Warren CG, Koblanski JN. Effect of therapeutic temperatures on tendon extensibility. Arch Phys Med Rehabil 1970;51:481.
28. Liberson WT, Holmquist HJ, Scot D, Dow M. Functional electrotherapy: stimulation of the peroneal nerve synchronized with the swing phase of gait of hemiplegic patients. Arch Phys Med Rehabil 1961;42:101.
29. Mannheimer JS, Lampe GN. Clinical transcutaneous electrical nerve stimulation. Philadelphia: FA Davis, 1984:249.
30. Melzack R, Wall P. The challenge of pain. New York: Penguin Books, 1982.
31. Michlovitz SL. Cryotherapy: the use of cold as a therapeutic agent. In: Michlovitz SL, ed. Thermal agents in rehabilitation. Philadelphia: FA Davis, 1990:63.
32. Michlovitz SL, Smith W, Watkins MP. Ice and high-voltage pulsed stimulation in treatment of lateral ankle sprains. Orthop Sports Phys Ther 1988;9:301.
33. Munsat TL, McNeal DR, Waters RL. Preliminary observations on prolonged stimulation of peripheral nerve in man. Arch Neurol 1976;33:608.
34. Newton RA. Contemporary views on pain and the role played by thermal agents in managing pain symptoms. In: Michlovitz SL, ed. Thermal agents in rehabilitation. Philadelphia: FA Davis, 1990:18.
35. Ray CD. Electrical stimulation: new methods for therapy and rehabilitation. Scand J Rehabil Med 1978;10:65.
36. Reid DC, Cummings GE. Factors in selecting the dosage of ultrasound with particular reference to the use of various coupling agents. Physiother Can 1973;63:225.
37. Rippe B, Grega GJ. Effects of 150 prenaline and cooling on histamine-induced changes of capillary permeability in the rat hind quarter bed. Acta Physiol Scand 1978;103:252.
38. Schaubel HH. Local use of ice after orthopedic procedures. Am J Surg. 1946;72:711.
39. Snyder-Mackler L. Electrical stimulation for pain modulation. In: Snyder-Mackler L, Robinson AJ, eds. Clinical electrophysiology, electrotherapy and electrophysiologic testing. Baltimore: Williams & Wilkins, 1989:203.
40. Snyder-Mackler L. Electrical stimulation for tissue repair. In: Snyder-Mackler L, Robinson AJ, eds. Clinical electrophysiology, electrotherapy and electrophysiologic testing. Baltimore: Williams & Wilkins, 1989:229.
41. Stralka SW. Protocol: neuromuscular electrical stimulation for postoperative knee patients. St. Paul: 3M, 1984.
42. Travell JG, Simons DG. Myofascial pain and dysfunction: the trigger point manual. Baltimore: Williams & Wilkins, 1983.
43. Winchester P, Montgomery J, Bowman B, Hislop H. Effects of feedback stimulation training and cyclical electrical stimulation on knee extension in hemiparetic patients. Phys Ther 1983; 63:1096.
44. Wright V, Johns RJ. Physical factors concerned with the stiffness of normal and diseased joints. Bull Johns Hopkins Hosp 1960; 106:215.
45. Ziskin MC, McDiarmid T, Michlovitz SL. Therapeutic ultrasound. In: Michlovitz SL, ed. Thermal agents in rehabilitation. Philadelphia: FA Davis, 1990:134.

Chapter 7

Joel A. Henry

# Manual Therapy of the Shoulder



Martin J. Kelley and William A. Clark: ORTHOPEDIC THERAPY OF THE SHOULDER.

The shoulder joint system allows the greatest range of motion in the human body. Because the joint design favors mobility at the expense of inherent stability, greater demands are placed on the supporting soft tissues to provide both static and dynamic stabilization.

The soft-tissue network of the shoulder complex is expansive, as necessitated by functional requirements. Striated muscle, along with its organizing areolar and dense connective tissue, forms a functionally inseparable composite termed *myofascia*. The attachments of myofascial components of the shoulder span the entire spine from occiput to pelvis and every level of the thoracic cage.[21] Sheaths of investing fascia, continuous beyond muscle origins and insertions, provide structural and functional integration between the shoulder and other anatomic regions.

The quantity of soft tissue and the multiple stresses placed on it make soft-tissue dysfunction a common occurrence at the shoulder. Rehabilitation therefore presents opportunities to employ techniques derived from a broad spectrum comprising the armamentarium of joint and soft-tissue mobilization techniques. These exist in a wide variety of formats derived from medical, osteopathic, and nonmedical sources and from within the profession of physical therapy.

The objective of this chapter is to familiarize the reader with several clinically useful concepts and techniques applicable to the management of shoulder dysfunctions that can be supported by the basic sciences and current anatomic and neurophysiologic principles.

It is the authors' hope that the reader will appreciate the inherent difficulties undertaken in attempting to learn manual therapy from written descriptions, skills that can only be acquired through practical experience. The reader therefore is encouraged to seek out training from those proficient in the techniques reviewed here.

Whether one chooses to perform a joint or soft-tissue mobilization technique to improve mobility, the tissues being affected (joint capsule, ligament, tendon, muscle, or fascia) are all forms of connective tissue. Therefore, an appreciation of its histochemical makeup, mechanical behavior, and response to injury and immobilization is paramount to effective intervention.

# Characteristics of Connective Tissue

## Histochemical Makeup

Ordinary fibrous connective tissue includes ligaments, tendons, synovial membrane, fascia, aponeuroses, and fibrous joint capsules. Ordinary connective tissue is comprised of cellular and fiber elements embedded in a gel-like ground substance.[21]

The primary cellular elements include fibroblasts, macrophage cells, mast cells, and undifferentiated mesenchymal cells. The fibroblasts are the main reproductive cells and are responsible for manufacturing the fiber components. Mature fibroblastic cells are also called *fibrocytes*. Histamine-releasing mast cells and phagocytic macrophage cells are commonly found in abundance throughout the connective tissues.

The fibers of connective tissue are of two primary types, collagenous and elastic. Collagen is the most abundant fiber element and is responsible for the tensile strength of the tissue. Collagen is a crystalline structure that is pliable but not very extensible. Collagen is composed of smaller unit fibers, held together by intra- and intermolecular cross-links, which increase in number to give collagen increased tensile strength as it matures. Elastin is a homogeneous fiber that varies in thickness and length and is rubbery and stretchable. Elastin provides extensibility to the tissue and is present in variable proportion to collagen, depending on the specific function of the tissue.

The ground substance is composed of 60 to 70 percent water, bound to glycoaminoglycans (GAG), which create a semifluid gel in which the cells and fibers are suspended.[1,14,21] The ground substance gives the tissue form and provides for movement and continuity. Four types of glycoaminoglycans have been identified in connective tissue: hyaluronic acid, chondroitin-4-sulfate, chondroitin-6-sulfate, and dermatin sulfate.[1,14] Hyaluronic acid, bound abundantly with water molecules, is thought to function as the primary lubricating substance, allowing for free fiber mobility.

Fibrous connective tissue is classified as either dense or loose depending on the density of the elements contained in the ground substance. Dense fibrous connective tissue is subclassified as organized or unorganized depending on the fiber orientation of the tissue. Organized dense fibrous connective tissues include tendons, ligaments, and aponeuroses, which have collagen fibers arranged in compact, parallel bundles that provide unidirectional tensile strength.

Unorganized dense fibrous connective tissues include joint and organ capsule, periosteum, dermis, dura mater, and fascial membranes.[21] In these tissues the fibers are found to be interwoven, not parallel, providing for multidirectional extensibility and tensile strength.

## Fascia

*Fascia*, from the Latin meaning "bandage" or "wrapping," is the term used in gross anatomy for all fibrous connective tissue not given a specific designation.[21] Fascia is an elastocollagenous tissue that exists in variable dense areolar and seromembranous forms depending on its local functional specialization. Three major subdivisions of the fascial system are the superficial, deep, and subserous layers. The superficial fascia covers the entire body immediately under the dermis. It is comprised of two distinct layers. The panniculus adiposus, or hypoderm, is the fatty outer layer that varies in thickness depending on the quantity of adipose tissue present. Under the hypoderm is the fibromembranous layer of superficial fascia, which is continuous with the hypoderm. In some areas, a potential space exists between the superficial and deep fascia.

The deep investing fascia is composed of dense, white, unorganized connective tissue. The deep fascias represent laminated, multilayered sheaths that divide to form body compartments, capsules of organs and viscera, and the wrappings of bone, nerves, and muscles. The deep fascial system extends with little interruption throughout the body.[21]

### FUNCTIONS OF FASCIA

Principal functions of fascia include defining anatomic shapes; binding and separating various tissue elements; forming anatomic compartments, capsules, and interstitial spaces; and providing structural support and protection, fluid regulation, and immune system functions.[21] Under nonpathologic conditions, the fascial investments allow free mobility and gliding between independent structures.

Fascia is subject to inflammation, erosion, calcification, and thickening during pathologic conditions. Fascia undergoes adaptation and remodeling in response to applied stresses. The shoulder complex is readily influenced by changes in fascial extensibility that occur in adaptation to postural influences. The multilaminal cervical fascia descends from the cranial base like a shawl draped over the whole of the shoulder yoke, being continuous with the clavipectoral, deltoid, and periscapular fascias. Portions of the fascial network may be found to be inextensible and shortened in the individual presenting with forward head postural dysfunction. Thickening and calcification occur at the insertion of the levator scapulae and rhomboid minor at the superomedial scapula angle. Distally, the dense, extremely strong lumbodorsal fascia can influence the shoulder through the latissimus dorsi and presents a commonly overlooked component of shoulder dysfunction.

## Myofascial Integration

Skeletal muscle is structurally and functionally integrated by fascia on both a macroscopic and a microscopic level. The description *myofascial* is quite accurate, since skeletal muscle, for all practical purposes, does not exist without fascia.

In the muscle interior, the sarcomere muscle cells are arranged linearly in tubes of elastic fascia, the *endomysium*. The contractile units are organized into fascicles or bundles by fibroelastic fascia, the *perimysium*, which is continuous with the *epimysium*, or outer layer of deep investing fascia that wraps the entire muscle.[21] Continuous fascial sheathing and bundling organizes the muscles into functional groups and compartments in the extremities. Fascial continuity from microscopic through macroscopic structural integration functions as a harness that effectively converts energy generated in the sarcomeres to function, providing for skeletal movement and stabilization.

The myofascial complex represents a functional integration of active and passive structural components (Fig. 7-1). The sarcomeres represent the active component, where contractile forces are generated by neurochemical action, influenced directly by alpha motor neuron, gamma efferent, and spinal reflex activity, and metabolic controls. Tendons and fascia represent the passive components along with the periosteal attachments and skeleton.[6] Tendons are arranged in series with the active elements, while the fascial harness is arranged in parallel. The

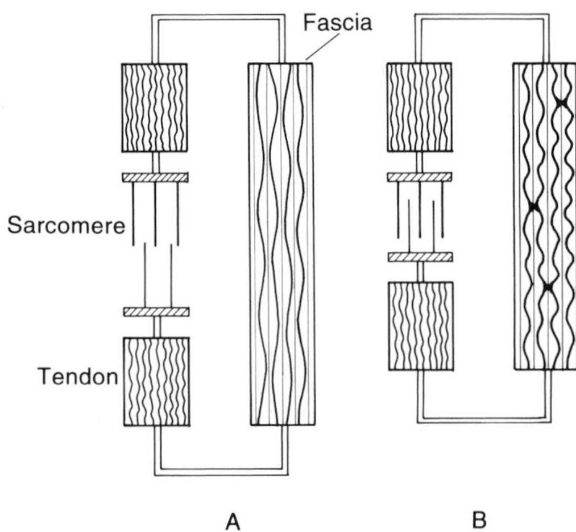


**Figure 7-1.** The myofascial complex. (a) Relaxed state. (b) Contracted state. The sarcomeres represent the active component; tendons and fascia represent the passive components along with the periosteal attachments and skeleton. Tendons are arranged in series with the active elements, while the fascial harness is arranged in parallel.

passive elements, while directly influenced by the active component, likewise influence the active elements via the muscle and connective-tissue receptor systems. Fascia, comprising muscle septa and wrapping, is similar in composition and mechanical properties to fibrous joint capsule, having unorganized fiber orientation. A relationship exists between the structural fiber constituents and their mechanical function. The proportion of collagen to elastin fibers determines the tissues mechanical response to extension or loading. The fascial system is always under some degree of load, being integrated with skeletal muscle and influenced by muscle tone and contraction.

## Mechanical Behavior of Connective Tissue

Bioengineering models explaining the mechanical behavior of collagenous tissues have been experimentally derived and are helpful in understanding the response of connective tissue to mechanical or manual therapy.

Dense ordinary connective tissues demonstrate elastic, plastic, and viscous properties. The degree to which the tissue will exhibit these biomechanical properties is in part a function of the proportion of cellular elements to extracellular water in the ground substance and the ratio of collagen to elastin fibers present. The composition will differ from tissue to tissue and during pathologic conditions, influencing the nature of mechanical response. Elastin, as the name implies, is readily extensible when loaded and possesses memory, allowing it to return to its original length when unloaded. Elastin provides for the elastic property of the tissue. In contrast, collagen is an inextensible fiber whose covalently bonded crystalline structure provides tensile strength. A higher proportion of collagen to elastin gives the tissue a more plastic nature.

The stress-strain graph is a useful model to express certain mechanical properties of connective tissue (Fig. 7-2). The stress-strain model can be applied similarly to explain the behavior of individual collagen fibers within the tissue or the elastocollagenous tissue complex such as ligament or fascia.

*Stress* is defined as load per cross-sectional area.[22,65] When a connective tissue is stressed initially, some degree of stiffness or resistance is encountered, which is influenced by the rate of stress application. A rapid load will encounter greater stiffness than a slowly applied load of the same magnitude. The elastin fibers engage early, offering low resistance, and attempt to restore the tissue to its original shape. When stress is applied and released without exceeding the elastic range (point $A_1$), the tissue will return to its original length (point $A_2$). The ability of the tissue to return to its original length over time when the stress is released is called a *hysteresis loop*. If stress loading continues beyond the elastic range, the tissue stiffens as the majority of col-

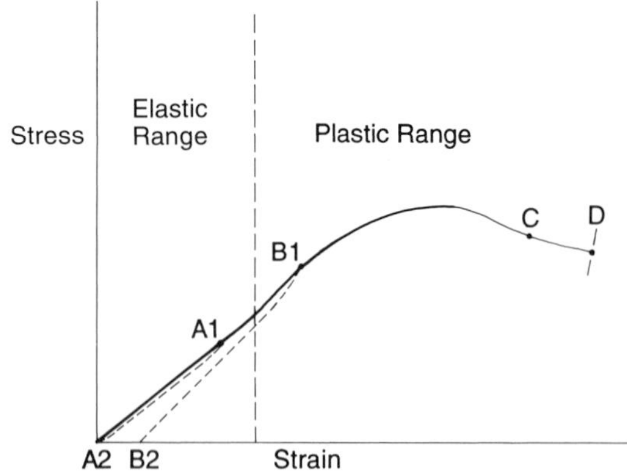


**Figure 7-2.** Stress-strain graph. Stress (load) applied and released without exceeding the elastic range (point $A_1$); the tissue will return to its original length (point $A_2$). If stress loading continues beyond the elastic range and then released ($B_1$), the tissue will shorten toward an unloaded state that differs from the original loaded state and assumes a new length (point $B_2$). Necking (*C*) represents structural weakening without any increase in the amount of stress applied. Strain of sufficient magnitude to produce structural failure of the tissue is represented by point *D*.

lagen fibers are engaged and straightened. The degree of extension will differ in individual fibers. When the load is released (point $B_1$), the tissue will shorten toward an unloaded state, that is, some degree less than the original loaded state, and assumes a new length (point $B_2$). When this occurs, the tissue is said to have undergone *strain*, which is defined as the degree of elongation per unit of original tissue length the tissue undergoes in response to stress, represented as the difference between points $A_2$ and $B_2$. The difference between the original and new length implies that some change has occurred in the structure of the tissue.

When elastocollagenous tissue such as fascia or ligament is subjected to loading held at a constant level, it will undergo extension and then relax as the initial stiffness is overcome. If the load is held constant over time, the tissue will continue to extend, or "creep," in response to the sustained load.[22] The process by which the degree of strain increases without increasing the stress load is referred to as *necking* (point *C*). Continuous loading of the tissue that exceeds the inherent tensile capacity results in structural weakening in the collagen fibers and tissue failure (point *D*). The rate of load application is significant to the ability of the tissue to accommodate the load or stress placed on it. Rapid, forceful loading of connective tissue that overwhelms the existing potential for load accommodation is a common mechanism resulting in structural failure and injury. The grade III acromioclavicular separation is a common example occurring at the shoulder where rapid loading results in elongation or strain to a destructive magnitude, typically referred to as *ligament sprain*. Repetitive cycle overloading, encountered in overuse injuries, can gradually weaken the tissue to a similar point of failure. Clinically, this is representative of certain cumulative trauma disorders.

The mechanical behavior of connective tissue demonstrated in experimental models must be appreciated in the clinical setting as the basis for the application of skilled manual therapy techniques, such as soft-tissue and joint mobilization, myofascial release, and other stretching procedures.

The stress-strain model used to describe the response of normal connective tissue also can be applied to connective tissue that has been traumatized. In the clinical setting, one recognizes the pathologic changes in the connective tissues by examination or evaluation. Once having detected the specific pathologic change or changes, the clinician can then select an appropriate intervention.

# Connective Tissue Dysfunction

## Myofascial Injuries

Glick[19] outlined a useful classification scheme, developed for the assessment of quadriceps injury, that is readily applicable to all myofascial structures.

Type I myofascial injury is typified by disabling pain from myofascial tearing. Four distinct grades of type I injuries are described:

*Grade I*: Small amount of muscle fiber damage with no fascial tearing, swelling, and pain with stretching.

*Grade II*: Moderate amount of muscle fiber damage, localized hematoma, but no fascial tearing.

*Grade III*: Large amount of muscle fiber damage, partial fascial disruption, and diffuse bleeding and ecchymosis.

*Grade IV*: Complete disruption of muscle and fascia, gross ecchymosis, palpable defect, and loss of function.

Type II myofascial injury is characterized by soreness or cramping during or immediately after exercise. In contrast to type I, pain will decrease with passive stretching.

Type III is typified by delayed-onset symptoms, occurring 24 to 48 hours after exercise, no swelling, and decreased pain with passive stretching. Significantly greater incidence of delayed-onset muscle soreness occurs following eccentric contractions. Several possible explanations exist to explain delayed-onset muscle soreness. Minute tears in muscle fibers, osmotic pressure changes with water retention, muscle spasms, and connective-tissue damage have been considered. There is some experimental evidence supporting muscle tearing and connective-tissue damage as a cause.[42]

## Myofascial Adhesions

Adhesion can develop following myofascial injury that is accompanied by inflammation, bleeding, and limited movement beginning 3 to 5 days following injury.[8, 65] When tearing of muscle or its fascia occurs, scarring helps restore function by reuniting the disrupted tissues. At the same time, intramuscular scar tissue adhesions can result in movement restriction by forming between adjacent fasciculi, limiting independent gliding of fiber bundles within the same muscle. The same process can adhere the muscle to neighboring muscle, fascia, skin, or bone. Adhesions can impose mechanical limitation of active and passive movement and act as an irritant that can result in loss of mobility because of pain during movement.

Adhesions of tendon can readily involve adjacent bursae, which normally possess freedom to glide, compress, or extend. Inflammatory processes involving the supraspinatus tendon and subacromial bursa can lead to tendon-bursa adhesions that alter the physiologic mobility of the tendon over the bursa that occurs during glenohumeral movement.

## Changes with Immobilization

Immobilization of fibrous connective tissues such as ligament, capsule, and fascia can result in matrix changes that decrease the mobility and extensibility of the tissue. Movement provides for potential functional organization of newly synthesized fibers and maintenance of lubrication and critical distance between the cells and fibers within the ground substance.[1,14,65] Studies by Akeson and Woo using animal subjects described the periarticular connective-tissue changes following immobilization of joints for a 9-week period. These changes in the matrix included a reduction in glycosaminoglycan (GAG) and extracellular water content and increased formation of interfiber cross-linkages. The increase in abnormal cross-links is a result of decreased critical fiber distance created by GAG depletion, particularly hyaluronic acid, and water loss. Immobilization deprives the tissue of movement necessary to orient the newly synthesized fibers along functional planes. The extensibility of the connective tissue is diminished by the presence of abnormal cross-links that limit collagen fiber movement, restricting the normal range of mobility and capacity for expansion specific to the function of that tissue (Fig. 7-3). The changes that occur in response to immobilization, summarized in the following list, occur similarly in all dense ordinary periarticular connective tissues, including ligament, capsule, tendon, and fascia.[14]

### EFFECTS OF IMMOBILIZATION

- Reduced collagen synthesis rate
- No net reduction of collagen content
- Random new fiber orientation
- Reduction in glycosaminoglycan content
- Loss of extracellular water volume
- Increased viscosity in ground substance
- Decreased distance between fibers
- Abnormal cross-linkage between new and mature fibers
- Diminished tissue extensibility

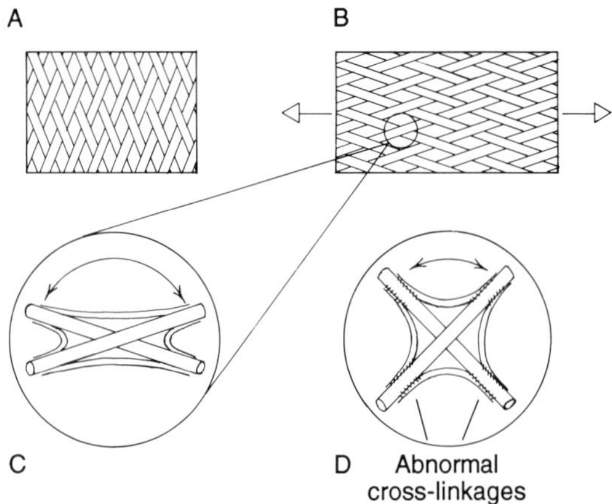

**Figure 7-3.** (a) Normal collagen fiber orientation in relaxed state. (b) Extended fiber alignment. (c) Magnified area of unrestricted fiber gliding when extended. (d) Abnormal cross-linkages limiting fiber gliding and tissue extensibility.

## Fibrositis and Chronic Inflammation

Chronic inflammation or fibrositis can occur in connective tissues following trauma, immobilization, or limited use during painful conditions. Adhesions, scar tissue, chemical exudates, and muscle tension can act as chronic irritants that retard the eventual resolution of the inflammation and healing process.[8,65] Low-grade inflammation can persist as long as some form of chronic irritant is present.[8]

Chronic myofascial inflammation can lead to fibrosis. Fibrosis involves changes in the connective-tissue matrix, including proliferation of collagen, increased fiber density, and interfiber cross-linkages that limit the extensibility of the tissue. Some degree of fibrositis and fibrosis may be found in the shoulder soft tissues in patients who present with capsular restrictions resulting from the same histopathologic connective-tissue changes. The upper trunk and scapular regions should be examined for the signs and symptoms of chronic inflammation or fibrositis, which can include generalized low-grade aching pain, warmth, sponginess, and redness, exaggerated histamine responses, and wheal formation. The resulting fibrosis is typified by loss of skin and superficial fascia mobility, tender subcutaneous nodules, and stringy myofascial texture. The nature of palpable nodules remains in question.

## Muscle Tone and Hypertonicity

Muscular tone is a product of the both active and passive elements of the myofascial complex. Tissue turgor, viscosity, and elasticity are components of tone as well as neuromuscular activity. A normal muscle at complete rest can be found to be electrically silent yet possess tone.[3] Likewise, muscles exhibiting hypertonicity also may be found to be in an electrically silent state at rest.

Spasm, conversely, is a consequence of neuromuscular reflexes triggering alpha motor discharge in response to stretch or pressure stimuli.[3] The term *spasm* is often used inappropriately to describe other manifestations of hypertonicity.

The interaction between pain, spasm, and dysfunction can be represented by the chain of events depicted in Figure 7-4. While this chain of events is typical of reflex somatic response to various pathologies, it offers an oversimplified representation of the various components of hypertonicity accompanying dysfunction typically encountered in the orthopedic setting.[49,50]

*Spasm* may be described more accurately as a brief involuntary neuromuscular response, reflexly triggered and typically perceived as painful. Spasm may occur repeatedly but is transient. Sustained spasmlike states can involve voluntary neuromuscular activity, fluid congestion, and histopathologic connective-tissue changes in addition to involuntary contraction. What is palpated and termed *hypertonicity* is an aggregate of involuntary, voluntary, fluid, and chemical holding influences perpetrated and sustained to some level of interaction. Paris[50] expanded the previously limited concept of the interactions among pain, spasm, and dysfunction as illustrated in Figure 7-4a to that demonstrated in Figure 7-4b.[50] A discussion of the chain of events can begin arbitrarily with the concept of involuntary muscle holding. The manual therapist regularly encounters involuntary holding when attempting to position the patient's arm for a passive mobilization technique and encounters resistance despite the patient's insistence that he or she is relaxed. The individual is unaware that a certain amount of contraction is present. Pain is not necessarily a component, but the individual experiences an altered perception of what constitutes a relaxed state of the muscle involved. Indeed, the muscle can be palpated or observed to be in a partially contracted state, even when the limb is passively supported. This situation is typically manifested in the trapezius, deltoid, and pectoralis muscles at the shoulder.

Because sustained partial contracture reduces the muscle's ability to pump venous and lymphatic fluids, a gradual buildup and retention of metabolites occur. Fluid congestion alters the palpable muscle tone, which superficially may be felt to be swollen but is firm and indurated upon deeper examination. Metabolite retention sensitizes the free nerve endings, alerting the nervous system (nociperception), thereby establishing awareness of discomfort and the potential for voluntary and neuromuscular reflex influences on tone. Chemical holding is accompanied by changes in pH in the local tissues, fibrotic changes, and eventual palpable tissue texture abnormalities.

Pain, being a highly individualized interpretation of its precursor, nociperception, is potentially the initiator, perpetrator, or result of this cycle of events depending on the etiology of the particular dysfunction. Adaptive shortening or contracture of the involved muscle is a consequence of sustained muscle holding, which represents a more permanent condition in that once it occurs, it will remain even after all perpetrating events have been eliminated. The clinical implications of such an arrangement consider the inseparable nature of the active and passive myo-

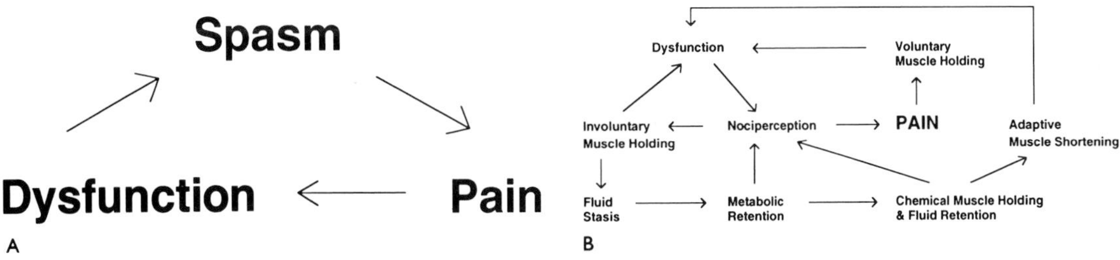


**Figure 7-4.** (a) Limited concept of reflex relationships between pain, spasm, and dysfunction. (b) Expanded perspective depicting the potential interrelationships of pain to various muscle holding states distinctly different by nature. (Reproduced with permission from Paris SV. Foundations of clinical orthopaedics. St. Augustine, Fla.: Institute Press, Division of Patris, 1989.)

fascial elements, whose dynamics are under combined neuromuscular, circulatory, metabolic, mechanical, and behavioral influences.

# Contracture and Adaptive Shortening

Adaptive shortening, myostatic contracture, and pseudomyostatic contracture represent subclassifications of myofascial shortening that are differentiated by the nature of their associated histopathologic mechanisms[8,9] (Fig. 7-5).

## ADAPTIVE SHORTENING

Adaptive shortening or lengthening of a muscle and its connective tissue is a slow, nonpathologic process occurring in response to the range of motion being utilized in the related joints. Under normal conditions, sarcomeres are continually being added or subtracted within a muscle in response to the mechanical stresses the muscle is subjected to. Skeletal muscle functions by contracting, or shortening, and relaxing. A muscle does not actively lengthen itself, although it is capable of actively controlling its rate of elongation in response to antagonistic or external forces. The balance of forces, then, tends to favor shortening over lengthening. Mechanical stress created within the muscle by regular elongation to its full length may serve as a stimulus for sarcomere and connective-tissue maintenance. Structural alterations can occur in its absence. Continuous functioning in a shortened range could reduce the mechanical stimulation necessary for tissue maintenance, resulting in functional adaptation and sarcomere depletion. (see Fig. 7-5b). Frequent strong contraction and shortening of a muscle, for example, not followed by stretching can lead to adaptive shortening. Certain muscles of the shoulder show a greater propensity for adaptive shortening. These are considered in more detail later in this chapter.

## MYOSTATIC CONTRACTURE

Myostatic contractures develop as a consequence of immobilization and represent structural adaptation of the muscle in response to changes in range of motion of the corresponding joint.[8,9] *Immobilization* here means the absence of mobilizing forces, either resulting from a period of casting or bracing, etc. or imposed by restriction of movement in the related joint. True myostatic contracture is thought to be accompanied by a reduction in the number of sarcomere units, which individually are found to maintain normal length. The muscle, however, is found to be some degree shorter than its normal physiologic length. When myostatic contracture develops following prolonged immobilization, the connective-tissue elements are found to be thinned and weakened, demonstrating up to 80 percent loss of tensile strength.[8,9] Clinically, this is encountered after casting or bracing. Care must be taken not to subject the myofascia in this situation to abrupt or vigorous stretch forces; prolonged low-load stretching is required. Connective-tissue weakening does not necessarily occur with nonpathologic adaptive shortening, where continued function suffices to maintain tensile integrity in the connective-tissue elements.

## PSEUDOMYOSTATIC CONTRACTURE

Pseudomyostatic contracture represents loss of extension secondary to dynamic changes that result in some decrease in individual sarcomere length, not from the reduction of their numbers

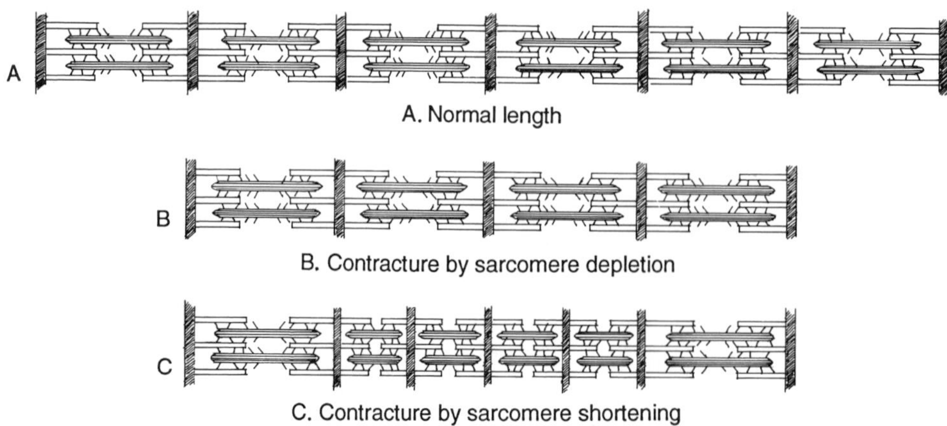


**Figure 7-5.** Subclassifications of contracture.

from the longitudinal arrangement[8,9] (see Fig. 7-5c). The exact mechanisms of pseudomyostatic contracture are unknown, but they may be related to abnormal extrafusal or intrafusal motor firing and may develop following tetanic muscle contraction.[9]

Pseudomyostatic contracture is not accompanied by structural changes initially, but its persistence can lead to sarcomere depletion consistent with myostatic contracture[9] (see Fig. 7-5b). Myofascial trigger points, thought to be an area in the muscle where the actin and myosin filaments in the involved sarcomeres remain chemically locked,[53,59] represent a mechanism of pseudomyostatic contracture.[9]

Stretching in the treatment of highly reactive conditions, for example, reflex spasm or active myofascial trigger points, can be enhanced by inhibitory techniques described in this chapter in the treatment of myofascial pain and dysfunction. Rapid reversal of pseudomyostatic contracture can occur from this type of treatment. However, if muscle shortening is a primary result of sarcomere depletion consistent with true myostatic contracture, inhibitory techniques operating via reflex pathways will be of little value in releasing the contracture.

## Functional Pathology of the Locomotor System

Muscle shortening and contracture are common components of postural and shoulder dysfunction. Shortened muscles do not allow a full range of active or passive movement of the related joint and can develop for different reasons. Janda[31] reports that certain muscles show a tendency to shorten and others a tendency to weaken under normal and pathologic circumstances. These muscle imbalances are associated with movement disturbances and altered joint precision, conceptualized by Janda as "functional pathology of the locomotor system."

In the absence of these muscle imbalances, muscle groups operating major joints will perform in a precise pattern demonstrated by initiation of movement by the phasic-acting protagonists and synergists, followed by the recruitment of synergistic tonic or postural stabilizing muscles. This is paired with concurrent reciprocal inhibition of the antagonists. In disturbances of the motor system, it is typical to find alterations of firing sequence and coordination.

Those muscles which typically shorten are usually the same muscles that develop spasticity in response to upper motor neuron lesions and are of primary postural function. These muscle groups do not necessarily correspond to specific muscle fiber type classification.[39]

The type of muscle shortening described by Janda as a component of functional pathology of the locomotor system is a form of myostatic contracture that does not show any spontaneous resting electrical activity and therefore is not maintained by active muscle contraction.[31] During movement, however, these muscles demonstrate hyperactivity, easy fatigue, impaired coordination, and difficulty with isolated, independent functions. Reciprocal inhibition can be disturbed, with tight muscles exhibiting lower firing thresholds and motor unit activity during primary functions of the paired antagonist, when it should be silent.

Tightness in tonic or postural muscles is accompanied by weakness or inhibition in the antagonistic and synergistic muscles that function in a dynamic or phasic fashion, termed *patterned pseudoparesis*. Movement disturbances occur at major joints as a consequence of altered muscle firing sequences and substitution of inhibited phasic muscles by postural or stabilizing muscles.

Muscles of the shoulder complex that tend to show tightness, shortening, and hyperactivity include the upper and middle trapezius, levator scapulae, pectoralis major and minor, biceps, sternocleidomastoid, and flexors of the arm. Muscles that tend to show concurrent weakness and inhibition include the deltoid, serratus anterior, triceps, rhomboids, and lower trapezius, and arm extensors.[31,39] Lewit[39] includes the supraspinatus and infraspinatus in the former group, while Janda[31] assigns the supraspinatus to the latter. Kendall[37] describes stretch-induced weakness of the middle trapezius as a typical finding in postural dysfunction accompanied by shortening of the anterior shoulder girdle muscles. Janda[31] reports that strengthening activities can result in increased muscle tightness of existing shortened muscles and limited strength gains in weak muscles.

Evaluation of reciprocal tightness and weakness involves passive mobility assessment of muscle length, manual muscle testing of strength, and dynamic movement assessment of muscle firing sequence and coordinated movement. Assessment of shoulder scapulohumeral rhythm during abduction is performed with the subject seated. The examiner observes the order of muscle recruitment and the resulting movement. With the elbow flexed, the patient is asked to elevate the arm slowly in abduction. The deltoid should be detected to initiate the motion by observation and palpation, followed by recruitment of the contralateral upper trapezius, the ipsilateral upper trapezius, the contralateral quadratus lumborum, and the ipsilateral middle and lower scapular stabilizers in that order. The movement should be repeated up to ten times to allow for palpatory examination of all component muscles and to assess the effects of fatigue on the quality of motion.

Up to 60 degrees, there should be no elevation of the shoulder girdle. Abnormal motion starts with shoulder girdle elevation before or simultaneous with scapulohumeral motion, when the ipsilateral upper trapezius fires early in the pattern of recruitment, substituting and inhibiting the deltoid.

Early recruitment or initiation of motion by muscles that function primarily as stabilizers is typical of the nature of pathologic locomotor disturbances.[31,39] Common shoulder dysfunctions such as subacromial impingement can be perpetrated by abnormal movement patterns; movement assessment should be included in shoulder evaluation, and correction of tight muscle components should be a primary consideration in the plan of treatment.

Janda demonstrated the value of stretching in reducing hyperactivity in shortened muscles and increased motor unit activity in weakened paired muscles; weak or inhibited muscles demonstrate increased strength and improvement of disturbed joint movement as a result of passive stretching of the tight components only, without engaging in strengthening. Janda[31] emphasizes the importance of releasing muscle tightness first, before engaging in strengthening or neuromuscular learning activities.[39]

## Facilitated Segment

The concept of segmental facilitation originated with Korr,[15,22,23] who described a neurophysiologic model to conceptualize the relationship between spinal somatic dysfunction and systemic pathology consistent with the osteopathic philosophy of health and disease. A *spinal segment* is defined as the adjacent halves of two vertebrae, the disk between, the related contents of the spinal canal and intervertebral foramen, the ligaments, joints, muscles, fascia, and skin that relate to that particular segment, and the shared nerve pathways common to all these structures.[56]

A segment is said to be facilitated when its sensory, motor, and autonomic input and outflow exhibit an increased central excitatory state, manifested by lower firing thresholds. A facilitated segment will react to a small-magnitude stimulus with exaggerated responses. This is thought to occur as a result of an increase in the number of abnormal afferent impulses reaching the segment from ascending, descending, and local stimuli. The "gain," or sensitivity, of the reflex and interneuron pathways is amplified, causing discharges from anterior horn cells along peripheral nerves to muscles and from lateral horn cells through sympathetic pathways to blood vessels and viscera. These abnormal efferent discharges are attributed to the increased central excitatory level at the segment producing exaggerated responses to any afferent input arriving there.

Neuromuscular function can be affected by misinformation within the muscle spindle–gamma efferent feedback loop and faulty interpretation of mechanoreceptor, proprioceptor, and other reflex mechanisms required for normal motor control.

The concept of the facilitated segment helps explain a reflex relationship between shoulder and cervical spine dysfunction in the absence of nerve pathology. For example, the rotator cuff musculature, biceps, and deltoid could all be influenced by facilitation at the C4–5 and C5–6 segment levels. A myofascial trigger point in the supraspinatus, then, can be perpetrated by facet joint irritation at the midcervical level without direct hard- or soft-tissue compromise of the exiting nerve root. By the same mechanism of segmental facilitation, the shoulder girdle is affected by the upper cervical spine through reflex pathways involving the sternocleidomastoid, omohyoid, or trapezius. Korr's facilitated segment concept is complemented by the model of spondylogenic syndromes in the following discussion.

## Spondylogenic Syndrome

Dvorak and Dvorak[15] link common soft-tissue dysfunction such as tendinitis with the activity of mechanoreceptors and nociceptors located in the fibrous capsules of the spinal apophyseal joints. Uninterrupted activation of type I mechanoreceptors in response to postural overloading or segmental dysfunction produces increased afferent input to the central nervous system. Abnormal reflexogenic pathways are established, delivering nervous misinformation through motor units to bundles of fibers within the muscles. Eventual histologic changes in muscle and tendon develop in response to long-standing hypertonicity, described as *myotendinosis*.[15] Myotendinotic changes are characterized by increased permanent tone and degenerative tissue changes resulting from hypoxia in the metabolically stressed muscle fibers and chronic tension in the musculotendinous and tendoperiosteal unit.

Tender or painful indurated tissue is found on palpatory examination of the involved fibers within the muscle, consistent with Travell[59,60] and Simon's[52,53] description of the taut band that harbors the myofascial trigger point. The clinical implications of myotendinosis in response to spondylogenic reflex mechanisms would emphasize the necessity to normalize cervical spine mechanoreceptor activity in the treatment of common soft-tissue pathology occurring at the shoulder. The forward head posture therefore can predispose the individual to subacromial impingement symptoms, for example, not only by altering the structural relationship of glenohumeral joint but also via myotendinotic changes in the rotator cuff produced by abnormal type I mechanoreceptor firing in the midcervical joints. The treatment plan, then, also must include establishment of orthostatic equilibrium of the cranium and cervical spine to normalize mechanoreceptor activity and eliminate reflexogenic neuromuscular influences at the shoulder.

# Myofascial Pain Syndrome

*Myofascial pain syndrome* is a nonsystemic disorder that results in referred pain and autonomic phenomena whose source is a trigger point located within a muscle or its fascia. This syndrome is frequently implicated in both acute and chronic shoulder pain and dysfunction.[59,60]

Janet G. Travell is widely recognized as the leading authority on myofascial pain syndromes. She adopted the term *myofascial* in 1952 after observing that pinching either the contractile tissue or the fascial covering of the infraspinatus during a muscle biopsy produced a referred pain pattern unique to the source.[59] Travell[59] identifies the potential occurrence of single muscle myofascial pain syndromes in every muscle of the shoulder complex.

Myofascial pain syndrome is recognized by certain characteristics that allow it to be identified as a distinct diagnostic entity. Mandatory of these characteristics is the occurrence of myofascial trigger points. A *myofascial trigger point* is defined as a hyperirritable spot, usually within a taut band of skeletal muscle or in the muscle's fascia, that is painful on compression and that can give rise to characteristic referred pain, tenderness, and autonomic phenomena.[59]

Trigger points can be either active or latent in nature. Active myofascial trigger points refer pain and sensory, motor, and autonomic phenomena to specific reference zones that can be far removed from the source and which do not coincide with peripheral nerve or dermatomal distributions.[59] Several models, convergence-projection, convergence-facilitation, sympathetic mediation, and peripheral branching of primary afferent nociceptors, help to explain the phenomenon of referred pain.[53,59] When considered singularly, none can fully account for all aggravating and alleviating mechanisms characteristic of trigger points. Most likely more than one pain relay is simultaneously active, resulting in misinterpretation of the exact somatic source. Active myofascial trigger points prevent full elongation of the host muscle and can refer pain while the muscle is at rest. Active contraction of the muscle is painful and reflexly weakened. Latent trigger points do not cause spontaneous symptoms but refer pain only upon localized pressure.[59] The patient may not be aware of symptoms caused by latent trigger points, which are only reproduced upon palpation. A distinction between a tender point and a latent trigger point is that the latter refers pain to a characteristic zone when stimulated.[59,60]

Satellite, or secondary, trigger points can develop in muscles located within the zone of reference of the primary trigger point.[59] Motoneurons supplying motor units within the reference zone of pain demonstrate decreased firing thresholds and easy excitability.[52] A trigger point located in the infraspinatus characteristically refers pain to the anterior shoulder, which may precipitate satellite trigger point development in the anterior deltoid (Fig. 7-6). Satellite trigger points are thought to occur as a consequence of increased motor unit activity during voluntary contraction of a muscle within the zone of reference.[52,59] Simons[52] electromyographically demonstrated bursts of motor unit action potentials upon deep palpation of deltoid trigger points located in the muscle reference zone. The taut band was demonstrated to be electrically silent until stimulated mechanically. The electrical response appeared to be specific to fibers within a palpable band and absent in band-free portions of the muscle.[52] The neurophysiologic relationship of trigger points to palpable bands is unknown but suggestive of hyperirritable spinal reflex mechanisms. Motor unit responses gradually diminished after repeated stimulation by digital snapping over a 45-minute period, helping to explain why trigger

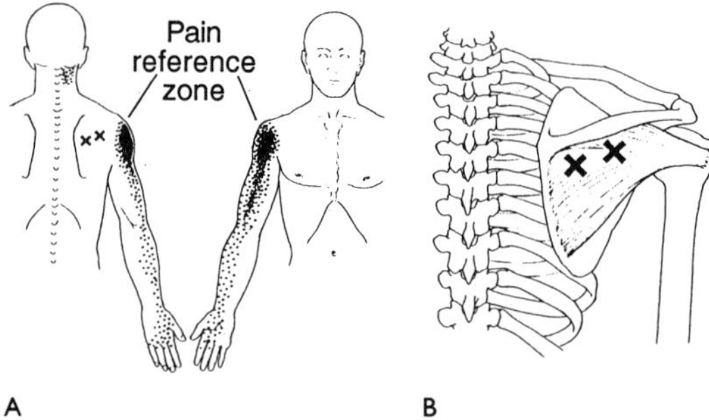


**Figure 7-6.** (a) Characteristic references zone of pain (b) from myofascial trigger points located in the infraspinatus. (Reproduced with permission from Travell JG. Myofascial pain and dysfunction: the trigger point manual. Baltimore: Williams & Wilkins, 1983.)

points are amenable to therapeutic application of deep pressure massage.

The electrically silent nature of taut fiber bands in the resting muscle is thought to be the result of sustained sarcomere shortening at the location of the trigger point.[52] Damage to the sarcoplasmic reticulum has been considered a possible mechanism that could account for this shortening.[52,59] Rupture of the sarcoplasmic reticulum would allow calcium leakage, which sustains contraction when present. The resulting increase in metabolic demand could deplete the available ATP required both to release the interlocked actin and myosin filaments and to power the sarcoplasmic calcium pump. Sustained contraction reduces circulation in the region, which in tandem with increased oxygen demand induces anemic hypoxia, metabolite retention, and subsequent activation of local nociceptor terminals. A trigger point in this model then represents a region of contractile tissue in metabolic distress.

Myofascial pain syndrome is perpetrated by mechanical, systemic, and psychological factors.[59,60] Single-episode and cumulative trauma, postural stress, and overuse injuries can precipitate trigger point development. Joint dysfunction has been identified as a potent perpetrator of trigger points and primary initiator of some myofascial pain syndromes.[59] Conversely, splinting and guarding accompanying pain of myofascial origin can accelerate muscle shortening, resulting in joint dysfunction or contracture.[8] Myofascial and articular dysfunction are frequently found to coexist; successful treatment of either requires identification and correction of both components and related perpetrating factors.

The following criteria will substantiate the diagnosis of an active myofascial trigger point:

1. A history of sudden pain onset following activities producing acute overload of the involved muscle or gradual onset resulting from exposure to cumulative overload
2. A pattern of pain that is characteristic of the specific muscle
3. Some degree of weakness in the involved muscle
4. Painful restriction of full physiologic range of motion to passive stretch or active contraction
5. A point of exquisite palpatory tenderness often located within a taut fiber band in the muscle
6. Reproduction or intensification of the reference zone upon application of brief digital pressure on the tender focus
7. A palpable and often visible local twitch response upon snapping or needling of the point
8. Alleviation of remote and local symptoms in response to specific therapy to the host muscle

# Soft-Tissue Mobilization

## Examination and Treatment Techniques

The various soft-tissue procedures reviewed in this section, regardless of the specifics of the technique, can all be assigned to two basic categories, namely, some form of massage or stretching.

Understanding the nature of myofascial injuries is important when planning appropriate manual treatment. Treatment planning and selection of soft-tissue techniques must consider and address the histopathologic changes specific to the dysfunction. Massage may produce rapid gains in length with pseudomyostatic shortening of a muscle but has limited effectiveness in the treatment of a myostatic contracture, which requires a course of stretching to produce gradual length gains. For example, an individual with restriction of full elbow extension secondary to the presence of an active trigger point in the brachialis muscle may recover full range of motion with a single, effective treatment of massage and stretching. The same muscle that has undergone shortening and structural change because of actual elbow joint contracture following fracture, inflammation, and immobilization will gradually lengthen over several weeks in response to daily stretching of both the joint and muscle contracture.

When treating any neuromusculoskeletal dysfunction, a comprehensive approach must be considered. Any one technique employed to the exclusion of another will not address the totality of the problem when joint, myofascial, and neuromuscular components are present.

The techniques and concepts reviewed here are typically used in conjunction with joint mobilization and therapeutic exercises, ensuring comprehensive management of shoulder dysfunction.

# Massage

*Massage* can be broadly defined as the manipulation of the soft tissues, performed with the hands, for the purpose of producing direct or indirect effects on the autonomic, somatic, and central nervous systems, on the circulatory and lymphatic systems, on muscle and connective tissues, and on psychological states.[5] Soft-tissue *mobilization* has been defined as "the forceful passive movement of the musculofascial elements through its restrictive direction(s) beginning with its superficial layers and progressing into depth while taking into account its relationship to the joints concerned."[24] Soft-tissue mobilization is massage by definition; however, the application of soft-tissue mobilization emphasizes the structural and functional relationship between articulations and the related soft tissues.

Many schools of thought exist, each presenting an approach to soft-tissue treatment that may differ more in philosophy than in the actual application of technique. The utilization of massage is quite varied between individual practitioners and clinics. Increased sophistication and mechanization of treatment modalities have had an impact on the methods and choices available in the treatment armamentarium. Certain practitioners develop technical expertise, but at the expense of neglecting manual skills; conversely, others rely on massage too heavily, which cannot substitute for joint mobilization, stabilization, or exercise. Others view massage as offering nothing more than a placebo effect and therefore not a worthwhile undertaking in the rehabilitation process.

Mennell[44] warns that it is "easier to rub a disability into a patient's mind than to rub it out of a limb." Overutilization of massage may lead the patient to believe the condition at hand is more serious than it actually is with respect to the degree of time and effort undertaken.

The appropriate utilization of massage must be determined by matching the intended treatment goals or purpose with what therapeutic effects a particular massage technique is capable of accomplishing. Consideration also must be given to treatment efficiency in the clinical setting, since there is usually more than one way to achieve the therapeutic response desired, for example, the application of moist heat instead of massage given for primarily general relaxation purposes.

## INDICATIONS

Several clinical uses of massage include exploration and assessment of soft tissue, analgesic effects and general relaxation, neuromuscular inhibition or facilitation, decongestion of fluid-holding states, reduction of tissue induration, fiber separation, elongation, connective-tissue mobilization, and influences on tissue remodeling.

Therapeutic massage is administered to alter the physiologic state of underlying tissues and reduce abnormal mechanical, fluid, and neuromuscular components of hypertonicity. Therapeutic massage is performed for specific effects and purposes; the types of strokes, amount of pressure, duration, and frequency are determined accordingly by what is necessitated by the nature of the dysfunction at hand and treatment response.

## CONTRAINDICATIONS

Contraindications for connective-tissue techniques presented in this chapter must be considered. A thorough diagnostic medical examination should always precede treatment to rule out organic pathology or assess the contribution of systemic diseases to somatic manifestations of related soft-tissue symptoms. Fever, active infections, osteomyelitis, cellulitis, acute circulatory conditions, hematoma, open wounds, and anticoagulant therapy present specific situations that restrict the use of manual therapy.

Caution must be emphasized in the presence of healing fractures, sutures and recent soft-tissue repair, paretic muscles, advanced diabetes, osteoporosis, malignancy, acute rheumatoid arthritis or advanced degenerative or trophic changes, and skin hypersensitivity. The potential risks, immediacy of need, and potential benefits of treatment must be considered in the presence of identifiable contraindications.

## HOW MASSAGE WORKS

James Mennell[44] writes, "there are four ways, and probably only four, in which massage can possibly work":

1. By reflex action
2. By mechanical means

3. By the reflex response of unstripped muscle to mechanical stimulation
4. By the formation of a histamine-like substance

The richly innervated integumentary system has long been appreciated as a therapeutic point of entry to influence physiologic and psychological functions. Numerous methods of massage and manual therapy take advantage of the direct and reflex neurophysiologic interactions of the skin with underlying muscle and organ systems.

The sensory role of muscle, however, is often overshadowed by its motor function. The manual therapist must appreciate the sensory, proprioceptive, and nocireceptor reflex influences on muscle tone in response to mechanical pressure, stretch, or force of contraction occurring within the muscle and fascia. These mechanical and reflex mechanisms are more or less active depending on the specific technique employed and are considered with the individual descriptions of treatment techniques in this section.

## EFFLEURAGE

Effleurage, as an introductory technique, offers a useful bridge between patient evaluation and treatment. Assessment of soft-tissue reactivity and tissue-texture abnormalities, performed by palpation, can begin with light effleurage to establish congenial contact. Skin sensitivity, temperature, moisture, congestion, and loss of elasticity are readily assessed.

Discovery of taut fiber bands and trigger points will be accompanied by pain. Soreness and tissue tenderness are a reflection of metabolite retention and chemical sensitization of free nociceptor nerve terminals in the local tissues. The recipient is found to offer better compliance to further examination if provocation of symptoms is tempered with the analgesic benefits of effleurage.

Effleurage employs light rhythmic stroking of the skin generally applied parallel to the underlying muscle fiber orientation. Some form of skin lubricant may be employed. Talcum powder, baby oil, and commercially prepared massage emollients are commonly used. Smooth, even timing and consistent stroke pressure on the skin and hypoderm can impart general sedation or reduce neuromuscular hypertonicity in those muscles sharing common innervation with the skin segments undergoing treatment. Deeper effleurage to the level of the outer layer of investing fascia can be used to gently elongate and stretch myofascia. Stroking can be applied with one or both hands but is always unidirectional. Effleurage is indicated to induce general relaxation and reduce guarding accompanying painful soft-tissue and joint conditions. These conditions usually exist following periods of immobilization associated with prolonged splinting in response to injury or following surgery. Effleurage is helpful in the reduction of local tissue congestion to some extent by passive mechanical movement of fluids; however, it provides an inefficient substitute for venous and lymphatic pumping produced by active muscle contractions. Mennell's "uncorking principle"[44] calls for the proximal portion of the limb to be treated before peripheral regions to decrease obstruction of drainage in the direction of venous and lymphatic return. The large anterior and posterior muscle groups of the shoulder should be worked first, with long strokes directed toward the axilla. The proximal arm should be treated before the forearm. Using the web space for contact, stroking is directed up the arm toward the shoulder only, never reflux toward the hand.

Lymphatic drainage massage employed in the treatment of upper limb obstructive edema is an extensive process requiring discussion and training well beyond the intended objectives of this presentation.

At first glance the typical application of massage demonstrated in Figure 7-7 may seem unrelated specifically to shoulder therapy. However, the entire superficial muscle layer of the posterior trunk is comprised of shoulder musculature, largely the latissimus dorsi and trapezius, which together originate from every spinal segment from occiput to pelvis.[21] The infraspinatus, teres minor and major, and posterior deltoid are also represented. Therefore, effleurage applied to the trunk and neck provides the opportunity for assessment of these tissues and their potential contributions to shoulder pain and dysfunction.

In general, effleurage is suitable early in the rehabilitation process and during acute states.

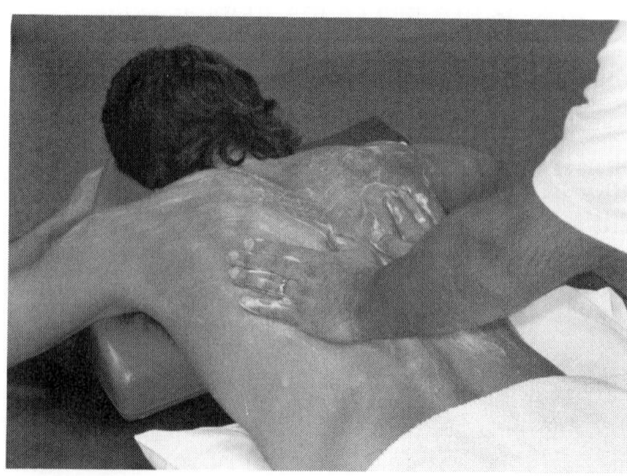

**Figure 7-7.** Effleurage.

Economical treatment will be better served by advancing to techniques that enhance functional restoration of movement and function as tolerated.

## PETRISSAGE

Massage is useful for circulatory benefits when muscle congestion and hypertonicity are present. Petrissage is a kneading technique that provides greater mechanical effect than effleurage and is better suited to the task of mobilizing fluid congestion within the muscle and fascia. Greater effect is also produced on the sensory receptor systems within the muscle and fascia which can participate in reflex reduction of neuromuscular hypertonicity and neuromodulation of nociceptor transmission. The petrissage technique involves squeezing, rolling, and lifting strokes, providing a deeper and greater mobilizing effect than the effleurage stroke. The thumb, index, and long fingers can be used effectively on the fusiform muscles of the upper limb (Fig. 7-8). Effort is made to create movement and space between individual muscles, for example, the biceps and underlying brachialis, as well as the individually partitioned muscle bellies. When working flat muscles such as found over the scapula and trunk, all the fingers of one or both hands can be utilized simultaneously. A typical massage session may begin with effleurage with gradual transition to petrissage strokes.

Active contract-relax cycles following massage are helpful to reactivate the muscle's venous and lymphatic pump and enhance tissue drainage.

# Connective-Tissue Mobilization

Connective-tissue mobilization employs short, hooking, and pulling strokes to restore extensibility in the skin and free gliding mobility between the dermis and underlying fascia. This technique is useful in the scapulothoracic region, where the subcutaneous adipose tissue is thin and the skin and superficial fascia can become bound to the deeper tissues overlying the ribs and scapulae.

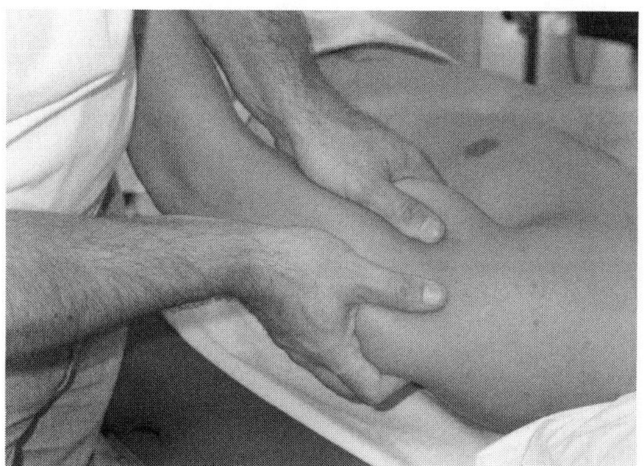

**Figure 7-8.** Petrissage.

The designation *connective-tissue mobilization* is used to distinguish the mechanical effect of the type of stroke, which is employed in the system of connective-tissue massage developed by Elizabeth Dicke known as *Bindegwebbsmassage*.[24,55] Dicke's connective-tissue massage emphasizes autonomic nervous system reflex interactions of the integumentary system with visceral and organic dysfunction. Treatment of these conditions is thought to be facilitated by correcting superficial connective-tissue changes sustained by sympathetic influences. Connective-tissue mobilization technique is considered here only for its usefulness in the treatment of localized soft-tissue changes manifested as a component of somatic dysfunction. Massage strokes can be applied directly in the directions of restriction with short excursion through the plane of the dermis. The recipient initially may report a sharp or cutting sensation. After a few minutes, the tissue loosens and discomfort diminishes.

## FASCIAL GLIDE

The soft tissues are examined for mobility by placing the finger pads and palm in light contact with the skin and gliding the tissues alternately in multiple directions. The skin and superficial fascia should possess multidirectional extensibility and glide freely on the underlying muscle. Assessment of fascial gliding is readily continued as treatment when restriction of extensibility is discovered. The slack is taken up and held at the motion barrier until the barrier releases. The rate of release is typically 1 in per 5 to 10 seconds.

## SKIN ROLLING

Skin rolling is a technique that is useful for both assessment and treatment[44] (Fig. 7-9). The dermis and superficial fascia are grasped between the thumbs and fingers, simultaneously rolling and lifting. The dermis and hypoderm should lift readily off the deeper myofascia. Fibrosis can restrict skin rolling and result in tissue-texture abnormalities. The skin in the area squeezed between the thumb and fingers can be found to have a characteristic "orange peel" appearance. Upon rolling, the tissues will feel stiff and somewhat leathery, accompanied by snapping, indicative of the pannicular state of the hypoderm. Skin-rolling technique is indicated to

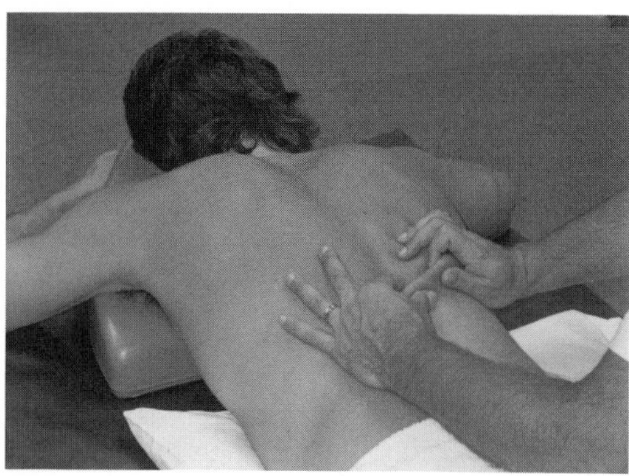

**Figure 7-9.** Skin rolling.

restore mobility, enhance circulation, and reduce pain. This technique is particularly useful for treatment of the latissimus dorsi, which should be examined and, if need be, treated along its extent. The greatest degree of restriction occurs in lumbar and pelvic portions of the muscle in the region of the thick lumbodorsal fascia.

## MYOFASCIAL MANIPULATION

Adaptive shortening of muscle and fascia is a common finding around the shoulder, typically occurring in the pectoral and axillary tissues and in the cervical and suprascapular regions. Upon examination, the muscles are found to be more rigid and solidified than supple or elastic, no longer able to return to a relaxed physiologic state. Not only is the length from origin to insertion affected, extensibility is also diminished to transverse and perpendicular forces. The independent mobility of muscle and fascial compartments is diminished, with the individual elements responding to manipulation in a congealer manner.

Myofascial manipulation imparts firm mechanical forces in the direction of restriction for the purpose of breaking up abnormal cross-linkages, loosening the connective-tissue weave, and restoring independent mobility to fascial compartments. Massage can be employed to restore independent mobility between muscle, fascia, and skin in areas of fascial thickening and binding that occur in response to chronic postural stresses or after trauma. Transverse massage can be applied over abnormal ropelike fascicles discovered within the muscle in an effort to tease apart tightly woven investing fascia. One or all finger pads, depending on the size of the area, can be used to apply firm strokes repeatedly across the tight strands in a washboard fashion.

The periscapular region is a common area to find changes in soft-tissue texture and tone, particularly the suprascapular fibers of the trapezius and at the insertions of the levator scapulae and rhomboids (Fig. 7-10). Transverse massage to the right trapezius and levator scapulae is initiated with the recipient positioned supine with the head supported on a low pillow and tilted toward the right enough to place the muscle on slack. Transverse strokes are given with the finger pads to the entire muscle, starting at the occiput and gradually progressing distally along the suprascapular fibers. The initial rhythm is slow with light pressure, one or two cycles per second. The contact and force are maintained even, not lifted from the surface, but drawn back and forth through the tissue. The entire structure is worked over once, noting particularly tight fibers, which are returned to for additional attention.

The individual's subjective verbal response serves as an accurate indicator to gauge appropriate pressure for the novice or experienced operator alike. Almost universally, the recipient describes this technique as a "good hurt" when applied correctly. Pressure that is too light fails to elicit this comment; too much force is easily determined by involuntary muscle contraction, voluntary withdrawal, and a distinctly different verbal response.

The side-lying position works equally well and gives greater access to the periscapular region. When this position is used, the head is propped on a folded pillow to allow the ipsilateral suprascapular tissues to be placed on slack. A pillow placed under the arm resting on the lateral thorax is desirable for additional comfort and stability. The prone position also can be used but is not preferred because of difficulty with optimal head and neck positioning in relation to the shoulder and arm.

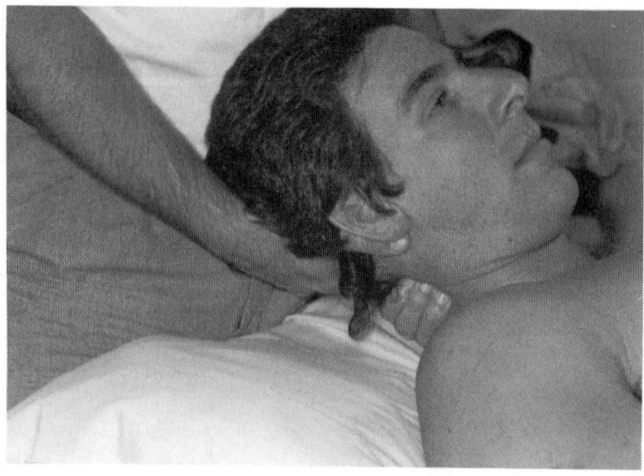

**Figure 7-10.** Transverse massage technique.

### BENDING TECHNIQUE

The supine position is used to treat the pectoral and axillary regions (Fig. 7-11). The ipsilateral arm is passively supported on a pillow, with enough abduction to gain access to the lateral pectoral border, but still allowing the muscle to remain slack. The operator uses the thumbs of one or both hands to grasp and lift the pectoral mass off the underlying pectorals minor and deep fascia. The hollow forming the armpit is created by traction on the suspensory ligament during abduction.[21] The suspensory ligament of the axilla is an extension of the clavipectoral fascia, which is the deep investing portion enveloping the pectoralis minor. Repetitive lift and release cycles are applied, taking up all the transverse slack so as to produce simultaneous bending and shearing force in the tissue. Manipulation in this manner is thought to break cross-fiber restrictions by application of perpendicular forces, much like a strong stick can be snapped across the thigh. In this instance, however, the thumbs function as the fulcrum with the pronated wrists moving into ulnar deviation. The technique should be carried out laterally along the course of the pectoralis tendon. A single thumb works well to get under and lift the tendon where it twists upon itself before the humeral insertion. The coracobrachialis and short head of the biceps and anterior fibers of the deltoid are also readily mobilized in this manner.

The posterior axillary wall formed by the subscapularis, teres major, and latissimus dorsi should be examined and treated when found to be restricted. The subscapularis is positioned superiorly but can be accessed by abducting the arm to the loose-pack position and drawing the scapula lateral on the thorax. The anterior portion of the teres major and latissimus dorsi are readily treated, forming the fleshy inferior mass of the posterior axilla.

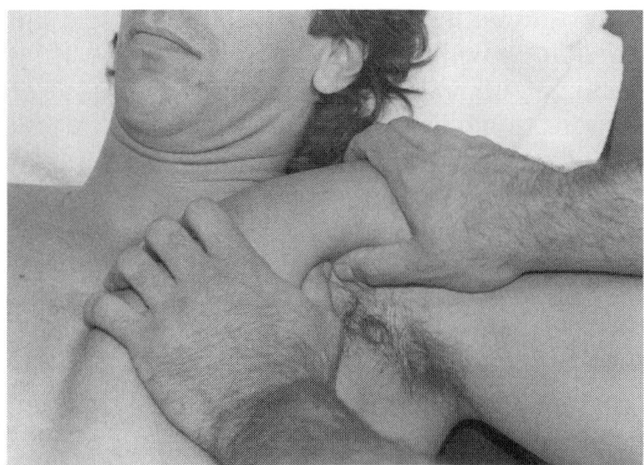

**Figure 7-11.** Bending technique, pectoralis major.

### PARALLEL SEPARATION

Further separation of individual muscles or fascicles within the muscle can be enhanced by the application of parallel oriented strokes to fascial clefts and muscle borders. An individual knuckle, the lateral edge of a finger, or even the point of the elbow can be used to draw or push along the myofascial structure, directed to stretch origin from insertion longitudinally. By working each pass progressively deeper, the tissues are spread apart, helping to restore free space and dimensional mobility. This type of myofascial manipulation is typically associated with what is called *rolfing*, after Ida Rolf, who developed a philosophy and method of body work called *structural integration*. It is not appropriate to refer to this type of manipulation as rolfing unless it is used in the context of what was developed by Ida Rolf and practiced by credentialed individuals engaged in the delivery of her specific system.

Application of deep parallel myofascial manipulation to the sternal portion of the pectoralis major is shown in Figure 7-12. The technique is initiated with the arm positioned to keep the muscle slack. After the entire length has been worked with several passes, the structure becomes more pliable, and increased depth is possible.

The arm is now repositioned to put the tissue on stretch by abducting and laterally rotating the shoulder. Passive stretching is enhanced by successive stroking starting at the sternal attachments and passing through the entire length to the humeral insertion.

## TRANSVERSE DEEP FRICTION MASSAGE

Deep friction massage is the application of concentrated, repetitive stroking directed perpendicularly to the fiber orientation in a localized area of tendon, muscle, fascia, or ligament at the site of scar, adhesion, or pain. Friction massage is used (1) to restore mobility between otherwise freely moving structures and (2) to render adhesions less capable of acting as a source of mechanical restriction and irritation.

### MODE OF ACTION OF DEEP FRICTION MASSAGE

1. Increase myotendinous scar pliability and facilitate proper collagen fiber orientation.
2. Enhancement of blood supply is thought to diminish pain by speeding the destruction of

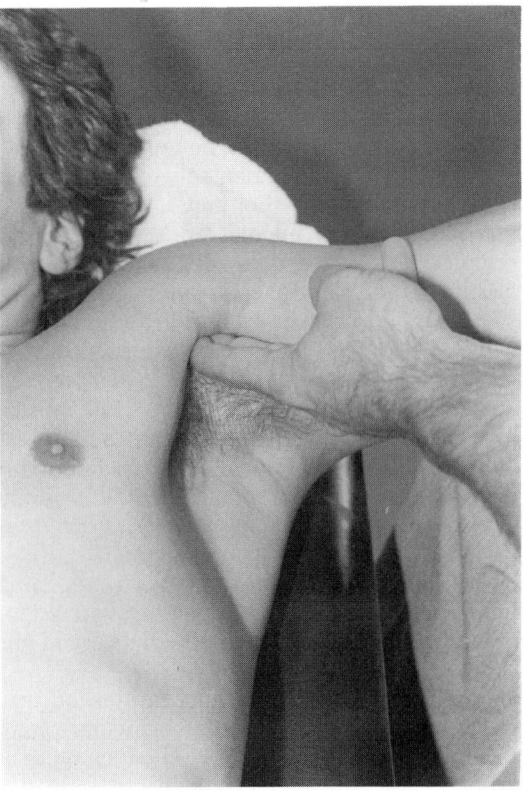

**Figure 7-12.** Parallel separation technique, sternal portion of pectoralis major.

substance P, thought to be the principal chemomediator of pain impulses from the periphery to the central nervous system. An appropriate dose of friction massage can result in a sustained period of posttreatment analgesia through depletion of substance P in the local sensory neurons. Additionally, increased tissue perfusion facilitates the removal of damaged tissue in preparation for new collagen production and wound repair.

3. Movement imparted through friction results in stimulation of mechanoreceptors which transmit impulses along large-fiber afferent pathways to the spinal cord, where they serve to decrease nociceptor transmission to higher pain centers. Movement may enhance the arrangement of newly synthesized collagen fibers to align so as to permit the restoration of physiologic mobility and pliability specific to the tissue in which the process of healing is taking place.

At this time, these proposed effects of friction massage have still not been substantiated by quality research, yet anecdotal and clinical results perpetrate its use.

## CONTRAINDICATIONS

Friction massage, or any mechanical technique, should not be applied to areas of active or acute inflammation due to bacterial action or infection.[11] Ossification or calcification in soft-tissue structures such as bursae, muscle, and tendon should not be disturbed with friction massage, which can perpetrate the condition or damage the adjacent healthy tissues. Friction massage to the capsuloligamentous complex is potentially harmful in the acute, subacute, and chronic stages of rheumatoid arthritis.

Deep friction massage is contraindicated in acute bursitis. The shoulder region contains numerous bursae that are often intimately involved with tendon pathology. Friction massage or deep pressure applied to an inflamed bursa would perpetrate additional pain and inflammation.

The expansive cap over the humeral head formed by the subacromial bursa requires that friction massage to the supraspinatus tendon and superior part of the long head of the biceps tendon be accessible largely through the overlying bursa. Caution is required with stage II and III subacromial impingement conditions, where the subacromial bursa is often inflamed and fibrotic. Caution also must be applied when treating the subscapularis, which frequently is found to have an underlying bursa at the capsule, occasionally opening into the joint.[21]

## EXAMINATION

A primary objective of examination is to determine whether the pain perceived originates from the local structures or is referred from some other source. Once it has been determined that the source of pain is located in the shoulder or surrounding tissues, it is necessary to isolate which tissue is at fault.

To this purpose, Cyriax[10,12] developed a system of "selective tissue tension" comprised of 12 primary examination maneuvers performed at the shoulder. Active movements indicate the individuals willingness (pain) and ability (mechanical restriction, weakness) to move. Inert tissues (capsules, ligaments, bursae) are tested by passive movement; contractile tissues (muscles, tendons) are assessed by midrange isometric resistance. The differential diagnosis and orthopedic evaluation are detailed in Chapter 5.

## INDICATIONS

### Intramuscular Lesions

Contraction of striated muscle is accompanied by broadening and separation of its fibers. This normal activity within the muscle can become restricted by the formation of scars or adhesions between individual fasciculi. Contraction in this situation can produce pain. Intramuscular scar tissue adhesions are more likely to limit function in multipennate muscles, for example, the deltoid, in which the fasciculi are relatively short.[8,11,21]

Transverse friction massage can be used in the healing phase in an effort to prevent scar tissue from binding separate fasciculi together and promote tissue mobility. Although scar tissue is required to join breached tissue, disorganized and thickened scar can be painful or functionally deficient. Massage strokes directed transversely can result in separation of fasciculi that have been bound to one another, and this type of soft-tissue mobilization will assist in promoting normal tissue mobility. Massage strokes directed longitudinally can lead to further separation of the healing breach. During the earliest stages of healing, this type of friction massage as well as passive stretching and resisted movements may strain the healing breach and thus should be avoided.[11] Friction massage can be followed by gentle active contractions with the muscle in a relaxed position to enhance fiber broadening and separation.

Mature lesions can impose significant restriction of muscle belly fiber broadening during contraction. Deep transverse massage is given for 5 to 10 minutes to the site of the scar, in an effort to tease apart adherent fibers and broaden the muscle passively. In this situation, massage is followed by maximal isometric contractions.

The lateral convergence of the clavicular, sternal, and costal fibers of the pectoralis major, medial to the tendon, is a common area of injury. Treatment of this clinical finding is outlined here (Fig. 7-13).

The recipient is supine with the arm in midrange of abduction and passively supported. Two or three fingers can be used to apply perpendicular frictions with firm enough pressure to penetrate the fiber bundle. Starting with the middle fiber portion, the operator's fingers are directed superiorly and medially. It may be helpful to give underlying support with the opposed thumb grasping the muscle mass. The hand technique must be modified according to the size of the individual as required. The degree of abduction can be altered as the massage progresses to engage fiber tension in various portions of the fanned arrangement.

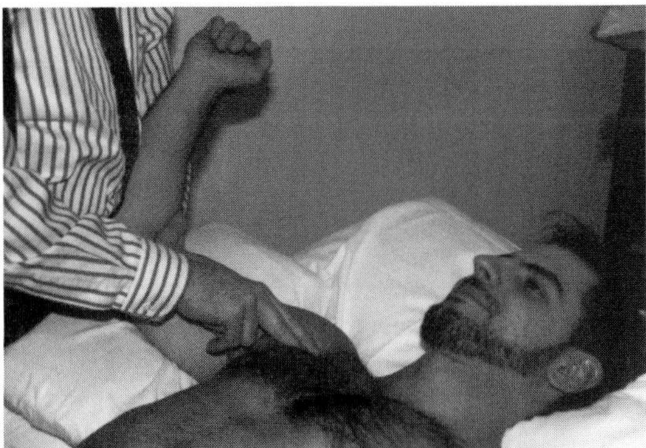

**Figure 7-13.** Transverse friction massage technique for intramuscular lesion in the pectoralis major muscle belly.

The lateral clavicular fiber portions are better approached with transverse strokes directed parallel to the inferior border of the clavicle. The arm can be positioned with some extension to better engage these more vertically oriented fibers.

**Tendinous Scar Tissue Adhesions**

Degenerative changes, overuse, or trauma can cause tendon fiber disruption. Tendinitis itself is considered by some to involve microtearing of tendon fibers. The rotator cuff tendons, particularly the supraspinatus and infraspinatus, in addition to the long head of the biceps, are vulnerable to tendinitis as well as partial- and full-thickness tears. Supraspinatus tears typically occur at the tenoperiosteal junction or within 1 cm of this junction. When scar tissue does develop, the painful or inflamed regions are considered to be at the scar and healthy tissue interface. Pain occurs as tension translates across these interfaces during active contraction or passive stretching. Transverse friction massage is utilized in these situations (1) to bring about proper collagen fiber orientation as the scar heals, (2) to mobilize the scar so that it is more pliable, and (3) to reduce the reactivity of this tissue to tensile forces.

These combined effects allow this immature tissue to behave more like a normal structure and improve its efficiency in force translation. What is interesting to note is that many supraspinatus partial-thickness tears occur on the articular side of the tendon. In this particular situation, the mechanical effects of transverse friction massage may be questionable.

Because rotator cuff pathology is sometimes difficult to distinguish with regard to tendinitis and actual tearing, a comprehensive physical examination is required to determine if friction massage is indicated. In the case of significant reactivity or suspected full-thickness tears, friction massage should be avoided because it could induce further irritation to the recently torn tissues. Also, a clinician should realize that subsequent to a full-thickness tear the tendon fibers retract from the bone and from one another.

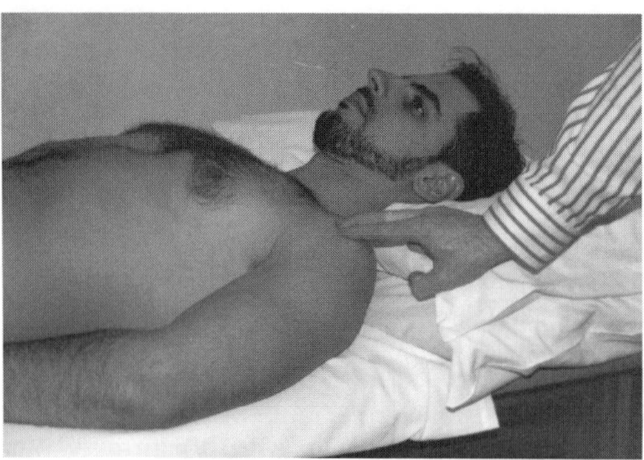

**Figure 7-14.** Transverse friction of the supraspinatus tendon.

**Supraspinatus Tendon**

The patient is positioned supine with the shoulder in extension, internal rotation, and adduction (Fig. 7-14). This position gives adequate body stabilization and access to the insertion and distal portion of the supraspinatus tendon, which is now positioned anterior to the acromion. The supraspinatus is placed on stretch in this position, which should be taken into consideration when structural weakness of the musculotendinous unit is suspected. When this is suspected, the technique can be modified to a sitting position, which may be better tolerated by the patient.

The therapist is positioned to the side and behind the ipsilateral shoulder and uses the index finger reinforced by the long finger's pad placed on the distal phalanx of the index finger. Transverse strokes of less than 1-in excursion are applied in a reciprocating fashion perpendicular to the tendon orientation. Sufficient pressure must be maintained to ensure that the skin overlying the tendon remains fixed to the fingerpad, imparting friction only to the tendon. The amount of pressure should not be so much as to make the patient guard or flinch. An initial dose of 2 to 3 minutes is adequate to assess the response to treatment. Analgesic benefits can be realized from this brief application in many cases. More chronic conditions where histologic changes are suspected may require longer sessions graduated to 10 minutes or more over 6 to 10 sessions. If the initial treatment produces a detectable inflammatory response or results in symptom exacerbation that persists more than several hours, additional friction massage should be delayed. In any instance, ice massage or cold packs can be utilized to alleviate post-treatment discomfort and control undesirable inflammation.

**Infraspinatus Tendon**

Access to the posterior capsule and infraspinatus tendon can be enhanced with the patient prone and propped up on the forearms, the humeri perpendicular, and the glenohumeral joint positioned in 90 degrees of flexion (Fig. 7-15). The involved arm is placed in some degree of adduction and then external rotation, with the hand holding the table edge. In this manner, the greater tuberosity and infraspinatus tendon are moved out from under the acromion.[11,12,63] The therapist places the index finger over the tendon just inferior to the posterior acromial edge, and transverse movement is applied to the musculotendinous unit.

**Long Head of the Biceps**

Tenosynovitis and adhesion are two potentially painful conditions affecting the tendon of the long head of the biceps for which transverse friction is useful. At the shoulder the tendon of the long head of the biceps is covered by the synovial sheath distal to the level of the transverse humeral ligament.[21] Adhesions can form between the tendon and sheath following an episode of bleeding or swelling. Tenosynovitis involves roughening of the synovial surfaces of a tendon possessing a sheath.[10,11] In this situation, pain can be provoked by movement of the tendon within its sheath, even in the absence of adhesion. Transverse friction is thought to be helpful to smooth the roughened surfaces of the tendon sheath and thereby alleviate the pain and associated dysfunction.[10,11]

The patient is positioned supine or semirecumbent, with the arm and elbow supinated and straightened, in slight external rotation, and extended beyond the table edge (Fig. 7-16). During transverse massage, the tendon is placed on stretch, which provides an immovable surface across which the sheath moves. Occasionally, the tendon is difficult to palpate at its proximal

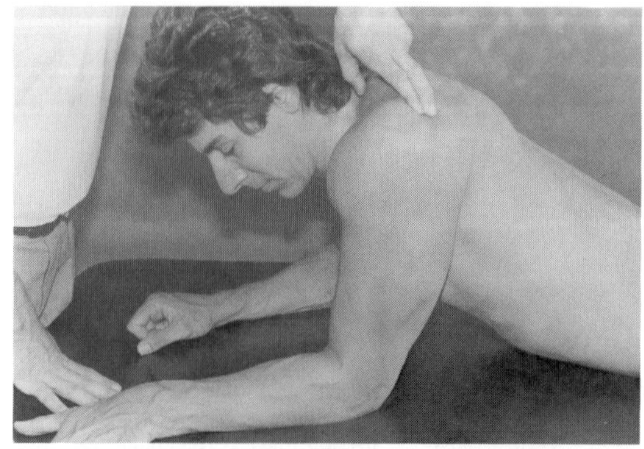

**Figure 7-15.** Transverse friction of the infraspinatus tendon.

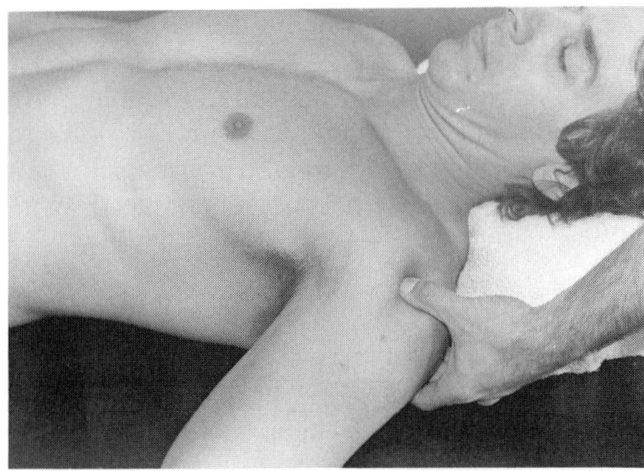

**Figure 7-16.** Transverse friction of the long head of the biceps.

extent. When this is the case, one can locate the tendon more easily in the distal groove between the crests of the greater and lesser tuberosities. The therapist places the treating thumb in line with and overlying the tendon at the level of the bicipital groove, with the thumb pad superior to the transverse ligament. The palm and fingers wrap around the proximal arm and give posterior support. Firm, short transverse strokes are then given by the thumb.

## MYOFASCIAL TRIGGER POINTS: EXAMINATION AND TREATMENT

Trigger points are physical signs detected by digital examination. They are often not located in the area of pain initially described by the patient. The notation of painful areas on a body drawing by the patient can give the clinician visual clues to the location of muscles suspected of harboring trigger points. Familiarity with specific pain patterns of individual muscles is therefore necessary. Intermittent pain not present at the time of examination may be reproduced by resisted contraction through a range of movement. When pain of myofascial origin is reproduced in this manner, it also may be relieved by repeating the resisted contraction while the examiner manually compresses the muscle during contraction or by squeezing a skin roll over the tested muscle. The exact location of a trigger point must be ascertained by palpation. The muscle to be examined should be positioned on some stretch just short of the painful range; an attempt should be made by the patient to allow the muscle to relax. If possible, the degree of stretch should engage the taut band but allow the uninvolved fibers to remain slack. Taut fiber bands typically feel like a cord 1 to 4 mm in diameter[59] and can be detected by drawing the finger pads transversely across the muscle perpendicular to the fiber orientation. Palpating along the taut band can reveal a firm, nodular focus of exquisite tenderness, the trigger point, which when pressed may evoke a wince or avoidance withdrawal by the subject, termed the *jump sign*.[59] Snapping the band may produce a transient, often visible contraction or localized twitch response of the fibers within it.[53,59]

Flat palpation is used in areas where the muscle can be pressed against underlying bone, for example, the infraspinatus. Muscles with accessible bellies (biceps, triceps, etc.) can be examined with pincer palpation by grasping the muscle between the thumb and fingers and then lifting and rolling the area, progressing along the entire length of the structure. Examining the patient can result in activation of significant and prolonged pain and therefore should not be undertaken unless immediate treatment is intended.

The principal objective of trigger point treatment is the restoration of full pain-free range of motion of the involved muscle during active contraction, active or passive lengthening, and while at rest. The primary method of treatment is the application of passive stretch, which is thought to disengage the actin and myosin filaments that have interlocked in the sarcomeres within the taut fiber band. To accomplish this, the painful trigger mechanism that is preventing full elongation of the muscle must first be deactivated. Trigger points can be managed clinically by different techniques, including vapocoolant spray, ischemic compression, deep massage, electrical stimulation, ultrasound, injection with local anesthetic, and dry needling. Their clinical effectiveness is attributed to interruption of transmission at the source and inhibition of reflex pathways at the spinal level.[59]

### SPRAY AND STRETCH

Vapocoolant spray for counterstimulation is thought to work in part by the gate-control mechanism of sensory modulation. Stimulation of skin touch and temperature receptors supplied by fast-conducting myelinated fibers is capable of interfering with nociceptor transmission, affording a brief period when the muscle can be stretched without provoking pain. Because the skin overlying the muscle containing the trigger point is supplied by afferent pathways regulated at segmental levels that also serve the involved muscle, stimulation of the skin can provide access to the neural feedback circuits involved in reflexly maintaining the dysfunction. To be effective, the stimulation must be in the range that activates only receptors that conduct pleasant sensations, without additional nociceptor activity. Of the vapocoolants commercially available, fluorimethane spray is well suited to provide the most effective sensory range for counterstimulation techniques. Ethyl chloride was used originally before fluorimethane was developed but is no longer recommended for several reasons: (1) it is combustible, and (2) it acts as a general anesthetic agent, limiting its safe use in treatment around the upper body, where it could be inhaled. Ethyl chloride produces a greater reduction in skin temperature to the degree that the transmission from the skin receptors is thermally blocked, rendering counterstimulation ineffective. This will occur when the temperature of the skin receptors drops to 10°C or 50°F.[59] The intention is to chill only the skin and not the underlying muscle, which could induce further contraction. The use of ice or a cold probe can be equally effective; extra care must be taken not to allow dripping and trickling of melted water, which could result in shivering and contraction.

Vapocoolant spray and stretch is the most frequently recommended and effective technique found to interrupt the trigger mechanism. Travell[59,60] emphasizes that "spray is the distraction, stretch is the action." A general protocol for treating myofascial trigger point dysfunction is applicable to treatment of all single-muscle myofascial pain syndromes: The treatment environment should be warm and free of drafts; the skin overlying the muscle to be treated and the reference zone of pain must be fully exposed. Prior to treatment, restriction of movement and location of pain are assessed.

The patient is positioned comfortably and is well supported, allowing for voluntary relaxation of the area to be treated. Positioning should allow one end of the muscle to be stretched while the other end is immobilized. In the relaxed position, the skin covering the entire muscle is covered once with unidirectional, parallel sweeps applied in the direction of the reference zone of pain.

The bottle is held approximately 18 in from the muscle; the jet stream should contact the skin at a 30-degree angle, moving unidirectionally at a rate of 4 in/s. Gentle stretch is initiated while the spray is applied with parallel sweeps, continuing beyond the muscle and covering the area of referred pain. The sequence is continued until full passive range is gained. No greater than three sweeps should be used over one area of skin without rewarming.

After a full range of passive stretch is achieved, the muscle is actively contracted concentrically and eccentrically for several repetitions through its complete range of motion.

The technique for treatment of the upper trapezius is demonstrated in Figure 7-17. The infraspinatus also can be treated from this position or from the lateral recumbent position, which allows better stabilization of the scapula.

## ISCHEMIC COMPRESSION

Ischemic compression is a convenient manual technique employed in the treatment of myofascial trigger points. The application of firm, sustained direct pressure to the point is thought to result in trigger point deactivation by creating a temporary nerve block induced by restricting circulation to the local nerve terminals. This technique is noninvasive but does involve a brief intensification of pain. It is best suited for use with latent trigger points and may not be well tolerated with higher levels of reactivity found with active trigger points.

The examiner attempts to locate the greatest focus of pain by digital palpation. Moderate but tolerable direct pressure is applied with a single finger or thumb, sustained for up to 1 minute in duration. An example of this type treatment technique is demonstrated in Figure 7-18. After the

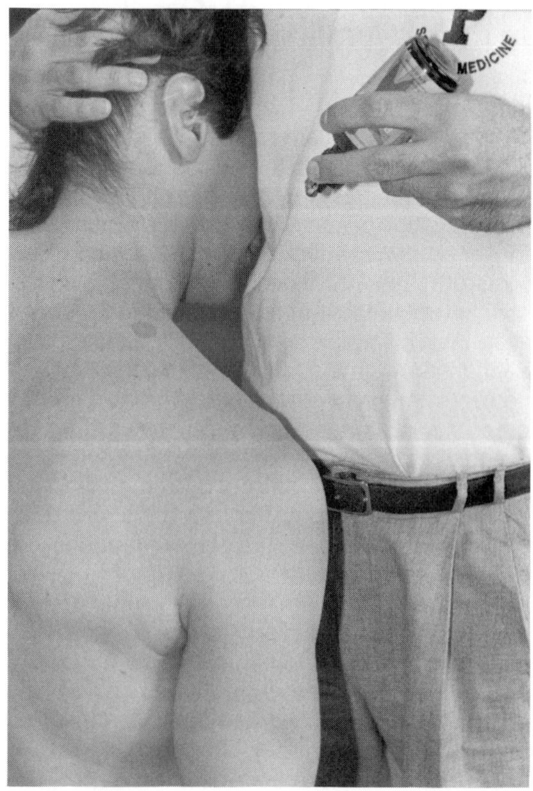


**Figure 7-17.** Spray and stretch of the upper trapezius.

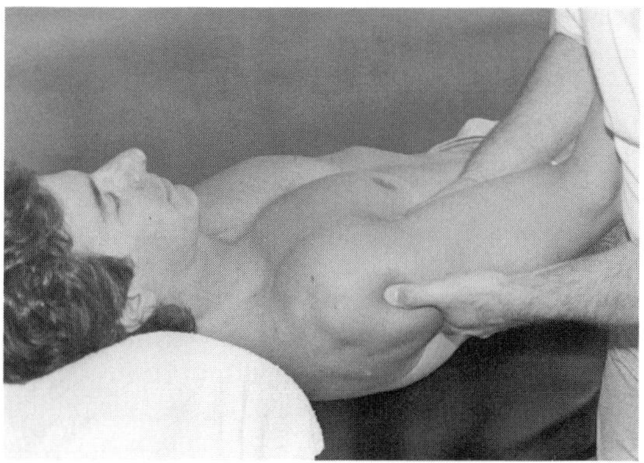

**Figure 7-18.** Ischemic compression of the deltoid.

initial discomfort is accommodated, from 5 to 15 seconds, the pressure can be increased gently. A therapeutic response is found when the pain diminishes while the pressure is maintained constant. An increasing pain gradient may result if the initial pressure is too strong or abrupt, and if this continues after appropriate adjustment of pressure, the technique should be terminated. Skin blanching followed immediately by reactive hyperemia is an expected response that accompanies ischemic compression. The production of hyperemia is thought to occur as well within the muscle and to be of therapeutic value.[53,60] The muscle is treated immediately by passive stretch and active contraction while the temporary nerve block is in effect.

### DEEP MUSCLE MASSAGE

The application of friction and stripping massage has been shown to result in pain relief, trigger point deactivation, and reduction of taut band tension in the muscles of myofascial pain patients.[53] The muscle to be treated is placed on slack, and the taut band is identified.

The technique is begun with firm bilateral thumb pressure applied longitudinally along the taut band and toward the muscle belly. After several passes, the band will begin to relax and then can be compressed firmly between the thumbs, effectively milking the region. The stripping massage action is continued until the regional tension approximates the tone felt in the adjacent tissue; usually 2 minutes will suffice to achieve this response. The taut fiber band, now being in a state of reduced reactivity, is amenable to elongation by reversing the direction, stroking away from the muscle belly. Transverse friction also can be employed at this time to help free up the involved fascicles. Deep muscle massage is augmented by immediate passive stretching, followed by active muscle contractions.

An example of this technique can be applied to the middle deltoid fibers which are situated at an anatomic disadvantage to undergo full elongation during physiologic motion. The distance through which the fasciculi can lengthen and shorten is less than found in the unipennate muscle design; therefore, restriction of free gliding may be more critical to the functional range. This is commonly the site of tender points, taut fiber bands, and trigger points that respond to deep massage techniques that can be used to separate and elongate the fibers (Fig. 7-19).

## Neuromuscular Stretching

Stretching can be performed as passive treatment, with participation of the patient, or as self-treatment. Stretching is indicated to produce mechanical and neuromuscular effects in the treatment of hypertonicity and shortening, including cramping, spasm, myostatic and pseudomyostatic contracture, and adaptive shortening. Each of these conditions represents a distinct mechanism of dysfunction that requires specific management. For example, treatment of true myostatic contracture requires imparting

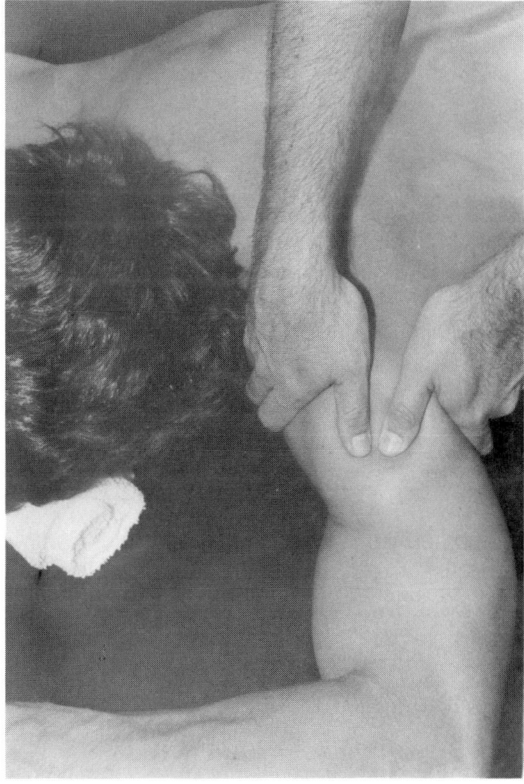

**Figure 7-19.** Deep massage of the deltoid.

some degree of strain or elongation to the passive connective-tissue components. However, subtle to overt resistance can be encountered from the active component when attempting passive stretch. Neuromuscular techniques to promote muscle relaxation preceding passive stretch would facilitate more effective passive stretching, but it is ultimately mechanical loading and elongation that are required to release a true contracture. In contrast, reflex muscle-holding states or pseudomyostatic contracture may be released by techniques used to enhance neuromuscular relaxation.

The term *neuromuscular stretching* offers a generic description that acknowledges the neurophysiologic basis of those stretch techniques which call for active muscle contractions by the patient as directed by the therapist. The treatment principles applied here are used in several therapeutic approaches including muscle energy, hold-relax and contract-relax proprioceptive neuromuscular facilitation (PNF), and postisometric relaxation. Optimal passive stretching can only be accomplished during periods of muscle relaxation, which is often promoted by interactive patient participation.

The integration of active contraction and passive stretching performed in tandem is thought to enhance muscle lengthening by several means. Strong voluntary contraction is immediately followed by a brief refractory period when the muscle cannot contract, providing a time when the muscle can be elongated without evoking the myotatic stretch reflex. This can last anywhere from milliseconds up to 10 or more seconds in pathologic conditions.[18]

A maximal voluntary contraction is more likely to result in a greater number of motor units being inhibited than occurs following submaximal effort, providing it is reasonably accommodated by the patient. Powerful isometric contractions exert considerable tension on the myofascial harness, augmenting fiber broadening and separation. Maximal contractions or strong stretch can activate the Golgi tendon organ system, which is inhibitory to neuromuscular activity in an attempt to protect the muscle from damage.

Maximal contractions are sometimes contraindicated in certain patients depending on the status of the involved soft tissues and joint structures. Patients who are apprehensive also may respond poorly to maximal contractions when attempting to optimize stretch. Voluntary relaxation of the muscle must first be promoted when stretching, and this can be achieved through submaximal contractions. Performing submaximal contractions allows patients to experience a cognitive and physical sense of when the muscle is contracted, helping them to differentiate a contracted from a relaxed state. Once they learn this distinction, optimal stretching can be achieved.

Effective stretching of myostatic contractures must overcome resistance encountered by increased tissue stiffness and viscosity to produce plastic deformation. This is better accomplished by lower loading over longer duration. The amount of time is more important to stretch effectiveness than the degree of force. This principle is extremely important for clinicians to grasp. Recognition of this helps to prevent unwanted injuries during the rehabilitation process, and it reduces unnecessary pain experienced on the part of patients. Some degree of soreness is predictable following stretch and exercise procedures that have produced changes in the connective tissues. Onset typically occurs within 12 hours and dissipates within 48 hours. Occasionally, posttreatment soreness lingers up to 72 hours; persistent discomfort is indicative of some degree of injury to the connective tissues.[42] Because the connective-tissue elements may be considerably weakened during long-standing myostatic contracture, care must be taken not to apply sudden loading. In calling for a maximal-effort contraction, the force should be ramped up gradually, reaching maximum over 6 to 10 seconds, and then eased off. This gives the connective tissues time to accommodate loading without failure. The force generated by the muscle will be less when initiated from its maximal length and the discomfort greater. Initiating the treatment by several cycles of contraction begun in midrange is often helpful to enhance the neuromuscular responses, increasing afferent activity and warming the muscle. Isometric contractions will produce increased compression in the corresponding joint. Preceding the technique with joint mobilization and distraction can reduce potential irritation. When possible, traction is maintained during the stretch.

When significant capsuloligamentous complex restriction is present, neuromuscular techniques are still required to enhance relaxation so that the mechanical effects of stretch can be imparted to the restricted capsuloligamentous complex through joint mobilization and prolonged stretch.

Manually resisted exercise in the available range preceding stretching or joint mobilization can enhance treatment effectiveness. Submaximal contractions against resistance performed through the available range works well to warm the tissues, increase afferent stimuli to reduce pain and guarding, and fatigue the muscle to reduce resistance to passive stretch.

## STRETCHING PRECAUTIONS

Stretch weakness can result when a muscle must continually operate in positions that elongate it beyond its optimal functional length. A muscle in this condition should not be subjected to vigorous stretching. The rhomboids and middle trapezius are typical examples where this condition is prevalent with anterior migration of the shoulder girdle accompanying forward head posture.

Paretic muscles that lack protective stretch reflex mechanisms must not be subjected to stretch or strain as the delicate connective-tissue elements are weakened and vulnerable to injury. Individuals with osteoporosis or other conditions where osseous structural weakening exists, for example, metabolic diseases, reflex sympathetic dystrophy, peripheral nerve injury, or following prolonged immobilization, requires caution when considering stretch intensity. Particular caution is in order in the presence of capsular laxity, hypermobility, or instability. Careful attention is required when stretching tight muscles around the shoulder after surgical repair.

In acute, painful situations, for example, the presence of active myofascial trigger points, where the neuromuscular reflex systems are facilitated, active patient participation is avoided due to diminished voluntary control. Voluntary contraction increases the likelihood of triggering further splinting or spasm. Contract-relax stretching can be employed once the trigger point is deactivated.

## INDICATIONS AND TECHNIQUE

Neuromuscular stretching is the primary treatment of myostatic contracture and adaptive shortening. The application of neuromuscular stretching technique is outlined for treatment of restricted abduction and external rotation commonly found at the shoulder. Other than the capsuloligamentous complex, the primary structures restricting motion-could include the pectoralis major, subscapularis, latissimus dorsi, teres major, as well as the anterior deltoid and coracobrachialis. A treatment technique for the pectoral muscle group is utilized here as an example.

The treatment sequence begins with the operator passively positioning the joint and muscle at the motion barrier. The patient is supine with the head in neutral alignment (Fig. 7-20). The humerus is positioned horizontally toward the coronal plane and in external rotation. The therapist, standing at the head, uses resistance applied with contact on the medial elbow. The therapist calls for resistance to match that which is applied. The patient may take and hold for 6 to 10 seconds a deep breath during contraction. The therapist, instructing the patient to relax and exhale and keeping the arm at the end range throughout the contraction, now takes up the slack with passive stretch held for 5 seconds, increasing up to 20 seconds through six or more successive cycles of alternating contraction and relaxation. The total time for the complete sequence is between 2 and 3 minutes.

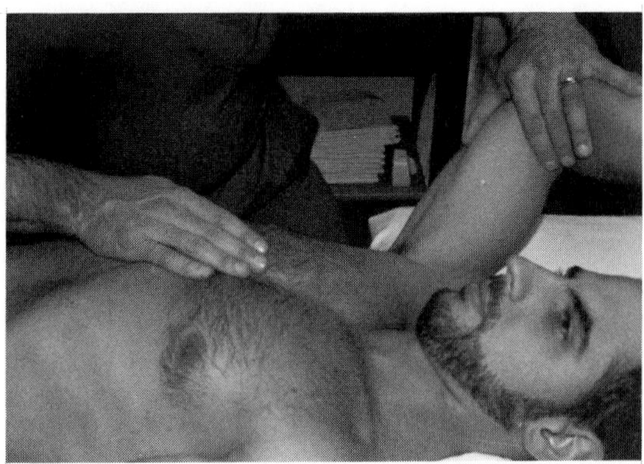

**Figure 7-20.** Neuromuscular stretch of the pectoral muscles.

Another useful neuromuscular stretch technique uses reciprocal inhibition of the muscle being stretched by stimulation of the antagonist muscle group.[16,18] Following completion of the neuromuscular stretch sequence, the therapist calls for contraction into the motion barrier. The therapist changes hand position to the posterior and lateral elbow. The therapist's other arm must stabilize the trunk to minimize substitution and maintain localization of forces to the glenohumeral joint. A series of six contractions, held from 6 to 10 seconds, is appropriate and can be followed by additional stretching. Incorporating reciprocal inhibition into the preceding sequence can enhance the effectiveness but may be difficult to demonstrate in this example. Additional treatment techniques utilizing neuromuscular stretching principles can be applied to other key muscle groups in the shoulder region. Several examples are demonstrated in Figures 7-21, 7-22, and 7-23. Stimulation of antagonists is helpful preceding neuromuscular stretching when contraction of the agonist is moderately painful.

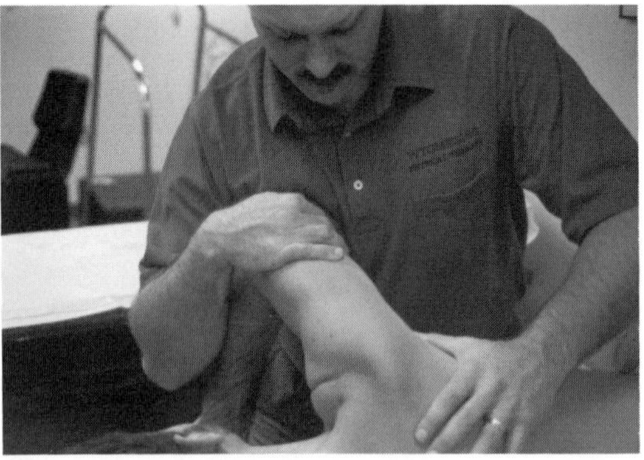

**Figure 7-21.** Neuromuscular stretch of the infraspinatus and teres minor.

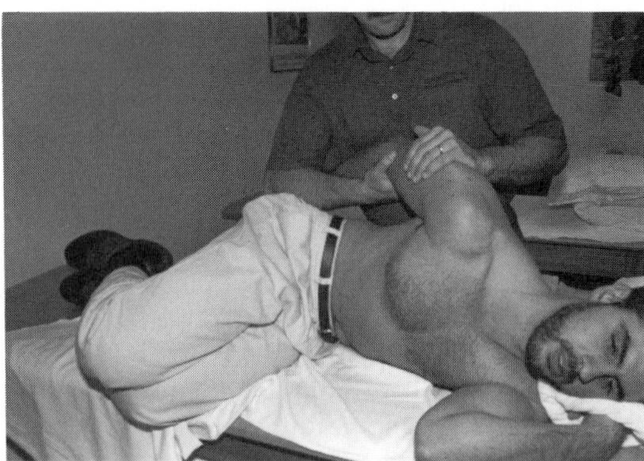

**Figure 7-23.** Neuromuscular stretch of the supraspinatus.

## PSEUDOMYOSTATIC CONTRACTURE

Submaximal effort neuromuscular stretching is indicated as the primary treatment of pseudomyostatic contracture and when strong contraction is painful. Treatment follows the neuromuscular stretching format previously outlined but calls for contractions of approximately 25 percent or even less to stimulate afferent input arising from the muscle within the range that can override nociception, reducing stretch-induced pain. Often, when a patient's apprehension level is a barrier to passive stretch, interactive treatment can enhance compliance, promote relaxation, and diminish guarding.

Passive stretching and scapulothoracic mobilization are indicated when scapular mobility is restricted as a result of pseudomyostatic contracture. The patient can be positioned side-lying with the ipsilateral shoulder upper most. The arm is positioned in glenohumeral medial rotation, with the elbow flexed and dropped behind the back. In the absence of restriction, the medial scapular border will readily move away from the thorax. The therapist grasps the medial border with both hands and gently lifts the scapula off the ribs. Rotation and gliding mobilization should be performed in all directions. This type of treatment technique can be applied while performing distraction of the scapulothoracic joint, as demonstrated later under joint mobilization (see Fig. 7-57).

When myostatic contracture of the serratus anterior accompanies scapular adductor muscles weakness, care must be taken not to subject the weakened muscles to vigorous stretch. The preceding technique is modified in the following manner.

The therapist places the hand flat on the thorax with the web space conforming to the distal medial scapular angle (Fig. 7-24). The other hand is cupped over the humeral head and applies pressure to glide the scapula medially over the hand. By working the scapula in this manner, the distal medial angle usually frees up enough to allow access to grasp the ventral surface for mobilization. The medial angle is pulled posteriorly away from the ribs, while the other hand

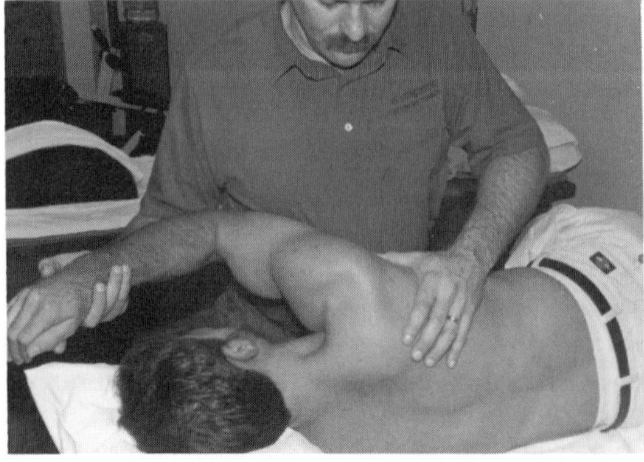

**Figure 7-22.** Neuromuscular stretch of the latissimus dorsi and teres major.

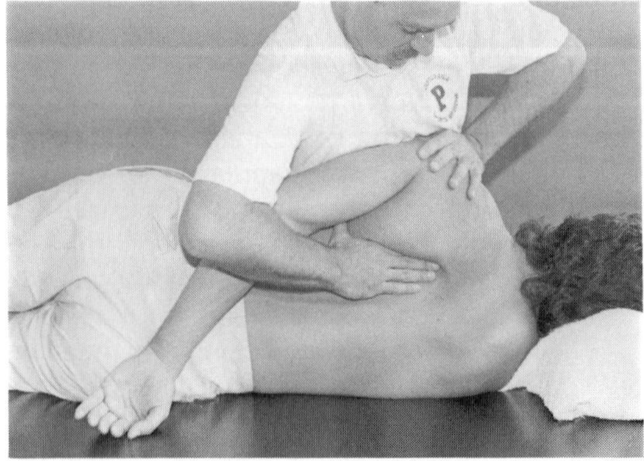

**Figure 7-24.** Modified stretch of the serratus anterior.

glides the scapula posteriorly and medially. Downward rotation of the acromion and upward rotation of the inferior angle are then introduced with alternating stretch and release.

### POST-ISOMETRIC MUSCLE RELAXATION

Lewit[38,39] advocates postisometric muscle relaxation to treat muscle tension and shortening associated with trigger points and pain-induced holding. This technique attempts to promote primarily relaxation, combining isometric contraction with inspiration and relaxation with expiration. The treatment procedure starts with taking out the slack in the muscle by positioning it at the maximal attainable length without introducing stretch. Applying this technique to the pectoral muscles is demonstrated in Figure 7-25. The patient simultaneously takes in and holds a breath while generating a mild isometric contraction against minimal resistance; the breath and contraction are held for 10 seconds, after which the patient is told to "let go." The patient is instructed to breath out slowly and fully, during which time the therapist monitors the relaxation-induced yielding of the motion barrier and passively takes up the slack to the new barrier. The sequence is repeated without interruption for three repetitions initially, and active range of motion is then reassessed. If the patient does not experience any difficulty with respiration, another three to five repetitions can be performed. A satisfactory result is evidenced by reduction of pain at rest and improvement of pain-free active movement. Passive stretch is not deemed essential, but merely the proof of successfully induced relaxation.[38]

Post-isometric relaxation is useful in self-treatment, and the patient can be instructed to perform the technique for home use substituting gravity for light isometric resistance.

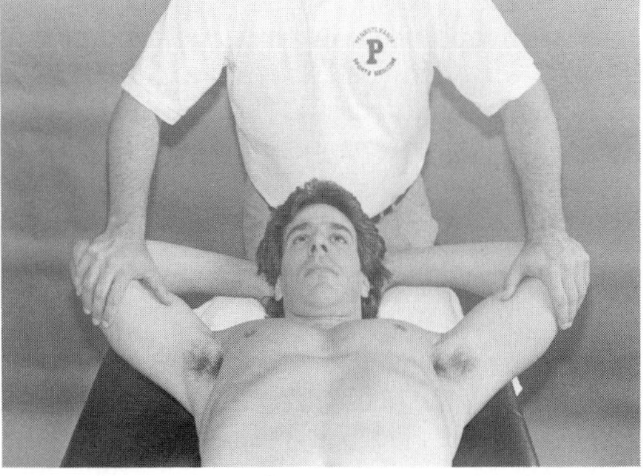

**Figure 7-25.** Postisometric relaxation of the pectorals.

## Osteopathic Approaches

Many of the techniques and treatment principles currently found in use in orthopedic physical therapy originated in or were derived from osteopathy. A. T. Still, the founder of osteopathic medicine, assigned prime importance to the role of connective tissue in both anatomic structure and physiologic function. The fascial system was recognized for its regulatory functions of circulation, consistent with his "law of the artery" philosophy of health and disease.

Advances in neurophysiology led to the eventual development of osteopathic techniques that took into account neuromuscular mechanisms of somatic dysfunction. Muscle energy, counterstrain, and myofascial release engage the muscle and connective-tissue proprioceptors via application of distinct mechanical forces to induce therapeutic changes in the neuromusculoskeletal system.

Muscle energy employs voluntary contractions, counterstrain uses passive positioning, and myofascial release applies pressure or stretch to influence sensorimotor regulation by altering mechanical input in the feedback loop. Consistent with Still's early emphasis on the role of fascia, it is the connective-tissue elements that function as the medium to convert mechanical to neuromuscular information in the muscle, tendon, and joint receptors.

### COUNTERSTRAIN PRINCIPLES

Osteopathic physician Lawrence H. Jones developed a nonmanipulative treatment approach to correct spinal lesions and somatic dysfunction by passive positioning of the involved segment.[32] Originally developed to address spinal column dysfunction, his concept of spontaneous release by positioning was further applied to the treatment of peripheral joints.

A primary principle of counterstrain technique is that protective muscle splinting, as a component of joint restriction, resists any motion away from the position of restriction, but returning to the original position reduces muscle activity. If that position is found in which the joint segments were in when the binding occurred and then further exaggerated, the neuromuscular component can relax or release the articular restriction.

Jones describes tender myofascial points that can be found to accompany joint movement restrictions when protective muscle splinting is the binding mechanism. The associated tender or trigger points can be correlated directly with specific lesions, and relief of pain and tenderness is accomplished only by relieving the causative joint lesion. Identifying the associated trigger point is important to technique application, during which it is monitored for reduction of sensitivity.

Shoulder muscle trigger points occur not only with localized glenohumeral or acromioclavicular dysfunction but also with mid-cervical or upper thoracic spine somatic dysfunction, probably through sympathetic reflex mediated pathways. Counterstrain technique can be used to treat painful restriction of glenohumeral abduction and external rotation by the following technique (Fig. 7-26) In this example, the right shoulder is treated with focus on the supraspinatus.

The patient is positioned supine, with the therapist seated on the ipsilateral side. A tender point in the right supraspinatus muscle belly may be found with deep palpation just above the midline of the spine of the scapula. The therapist maintains contact with the tender point with gentle but firm pressure applied with the index or long finger, which monitors for changes in tension and reactivity throughout the technique. Using the right arm, the therapist passively positions the limb in 45 degrees of abduction and flexion and then moves slowly toward full lateral rotation. The therapist can fine-tune the position, sensing for a reduction in tissue tension and listening for the patient's verbal report of reduced tenderness. Gentle traction or compression also can be included in the application of counterstrain techniques. Typically, the desired response takes 90 seconds to complete after the correct position has been localized and is thought to be mediated by the Golgi tendon reflex mechanisms.

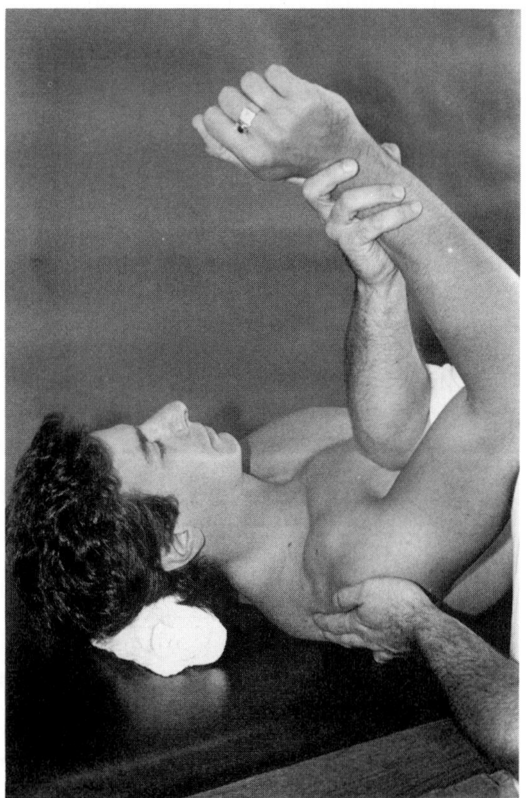

**Figure 7-26.** Counterstrain technique for the supraspinatus.

The prone position can be used to treat the deltoid or teres major. The arm is extended and abducted to varying degrees as the therapist searches for the position of release while monitoring the involved muscle.

## MYOFASCIAL RELEASE

Myofascial release relates to muscle as well as connective-tissue relaxation that is brought about by the appropriate application of stress on that tissue.[6] Myofascial release techniques involve the application of traction or elongation combined with some degree of simultaneous shearing, twist, and often compression, depending on the specific technique. Both mechanical and reflex mechanisms are involved in this release process.[6,23] The perception of "release" is by nature an experiential event, perceived as yielding of tension and resistance in response to pressure or traction.

A common area where these techniques have been described and employed are in the lumbodorsal region. The lumbodorsal fascia is functionally related to the shoulder via the latissimus dorsi, into which it is incorporated by thick, white aponeurosis.[21] Binding down and shortening of the latissimus dorsi can occur in response to reduction of joint mobility either in the lower spine or at the shoulder, particularly when a capsular pattern of restriction is present. This technique is derived from the system of myofascial release practiced by Robert Ward.[6,23]

Ward's approach involves the induction of force-application load to produce mechanical deformation in the tissue. His POET concept refers to the *point of entry* being where the greatest degree of soft-tissue tension is detected. The T represents the combined forces of twist, tension, and traction applied initially at the point of entry, producing three-dimensional loading.

To apply this technique to the lumbodorsal fascia, the patient is positioned prone with the arms by the side in the neutral position and head in the midline (Fig. 7-27). The therapist places the thumbs parallel to the lumbar spine bilaterally over the sacrospinalis mass. The remain-

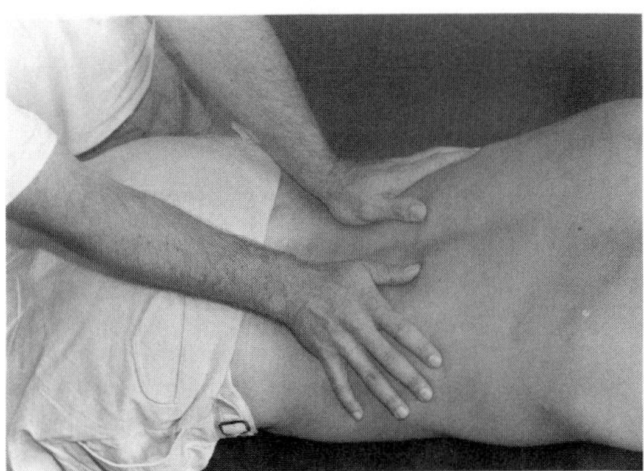

**Figure 7-27.** Myofascial release of the lumbodorsal fascia.

ing hand is placed in full contact with the fingers oriented longitudinally to the latissimus fibers. The slack is taken out with lateral movement away from the spine. the skin should turn white between the thumbs, indicating sufficient application of tension. Simultaneous compression is applied, deep enough to deform the myofascial mass but not so much as to load or impart passive movement of the lumbar spine. The release process begins rapidly, within 10 seconds after the initial engagement of the motion barrier, and is signaled by spontaneous movement in the tissues. Inherent tissue motion is believed to be produced by changes in tonic and phasic activity of the muscle at the level of the annulospiral system that occur as a consequence of alpha motor neuron and gamma efferent input from the central nervous system.[6] The initial tissue relaxation therefore occurs in the active or neuromuscular component. When the active component ceases to offer resistance, the mechanical forces can begin to affect the passive connective-tissue elements. The therapist follows along behind the inherent movement, maintaining consistent force of application and often engaging a series of barriers and subsequent releases, which can be perceived as rapid oscillations or pulsations occurring within the tissue. The technique is continued without interruption until the inherent motion dissipates, typically after 30 to 90 seconds, depending on the magnitude of restriction.

Significant releases are accompanied by the production of heat and blushing of the skin in the region, thought to be in part an indicator that changes in the tissue have occurred involving hysteresis and dissipation of stored energy. The release then is thought to affect the passive components by breaking abnormal cross-links and reducing higher-viscosity levels in the ground substance within the region of fascial dysfunction. Some degree of pulsing and increased tissue temperature may be detected, thought to be related to energy release from cross-linkage disruption.[6] The procedure is then repeated with the arm repositioned elevated and supported on the treatment table with the latissimus dorsi on stretch.

Once the transverse plane of restriction is released, the longitudinal component is addressed. Oblique restrictions also occur but are encountered and corrected in the preceding and following technique.

The therapist places one hand flat and in full contact over the lumbosacral junction and the other over the thoracolumbar region, in the midline with the fingers pointed caudally. The proximal hand draws the fascia cranially, taking out the slack, and the distal hand applies pressure on the sacral base caudally and anteriorly. The procedure is the same as previously described and is performed with the latissimus first on slack and then on stretch.

## DEEP PRESSURE APPLIED AT TENDON OR MUSCLE BELLY

Sustained pressure applied to the tendon area can be beneficial for reduction of muscle tension and related pain. Although very similar in application to ischemic compression applied to myofascial trigger points, the probable underlying therapeutic mechanism is by Golgi tendon organ stimulation and resulting reduction of neuromuscular sensitivity to pressure and stretch. Myofascial trigger points, in contrast, are typically found in the muscle belly, not in or very near the tendon.[59]

This technique works well over broad, flat tendons adjacent to or over the osseous junction, for example, the cranial attachments of the trapezius and semispinalis capitis, or muscles such as the pectoralis major or latissimus dorsi. Sustained pressure is applied with the fingertips directly perpendicular to and into the tendon; the muscle is placed on enough tension to engage the first resistance barrier without additional stretch. Pressure is maintained constant for 60 to 120 seconds, during which time softening of the tissues can be felt, indicating neuromuscular relaxation.

The technique can be enhanced by performing deliberate slow deep breathing with emphasis on long exhalation. Once the patient and the soft tissues are in a relaxed state, it is advantageous to immediately follow the technique with passive and hold-relax stretching and active range of motion.

After the superficial muscles relax, pressure can be directed into the deeper layers, where the short, suboccipital muscle group is located. Pressure applied into the muscle belly also can produce neuromuscular relaxation, probably by altering the mechanical tension in the gamma spindle loop, which is not accompanied by dynamic change in muscle length or position.

## THORACIC INLET RELEASE

Upledger[62] describes a myofascial release technique included in his system of craniosacral therapy that is useful for restoring myofascial mobility and reducing soft-tissue tension. This technique can prove beneficial for treatment of holding states associated with pain and reflex hyperirritability compatible with Korr's facilitated segment concept. Physical alterations of the connective tissue such as adhesion lysis are probably not a direct result of this particular release technique.

The soft tissues of the anterior and posterior thoracic inlet are examined for free fascial gliding by placing the palmar surface of the hand and fingers flat on the region, with light pressure, enough to provide adherence. The therapist then deliberately glides the skin and superficial fascia in one direction, noting the quality of free gliding and extensibility. This gliding motion is repeated in each direction, feeling for gliding restriction.

The release technique involves gentle compression, less than 1 oz of pressure, with the flat hand, now without inducing voluntary motion, as performed with mobility assessment of fascial glide. Hand placement is posterior at the cervicothoracic junction and anterior over the manubrium and sternoclavicular joints.

The application of gentle pressure may facilitate release, perceived as motion under the hand of a floating nature. Ward attributes this inherent tissue mobility to central nervous system regulation of alpha motor neuron and gamma efferent discharge affecting the tonic and phasic activities of the muscle at the level of the annulospiral system.[6] This motion typically starts within 10 seconds and lasts up to 1 minute or more. The therapist allows the tissue to release in the direction of spontaneous motion.

This type of reflex-mediated myofascial release can be followed by connective-tissue mobilization to address remaining mechanical restrictions of fascial and skin mobility.

## ARM TRACTION TECHNIQUE

This technique is useful to enhance mobility of the shoulder and upper extremity by releasing the regional fascia, thereby affecting restrictions not addressed fully by specific muscle stretching (Fig. 7-28). It is effective in the treatment of myofascial pain and other mechanisms of pseudomyostatic contracture and immobilization.

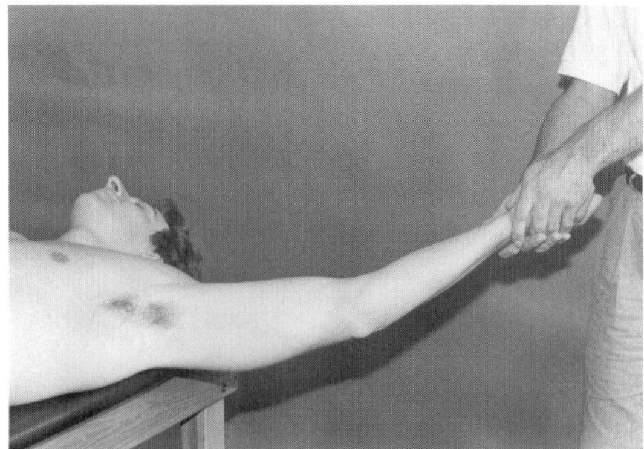

**Figure 7-28.** Arm traction technique.

The mechanisms of release here are both mechanical and neuromuscular. The introduction of twisting and shearing forces combined with traction loads the fascia in an attempt to break up mechanical restrictions. In essence, the fascial component is effectively wrung out, facilitating drainage of the interstitial compartments and spaces in the arm, shoulder, and axilla. Sustained traction can activate Golgi tendon organs situated in the muscle tendons and in the fascial intermuscular septum, producing neuromuscular relaxation.

The patient is positioned supine with the shoulder to be treated at the edge of the table. The therapist grasps the patient's wrist with one hand and introduces light traction, enough to take out the slack in the fascial sleeve. The starting position is from anatomic neutral. The arm is elevated in abduction, and some twisting is introduced in the direction of external rotation; traction is maintained throughout. The therapist attempts to continually engage the elastic tissue barrier and perceive the induced relaxation, which will dictate the pace of passive motion provided by the therapist. The technique is continued through a full range of circumduction, allowing the head of the humerus to rotate with physiologic motion. Elapsed time should be in the range of 2 minutes for maximum benefit. Immediate active exercise is recommended, which reestablishes neuromuscular communication.

The therapist must appreciate that this type of release is not purely mechanical; forceful traction must not be used, and there should be no pain, perhaps only stretch discomfort. Movement is never forced through a barrier, at which passive motion is held once encountered. Stiffer elastic barriers are felt with myostatic contracture, and a hard end feel is indicative of undesirable acromiohumeral approximation. When the restriction is accompanied by a firm, capsular end feel, the following technique can be employed.

### CAPSULAR TWIST TECHNIQUE

Significant changes in the connective-tissue matrix exist in the frozen and thawing phases of adhesive capsulitis or "frozen" shoulder. Increases in collagen fiber density and in interfiber cross-links can involve the full depth and extent of the capsule, resulting in capsular shrinkage and significant multidirectional motion restriction.[8,10]

The capsular twist technique is a modification of the arm traction technique, which localizes forces to the capsule by moving the grip proximally to the humerus (Fig. 7-29). The motion barrier in this case will be considerably more firm. Twisting and stretch are introduced in an attempt to break up and stretch out these restrictions and increase free gliding between fibers. Some localized pain of a diffuse tingling or burning, typical of capsule or fascia, can occur and may be accompanied by some perception of heat. Both are indicative of structural changes in the connective-tissue matrix and lysis of abnormal cross-links resulting from induced strain on the fiber elements, hysteresis, and energy release.

The patient is positioned prone. The therapist stabilizes the scapula with one hand and with the other grasps the humerus above the elbow. While maintaining strong longitudinal traction, the arm is twisted into medial rotation. Extension is then slowly introduced. The arm is slowly brought into abduction to the next barrier, held 30 to 60 seconds, and then unwound into lateral rotation to the barrier and held another 30 or more seconds. Total time should be approximately 2 to 3 minutes employing low continuous load throughout.

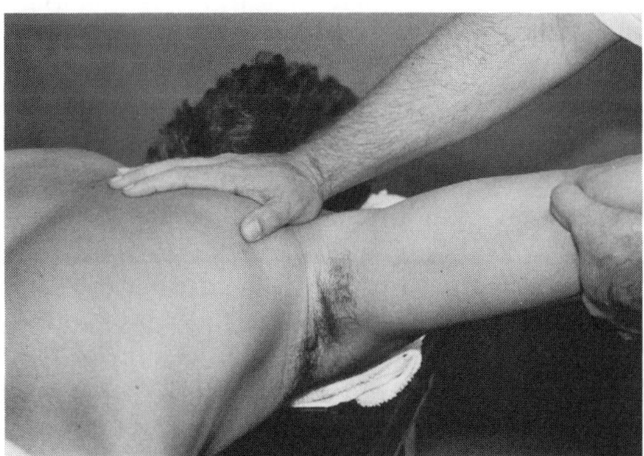

**Figure 7-29.** Capsular twist technique.

When a capsular pattern of restriction exists, the inferior capsule may be the primary site of adhesion, where binding between the capsular folds will limit its extensibility, particularly during glenohumeral abduction and lateral rotation. Specific joint-mobilization procedures in this case are indicated to restore joint play and normal arthrokinematics.

## MUSCLE ENERGY

The "muscle energy" approach was developed by osteopathic physician Fred Mitchell, Sr. Muscle energy techniques are described in the osteopathic literature as being alternatives to joint manipulations used to correct somatic dysfunction and articular positional faults.[23,46] Muscle energy attempts to improve muscle function and joint control by resetting the faulty gamma system gain to the muscle spindle.

It is an interactive approach in that the therapist passively positions the segment or joint at the motion barrier and calls for active contraction of the prime movers of that joint executed against a distinct counterforce given by the therapist. In this respect, muscle energy is synonymous with isometric joint manipulation, since the patient's "muscle energy" provides the corrective force. Both direct and indirect techniques can be used. Direct technique calls for active contraction away from the barrier, followed by the therapist taking up the slack after the contraction and repositioning the joint at the new limit of motion. The technique is similar to hold-relax stretching but may be less forceful, depending on the application. The contraction is held for several seconds and is typically submaximal, with the amount of force and counterforce evenly matched. The intensity is adjusted as necessary at the therapist's discretion and with respect to the patient's condition and level of reactivity.

Muscle energy can be used to influence either muscle activity or joint position and mobility. The principles applied in muscle energy therapy are similar to those of PNF techniques employed to release tight myofascia and to reeducate neuromuscular functions and joint control. Treatment of shoulder dysfunction can be enhanced by muscle energy principles but offers no distinct advantage over neuromuscular stretching techniques described earlier in this chapter.

The arthrokinematics of the glenohumeral joint are determined principally by the articular surfaces and the capsuloligamentous complex, not by muscle contraction. Mennell[45] describes joint play as the mobility normally present in synovial joints that is not under voluntary muscle control. Therefore, muscle energy techniques cannot substitute for joint mobilization techniques directed at the glenohumeral joint for the purposes of restoring lost joint play. Utilization of muscle energy techniques for joint mobilization and repositioning is more appropriate to treatment of the spine and pelvic articulations. Some techniques could be applied to scapulothoracic and acromioclavicular joints. An example involving the acromioclavicular joint is described as well as two techniques for the thoracic outlet.

An application of muscle energy at the acromioclavicular joint calls for the clavicular fibers of the trapezius to provide superior translation and decompression of the acromioclavicular articulation.[16] Indications include palpatory tenderness, restriction of passive motion, and pain during abduction.

The patient is seated upright, with the therapist standing behind. The therapist positions the cranium in rotation with the chin turned away from the shoulder to be treated. The therapist stabilizes the occiput with one hand at the insertion of the trapezius and places the other forearm on the ipsilateral clavicle. The therapist calls for and isometrically resists elevation of shoulder shrug, performed simultaneously with inhalation. Each contraction is held 6 to 10 seconds and repeated three to five times. The passive and active movements are then reassessed.

### THORACIC OUTLET TECHNIQUES

Muscle energy can be applied to treat first rib elevation and thoracic kyphosis in the management of Thoracic Outlet Syndrome when soft-tissue reactivity prohibits direct pressure over the first rib during mobilization. An effective technique for mobilizing the first rib and restoring mobility in the upper thoracic region utilizes muscle energy principles by employing the action of those muscles which attach to the first rib to facilitate combined upper thoracic back bending and first rib depression.

The iliocostalis thoracis attaches to the superior border of the costal angle of the first rib. It acts to back bend and laterally flex the trunk, drawing the first six ribs caudally.[21] The upper slips of the serratus anterior attach to the first rib along the superior outer border and pass posterior to attach on the ventral surface of the superomedial scapula. When the shoulder girdle is fixed, the serratus can function as an accessory muscle of deep inhalation. By employing the serratus anterior during inhalation and the iliocostalis thoracis during exhalation, an effective mobilization force can be attained without direct pressure on the rib or spinal articulations.

To perform the technique unilaterally on the left, the patient is seated upright in a chair with both feet on the floor (Fig. 7-30a). The scalenes are put on slack by left-side bending until the ipsilateral cervical fascia and scalenes are felt to relax. This helps to reduce scalene contraction during deep inspiration. With the patient's elbow flexed, the ipsilateral arm is elevated in the plane of the scapula, taking up the slack. This positions the scapular attachment of the upper slips of the serratus below the first rib and places the upper fibers on stretch. The therapist, standing on the same side, places his or her left hand at the point of the flexed elbow. The therapist's right hand is now moved from the patient's head to the apex of the thoracic kyphosis and guides the trunk into the fully erect position (see Fig. 7-30b). The patient is asked to take a deep, full inhalation, and the therapist simultaneously takes up the slack into further trunk erection and upper thoracic back bending. After a brief pause, the patient is asked to perform a prolonged, forceful exhalation, and simultaneous isometric resistance of scapular protraction is given, not allowing the scapula to move from the fixed position. The upper fibers will then exert a pulling force on the first rib, creating depression. Forced exhalation is helpful to further relax the scalenes via reciprocal inhibition. During exhalation, the therapist assists upper thoracic back bending coupled with some ipsilateral side bending and rotation localized to the upper segments. This sequence is repeated three to six times as tolerated. The therapist should verbally monitor the occurrence or reproduction of symptoms into the upper extremity. An alternate position for those who cannot tolerate arm elevation is horizontal adduction of the ipsilateral arm with the elbow brought to the midline and pointing anteriorly. This technique is readily adaptable to the side-lying position, which provides additional trunk stabilization (Fig. 7-31). In this position, pillows are used to position the head and neck in side bending.

Muscle energy technique is also effective for restoring upper thoracic mobility in the treatment of kyphosis accompanying forward head posture. In this instance, the patient folds the arms across the chest, and the therapist supports them from beneath, elevating them to take up the slack. The patient rests the forehead against the folded arms and maintains this contact throughout the procedure. This helps position the scalenes on slack. The therapist guides the up-

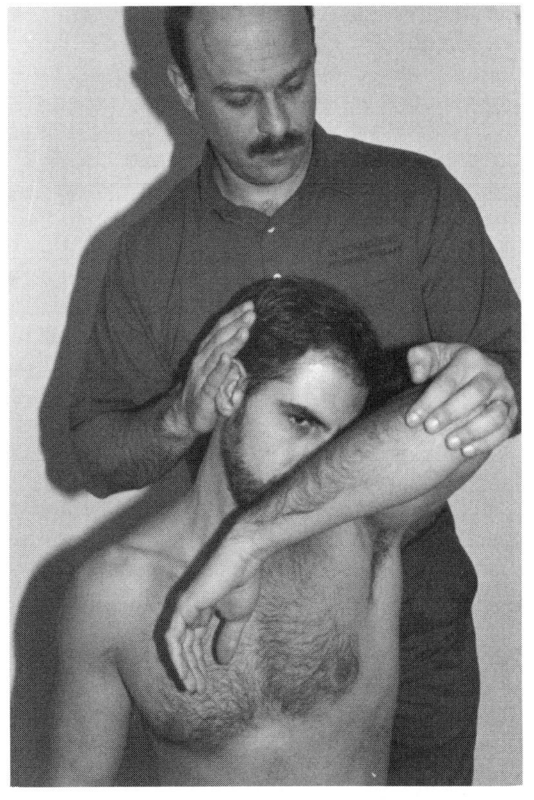

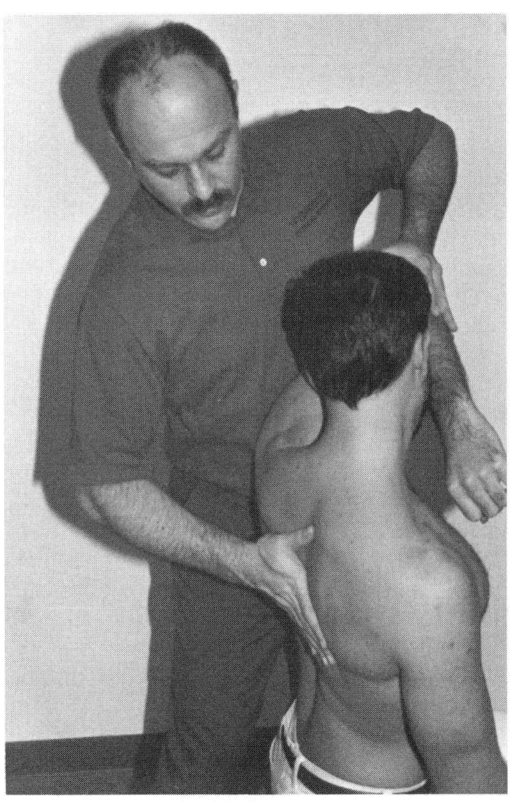

A B

**Figure 7-30.** Muscle energy technique for the first rib. (a) Starting position. (b) Thoracic extension position.

per trunk into erection and back bending during inhalation and maintains the position during forced exhalation as above. Oscillations directed from posterior to anterior in the sagittal plane can be given.

## Summary

Shoulder function is demanding on the supporting soft-tissue network, making dysfunction common. Soft-tissue pathology includes mechanical, neurophysiologic, circulatory, and reflexogenic mechanisms. The reflex influences to shoulder dysfunction may not be fully appreciated in the clinical setting; therefore, a review of some of these mechanisms was included as appropriate for the discussion of evaluation and treatment.

Optimal treatment outcomes necessitate knowledge in the evaluation and correction of related dysfunction; therefore, the scope of treatment of the glenohumeral joint and shoulder was expanded to address other anatomic regions to which the shoulder is structurally and functionally interrelated.

Myofascial and articular dysfunction typically coexists to some extent. Each component of dysfunction requires its own set of examination and treatment techniques specific to the tissue. Treatment of one does not substitute for the other, although they are functionally inseparable, for all practical purposes.

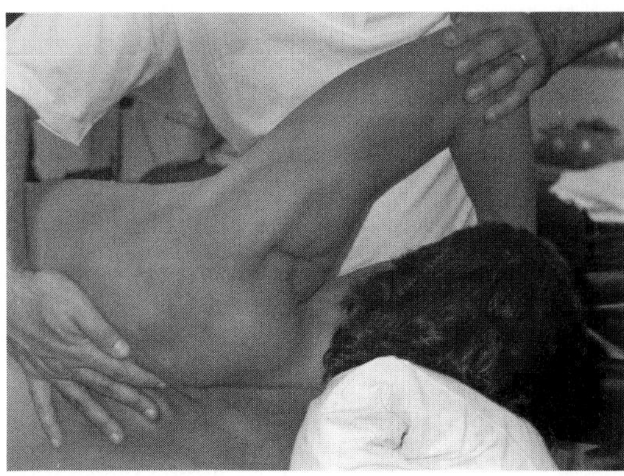

**Figure 7-31.** First rib technique, alternate side-lying position.

# Joint Mobilization and Manipulation

Treatment of the articulations of the human body by manipulation has been practiced since the days of Hippocrates and by various cultures from ancient times to the present. Presently, the use of manipulative therapy endures and is enjoying increased acceptance among physicians and physical therapists throughout the international community.

The use of manipulation by physical therapists was slower to gain momentum in the United States than abroad, propagated largely by physical therapy and medical practitioners from other nations, primarily Norway, England, New Zealand, and Australia. Osteopathic concepts and techniques, for example, muscle energy or counterstrain, are increasingly employed by physical therapists; the influences derived from chiropractic are inconsiderable, particularly in the application of manipulative therapy to the appendicular articulations.

## Schools of Thought

Contemporary manipulative therapy specific to the shoulder has been strongly influenced by concepts popularized by certain individuals, most notably James Cyriax, Freddy Kaltenborn, Geoffrey Maitland, John Mennell, and Alan Stoddard. Some of their individual contributions are hear briefly acknowledged. It is interesting that James Cyriax, a certain proponent, makes diminutive use of manipulation in application to shoulder treatment. Dr. Cyriax's significant contributions include the concept of "end feel" and the classic "examination by selective tissue tension" that has emerged as the foundation for extremity joint assessment, perhaps with best application at the shoulder. Treatment by injection and massage and stretching are more often utilized, however; Cyriax offers a singular mobilization technique, lateral distraction of the humeral head from the glenoid, to restore accessory movement but credits physiotherapist Jennifer Hickling as the originator.[11]

John McM. Mennell and his father, James, along with James Cyriax, belong to the very small fraternity of medical practitioners to champion the use of manipulation in treatment of the musculoskeletal system. John Mennell defined what he termed *joint dysfunction* as a loss of accessory or joint-play movement, which is movement that is normally present in the joint but not under voluntary muscle control.[45] Mennell recognized joint dysfunction as a pain-producing pathologic condition that caused loss of movement. Joint dysfunction was detected by passive movement examination, which should be pain-free and unrestricted in all maneuvers ascribed to the particular joint. Treatment is aimed at restoration of joint play as a means to restore full, pain-free voluntary movement.

Freddy Kaltenborn (physical therapist) applied the earlier work of M. A. MacConaill, who described convex-concave and close-pack, loose-pack joint relationships, to the treatment of joint dysfunction, with particular detail to the arthrokinematics of individual articulations.[33,34] Kaltenborn's focus was on the movements taking place within the capsule of the joint, the arthrokinematics, and the relation of the articular motion to the direction of bone motion, the osteokinematics. The osteokinematics and arthrokinematics at a specific joint may be in the same or in opposite directions, depending on the joint design. For example, at the glenohumeral joint during abduction, the humeral head presents a convex surface moving caudally within the glenoid fossa, which represents a relatively fixated concave surface, while the humeral shaft moves opposite. Accordingly, Kaltenborn would use the technique of caudal glide of the humeral head in the treatment of restricted glenohumeral abduction with hypomobility.[33] More recent research has challenged these rules, and this will be addressed in more detail later in this chapter.

Geoffrey Maitland (physical therapist), departing from the biomechanical model, advocated treatment of painful restricted joints by oscillatory passive movements that provide a neurophysiologic and mechanical therapeutic effect. He devised a graded system for applying passive movements throughout the extent of the joint's range, comprised of four grades differing in amplitude and excursion.[41] Maitland's grading system is defined further under general principles of mobilization, since these grades can be applied to all types of joint mobilization regardless of the school of thought.

Stanley Paris (physical therapist) can be credited with organizing and promoting manipulative therapy in the United States to the medical community as a primary modality in the treatment of musculoskeletal dysfunction. Paris recognized the physician's role to be the diagnosis and treatment of disease, whereas the primary role of the physical therapist is the evaluation and treatment of dysfunction.[50] As defined by Paris, dysfunction differs from Mennell's description, which focuses on painful hypomobility. To Paris, joint dysfunction is "a state of altered mechanics, either an increase or decrease from the expected normal, or the presence of an aberrant motion."[50] Passive movement examination is rated on a seven-level scale, with 3 representing normal mobility, 0 being no mobility, and 6 denoting instability. The selection of appropriate treatment is enhanced by this assessment.

Paris expanded Cyriax's end-feel classification from 3 normal and 3 abnormal to 5 normal and 10 abnormal states.[49,50] He practices an integrated approach to evaluation and treatment of extremity dysfunction, drawing from the work of those individuals mentioned here and others.

## Mobilization: Concepts and Terminology

Mobilization has been called "intelligent range of motion." Mobilization and manipulation are defined differently, depending on the source. The official terminology offered by the Orthopaedic Section of the American Physical Therapy Association defines *manipulation* as "any manual procedure used for the purpose of examination, correction, or modification of an articular or soft tissue dysfunction," and *mobilization* is defined as "the act of imparting movement, either actively or passively, to a joint or soft tissue."[56] Paris[50] defines *manipulation* as "the skilled passive movement to a joint, either within or beyond its active limits of motion."[50] Maitland[41] distinguishes manipulation from mobilization, describing the former as "a sudden small-amplitude thrust delivered at a speed which renders the patient powerless to prevent it." Manipulation is represented by Maitland as grade V passive movement, delivered at and through the pathologic limit of range. Mobilization is depicted as either passive oscillatory movements or sustained stretch at the limit of range. To Kaltenborn,[33] mobilization as a component of manual therapy refers to any procedure that increases mobility of the soft tissues and/or of the joints. Paris[50] places mobilization under the larger definition of manipulation, describing it more specifically as "therapeutic maneuvers applied to a joint demonstrating dysfunction in an attempt to restore arthrokinematics." Mobilization, then, is a form of manipulation, but the term *mobilization* is found more acceptable to many because of the negative associations ascribed to manipulation in the medical community. The term *manipulation*, then, can represent a spectrum of passive movements ranging from the rather crude stretching performed on the shoulder under anesthesia to break adhesions to tiny oscillatory pressures "so gentle as not to bend the legs of a fly when applied to his back," to paraphrase Maitland, whereas *mobilization* would apply only to the latter example.

## Kinematics

*Kinematics* is the study of movement. *Osteokinematics* pertains to the overall movement of bones. These classic movements are referred to as flexion, extension, abduction, adduction, and internal and external rotation. *Arthrokinematics* pertains to the movement of one articular surface in relation to its partner, described by spin, roll, or glide.[33,50,56]

## Accessory Movements

*Accessory movements* are those motions which accompany the classic movements and are necessary for normal function but are not under voluntary neuromuscular control.[45,50,56] Two categories of accessory movements exist: joint play and component motion.

1. *Joint play*: a type of accessory movement where intraarticular movement occurs in response to an outside force, for example, the additional passive range that exists in normal synovial joints beyond the maximal active range. At the shoulder, lateral distraction of the humeral head away from the glenoid fossa represents a primary joint-play movement of the glenohumeral joint.[45] At the acromioclavicular joint, anteroposterior play is present. The sternoclavicular joint possesses superoinferior joint play. At the scapulothoracic joint, the scapula possess joint play with distraction away from the thorax.[45]

2. *Component motion*: a type of accessory movement that is directly associated with the production of osteokinematic movement or motion that takes place in a joint complex or related joint to facilitate a specific active motion.[50] For example, the scapula not only rotates and elevates, but it also tilts posteriorly during abduction.[51] During functional internal rotation, the scapula is required to tilt anteriorly and elevate.

Mennell[45] describes traditional component motions of the glenohumeral joint with reference to the active movement during which they occur:

1. Inferior and posterior glide of the humeral head during sagittal flexion
2. Inferior glide of the humeral head during elevation in the scapular plane

3. Inferior and posteroanterior glide during coronal abduction.
4. Anterior glide of the humeral head during external rotation.
5. Posterior glide of the humeral head during internal rotation.

These component motions are also referred to as *arthrokinematic motions*.

## Arthrokinematics

MacConaill was one of the first to "investigate" arthrodial movement. His work is based on osteokinematics and "perceived" movement of the articular surfaces from direct observation and empirical mathematical calculations. *Rolling* is defined by multiple equidistant contact points on the moving surface meeting multiple equidistant contact points on the stationary surface. Rolling is considered never to occur alone, since it would cause abnormal compression and disarticulation. *Gliding* occurs when a fixed point on the moving surface contacts new multiple points on the stationary surface. Pure gliding is considered to occur only between congruent flat surfaces. Kaltenborn[33,34] stated that gliding occurring between congruent curved surfaces is rotation. However, Kaltenborn states, "no joints in the body have completely congruent surfaces" and no pure rotation (gliding) occurs."[33,34] Therefore, motion at the glenohumeral joint is between incongruent surfaces in a roll-gliding movement. *Rotation* or *spin* is defined as multiple contact points on the moving surface contacting the same fixed point on the stationary surface (Fig. 7-32).

Based on MacConaill's observations, the convex-concave rule was developed and became a pivotal concept in determining mobilization rationale. Simply stated, "if a bone motion takes place in one direction, the rolling that accompanies this motion takes place in the same direction. However, the translatoric gliding in the joint which accompanies this motion takes place (1) in the opposite direction if the moving joint surface is convex and (2) in the same direction if the moving joint surface is concave."[34] Given this rule, the arthrokinematics that take place can be described as follows: (1) when a concave surface moves on a convex surface, roll and glide occur in the same direction, and (2) when a convex surface moves on a concave surface (as at the glenohumeral joint), roll and glide occur in opposite directions.

### CURRENT LITERATURE

Current orthopedic research utilizing more sophisticated measurement tools and designs have studied the articular relationships within the glenohumeral joint. Poppen and Walker[51] noted a 1- to 2-mm inferior and superior excursion of the humerus during abduction in the scapular plane. Howell et al.[29] radiographically determined that the humeral head normally translates *posteriorly* (4 mm), not anteriorly, in the combination position of 90 degrees of abduction, external rotation, and horizontal abduction. Using telemetry in cadavers, Harryman et al.[27] found 0.7 and 0.8 mm of superior glide during abduction and flexion, respectively. In addition to superior glide, anterior gliding of 3.8 and 5.3 mm was found during flexion, and 5.0 mm of posterior gliding occurred during extension.[27] *Posterior*, not anterior, gliding was found with external rotation, and anterior, not posterior, gliding was found with internal rotation.[27] Both Howell et al.[29] and Harryman et al.[27,28] concluded that the direction of humeral head translation is *opposite* the side of primary capsuloligamentous complex tightening. These current findings are in direct contrast to traditional teachings of humeral head motion.

Kelkar et al.,[36] using sterophotogrammetry, found 0.94 mm of superior glide during the initial 30 degrees of scapular abduction; subsequent elevation resulted in negligible gliding. This study also suggests that based on the proximity of the helical axes to the center of the humeral sphere, "the humeral head performs a pure rotation about the center of curvature of its articular surface during abduction in the scapular plane." Soslowsky et al.,[54] using the same technique, found that the average radii of curvature of the humeral head and glenoid cartilage surface was

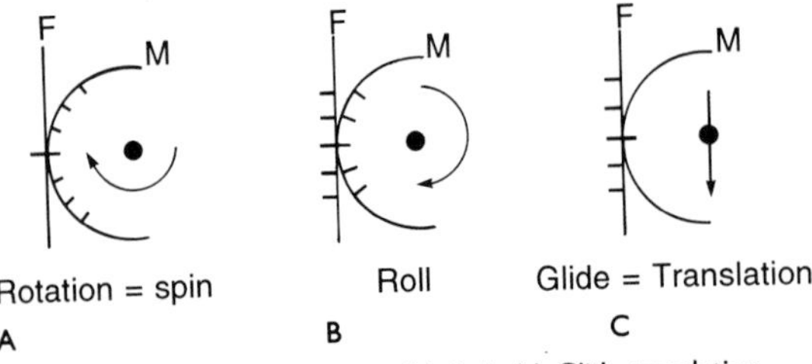


**Figure 7-32.** (a) Spin-rotation. (b) Roll. (c) Glide-translation.

26.85 and 26.37 mm, respectively, for male specimens. The average ratio of radii of curvature between the humeral head and glenoid was 0.99 ($<0.05$), indicating motion that is pure rotational. These two studies conclude that the glenoid and humerus are no longer considered incongruent but congruent surfaces. In fact, they are considered "essentially identical" in their radii of curvature, which contradicts the findings discussed previously by Kaltenborn and MacConaill regarding curved congruent surfaces not being present in the body.

## FUNCTIONAL UNIT

To fully appreciate the arthrokinematics of the glenohumeral joint, the role of the capsuloligamentous complex must be understood. A review of the literature regarding glenohumeral stability reveals information about the restricting capabilities of the capsuloligamentous complex. Turkel et al.[61] and Oversen et al.[48] performed sequential incising studies on the capsuloligamentous complex. Both these studies concluded that anterior stability was not only the responsibility of the anterior capsuloligamentous complex but, in part, the responsibility of the posterior capsuloligamentous complex, and vice versa. O'Brien et al.[47] identified the thickened anterior and posterior bands of the inferior glenohumeral ligament complex. They determined that this ligament complex prevented anterior and posterior translation when the humerus was externally and internally rotated, respectively. From these findings one could easily see how this structure, if contracted, could limit elevation, internal rotation, and external rotation. Harryman et al.[28] evaluated the effects of imbricating and incising the rotator cuff interval. This interval is comprised of the superior glenohumeral ligament and, mostly, the coracohumeral ligament. In summary, this investigation demonstrated that imbrication of the rotator interval led to a loss of inferior, anterior, and posterior glide of 8, 5, and 8 mm, respectively, when evaluated at neutral.[48] When glenohumeral motion was evaluated at 60 degrees of scapular plane abduction, loss of anterior and posterior gliding was negligible (inferior gliding was not evaluated). When the interval was imbricated, motion in external rotation at zero elevation, extension, and flexion was reduced by 38, 18, and 8 degrees, respectively. Terry et al.[57] performed a strain-gauge study monitoring tension-sharing relationships of the different ligaments and capsular regions encasing the glenohumeral joint during various isolated and combination movements of the shoulder. Their results, of which there were many, found significant tightening of the coracohumeral ligament during flexion, extension, and external rotation at zero elevation.

From the preceding studies on the capsuloligamentous complex we can draw several conclusions. First, specific capsuloligamentous complex structures are primarily responsible for limiting certain motions. Second, the overwhelming conclusion is that the capsuloligamentous complex is a single contiguous unit whose varying regions are position-dependent in their responsibility to limit motion, yet these regions (ligaments) are completely *inter*dependent. In essence, limitation of one region affects the unit as a whole. Third, the direction of humeral head translation is dictated by, and *opposite* to, the side of capsuloligamentous complex tightening. A fourth interesting conclusion is the importance of the rotator cuff interval (coracohumeral ligament and superior glenohumeral ligament) and its influence on various motions. Therefore, it is apparent that attention also needs to be directed toward the superior capsule in conditions where passive mobility is impaired.

To summarize, the clinician needs to reconsider traditional concepts regarding glenohumeral arthrokinematics and the capsuloligamentous complex. Critical analysis of the rationale for joint mobilization, based on the new literature, is also required. For instance, joint mobilization is believed to work by reestablishing proper component motion, that is, if external rotation is limited, treatment using anterior glide mobilizations should be performed, since anterior gliding occurs during external rotation. However, the new literature concludes that a *posterior* glide, not an *anterior* glide, occurs with external rotation; thus should a *posterior* glide be performed? As we shall see, the new literature does not contradict the "use" of an anterior glide to regain external rotation motion but does challenge the concept of "why" the anterior glide is used.

In recognition of these current concepts regarding glenohumeral arthrokinematics, we are not invalidating the effectiveness of joint mobilization, since it has been a clinically proven technique for over 50 years. Rather, we support the following concepts: (1) mobilization is a form of stretching, and (2) the capsuloligamentous complex is a functional unit, and stretching any portion of the complex results in increased extensibility to the unit as a whole; as a result, motion is improved in all planes. To further illustrate this concept, an example will be used.

A patient presents with a capsular pattern, significantly restricted external rotation and abduction and less restricted internal rotation. Glenohumeral glides are reduced in all directions. Reactivity is mild, with pain felt with overpressure at end range. Based on traditional beliefs, anterior glides should be performed to reestablish external rotation, since anterior gliding occurs with this motion. Also, inferior gliding should be performed to regain normal inferior gliding or "depression" during abduction. Let us say that both these glides are carried out over several treatment sessions, and indeed, an increase in glenohumeral external rotation and abduction motion is noted on reevaluation. If we accept the new literature, which concludes that posterior gliding occurs with external rotation and more superior gliding occurs with abduction, then how do we explain that mobilizations (gliding anteriorly and inferiorly) opposite to the true component motion brought about an increase in physiologic motion? The answer is because the anterior glide *stretched* the anterior capsuloligamentous complex and the inferior glide *stretched* the inferior capsuloligamentous complex by displacing the insertions of that particular region's soft-tissue elements, both which resulted in a complex with overall greater extensibility. Therefore, greater range of motion was noted.

In viewing mobilization in this manner, one can appreciate its potential therapeutic benefits and not be overly concerned with determining which research is most accurate. What is important to recognize is that justifying one's choice of direction in which to apply a mobilization force cannot be based *solely* on previous rules regarding arthrokinematics or on the more recent sophisticated research on articular relationships within the glenohumeral joint. In time and with clearer interpretation, the contradictions in research and possibly terminology will be resolved. In the mean time, it is important to recognize that restoration of capsuloligamentous extensibility is paramount to improving passive joint range of motion. Joint mobilization of a mechanical nature places sufficient tension on the capsuloligamentous complex and by doing so alters the mechanical behavior and elasticity of this structure. These concepts support the mechanical effects of joint mobilization and substantiate its use in the treatment of glenohumeral joint dysfunction.

## Articular Neurology

Familiarization with the types and functions of mechanoreceptors located in the shoulder joint and surrounding tissues will aid the understanding of neurophysiologic responses to injury and neurophysiologic effects of joint mobilization. Mechanoreceptors are neural sensory organs that convert mechanical energy to nerve action potentials when stimulated by some degree of mechanical deformation or movement. Mechanoreceptors report a number of sensations arising from the superficial and deep tissues to the central nervous system, which include touch, vibration, tickle, pressure, and position.[26] The mechanoreceptors contribute largely to proprioception by providing information on rate of movement, tension, pressure, and position. Each mechanoreceptor type is very highly sensitive to a specific type of stimulus, depending on its morphologic construction. All mechanoreceptors possess a varying degree of firing adaptation, specific to the receptor's nature and sensory role. Rates of adaptation can range from milliseconds to several hours.[26]

The contributions of Wyke[68] to articular neurology provide evidence to support a neurophysiologic basis by which manipulation works to alleviate pain or restore joint function. Wyke classified four types of synovial articular mechanoreceptors with respect to morphology, behavioral characteristics, and function. Important from his work is evidence of mechanoreceptor effects on static and dynamic reflex controls of the skeletal musculature during both normal and dysfunctional states.

Type IV receptors are high threshold and nonadapting, with nociceptive function. When stimulated by mechanical deformation or inflammation, they produce tonic reflexogenic effects on neck, limb, jaw, and eye muscles.

Type III mechanoreceptors are similar in design and function to the Golgi tendon organ and serve a protective role. Type III receptors are fired by sustained pressure, strong stretch, or high-velocity thrust manipulations. When stimulated, these have reflex inhibitory effects on the motoneuron pool, in particular the prime movers of the same joint. Very slowly adapting, the inhibitory effects can last several hours.[26,68]

Type II articular receptors, rapidly adapting and responsive to rapid movement and vibrations, can be fired by oscillations or repetitive stretches. When stimulated, they produce phasic and reflexogenic effects on neck, limb, jaw, and eye muscles and transitory inhibition of nociceptive activity of the joint capsule.[15]

Type I receptors are slowly adapting postural receptors that monitor the tension or change in tension of the outer layers of the joint capsule. Type I receptors differ to some degree in the individual firing thresholds and provide both static and dynamic proprioceptive monitoring of joint position.

When fired by oscillatory motion or static tension, these produce tonic reflexogenic effects on the motoneurons of the neck, limb, jaw, and eye muscles and transsynaptic inhibition of the nociceptive afferent receptors.[15]

## MECHANORECEPTOR REPRESENTATION AT THE SHOULDER

Based on Wyke's[68] studies of spinal articular neurology, it is hypothesized that all other synovial joints in the body are provided with a mixture of tonic, phasic, and nociceptive mechanoreceptors.[68] Vangsness and Ennis[64] confirmed the same mechanoreceptor representation to be present at the glenohumeral articulation.

*Pacinian corpuscles* are viscoelastic organs located both in the superficial fascial layers beneath the skin and in the deep fascial layers and ligaments.[26] Phasic or very rapidly adapting, from hundredths to a few thousandths of a second, they are well suited to detect vibrations and rapid changes in the mechanical state of the tissues. At the shoulder, pacinian corpuscles are identified in the superior, middle, inferior, and posterior portions of the glenohumeral ligaments and in lesser concentrations in the conoid, trapezoid, and coracoacromial ligaments.[64] Pacinian corpuscle mechanoreceptors are also referred to as *type II articular receptors*, after Wyke.[68]

*Ruffini end organs*, located in deep dermis, joint capsule, ligament, and fascia, are tonic or slowly adapting receptors that can continue to transmit information for several hours, providing information on position, joint angle, tension, and load. Two types of Ruffini endings have been identified in the shoulder ligaments.[64] The first, the classical Ruffini end organ, has a lower firing threshold and responds to slight changes in tension. It is the most abundant mechanoreceptor represented in the shoulder ligaments and equates to the type I receptor described by Wyke.[68] Another slowly adapting end organ is also present, resembling a small Golgi tendon organ, and, similar to it, may possess a higher firing threshold level than the first. This type, corresponding to Wyke's type III classification, is found mostly in the acromioclavicular ligaments and only sparsely in the capsule and is less numerous than the classical Ruffini or the pacinian mechanoreceptor.

*Free nerve ending mechanoreceptors* are located throughout the connective tissues. These are synonymous with type IV receptors in Wyke's classification. Very slow or nonadapting, they subserve the body's protective senses to signal potentially injurious levels of tissue deformation. Free nerve endings are the only mechanoreceptors present in the glenoid labrum, but they appear only in the peripheral half.[64]

## IMPLICATIONS FOR DYSFUNCTION AND TREATMENT

The influences of mechanoreceptor activity on neuromuscular control explain the reflex weakening typically found when hemarthrosis exists in the joint or following glenohumeral arthrograms. Distension of the capsule produces firing of the type III receptors, which are inhibitory to the joint musculature. Because type III receptors are not well represented in the glenohumeral ligaments, resulting inhibition may occur from the receptors located in the tendinous portions of the rotator cuff musculature that are intimate with the capsule. The ample quantity of type III receptors in the acromioclavicular ligaments implicates neurophysiologic influences on the glenohumeral joint and shoulder complex derived from acromioclavicular mechanical dysfunction.

Damage and disruption of the mechanoreceptor reporting system can result from sprain or dislocation, resulting in proprioceptive deficits. The glenohumeral joint is particularly vulnerable to diminished proprioceptive reflexes, requiring a high degree of neuromuscular precision for functional dynamic stability. Retraining proprioceptive functions is of primary importance in rehabilitation of shoulder joint laxity or instability.

# Examination Principles

## RULES OF EXAMINATION

Assessment of joint play to detect dysfunction requires the application of passive motion imparted by the examiner in duplication of the joint-play motion under scrutiny. General rules of joint play as instructed by Mennell[45] include the following:

1. The patient must be relaxed, and the joint being examined must be supported in a way to allow for comfort and prevention of spasm or painful, unguarded movement.
2. The examiner must be relaxed and use firm, controlled, nonpainful contact.
3. Only one joint is examined at a time.
4. Only one movement at each joint is examined at a time.
5. Only one component of the joint is mobilized; the other must be stabilized.

6. No forceful movement is ever used.
7. Movement is stopped if pain is evoked.
8. No examination is performed to an obviously inflamed or diseased joint.

## END FEEL

The term *end feel* refers to the nature of movement limitation experienced by the examiner and occurring with assessment of either joint play or passive physiologic range of motion. *End feel* has been defined as the "sensation imparted to the examiner's hands during passive movement of a joint at the extremes of possible range."[56] Testing the end feel provides diagnostic information on the quality-of-motion limits, in contrast to standard range-of-motion measurement, which quantifies movement.

Cyriax[12] identifies three normal and three abnormal end feels for synovial joints, determined by the individual articular design and specific periarticular soft-tissue components. Normal end-feel descriptors include hard, soft, and elastic. Abnormal end feels include empty, spasm, and springy. Paris[49,50] elaborated on these descriptions by defining 5 normal and 10 abnormal end feels. The 5 normal end feels include soft-tissue approximation, muscular, ligamentous, cartilaginous, and capsular. The 10 abnormal end feels include chronic inflammatory and acute inflammatory capsular, adhesions and scarring, bony block, bony grate, springy rebound, pannus, loose, empty, painful, and muscle. The normal end feel experienced at the shoulder under Cyriax's classification would be defined as elastic. Under Paris's classification, the end feel might be described as muscular, ligamentous, or capsular. In both classifications, the mechanical property of elasticity is present. This holds true in the clinical setting due to the fact that the restraints to motion are a combination of capsular, ligamentous, and musculotendinous elements. Some consideration must be given to the nature of end feels experienced during physiologic motion versus joint-play assessment of the same glenohumeral joint. For example, anterior glide of the humeral head performed in the loose-pack position is thought to predominately engage resistance from the anterior capsuloligamentous complex. The end feel experienced, then, is primarily a function of the capsule. The same joint examined for end feel of external rotation from anatomic neutral, also thought to be limited by the anterior capsular structures, may demonstrate a different end-feel quality. The difference in the latter can be accounted for by the composite influences of the subscapularis musculotendinous unit plus scapulothoracic joint-play motion.

Recognition of an abnormal end feel determines in part the appropriate selection of treatment techniques. An empty end feel is rarely encountered, but when present, it is suggestive of underlying serious pathology such as a hemarthrosis, fracture, neuropathologic disorder as in a charcot joint, or malignancy. Likewise, a loose end feel, indicative of instability, is a contraindication to mobilization of a mechanical nature. More often than not, the type of abnormal end feels encountered at the glenohumeral joint include painful muscular guarding of an involuntary or voluntary nature, tight capsular restrictions of both an acute and chronic nature, adhesions and scarring, and looseness. With the exception of a loose or empty end feel, all the others offer an opportunity for treatment by mechanical mobilization. What is challenging about the glenohumeral joint is the difficulty in distinguishing between a true capsular end feel and a true muscular end feel. The reasons for this are several. First, restrictions in these two tissues are often present at the same time, especially in a highly reactive shoulder joint. In addition to this, the intimate relationship that exists between the glenohumeral joint capsule and the rotator cuff tendons necessitates that stress applied to one is applied to both. Furthermore, the biomechanical function of the rotator cuff musculature is to assist the capsule and labrum in providing limitations to movement between the humeral head and glenoid cavity. Thus, when one evaluates the end feel of certain component or joint-play motions, the findings are often indistinguishable. The key to treating the glenohumeral joint successfully is to reduce the influence of the muscular components through neurophysiologic techniques and then proceed with mechanical techniques directed more specifically at the restricted capsular structures.

## INDICATIONS AND CONTRAINDICATIONS FOR JOINT MOBILIZATION

It is perhaps easier to state the indications for joint mobilization than the opposite. In a broad sense, mobilization is indicated to restore mobility to a joint when it is found to be limited. Mobilization can produce mechanical, neurophysiologic, and psychological effects. In vivo, however, it is often difficult to attribute the primary therapeutic response to any singular mechanism. Absolute contraindications are few, such as a newly displaced fracture, but conditions that require careful forethought and consideration before proceeding are abundant. Any situation that calls for immobilization requires precautionary measures. Hemarthrosis or inflammatory distension of the capsule requires rest, not mobilization. Active disease processes can result in pain and loss of mobility. Under these circumstances, with certain discretion, pain may be treated with mobilization, but restoration of movement should not be attempted until active disease has abated.

The clinician must approach the selection of appropriate techniques based on matching the potential benefit to the nature of the particular dysfunction currently at hand. For example, joint mobilization at first glance would seem inappropriate to include in the treatment plan of the patient presenting with symptomatic multidirectional glenohumeral instability. True, but only for the introduction of significant mechanical stress to the capsuloligamentous complex. In this instance, mobilization for neurophysiologic effects may be indicated to reduce pain and spasm before performing stabilization exercises.

The reactivity level at any given time will necessitate what particular techniques are indicated. Reactivity level can be arbitrarily graded as level one, two, or three.[50] Level one reactivity is typified by pain at rest or pain occurring in advance of engaging any mechanical resistance. The end feel is empty. Mobilization for neurophysiologic effects can be considered, but stretch is contraindicated. Level two reactivity occurs when the onset of pain coincides with end-feel resistance interpreted as capsular, not spasm. Gentle grade III mobilization advancing to grade IV as tolerated, provides combined neurophysiologic and mechanical effects. Level three demonstrates engagement of capsular end feel with little or no pain. Some predictable stretch-related discomfort can occur as the capsuloligamentous complex is stressed. Grade III and IV oscillations and sustained grade IV techniques can be used.

# Mobilization Techniques

## GENERAL DISCUSSION

The particular techniques one selects to utilize for joint mobilization vary from one school of thought to another. If one chooses to follow the techniques instructed by Kaltenborn, then mobilization movements are performed based on the convex-concave rules and in recognition of arthrokinematic principles of roll and glide. With respect to the glenohumeral joint, movements of anterior and posterior glide are performed with the therapist using both his or her hands to produce a translatory movement in the same direction simultaneously. In contrast to Kaltenborn's instructions, Mennell, Paris, Maitland, and others produce motion with one hand and provide positioning and/or stabilization with the other. Regardless of the particular technique used or the school of thought one chooses to follow, the end result of the mobilization treatment remains the same, that being a decrease in pain and/or an increase in mobility.

The grades of mobilization as described by Maitland can be applied universally regardless of the technique one employs. Grade I movement is defined as a small-amplitude movement performed at the beginning of the range. Grade II is a large-amplitude movement performed anywhere within but not reaching the limit of the range. A grade III movement is also of large amplitude but is carried to the full extent or pathologic range limit. Grade IV consists of small-amplitude movement performed at the limit of the range. By this definition, grade I and II movements work primarily by neurophysiologic means, firing mechanoreceptors that influence the neuromodulation of pain. Grade III and IV movements stretch the capsule and adjacent soft tissues to some extent, providing both mechanical and neurophysiologic effects. Maitland[41] applies these passive movements both in the direction of physiologic motion (Fig. 7-33a) and in the arthrokinematic planes (see Fig. 7-33b). From a mechanical perspective, mobilization is simply a form of stretching. Grade III and IV mobilizations, as defined by Maitland,[41] produce stretch to some part of the capsuloligamentous complex as directed by the therapist with the intention of increasing extensibility in an area that is perceived to be restricted. This can be performed in imitation of physiologic motion as well as pure translation or joint-play motion. Techniques described by Kaltenborn occasionally make use of straps, sandbags, wedges, and towel rolls to assist in stabilization and direction of mobilizing forces. Where these devices assist one in producing more effective mobilization, they are advocated.

The techniques presented here should be viewed as a treatment progression. Initially, techniques are applied to the glenohumeral joint in a loose-pack position and are unidirectional so as to minimize the degree of strain placed on the soft tissues and articular structures. As the patient demonstrates improvement in mobility and a decrease in reactivity, then advanced tech-

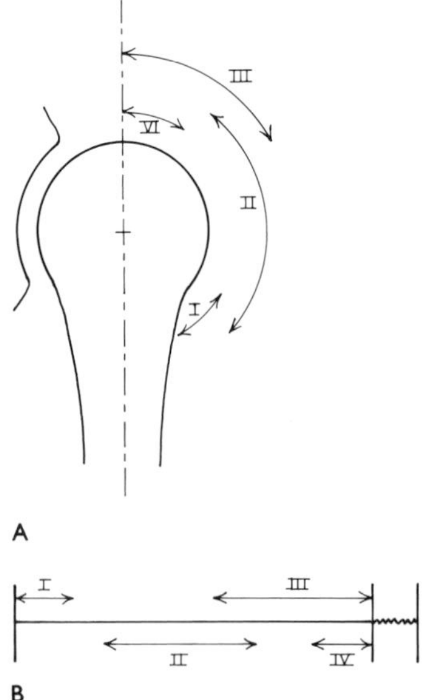


**Figure 7-33.** Grades of mobilization. (a) Physiologic motion. (b) Translation.

niques are advocated. The advanced techniques place the glenohumeral joint in more demanding positions combining positions of elevation with rotations. In so doing, the dynamic and static stabilizers are lengthened to the point of or near the point of pathologic limit. Thus, when mobilization is applied, the mechanical effects are enhanced.

## OSCILLATIONS

Mobilization movements are commonly delivered in an oscillatory fashion at a rate of two to three per second, typically of 15 to 30 seconds' duration, followed by reassessment. This applies equally to any of Maitland's four grades of movement. The oscillatory rhythm can be delivered evenly or modulated to enhance neurophysiologic effects. Grade III or IV mobilization can be given with progressively longer duration end-range force, for example, advancing in sequence from 1 or 2 seconds to 10 or 15 seconds. Grade IV mobilization also can be given as sustained end-range force for up to 60 seconds or more.

## TRACTION AND DISTRACTION

*Traction* is separation of the joint surfaces by movement in a longitudinal direction. *Distraction* is separation of the joint surfaces by movement directed perpendicular to the long axis of the bone. Some mobilization techniques are performed as primary distraction, which imparts greater separation of the joint surfaces. Most mobilization techniques are combined with some degree of traction, graded as follows[33,49]:

Grade I: The joint surfaces are just barely unweighted.
Grade II: The slack in the capsule is taken out but not stretched.
Grade III: The capsule and ligaments are stretched.

Simply stated, the three stages of traction or distraction are (1) loosen, (2) tighten, and (3) stretch[34] (Fig. 7-34). Grade I traction is sometimes referred to as *piccolo traction*. Grade I would impart primarily neurophysiologic effects, grade II would produce some mix of mechanical and neurophysiologic, and grade III would produce primarily mechanical effects.

Most techniques can be performed in several different positions, each with their own advantages and disadvantages. The therapist is encouraged to become familiar with the techniques presented, adapting them when necessary to accommodate patient or therapist needs. Consideration should be given to the degree of stabilization, accessibility, and ergonomic efficiency afforded, as well as the ability to interchange different techniques without repositioning.

The following manual therapy procedures represent useful techniques from many sources and do not adhere to any individual school of thought, of which many exist. It is therefore inevitable that some of this information will be contrary to some teachings, although a core exists of fundamental principles common to all approaches. A generic approach is offered to pro-

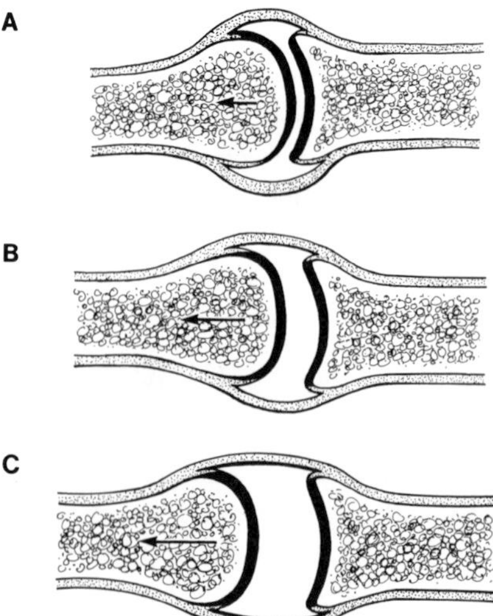


**Figure 7-34.** Grades of traction. (a) Grade I, loosen. (B) Grade II, tighten. (c) Grade III, stretch.

vide tools of clinical value from several experts without exclusion. While the novice therapist is encouraged to acquire skills through qualified instruction, the experienced therapist should find this section to be clinically practical.

## GLENOHUMERAL JOINT

### OSCILLATIONS, LOOSE-PACK POSITION (FIG. 7-35)

*Patient position*: Supine, arm in 55 degrees of scapular plane abduction, 30 degrees of forward flexion, neutral rotation, with elbow at 90 degrees.

*Therapist position*: Proximal hand supports arm at humerus just above elbow; distal hand controls the limb at the wrist.

*Action*: Rapid grade II oscillations, 4 per second, are given into internal rotation and external rotation.

*Primary tissue affected*: Mechanoreceptors in the capsuloligamentous complex.

*Comments*: Good introductory technique that is helpful to stimulate the synovium and enhance joint lubrication. Also promotes relaxation and analgesic benefits.

### OSCILLATIONS IN ELEVATION (FIG. 7-36)

*Patient position*: Supine.

*Therapist position*: Standing at the head of the table, behind the patient. The therapist's knee is placed on the table directly behind the involved shoulder. The proximal hand controls the patient's flexed elbow at the olecranon; the distal hand (or both) supports the wrist. The therapist's thigh is positioned to act as a stop before the painful portion of the elevation range.

*Action*: The arm is raised and lowered with large-amplitude grade II movement. The therapist's thigh is repositioned to permit increased elevation as tolerated. The painful range is approached but not engaged.

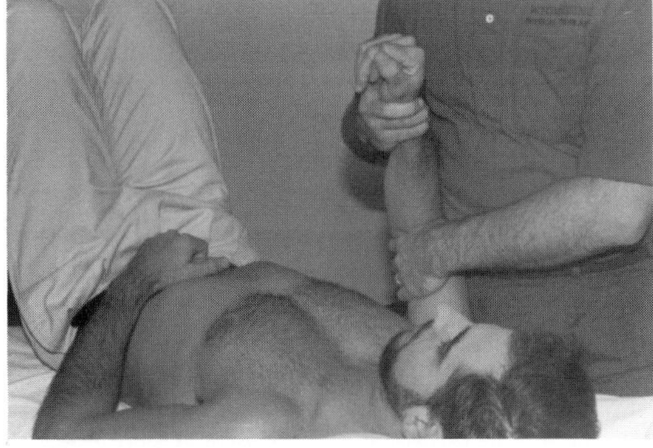

**Figure 7-35.** Oscillations, loose-pack position.

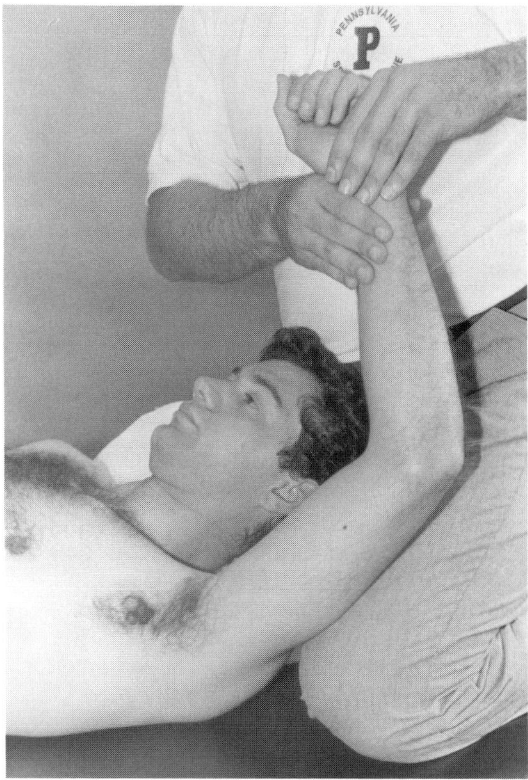


**Figure 7-36.** Oscillations in elevation.

*Primary tissue affected*: Mechanoreceptors in the capsuloligamentous complex.

*Comments*: Useful to promote relaxation and decrease painful movement restriction. Also can be applied to quadrant position by redirecting the line of movement from the sagittal plane to an oblique line. In this instance, the therapist uses the outside thigh as the stop.

### ANTERIOR GLIDE, LOOSE-PACK POSITION (SUPINE) (FIG. 7-37)

*Patient position*: Supine, arm in 55 degrees of abduction and 30 degrees of forward flexion.

*Therapist position*: Both hands contact the posterior aspect of the proximal humerus, the distal arm stabilized between the therapist's body and forearm.

*Action*: Grade I long-axis distraction is applied. The humeral head is glided anteriorly and medially, perpendicular to the scapular plane.

*Primary tissue affected*: Anterior capsuloligamentous joint.

*Comments*: The supine position is advantageous for arm accessibility so that other directional glides or combination motions can be easily performed. Scapular stabilization is compromised, however, when performing grade III or IV mobil-

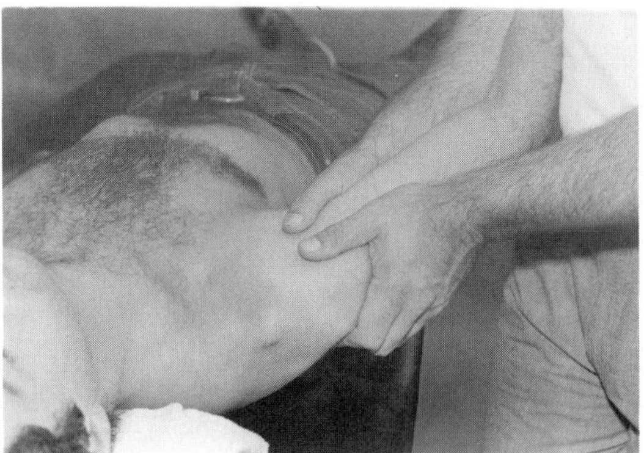

**Figure 7-37.** Anterior glide, loose-pack position (supine).

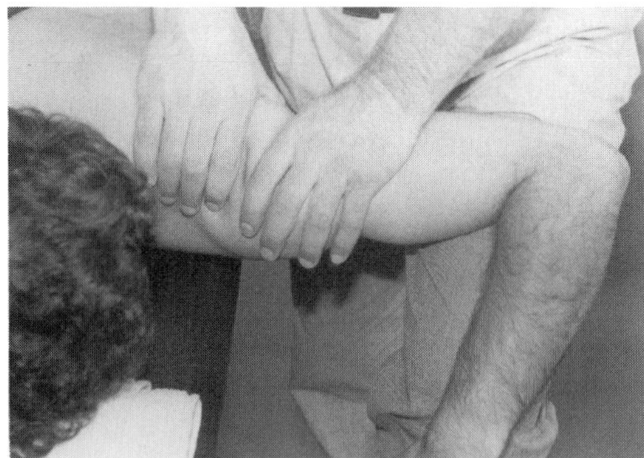

**Figure 7-39.** Anterior glide, combination external rotation/abduction (prone).

ization unless a stabilizing belt or one hand (proximal) stabilizes scapula.

### ANTERIOR GLIDE, LOOSE-PACK POSITION (PRONE) (FIG. 7-38)

*Patient position*: Prone, with arm in 55 degrees of abduction, 30 degrees of forward flexion. Towel roll or wedge can be positioned anteriorly over the coracoid.

*Therapist position*: Proximal hand contacts posterior proximal humerus; distal hand controls humerus superior to elbow.

*Action*: Grade I long-axis traction is applied. The humeral head is glided anteriorly and medially, perpendicular to the scapular plane.

*Primary tissue affected*: Anterior capsuloligamentous complex.

*Comments*: Prone position affords greater scapular stabilization; however, patient comfort must be considered.

### ANTERIOR GLIDE, COMBINATION EXTERNAL ROTATION/ABDUCTION (PRONE) (FIG. 7-39)

*Patient position*: Prone, with glenohumeral joint abducted in coronal plane to initial barrier and then combined with external rotation to next barrier. The forearm can rest on therapist's thigh.

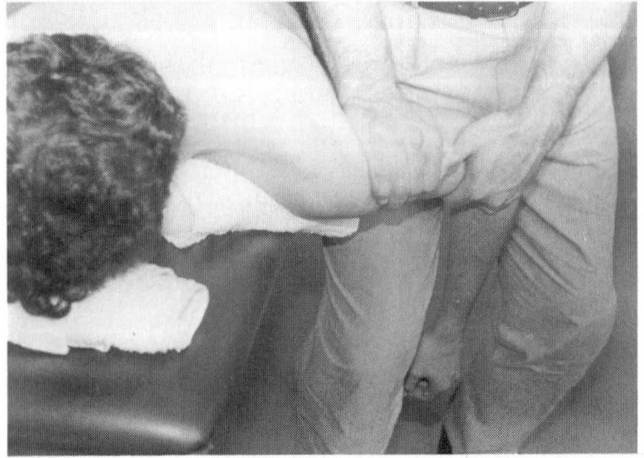

**Figure 7-38.** Anterior glide, loose-pack position (prone).

*Therapist position*: Standing with leg placed on chair or stool to support patient's forearm. Proximal hand contacts posterior proximal humerus. Distal hand can control the humerus at the elbow so that humeral rotation and horizontal abduction can be modified.

*Action*: Grade I long-axis distraction is applied by distal hand. The humeral head is glided anteriorly and slightly medially depending on scapular orientation.

*Primary tissue affected*: Anterior and inferior capsuloligamentous complex.

*Comments*: This is an advanced position, best utilized in grade III and IV mobilizations. It affords good mechanical advantage (since the scapula is stabilized against the thoracic wall) and therapist control when strong prolonged stretching is indicated. Further external rotation or horizontal abduction can be incorporated individually or in combination to increase the stretch effect.

### INFERIOR GLIDE, SLIGHT ABDUCTION (SUPINE) (FIG. 7-40)

*Patient position*: Supine at edge of table, with glenohumeral joint in 10 to 20 degrees of abduction and neutral rotation.

*Therapist position*: Standing, situated between patient's body and arm. Proximal hand controls and stabilizes lateral border of scapula near glenoid. The distal hand contacts the humerus superior to the elbow and against the therapist's body.

*Action*: Grade I lateral distraction is applied. The humeral head is glided inferiorly by the distal hand displacing the humerus downward as the proximal hand stabilizes the scapula.

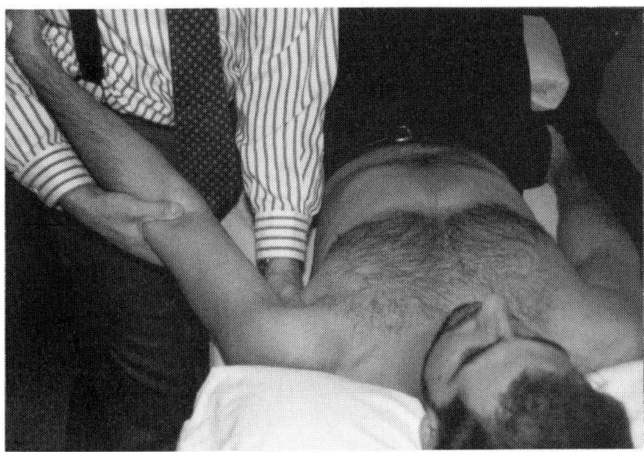

**Figure 7-40.** Inferior glide, slight abduction (supine).

*Primary tissue affected*: Superior capsuloligamentous complex.

*Comments*: Readily adaptable to side-lying position.

### INFERIOR GLIDE, LOOSE-PACK POSITION (SUPINE) (FIG. 7-41)

*Patient position*: Supine, with arm in 55 degrees of abduction and 30 degrees of forward flexion.

*Therapist position*: Proximal hand contacts the superior proximal humerus; distal hand controls humerus superior to the elbow.

*Action*: Grade I long-axis distraction is applied. The proximal humeral head is glided inferiorly and slightly laterally.

*Primary tissue affected*: Inferior capsuloligamentous complex.

*Comments*: Lateral direction is incorporated due to inclination of the glenoid. Depending on the degree of lateral scapular rotation, the direction of lateral force must be adjusted to parallel the glenoid surface.

### INFERIOR GLIDE, LOOSE-PACK POSITION (SITTING) (FIG. 7-42)

*Patient position*: Seated upright, with trunk support as necessary. Glenohumeral joint in 55 degrees of abduction and 30 degrees of forward flexion.

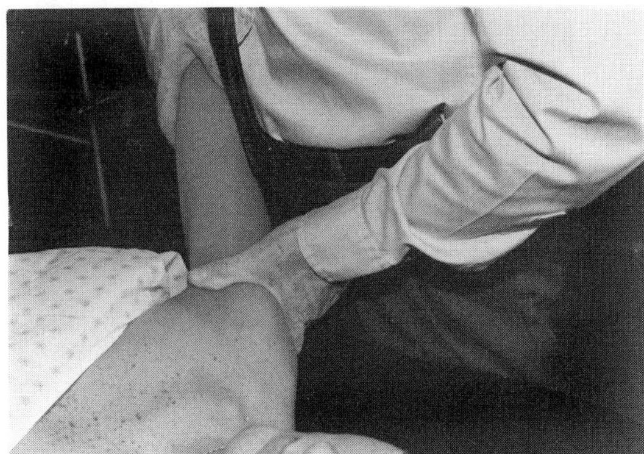

**Figure 7-41.** Inferior glide, loose-pack position (supine).

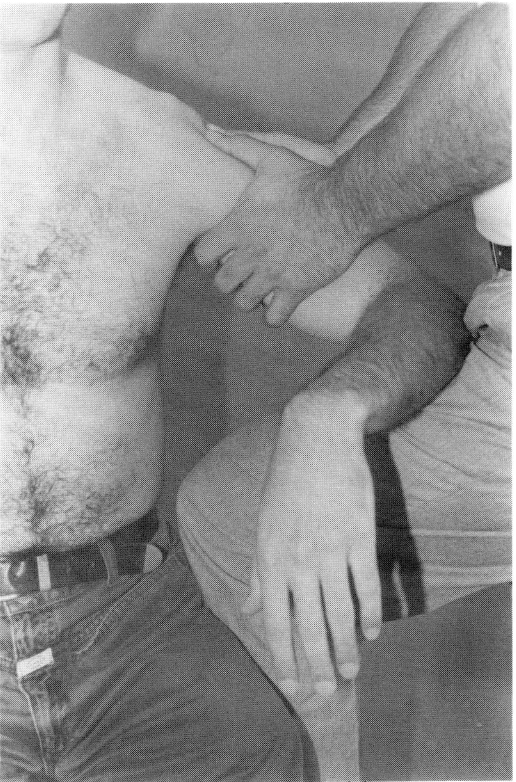

**Figure 7-42.** Inferior glide, loose-pack position (sitting).

*Therapist position*: Proximal hand contacts over superior proximal humeral head with one or both hands. Distal humerus controlled with other hand or stabilized on the therapist's thigh.

*Action*: Grade I long-axis distraction is applied. The humeral head is glided inferiorly and slightly laterally.

*Primary tissue affected*: Inferior capsuloligamentous complex.

*Comments*: Affords therapist a mechanical advantage in directing forces inferiorly.

### INFERIOR GLIDE AT GLENOHUMERAL END RANGE (SITTING) (FIG. 7-43)

*Patient position*: Sitting at edge of treatment table, with glenohumeral joint abducted in scapular plane to initial barrier. Distal humerus resting on therapist's shoulder with arm in neutral rotation.

*Therapist position*: Standing facing joint to be treated, with both hands placed over proximal humerus.

*Action*: Grade I long-axis distraction is applied. The humeral head is glided inferiorly and slightly laterally.

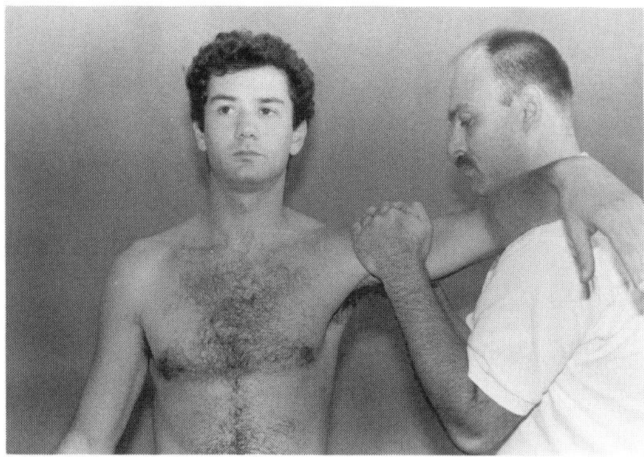

**Figure 7-43.** Inferior glide, at glenohumeral end range (sitting).

*Primary tissue affected*: Inferior capsuloligamentous complex.

*Comments*: Affords good mechanical advantage and therapist control when strong prolonged stretch is indicated. Direction of lateral glide is dependent on degree of scapular rotation.

### INFERIOR GLIDE, COMBINATION ADDUCTION AND EXTERNAL ROTATION (SUPINE) (FIG. 7-44)

*Patient position*: Supine, with arm adducted with towel roll in axilla and elbow bent to 90 degrees.

*Therapist position*: Proximal hand contacts the proximal forearm; distal hand controls at the wrist. Proximal hand stabilizes (modified) the scapula in axilla; distal hand controls at the proximal forearm.

*Action*: The axillary towel roll (or proximal hand) provides a lateral distraction force with the arm adducted. The humeral head is glided inferiorly to the first barrier and then is externally rotated to the next barrier.

*Comments*: This is an advanced position and an excellent technique for isolating the superior capsuloligamentous complex, particularly the coracohumeral ligament.

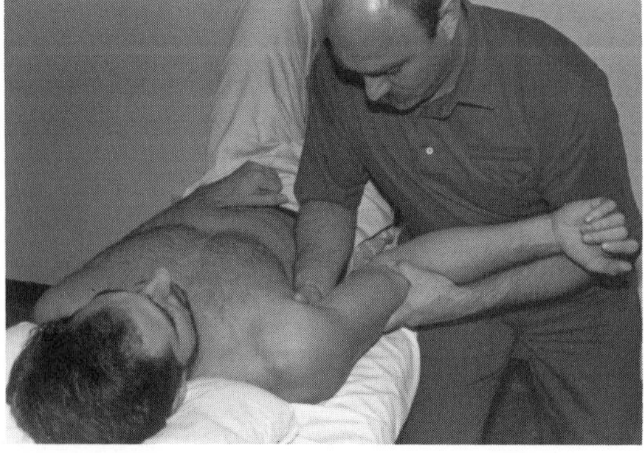

**Figure 7-44.** Inferior glide, combination adduction/external rotation (modified).

### INFERIOR GLIDE, COMBINATION ADDUCTION AND INTERNAL ROTATION (SIDE LYING) (FIG. 7-45)

*Patient position*: Side lying, with arm adducted.

*Therapist position*: Standing at patient's back. Proximal hand stabilizes lateral border of scapula near glenoid; distal hand contacts the distal humerus.

*Action*: Grade I lateral distraction is applied. The humeral head is glided inferiorly to barrier and then is internally rotated to next barrier.

*Primary tissue affected*: Superior capsuloligamentous complex.

*Comments*: This is an advanced position in which the therapist can incorporate extension and adduction to stretch the supraspinatus.

### INFERIOR GLIDE, COMBINATION ABDUCTION AND EXTERNAL ROTATION (SUPINE) (FIG. 7-46)

*Patient position*: Supine, with glenohumeral joint elevated in abduction to initial barrier and then combined with external rotation to next barrier.

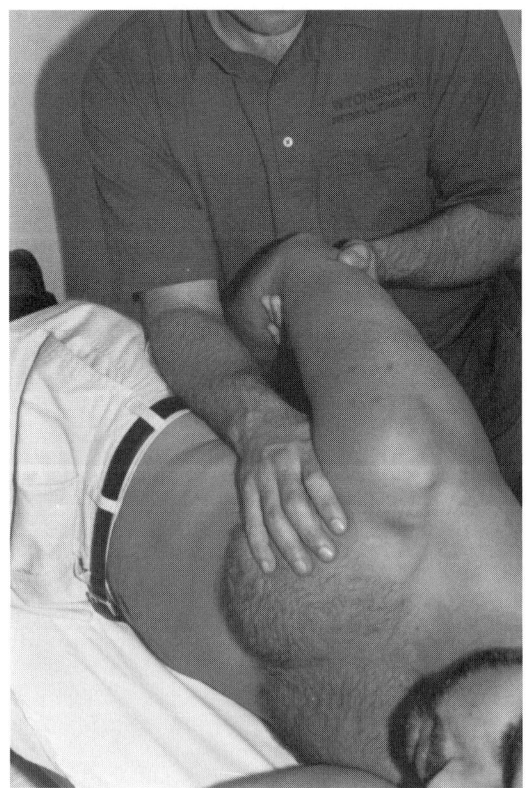

**Figure 7-45.** Inferior glide, combination adduction/internal rotation.

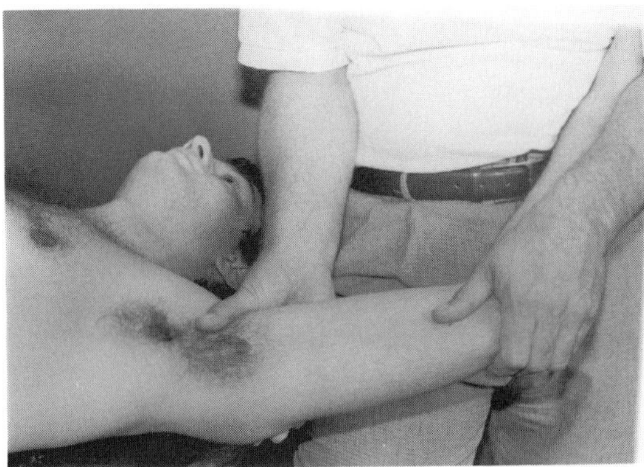

**Figure 7-46.** Inferior glide, combination abduction/external rotation (supine).

*Therapist position*: Proximal hand contacts over superior proximal humerus; distal hand over olecranon and therapist's distal forearm over patient's forearm so that humeral rotation and horizontal abduction can be modified.

*Action*: Grade I long-axis distraction is applied by distal hand. The humeral head is glided inferiorly and laterally depending on scapular rotation.

*Primary tissue affected*: Inferior and anterior capsuloligamentous complex.

*Comments*: This position is best utilized in grade III and IV mobilizations. It affords good mechanical advantage and therapist control when strong prolonged stretching is indicated. Further external rotation or horizontal abduction can be incorporated into the stretch individually or in combination.

### POSTERIOR GLIDE, ADDUCTED (SUPINE) (FIG. 7-47)

*Patient position*: Supine, with arm at side and glenohumeral joint in neutral rotation. Towel roll, or therapist hand wedge can be positioned posteriorly under the scapula. A towel roll is also placed in the axilla.

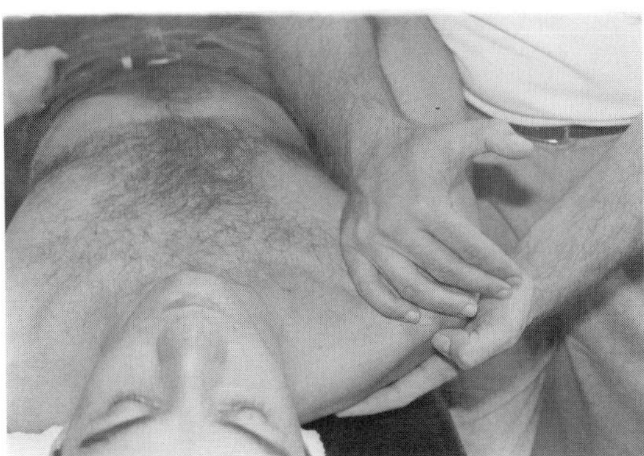

**Figure 7-47.** Posterior glide, adducted (supine).

*Therapist position*: Proximal hand contacts anterior proximal humerus; other hand stabilizes scapula.

*Action*: The axillary towel roll provides a lateral distraction force with the arm adducted. The humeral head is glided posteriorly and laterally, perpendicular to the scapular plane.

*Primary tissue affected*: Posterior capsuloligamentous complex.

*Comments*: Comfortable position with good scapular stabilization provided by wedge, roll, or therapist hands. Works well for grade III and IV. As mobility is improved, internal rotation can be used to produce a greater stretch

### POSTERIOR GLIDE, LOOSE-PACK POSITION (FIG. 7-48)

*Patient position*: Supine, with glenohumeral joint in 55 degrees of abduction and 30 degrees of forward flexion. Towel roll or wedge can be positioned posteriorly under the scapula.

*Therapist position*: Proximal hand contacts anterior proximal humerus; distal hand controls humerus superior to elbow and between therapist's arm and body.

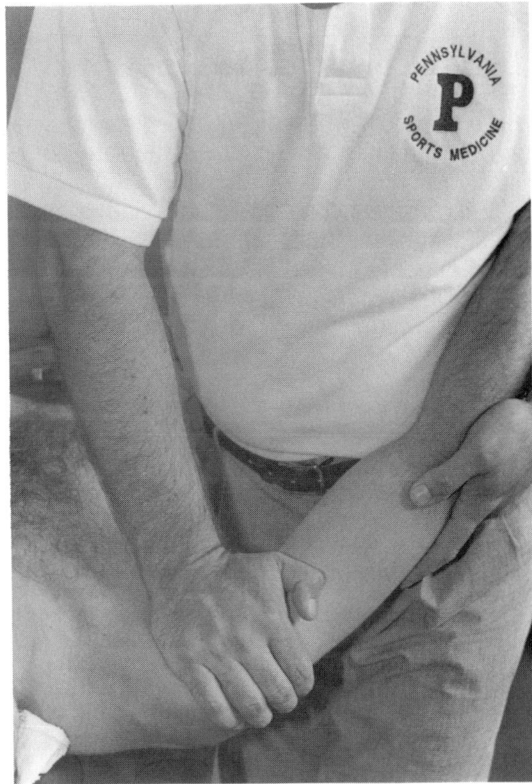


**Figure 7-48.** Posterior glide, loose-pack position.

*Action*: Grade I long-axis distraction is applied. The humeral head is glided posteriorly and laterally, perpendicular to the scapular plane.

*Primary tissue affected*: Posterior capsuloligamentous complex.

*Comments*: Supine position affords good scapular stabilization.

**POSTERIOR GLIDE IN FLEXION (SUPINE) (FIG. 7-49)**

*Patient position*: Supine, with the humerus at 90 degrees of flexion and slight horizontal adduction and elbow flexed beyond 90 degrees, with hand resting on patient's chest. Towel or wedge can be positioned posteriorly under the scapula.

*Therapist position*: Therapist places the distal hand over the distal humerus, with the point of the elbow cradled between arm and chest. The proximal hand contacts the posterior scapula near the glenoid.

*Action*: Proximal hand provides scapular stabilization. Therapist's body applies a posterolateral force through the long axis of the humerus, gliding the humeral head posteriorly.

*Primary tissue affected*: Posterior capsuloligamentous complex.

*Comments*: Affords strong stretch localized to posterior capsuloligamentous complex. Further internal rotation or horizontal adduction can be incorporated individually or in combination to increase the stretch effect.

**LATERAL DISTRACTION, ADDUCTED (SUPINE) (FIG. 7-50)**

*Patient position*: Supine, with glenohumeral joint in adduction and neutral rotation and elbow flexed to 90 degrees.

*Therapist position*: Proximal hand contacts medial proximal humerus in the axilla; distal hand controls humerus superior to elbow; and patient's forearm controlled between therapist's arm and body.

*Action*: The humeral head is laterally distracted from the glenoid in the scapular plane.

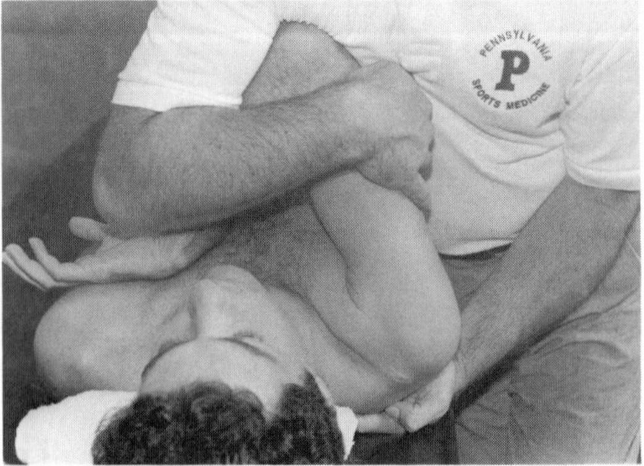


**Figure 7-49.** Posterior glide in flexion (supine).

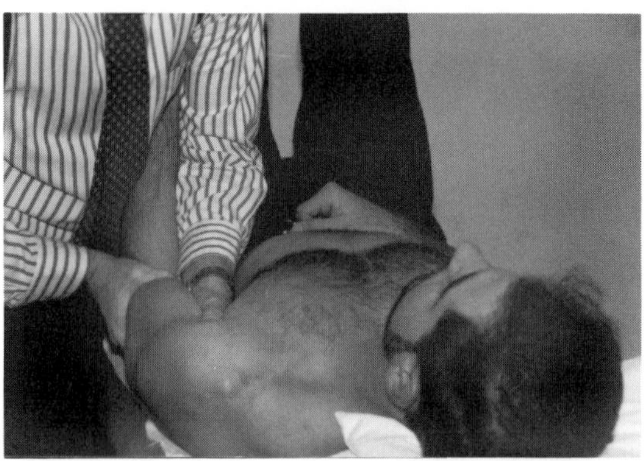

**Figure 7-50.** Lateral distraction, adducted (supine).

*Primary tissue affected*: Superior capsuloligamentous complex.

*Comments*: Excellent technique for stretching the superior capsuloligamentous complex, although can be physically demanding.

**LATERAL DISTRACTION IN FLEXION (FIG. 7-51)**

*Patient position*: Supine, with the humerus at 90 degrees of flexion and slight horizontal adduction.

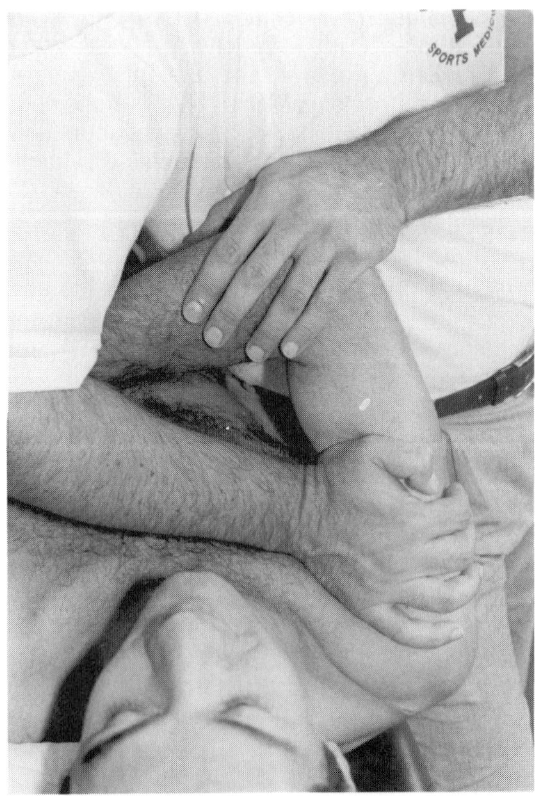

**Figure 7-51.** Lateral distraction in flexion.

*Therapist position*: The proximal hand contacts the proximal medial humerus; the distal hand controls the humerus superior to the elbow.

*Action*: The humeral head is laterally distracted from the glenoid toward the coronal plane.

*Primary tissue affected*: Superior and posterior capsuloligamentous complex.

*Comments*: Affords strong stretch localized to the superior and posterior capsuloligamentous complex. Further internal rotation or horizontal adduction can be incorporated individually or in combination to increase the stretch effect. Can combine with inferior glide by distal hand control.

## QUADRANT POSITION (FIG. 7-52)

*Patient position*: Supine, with involved arm in full scapular plane abduction and external rotation and elbow at 45 degrees.

*Therapist position*: Standing on the ipsilateral side, with the proximal hand placed under the shoulder. The distal hand controls at the olecranon.

*Action*: For assessment, the elbow is moved toward the floor with gentle overpressure at the limit of range. A small arc of movement can be produced by adding a small amount of abduction. Symptom reproduction is noted. The therapist should observe the range of movement in the sagittal plane. Comparison is made with the uninvolved shoulder. Anteroposterior oscillations of grade III or IV are given with the distal hand at the elbow, while the proximal hand stabilizes the scapula.

*Primary tissue affected*: Anterior and inferior capsuloligamentous complex.

*Comments*: Internal and external rotation can be added as necessary. Grade IV should be given as small-amplitude oscillations, avoiding sustained or aggressive stretch. The quadrant position should be utilized when the patient has minor degrees of movement restriction or when the functional range of motion is apparently normal yet symptoms persist.

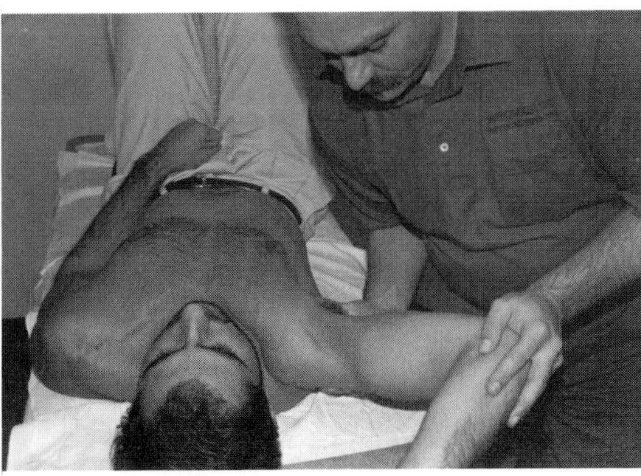

**Figure 7-52.** Quadrant position.

## GLENOHUMERAL STRETCH (FIG. 7-53)

The following technique is useful as a passive stretch or can be combined with the interactive contract-relax technique. As a passive stretch, it provides the patient with some distraction, which can be helpful in reducing voluntary

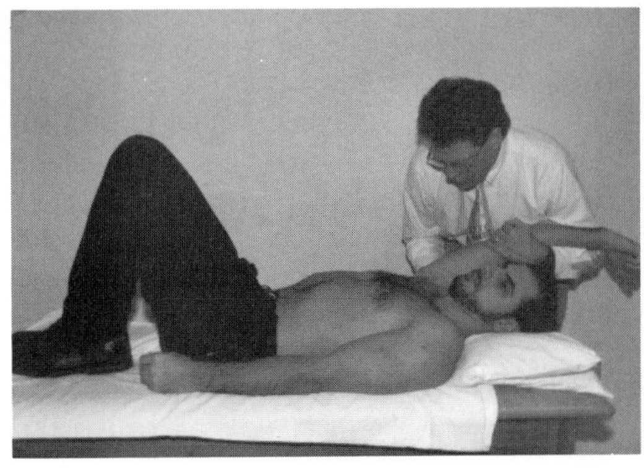

A

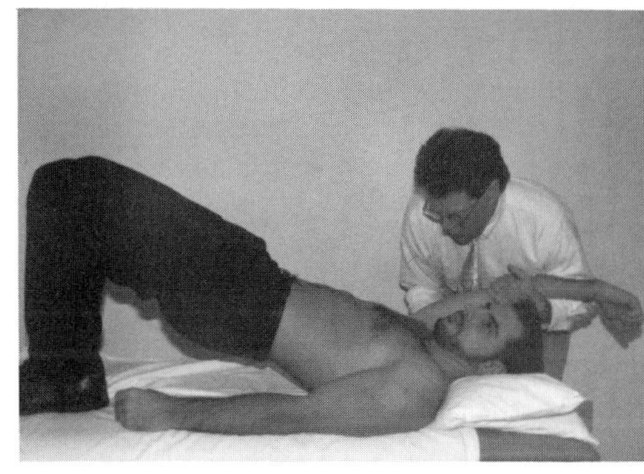

B

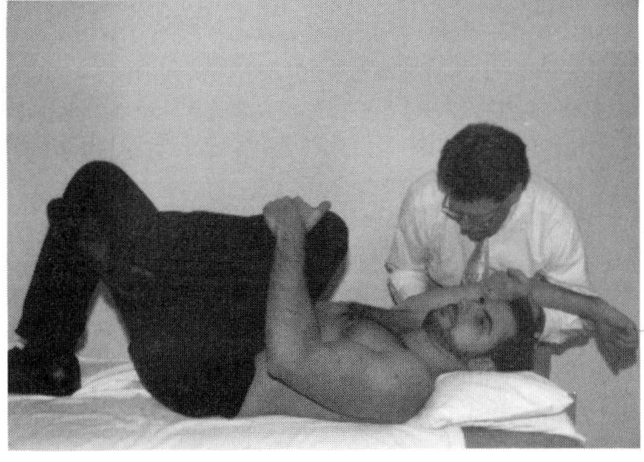

C

**Figure 7-53.** Glenohumeral stretch.

guarding. This technique is best suited for use in the presence of low-level reactivity (grade III), where patient discomfort is primarily a consequence of the application of stretch at the mechanical limits of the range.

The therapist stands at the head of the table. The patient is supine, with knees and hips flexed and feet resting on the table.

1. The involved arm is elevated to its limit of range without overpressure. The therapist controls the arm, with the distal hand contacting the distal posterior humerus. The proximal hand is placed over the superoposterior aspect of the glenohumeral joint. (See Fig 53a.)
2. The patient is instructed to bridge the trunk by elevating the pelvis and lumbar spine vertically from the table. Simultaneously, the therapist takes up the slack by further elevating the glenohumeral joint. The patient will not feel any substantial stretch while the trunk is elevated from the table. (See Fig. 53b.)
3. The patient is instructed to lower the body to the table slowly, which will introduce stretch to the glenohumeral joint while the humerus remains fixed.
4. At this point, the patient is instructed to bring the knee to the chest on the contralateral side to stabilize the trunk in posterior pelvic rotation with the lumbar spine flattened to the table. The shoulder is now positioned in a manner that will allow for good localization of stretch to the glenohumeral soft tissues with the trunk stationary and controlled. This in essence creates two long levers, one the humerus and the other the trunk. The fulcrum of the stretch is then directed at the glenohumeral joint. (See Fig. 53c.)
5. The therapist can deliver passive stretch by several means: The proximal hand can perform oscillatory stretch directed inferiorly and laterally, the proximal hand can be repositioned so that the lateral border of the scapula is stabilized while the stretch is given by further elevation of the arm by the controlling hand on the distal posterior humerus, hold-relax or contract-relax technique can be combined with this technique, and/or the quadrant position can be localized when the therapist places the proximal hand underneath the scapula and repositions the axis of the humerus from a vertical to an oblique orientation.
6. Sequences 1 through 5 are repeated as indicated.

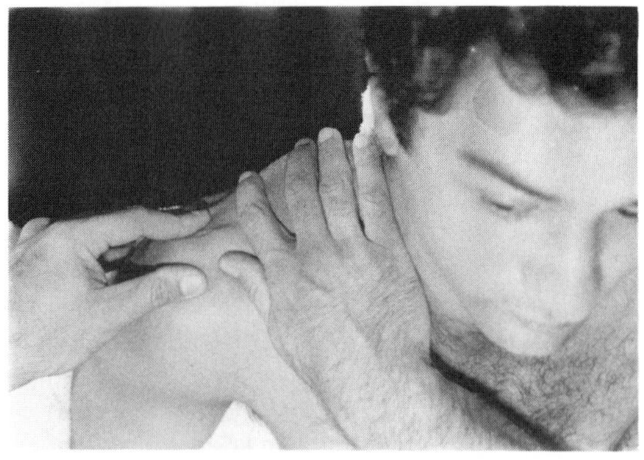

**Figure 7-54.** Anterior/posterior glide acromioclavicular joint.

## ACROMIOCLAVICULAR JOINT

### ANTERIOR/POSTERIOR GLIDE (FIG. 7-54)

*Patient position*: Supine, with the arm passively supported in a relaxed position.

*Therapist position*: Standing; proximal hand contacts distal clavicle with thumb placed anteriorly and index finger pad on posterior surface; distal hand stabilizes scapula with thumb and index finger on acromion.

*Action*: Posterior or anterior unidirectional translation.

*Primary tissue affected*: Acromioclavicular ligament and articular capsule.

*Comments*: Alternate position prone. Supine position better for scapular stabilization with posterior glide.

## STERNOCLAVICULAR JOINT

### POSTERIOR GLIDE (FIG. 7-55)

*Patient position*: Supine, with arm supported in a relaxed position.

*Therapist position*: Thumb pad over anterior sternal end of clavicle. No stabilization is required.

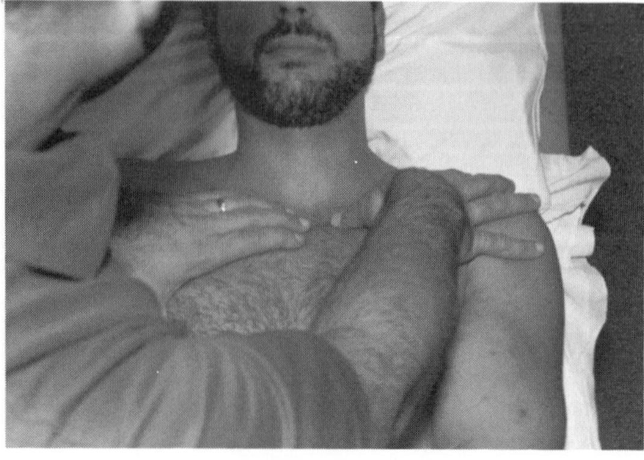

**Figure 7-55.** Posterior glide sternoclavicular joint.

*Action*: Thumb gently oscillates clavicle in posterior direction.

*Primary tissue affected*: Articular capsule, posterior sternoclavicular ligament.

*Comments*: Passive movement directed anteriorly is not easily imparted in this technique. Posterior force applied to the distal clavicle will produce anterior tilt at sternoclavicular joint through fulcrum effect. Stabilization of manubrium with thumb is helpful.

### SUPERIOR GLIDE (FIG. 7-56)

*Patient position*: Supine, with arm supported in a relaxed position.

*Therapist position*: Thumb placed on inferior surface of proximal clavicle. No stabilization is necessary.

*Action*: Clavicle is directed superiorly and medially, parallel to sternal articular surface.

*Primary tissues affected*: Articular capsule, interclavicular ligament, costoclavicular ligament.

*Comments*: Useful as additional technique to assist restoration of sternoclavicular rotation and anteroposterior glide. A small degree of superior glide accompanies shoulder girdle depression.

## SCAPULOTHORACIC ARTICULATION

### DISTRACTION (FIG. 7-57)

*Patient position*: Side lying at edge of table, with glenohumeral joint in adduction.

*Therapist position*: Both hands grasp medial border of scapula.

*Action*: The medial border of the scapula is gently separated from the posterior thorax. Intermittent stretch and release are used to release muscular resistance.

*Primary tissues affected*: Serratus anterior, rhomboids.

*Comments*: Once the medial scapula can be distracted adequately, upward and downward rotation, anteroposterior tilt, and gliding can be added.

*Alternate position*: Glenohumeral joint in internal rotation with the arm behind the back.

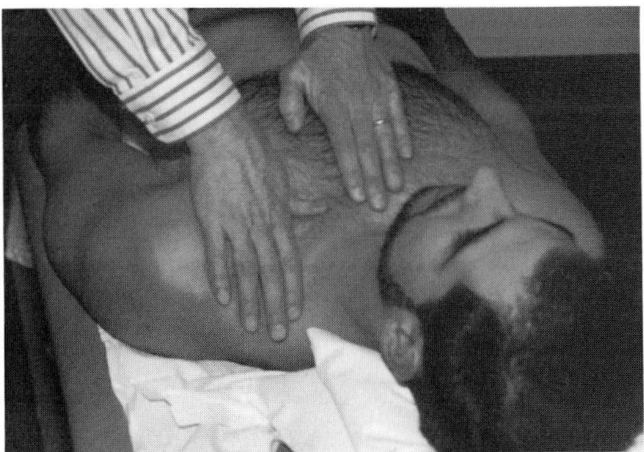

**Figure 7-56.** Superior glide sternoclavicular joint.

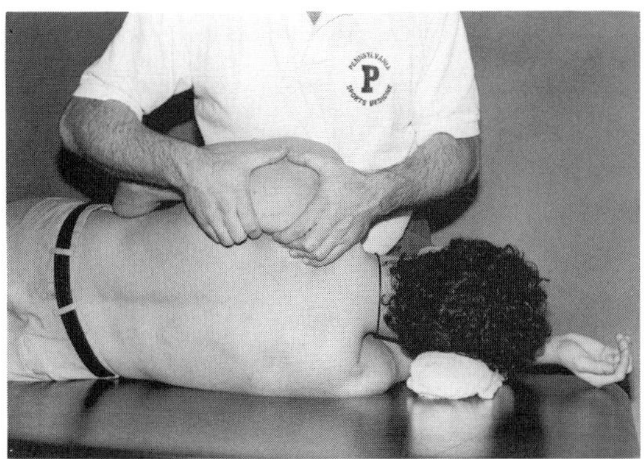

**Figure 7-57.** Scapulothoracic articulation/distraction.

## References


1. Akeson WH, Amiel D, Mechanics GL, et al. Collagen cross-linking alterations in joint contractures: changes in the reducible cross-links in periarticular connective tissue collagen after nine weeks of immobilization. Connect Tissue Res 1977;5:15.
2. Barnes JF. Myofasical release seminar, course manual. Paoli, Pa.: Rehabilitation Services 1984.
3. Basmajian JV. Muscles alive. 4th ed. Baltimore: Williams & Wilkins, 1979.
4. Basmajian JV. Manipulation, traction and massage. Baltimore: Williams & Wilkins, 1985.
5. Bourbon B. Physical agents (course). Philadelphia: University of Pennsylvania Physical Therapy Curriculum, 1977.
6. Burkhart SL, Ward RC. Myofascial release techniques: scientific and clinical rationale in the management of low back pain. Pittsburgh: AREN publication/video conference, 1986.
7. Chiatow L. Soft-tissue manipulation. London: Thorsons Publishers, 1987.
8. Cummings CG, Crutchfield CC, Barnes BM., Orthopedic physical therapy series volume 1: Soft tissue changes in contractures. Atlanta: Stokesville, 1983.
9. Cummings GS. Change in soft tissue mobility: implications for treatment. Lecture presented at APTA national convention, Las Vegas, 1988.
10. Cyriax J. Textbook of orthopaedic medicine. Vol. 1: Diagnosis of soft tissue lesions. London: Bailliere Tindall, 1978.
11. Cyriax J. Textbook of orthopaedic medicine. Vol. 2: Treatment by manipulation, massage and injection. London: Balliere Tindall, 1984.
12. Cyriax J, Cyriax P. Illustrated manual of orthopaedic medicine. London: Butterworth, 1984.
13. DiLorenzo CE. The importance of shoulder and cervical dysfunction in the etiology and treatment of athletic elbow injuries. J Orthop Sports Phys Ther 1990;11:402.
14. Donatelli R, Burkhart H. Effects of immobilization on the extensibility of periarticular connective tissue. J Orthop Sports Phys Ther 1981;3:67.
15. Dvorak J, Dvorak V. Manual medicine diagnostics. New York: Thieme-Stratton, 1984.
16. Dvorak J, Dvorak V. Manual medicine therapy. New York: Thieme-Stratton, 1988.
17. Ebner M. Connective tissue massage: theory and therapeutic application. Huntington, N.Y.: Robert E Knieger Publishing, 1985.
18. Evjenth O, Hamberg J. Muscle stretching in manual therapy: a clinical manual. Sweden: Scand. Book AB Sweden, 1985.

19. Glick JM. Muscle strains: prevention and treatment. Phys Sports Med 1980;8:73.
20. Goodridge JP. Muscle energy technique: definition, explanation, methods of procedure. Journal of the American Osteopathic Association 1981;81:67.
21. Goss CM. Gray's anatomy. 29th ed. Philadelphia: Lea & Febiger, 1973.
22. Greenman PE. Concepts and mechanisms of neuromuscular functions. New York: Springer-Verlag, 1984.
23. Greenman PE. Principles of manual medicine. Baltimore: Williams & Wilkins, 1989.
24. Grodin AJ. Myofascial manipulation. St. Augustine, Fla.: Institute Press, Division of Patris, Inc., 1991.
25. Grodin AJ. Soft tissue mobilization, course material. New York: Institute of Graduate Health Sciences 1983.
26. Guyton AC. Textbook of medical physiology. Philadelphia: WB Saunders, 1986.
27. Harryman DT, Sidles JA, Clark JM, et al. Translation of the humeral head on the glenoid with passive glenohumeral motion. J Bone Joint Surg 1990;72A:1334.
28. Harryman DT, Sidles JA, Harris SZ, Matzen FA III. The role of the rotator internal capsule in passive motion and stability of the shoulder. J Bone Joint Surg 1992;74A:53.
29. Howell SM, Galinat BJ, Renzi AJ, Marone PJ. Normal and abnormal mechanics of the glenohumeral joint in the horizontal plane. J Bone Joint Surg 1988;70A:227.
30. Jacobson EC, Lockwood MD, Hoefner VC, et al. Shoulder pain and repetition strain injury to the supraspinatus muscle: etiology and manipulative treatment. Journal of the American Osteopathic Association 1989;89:1037.
31. Janda V. Muscle function testing. London: Butterworth, 1983.
32. Jones LH. Spontaneous release by positioning. The D.O., January 1964:109.
33. Kaltenborn FM. Manual therapy for the extremity joints. Oslo: Olaf Bokhandel, 1976
34. Kaltenborn FM. Mobilization of the extremity joints: examination and basic treatment techniques. Oslo: Olaf Bokhandel, 1980.
35. Kapandji IA. The physiology of the joints. Vol. 3: The trunk and vertebral column. New York: Churchill Livingstone, 1974.
36. Kelkar R, Flatow EL, Bigliani LU, et al. A stereophotogrammetric method to determine the kinematics of the glenohumeral joint. In Advances in bioengineering. 1992:19.
37. Kendall HO, Kendall FP. Posture and pain. New York: Robert E Krieger Publishing, 1975.
38. Lewit K, Simons DG. Myofascial pain: relief by post-isometric relaxation. Arch Phys Med Rehabil 1984;65:452.
39. Lewit K. Manipulative therapy in rehabilitation of the motor system. London: Butterworth, 1985.
40. MacConail MA, Basmajian JV. Muscles and movements: a basis for human kinesiology. Baltimore: Williams & Wilkins, 1969.
41. Maitland GD. Peripheral manipulation. 2nd ed. London: Butterworth, 1977.
42. McArdle W, Katch F, Katch V. Exercise physiology, energy, nutrition, and human performance. Philadelphia: Lea & Febiger, 1986.
43. Melzack R. Myofascial trigger points: relation to acupuncture and mechanisms of pain. Arch Phys Med Rehabil 1981;62:114.
44. Mennell JB. Manual therapy. Am Lect Phys Med Publ 85, 1951.
45. Mennell JMcM. Joint pain: diagnosis and treatment using manipulative techniques. Boston: Little, Brown, 1964.
46. Mitchell FL, Moran, PS, Pruzzo, NA. An evaluation and treatment manual of osteopathic muscle energy procedures. St. Louis: Mitchell, Moran and Pruzzo, 1979.
47. O'Brien SJ, Neves MC, Arnoczky SP, et al., The anatomy and histology of the inferior glenohumeral ligament complex of the shoulder. Am J Sports Med 1990;18:449.
48. Ovesen I, Nielsen S. Anterior and posterior shoulder instability. Acta Orthop Scand 1986;57:324.
49. Paris SV, Patla C. Extremity dysfunction and manipulation. St. Augustine, Fla.: Institute Press, Division of Patris, 1988.
50. Paris SV. Foundations of clinical orthopaedics. St. Augustine, Fla.: Institute Press, Division of Patris, 1989.
51. Poppen NK, Walker PS. Normal and abnormal motion of the shoulder. J Bone Joint Surg 1976;58A:195.
52. Simons DG. Electrogenic nature of palpable bands and local twitch response associated with myofascial trigger points. Adv Pain Res Ther 1976;1:913.
53. Simons DG. Myofascial pain syndrome due to trigger points. Int Rehabil Med Assoc Publ 1, 1987.
54. Soslowsky LJ, Flatow EL, Bigliani LU, Mow VC. Articular geometry of the glenohumeral joint. Clin Orthop (in press).
55. Tappan FM. Healing massage techniques: classic, holistic and emerging methods. Reston, Va.: Reston Publishing Co., 1978.
56. Terminology of orthopaedic physical therapy. Alexandria: Official Publication of the Orthopaedic Section, APTA, 1987.
57. Terry GC, Hammon D, France P, Norwood LA. The stabilizing function of the passive shoulder restraints. Am J Sports Med 1991;19:26.
58. Tollison CD. Handbook of chronic pain management. Baltimore: Williams & Wilkins, 1989.
59. Travell JG. Myofascial pain and dysfunction: the trigger point manual. Baltimore: Williams & Wilkins, 1983.
60. Travell JG. Chronic myofascial pain syndromes. Adv Pain Res Ther 1990;17:
61. Turkel SJ, Panio MW, Marshal JL. Stabilizing mechanisms preventing anterior dislocation of the glenohumeral joint. J Bone Joint Surg 1981;63A:1208.
62. Upledger J. Craniosacral therapy. Seattle: Eastland Press, 1983.
63. Vaes PH, Annaert JM, Claeys PH, et al. Shoulder position and access for palpation to the rotator cuff tendons: an anatomical and kinesiological study. I.F.O.M.T. 5th Annual Conference, Vail, Colo., June 1992.
64. Vangsness CT, Ennis M. Neural anatomy of the human shoulder ligaments and the glenoid labrum. C. Thomas Vangsness, Jr., M.D., Healthcare Consultation Center, 1510 San Pablo Street, No. 322, Los Angeles, Calif. In press.
65. Woo S, Buckwalter JA. Injury and repair of the musculoskeletal soft tissues. Savannah: American Academy of Orthopaedic Surgeons Symposium, 1987.
66. Wood EC, Becker PD. Beard's massage. 3rd ed. Philadelphia: WB Saunders, 1981.
67. Woodman R. Pittsburgh: AREN Publications/Video, 1985.
68. Wyke BD. The neurology of joints, Ann R Coll Surg 1967;41:2550.

Christopher A. Arrigo
Kevin E. Wilk

Chapter 8

# Shoulder Exercises: A Criteria-Based Approach to Rehabilitation



Rehabilitation following a shoulder injury or surgery should progress through an integrated multiphased process that is sequential and progressive in nature. The ultimate goal of this entire process is returning the injured individual to unrestricted, symptom-free functional activity as quickly and safely as possible. The purpose of this chapter is to describe and illustrate various types of exercises for the shoulder complex and its related pathologies, both surgical and nonsurgical. These exercises will include isometrics, isotonics, isokinetics, plyometrics, neuromuscular control exercises, and closed kinetic chain exercises presented in a logical and sequential nature to provide a comprehensive approach to rehabilitation of the shoulder complex.

To effectively implement a proper therapeutic rehabilitation program, Kisner and Colby[77] outlined four basic necessities. First, the clinician must possess a thorough working knowledge of both the principles and effects of all treatment interventions used. Second, the clinician must be able to perform and properly interpret a functional physical examination of the client. Next, the clinician must thoroughly understand the interrelationships between the anatomy, biomechanics, and pathomechanics of the affected body part. Finally, the clinician must have an understanding of the state of the disability as well

Martin J. Kelley and William A. Clark: ORTHOPEDIC THERAPY OF THE SHOULDER.

as of its rehabilitation potential, complications, precautions, and treatment contraindications.

# Physiologic Responses to Exercises

Proper implementation of a progressive therapeutic rehabilitation program has been shown to enhance the restoration of normal muscular strength and endurance, flexibility and mobility, and the coordination and skill of the injured area. *Wolf's law* states that the musculoskeletal system of the human body reacts, adapts, and develops in response to the forces and stresses applied to it. Both the absence of normal stress and the presence of abnormal stress can produce musculoskeletal deformity, injury, disease, pain, and dysfunction.[77] Utilization of a progressive, criteria-based rehabilitative exercise program places positive stresses and forces on healing tissue, thus maximizing the client's return to functional activities as quickly and safely as possible.

## Muscular Strength

*Muscular strength* can be defined as the maximum force or tension generated by a muscle or group of muscles.[91] Improving muscular strength is a primary goal of most therapeutic rehabilitation programs.

Six interdependent factors influence the strength of normal muscle tissue.[7] First is the cross-sectional area of the muscle, in that the larger the muscle is in diameter, the greater is its potential force-generating capability. Because muscle tissue generates the greatest amount of force when it is placed on a slight stretch at the time of contraction, the second factor is the length-tension relationship of the muscle at the time of contraction. The third factor relates to the number of motor units recruited, in which the force output generated is directly related and proportional to the number of motor units firing. The fourth factor is the type of muscle contraction produced. Muscle tissue produces the greatest amount of force when contracting eccentrically against resistance, followed by less force with an isometric contraction, and the smallest amount of force during a concentric contraction. The fifth factor cited is the speed of the muscular contraction; the greatest muscle torques are produced at slower contractile velocities because of enhanced motor unit recruitment. Finally, a patient must put forth a maximal effort to elicit maximal strength, and thus motivation is a significant factor influencing normal strength.

The two most cited significant changes in the neuromuscular system that lead to improvements in muscular strength are hypertrophy and motor-unit recruitment.[77] Hypertrophy is a complex physiologic phenomenon that results in an increase in myofibril size. Because the strength-generating capacity of muscle tissue is directly related to its cross-sectional area, hypertrophy leads to muscular strength gains.[77] Strength gains also can be made without tissue hypertrophy because the greater the number of motor units firing, the greater is the force-generating capacity of the muscle. To elicit these types of adaptive infrastructure changes within the muscle, it must be exercised to the point of fatigue.[77]

## Muscular Endurance

*Endurance* is best defined as the ability to perform work over a period of time.[77] Therefore, *muscular endurance* is the ability of a muscle or muscle group to repeatedly contract and sustain tension over a period of time.[77]

Improved muscular endurance from exercise is a result of both immediate and long-term changes. Increased blood flow, heart rate, arterial pressure, oxygen demand and consumption, and the rate and depth of respiration are the most significant immediate changes during exercise that lead to improved muscular endurance.[77] The long-term muscular change that enhances endurance is the increased vascularization of the muscle tissue, which makes greater amounts of oxygen available for utilization.[77]

Muscular endurance will improve with the implementation of exercise activities designed to improve muscle strength, because active repetitive exercise to the point of fatigue will enhance endurance.[77] General or total-body endurance is related to the aerobic capacity of the patient. Exercises that stress the oxygen transport system of the body will improve endurance, aerobic capacity, and cardiopulmonary fitness.[77] This type of exercise program is usually directed toward large muscle groups and performed for a minimum of 20 to 40 minutes three times a week to be effective.[77,91]

## Flexibility and Mobility

Adequate flexibility and mobility of the joints of the musculoskeletal system and its surrounding soft tissue are required to perform normal, unrestricted functional movements. Soft-tissue and joint restrictions can cause pain, weakness, and/or inflammation, as well as impairing mobility.[77]

*Soft-tissue mobility* refers to the elastic components of muscle, connective tissue, and skin. Immobilization in one position for any length of time results in a loss of soft-tissue flexibility and/or contracture because of the contractile properties of muscle tissue. Restoration of muscular flexibility may be accomplished by means of active and/or passive therapeutic exercise activities. Connective tissue, composed of collagen and ground substance, will elongate slowly with long-duration stretching and adaptively shorten when immobilized.[77] *Skin mobility* is also required for normal motion. Burns, incisions, or lacerations may lead to tightness and limitations in the suppleness of the surrounding skin and therefore also must be properly mobilized.[77]

*Joint mobility*, the proper arthro- and osteokinematics of a joint, is required for normal motion. This includes adequate capsular laxity between joint surfaces to allow for the normal rolling, gliding, and spinning accessory joint motions to occur.

The four most common mobility exercise categories include passive and active stretching, flexibility exercises, and joint mobilization. Passive stretching includes manual, mechanical, or positional soft-tissue stretches where force is applied in the opposite direction of the shortening without any active patient involvement.[77] Active stretching techniques utilize neurophysiologic treatment principles to reflexively inhibit antagonistic muscle tissue to produce soft-tissue elongation.[77] Flexibility exercises, on the other hand, are general techniques performed without therapist assistance to actively or passively elongate soft tissue. Joint mobilization techniques are passive traction and/or gliding motions manually applied to joint surfaces to restore the normal joint mechanics required for unrestricted motion and function.[73,77,83]

## Coordination and Skill

*Coordination* is the basis of smooth, efficient, and effective movement patterns and refers to using the right muscles at the right time with the right intensity.[77] Therapeutic exercise techniques used to enhance neuromuscular coordination involve the use of constant repetition with proper sensory cuing and an increase in the speed of the activity over time.[77]

# Rehabilitative Considerations

Previously, with shoulder injury or surgery, the initiation of rehabilitative interventions was usually postponed for several weeks to allow for healing of the repaired or injured tissues. It has been common to see 4 or 6 weeks of immobilization followed only by passive motion as the postoperative rehabilitative management following rotator cuff repair, open acromioplasty, or shoulder stabilization procedures.[16,18,35,61] This type of rehabilitative approach may frequently result in a significant amount of shoulder girdle muscular atrophy, scapular muscle compensations during arm elevation motions, and extended complaints of shoulder pain and dysfunction.

It has been demonstrated that rehabilitation programs that stress early motion and strengthening have a lower incidence of recurrent subluxations and dislocations of the glenohumeral joint when compared with programs advocating several weeks of strict immobilization.[12,63,154] Strict immobilization can result in functional instability of the shoulder complex due to a loss of dynamic stability via rotator cuff inhibition, muscular atrophy, and poor neuromuscular control.

Current rehabilitative trends lean toward earlier protected motion and strengthening activities in conjunction with appropriate stabilizing exercises for the rotator cuff musculature to reestablish involuntary stability of the humeral head within the glenoid. These earlier progressive rehabilitative efforts are possible because of the improved surgical techniques[19,59,96,144] and arthroscopic advancements[3–7,9,10,27,28,56,84,92,141,144] that have decreased the amount of tissue morbidity and deltoid resection required during surgery. This has allowed for earlier and more progressive rehabilitation programs, including active assisted motion immediately following rotator cuff repairs and capsular stabilization procedures.

Consideration also must be given to the patient variables that influence rehabilitation potential following shoulder injury or surgery. These variables include the tissue integrity of the patient, the type and severity of the injury, the age of the patient, the individual's desired activity level, and the type of surgical procedure performed. Tissue integrity often determines the inherent stability of the glenohumeral joint and is directly related to the degree of rehabilitative aggressiveness following surgical intervention. The more compromised or lax the tissue, the less aggressive interventions should be initially. Specific injuries and pathologies have identifiable healing constraints and rehabilitative restrictions. These include but are not limited to post-operative rotator cuff repair and shoulder stabilization procedures. Patient age must be considered to ensure that exercises are properly adapted and tailored to both challenge younger athletic patients and maximize symptom-free function in more sedentary or elderly individuals. Successful rehabilitation in practice is the proper implementation of appropriate exercises to the individual patient, remembering that not every exercise is always correct for every patient. The individual's desired activity level also plays a part in the rehabilitative process. Program alterations can be made to satisfactorily challenge the overhead athlete and worker, as well as to ensure adequate strength in those individuals only requiring the performance of routine daily activities.

## Anatomic Considerations

The shoulder is a tremendously complex unit that requires integrated motion from the glenohumeral, scapulothoracic, acromioclavicular, and sternoclavicular joints, as well as from the spine, to ensure the performance of unrestricted functional and/or athletic activities. Three separate anatomic systems combine to provide glenohumeral joint stability: (1) the osseous geometric configuration of the joint, (2) the ligamentous structures, and (3) the neuromuscular system. The interaction of these three anatomic components provides functional stability for the entire shoulder complex.

Dynamic glenohumeral joint stability is provided via the neuromuscular system. There are 26 muscles controlling the shoulder girdle; however, only a third are believed to play a significant role in dynamic stability of the glenohumeral joint.[124] The primary role of the rotator cuff musculature is to dynamically stabilize the humeral head in the glenoid fossa through the muscles of the shoulder working in a force-couple fashion.[87,95,97,98,113] This results in a co-contraction of the rotator cuff musculature, thereby balancing the forces across the shoulder applied by the prime movers of the arm. The primary force couples of the glenohumeral joint are the subscapularis counterbalanced by the infraspinatus and teres minor and the anterior deltoid and supraspinatus counterbalanced by the infraspinatus and teres minor. Equilibrium of these force couples is critical for normal shoulder function.

The shoulder musculature combines to provide dynamic joint stability via four mechanisms (Table 8-1). First, the muscles of the shoulder provide passive glenohumeral joint tension.[79] This serves to improve joint stability by increasing the area of contact between the articulating surfaces. The second element of joint stability is via active articular surface compression through rotator cuff muscular activity.[64] When arm movement is initiated, the muscular force couples contract to center the humeral head within the glenoid fossa. This serves to maximize muscular efficiency so that functional arm movements can occur. The next element of stability is provided through the cross-sectional area of the muscle fibers that blend with the anterior joint capsule. The subscapularis muscle exhibits a large attachment to the anterior joint capsule and is believed to provide a large anterior stabilizing effect through its contraction.[38,39,125] The infraspinatus and teres minor muscles function in a similar fashion posteriorly to stabilize the glenohumeral joint. Lastly, the neuromuscular system provides joint stability through proprioceptive awareness. Smith and Brunolti[121] reported a deficit in shoulder kinesthesia following glenohumeral dislocation. Thus training the proprioceptors of the shoulder and improving neuromuscular control may be beneficial in improving the overall dynamic stability of the glenohumeral joint.[148]

The rotator cuff musculature (subscapularis, supraspinatus, infraspinatus, teres minor), long head of the biceps brachii, and the deltoid combine to provide most of the dynamic stability afforded the glenohumeral joint. Because the rotator cuff musculature blends with the glenohumeral joint capsule, it provides a tendoligamentous structure that acts together to provide stability via active-passive tension theories.[32,37,67,87,115]

**Table 8-1**

**Dynamic Stabilization of the Glenohumeral Joint Complex**

1. Passive muscle tension
2. Muscular co-contraction (increasing joint contact pressures)
3. Cross-sectional contact area to capsule
4. Neuromuscular control (reactive control)

An example of this system occurs during shoulder external rotation. As the prime movers (the teres minor and infraspinatus) produce this motion actively, the other rotator cuff muscles contract to stabilize the humeral head within the glenoid. This causes the capsule to become taut, increasing joint contact pressure and thus stability. This rotator cuff force couple serves to center the humeral head in the glenoid fossa, maintain proper muscular length-tension relationships, and allow unrestricted symptom-free glenohumeral function. During other arm movements, such as elevation or horizontal abduction, a similar muscular contraction pattern occurs between the humeral head stabilizing muscles and the prime movers. Thus it would appear that a strong, intact rotator cuff and surrounding shoulder complex musculature are vital to normal shoulder function. The efficiency and neuromuscular control of these force-couple mechanisms of the glenohumeral joint appear to greatly affect the overall functional ability of the shoulder.

## Criteria-Based Rehabilitative Phases

Six basic rehabilitative principles serve as the foundation for developing a sequential and progressive treatment approach for the injured shoulder. These basic principles must be considered throughout the rehabilitative process. They serve to guide patient progression and allow the integration of exercise techniques that build from one level to another throughout the entire treatment process. First, the effects of immobilization must be minimized. Second, healing tissue must never be overstressed. Third, the patient must fulfill specific criteria to progress successfully through the rehabilitative program. Fourth, the rehabilitative program must be based on current clinical and scientific research. Fifth, the program must be adaptable to all patients and their specific goals. Sixth and finally, these basic treatment principles should be followed throughout the entire rehabilitative process for both surgical and nonsurgical shoulder conditions.

To enable the sequential progression of shoulder rehabilitation, a continuous, four-phased rehabilitative approach has been developed. Table 8-2 illustrates a logical rehabilitation progression utilizing these basic principles and this multiphased approach, as well as a continuum for progression of various exercise activities for the shoulder. Specific objective and functional criteria are preestablished for each phase of the rehabilitation program to both guide and ensure a proper rate of progression during the rehabilitative process. This type of approach requires consistent fulfillment of minimal objective standards before higher levels of function and exercise are attempted. This allows the adaptation of these rehabilitative phases to a wide variety of nonsurgical as well as surgical pa-

**Table 8-2**

**A Continuous Four-Phased Rehabilitation Approach**

| | Criteria-Based Phases of Shoulder Rehabilitation | Continuum of Shoulder Strengthening Activities |
|---|---|---|
| Phase I: | Immediate motion exercises<br>Active assisted motion<br>Stretching<br>Isometrics<br>Weight bearing | Multiangle isometrics<br>↓<br>Isotonics short range<br>↓ |
| Phase II: | Intermediate exercises<br>Isotonics<br>Stretching<br>Manual resistance<br>Neuromuscular controls | Isotonics full range<br>↓<br>Submaximal isokinetics (modified neutral position)<br>↓<br>Exercise tubing neutral position)<br>↓ |
| Phase III: | Advanced strengthening exercises<br>Constant loading<br>Isokinetics<br>Plyometrics<br>Neuromuscular | Maximal isokinetics (modified neutral position)<br>↓<br>Exercise tubing (90°/90° position)<br>↓<br>Maximal isokinetics (90°/90° position)<br>↓<br>Plyometrics<br>↓ |
| Phase IV: | Return-to-activity exercises/drills<br>Interval sport programs<br>Work-simulation programs<br>Constant loading<br>Isotonics | Resistive functional exercise<br>↓<br>Unrestricted functional activities |

thologies. Because specific predetermined criteria must be fulfilled for progression, patients advance at an individualized pace related to their individual age, injury, tissue type, and surgical procedure.

There are certain specific healing constraints, precautions, and contraindications during the rehabilitation of various surgical procedures that must be considered. Keeping in mind that various pathologies and surgical procedures have variations in exercise activities, positioning, and progression based on the type of procedure performed, the healing constraints involved, and the tissues stressed during rehabilitation, this chapter will present a general overview of this multiphased criteria-based rehabilitative program. This can then be applied, with adaptations, to numerous situations as long as strict adherence to progression is followed within the objective criteria established. This program provides the reader with the generalized principles of a progressive shoulder rehabilitation program.

## Phase I: Immediate Motion Exercises

The goals of this initial phase are to reestablish a nonpainful range of motion, retard muscular atrophy, and decrease pain/inflammation.

Immediately following a shoulder injury or surgery, motion is allowed in a protected, nonpainful arc. By allowing immediate motion, the deleterious effects of immobilization, such as articular cartilage degeneration, muscular atrophy, and adverse collagen tissue formation, may be minimized.[1,36,45,46,101,106,116,117] In addition, early motion also may align collagen fibers according to their appropriate patterns of stress.[1,153] These early motion exercises are accomplished through active assisted range of motion (AAROM) movements with a stick, wand, or T-bar device and/or rope and pulley. The movements emphasized include pain-free shoulder elevation in the sagittal or scapular plane, external rotation, and internal rotation. Stick or wand and rope and pulley shoulder flexion activities should be performed while leading with the thumb to clear the greater tuberosity from under the coracoacromial arch (Fig. 8-1). Shoulder external/internal rotation is often initiated at 0 degrees of abduction, then to 45 degrees (Fig. 8-2), and ultimately to 90 degrees of abduction (Fig. 8-3). Performing these exercises in the scapular plane is often advantageous due to decreased tension on the capsuloligament-tendon complex. In some cases, such as following rotator cuff repair under tension, rotation exercises should be initiated at 45 degrees of abduction to minimize tension across the repair. With all these active assisted activities, the noninvolved arm controls the movement of the involved arm. Motion is taken to the point of a mild stretch, held for 2 to 3 seconds, and then relaxed. These activities begin with one to two sets of 10 repetitions, allowing the patient to progress to four to five sets as tolerated. Capsular stretches are also employed during this

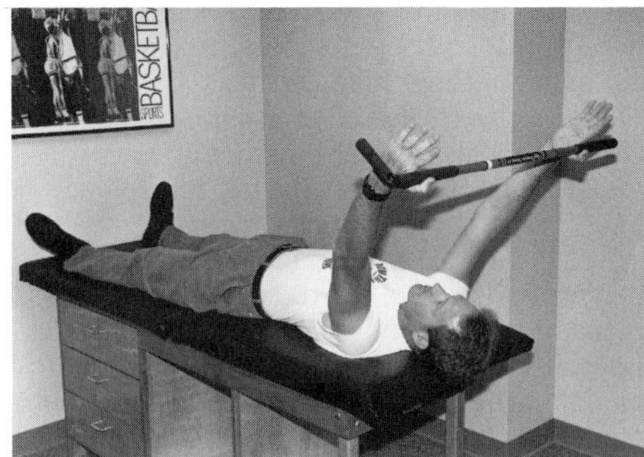


**Figure 8-1.** Active assisted shoulder flexion movement performed with a T-bar.

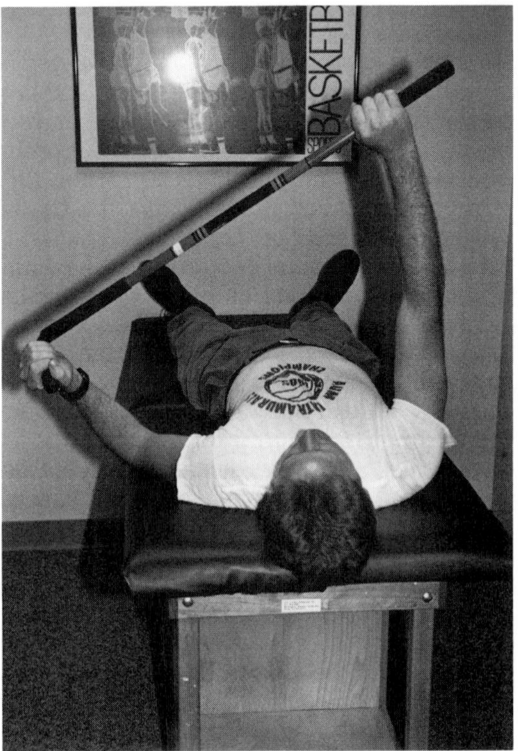


**Figure 8-2.** Active assisted shoulder external rotation movement at 45 degrees of abduction.

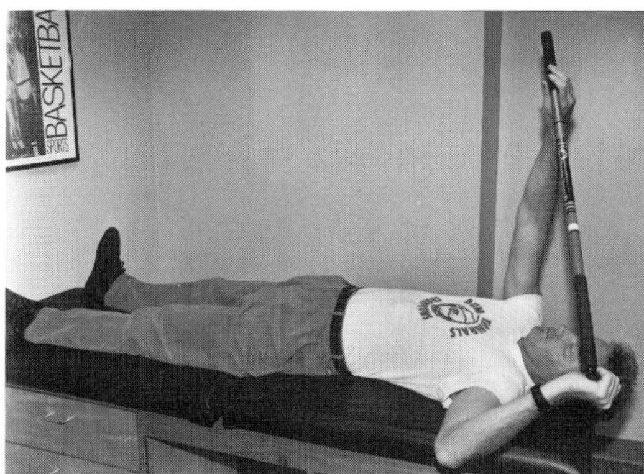


**Figure 8-3.** Active assisted shoulder external rotation movement at 90 degrees of abduction.

**Table 8-3**

**Humeral Head Stabilizing Exercises**

I. Submaximal isometrics
   1. Abduction at 30° and 60°
   2. Supraspinatus at 30° and 60° (empty-can position)
   3. ER at 0° abduction
   4. IR at 0° abduction
   5. Biceps isometrics

II. Short-arc isotonics
   1. Abduction 30° to 90°
   2. Supraspinatus 30° to 90°
   3. Flexion 30° to 90°
   4. ER at 30° with towel roll with tubing
   5. IR at 30° with towel roll with tubing
   6. Biceps isotonics tubing at 35° to 40° flexion (shoulder)
   7. D2 flexion RS at 30°, 60°, 90°, and 120°

III. Rotator cuff dynamic stabilizing sets (begin with no weight program to 1 lb and then gradually increase)
   1. Arm elevation from 0° to 60° isometric hold 2 seconds (2 points)
   2. Arm elevation from 60° to 120° isometric hold 2 seconds (2 points)
   3. Supraspinatus from 0° to 60° isometric hold 2 seconds (2 points)
   4. Supraspinatus from 0° to 90° isometric hold 2 seconds (2 points)
   5. D2 flex UE, RS and SRH at 0°, 60°, 120°, and 160°
   6. Tubing D2 flex with isometric holds

rehabilitative phase for the inferior, posterior, and anterior portions of the glenohumeral joint capsule, as appropriate. Performing joint-mobilization techniques and contract-relax-stretch procedures with patients in the early stages of rehabilitation is quite often facilitated by using the scapular plane for both types of stretches. Furthermore, a general guideline to use to judge the appropriate force of stretching is that the patient should feel slight discomfort during the stretch but no pain or discomfort once the stretch is removed. Rather, the patient should note an improvement in range of motion and a decrease in pain. An increase in the complaint of pain or a decrease in range of motion can indicate that one is being overly aggressive, and appropriate modifications need to be implemented.

Immediately following a shoulder injury or surgery, it is common to observe a functional decrease in the strength of the rotator cuff musculature secondary to pain, swelling, and/or injury. Because the primary function of the rotator cuff is to dynamically stabilize and steer the humeral head during arm movements, it is critical to reestablish voluntary control and pain-free function of these muscles as quickly and safely as possible following trauma. Restoring one's voluntary control of the rotator cuff is imperative to prevent excessive uncontrollable humeral head migration.[144] Pain-free, submaximal, isometric muscular contractions are often utilized during this phase to reinitiate rotator cuff function. Eliminating inflammation as a cause of pain and neuromuscular inhibition of the rotator cuff is the first priority. Then incorporation of a submaximal isometric exercise program is the first of three phases used to restore functional humeral head stabilization[144] (Table 8-3). These contractions should be performed submaximally, at multiple angles, and in a pain-free fashion. The muscles to emphasize include the external/internal rotators at 0 to 30 degrees of abduction and in 0 to 30 degrees of rotation (Fig. 8-4), the abductors at 30 and 60 degrees of shoulder elevation (Fig. 8-5), the supraspinatus in the scapular plane (empty-can position/"scaption") at 30 and 60 degrees of elevation (Fig. 8-6), and the elbow flexors. Supraspinatus strengthening exercises in the scapular plane with internal rotation (scaption) may not be appropriate for all individuals, particularly elderly patients. This particular exercise is often criticized for increased shear forces and the production of pain in certain individuals. In these situations, this exercise should be avoided. Each isometric contraction should be held for 6 to 8 seconds. Patients should again progress from one to two sets of 10 to 15 repetitions up toward four to five sets as tolerated. These exercises should be performed two to three times daily in conjunction with the active assisted range of motion exercises previously described.

These isometric contractions serve to reinitiate dynamic control of the humeral head and are vital to successful rehabilitation. Often patients

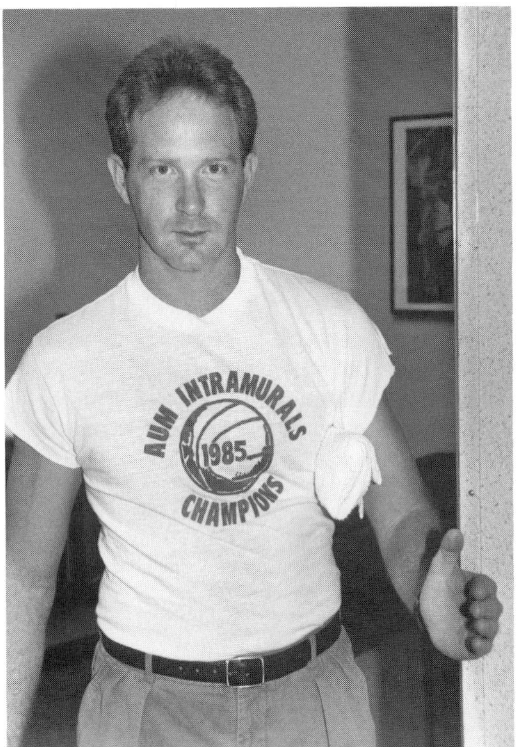


**Figure 8-4.** Isometric muscular contraction of the shoulder external rotators at 30 degrees abduction.

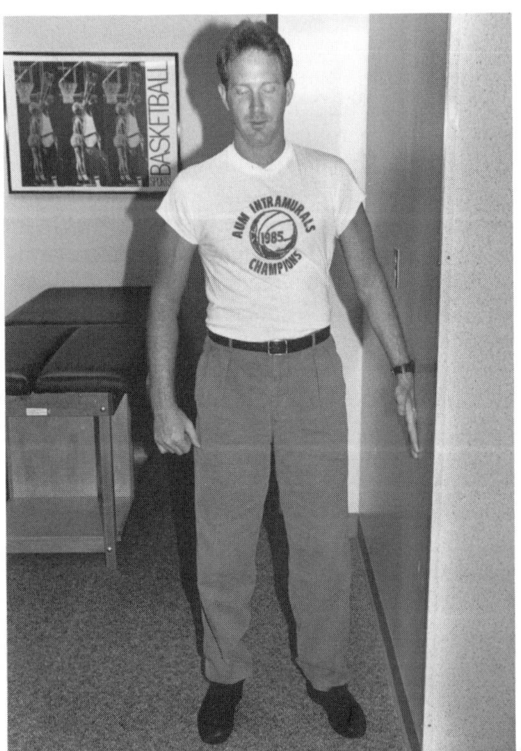


**Figure 8-5.** Abduction movement with isometric resistance at 30 degrees of abduction.

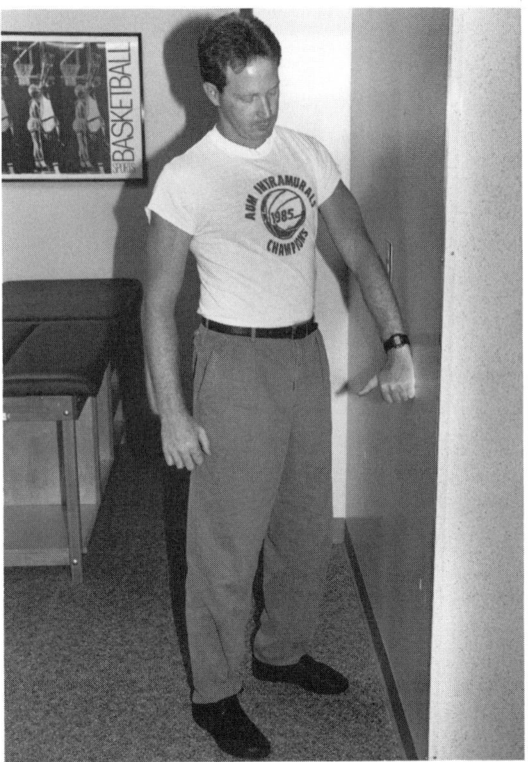


**Figure 8-6.** Isometric muscular contraction of the supraspinatus muscle with the arm elevated to 30 degrees and in the scapular plane.

who exhibit pain with AAROM exercises do so secondary to poor strength of their humeral head depressors and stabilizers. Frequently, this can be observed with pain occurring during arm lowering at between approximately 70 and 45 degrees of shoulder flexion. If this occurs, the humeral head stabilizing exercises previously referred to are emphasized throughout the rehabilitative process. The restoration of dynamic humeral head stabilization is imperative to the rehabilitative process. These three phases, beginning with submaximal isometrics, progressing to short-arc isotonics, and finally to rotator cuff dynamic stabilizing sets, as outlined in Table 8-3, have been extremely beneficial in the restoration of dynamic humeral head control and in preventing rotator cuff "shutdown" following injury or surgery.

In addition, weight-bearing exercises are incorporated to facilitate cocontractions around the shoulder joint. These are performed with the patient standing or kneeling placing a proportionate amount of body weight through the hands as tolerated. The patient is instructed to shift his or her weight from side to side, forward to backward, and diagonally on and off the affected side. As the patient improves, this type of exercise can be progressed using manual resistance, a large ball, and finally a smaller ball. Hand placement can be progressed from the sides of the ball to the top of the ball and finally to one hand on top of the other in increasing amounts of difficulty.

Before a patient can be progressed from phase I to phase II exercises, specific criteria must be exhibited on physical examination. These criteria are (1) full nonpainful range of motion, (2) minimal tenderness and pain on clinical examination, and (3) good strength (a manual muscle test grade of 4 out of 5) of the shoulder internal and external rotator and flexor muscles.

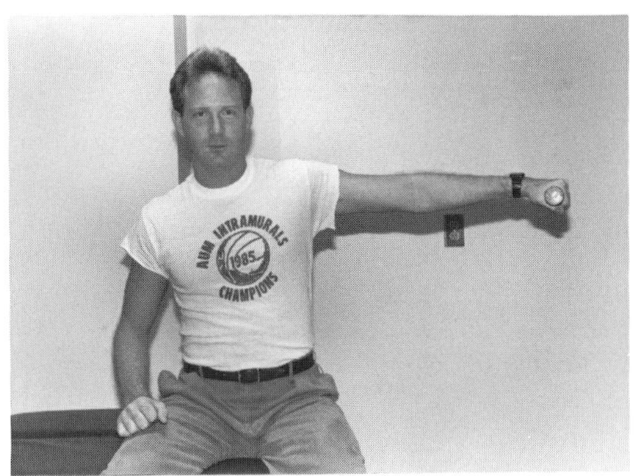

**Figure 8-7.** Shoulder abduction to 90 degrees of elevation in neutral rotation with a dumbbell.

# Phase II: Intermediate Exercises

Phase II strengthening exercises are progressed from submaximal isometric muscle contractions to submaximal isotonic muscle contractions. The goals of this phase are to improve the muscular strength and endurance, as well as the neuromuscular control of the entire shoulder complex. During this phase, scapulothoracic stabilization exercises are also emphasized or initiated if they have not already been initiated during the first phase.

Initially, the exercises incorporated during this phase are submaximal isotonic muscle contractions for the glenohumeral and scapulothoracic musculature. Low-weight submaximal contractions are utilized, because most functional contractions about the shoulder are submaximal in nature. The concept of lighter weights with longer isometric holds is employed to emphasize the glenohumeral "steering" and stabilizing muscles, the supraspinatus, infraspinatus, and subscapularis, while slightly larger weights and greater resistance are utilized to strengthen the "prime mover" muscles of the shoulder complex, the pectoralis major, deltoid, latissimus dorsi, and teres major and minor.[108, 114, 115] In most situations, this progression begins without weight at two sets of 10 repetitions. The patient then works to five sets of 10 repetitions. Upon successful attainment of this goal in a pain-free fashion with good technique, a progressive resistance exercise approach is incorporated. Patients progress at 1- to 2-lb intervals to 5 to 10 lb, five sets of 10 repetitions as tolerated.

The rotator cuff exercises used are expanded from the short-arc isotonic and dynamic stabilizing sets highlighted in Table 8-3 to full-arc isotonics as dynamic humeral head stability is enhanced. Standing shoulder abduction to 90 degrees with the arm in slight internal rotation (palm down) (Fig. 8-7) is used to strengthen the deltoid complex. If this exercise provokes a painful response, the exercise can be modified so that elevation is performed in the scapular plane either with internal rotation or in neutral. Prone shoulder extension with the thumb in the neutral position is used to strengthen the infraspinatus and teres minor. Additionally, for the infraspinatus and teres minor muscles, external rotation is performed in either a side-lying position with a dumbbell or in a standing position with exercise tubing (Fig. 8-8). Some patients will be more comfortable if a towel roll is inserted between their upper arm and thorax during these exercises (Fig. 8-9). This modification likely reduces strain on the superior capsule and cuff and also may improve vascularity of the supraspinatus tendon. The subscapularis muscle is exercised during resisted internal rotation move-

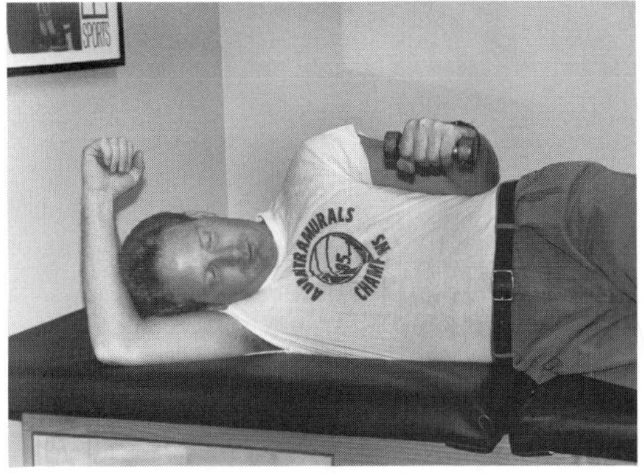

**Figure 8-8.** Isotonic muscular contraction of the external rotators in sidelying using a dumbbell for resistance.

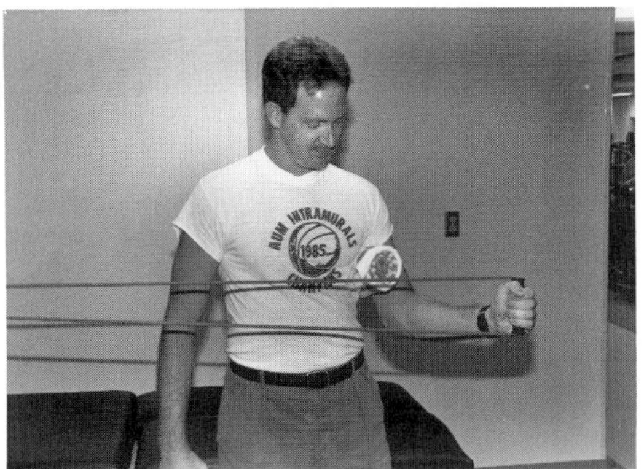

**Figure 8-9.** Isotonic muscular contraction of the external rotators in standing position utilizing exercise tubing with a towel roll between humerus and side to improve dynamic isometric stability.

ments, again using either the side-lying or standing position. If a patient exhibits poor humeral head stabilizing capacity of the glenohumeral musculature (pain with exercise activity), again a towel roll may be placed between the medial arm and thoracic cage during internal/external rotation strengthening movements with exercise tubing. This will elicit a muscular cocontraction about the glenohumeral joint and may produce improved humeral head stabilization. Additionally, it has been reported by several authors[80,81,93,109,111,120] that supraspinatus vascularity may be enhanced with shoulder abduction. Rathbun and Macnab[109] have described a zone of increased rotator cuff avascularity with the arm in 0 degrees of abduction. They reported that the supraspinatus may experience a pathologic "wringing out" in this position.[109] Therefore, during internal and external rotation exercises in certain patients, especially those with compromised rotator cuff integrity, clinicians might prefer a position of glenohumeral abduction between 30 and 45 degrees and forward flexion between 30 and 45 degrees, thus placing the glenohumeral joint within the scapular plane. Use of this position may serve to facilitate increased muscular cocontraction, improved vascularity, and reduced tension on the rotator cuff and capsule. Use of the scapular plane during shoulder rotation strengthening exercises also may serve to enhance biomechanics within the glenohumeral joint by allowing the tendons of the rotator cuff to exert direct forces on the humeral head while in an optimal length-tension relationship. Blackburn et al.[20] reported increased electromyographic (EMG) activity in the supraspinatus during arm horizontal abduction to 100 degrees in external rotation while in the prone position. Therefore, this exercise may be incorporated with one modification. The hand position used is the neutral or palm-down position to decrease the amount of stress placed on the anterior capsule during the performance of this exercise. Subacromial tissue tolerance is obviously required to attain this position. When appropriate, elevation in the scapular plane with the glenohumeral joint in internal rotation ("scaption") to 90 degrees is incorporated for strengthening the supraspinatus muscle (Fig. 8-10).

Several authors have reported that the supraspinatus muscle plays an important role in normal glenohumeral function by depressing the humeral head during elevation.[39,132,138] However, MacConaill and Basmajian[90] have noted that the supraspinatus was not necessary for normal shoulder function by demonstrating that its complete paralysis only served to reduce the force of active shoulder abduction. The primary depressors of the humeral head during shoulder elevation are the infraspinatus, teres minor, and subscapularis muscles, not the supraspinatus. Because the infraspinatus is involved in two critical force couples about the glenohumeral joint, the quality of shoulder motion is directly related

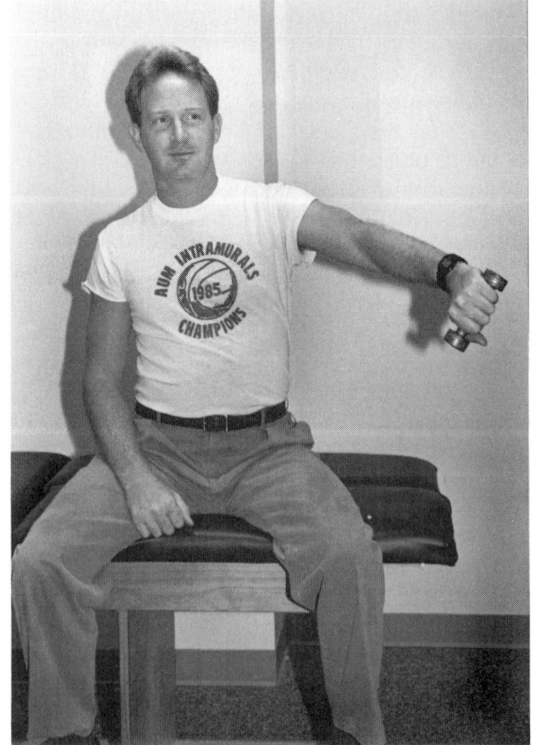

**Figure 8-10.** Arm elevation with internal rotation in the scapular plane ("scaption").

to its function. More often, massive rotator cuff tears extend posteriorly into the infraspinatus rather than anteriorly, rendering the infraspinatus incapable of offsetting the force movements produced by the anterior deltoid and the subscapularis. Therefore, dynamic glenohumeral joint stability is not solely the function of the supraspinatus but is directly related to the integrity of the entire rotator cuff. Because the load-sharing capacity of the rotator cuff muscles is altered when one of the muscles is injured or torn, an increased amount of stress is placed on the remaining healthy tissue, which may ultimately result in tissue failure. Therefore, using elevation in the scapular plane with internal rotation is not appropriate for all patients. Clinically, elderly, sedentary patients and those with rotator cuff disease should avoid strengthening activities with this exercise when painful.

Strengthening of the scapulothoracic musculature and neuromuscular control drills for the shoulder complex are imperative for normal glenohumeral joint function and successful rehabilitation. The scapulothoracic articulation must provide a stable base of support ensuring proximal stability to allow for distal mobility of the arm. For full unrestricted elevation of the arm, the scapula must be able to rotate upwardly approximately 60 degrees on the thoracic wall.[65,74,108] This upward rotation of the scapula is due in part to a conjunct rotation at the acromioclavicular joint caused by distal clavicular elevation.[74] As the clavicle elevates, passive tension is created in the conoid ligament. Because of this ligamentous orientation, a posterior conjunct rotation of the clavicle is produced during arm elevation. This clavicular rotation is necessary for unrestricted scapular mobility. The scapulothoracic musculature plays a significant role in providing adequate scapular mobility. More important, this musculature provides a stable proximal scapular base for the arm to function from. Therefore, the primary function of the scapula is to provide stability during changing positions of the arm, thereby maintaining a consistent length-tension relationship of the rotator cuff muscles to ensure maximal force-couple function.

Moseley and coworkers,[94] through the use of EMG, studied the scapulothoracic muscles during various exercises. Utilizing their data, several exercises to isolate the scapulothoracic musculature can be identified. Prone horizontal shoulder abduction (neutral arm position) is incorporated to strengthen the rhomboideus major and minor muscles and the middle trapezius fibers.[94] A progressive push-up exercise provides for the serratus anterior and pectoralis minor muscles.[129] Push-ups are initiated into a wall, with the hands internally rotated approximately 45 degrees, then progressed to table height, and finally to the floor for increasing resistance. A prone rowing maneuver with an isometric hold also has been shown to strengthen the upper trapezius and levator scapulae muscles.[94] An isometric press-up (Fig. 8-11) has been shown to create high EMG activity for the pectoralis major, latissimus dorsi, and pectoralis minor muscles as well. Moseley et al.[94] reported that four exercises appeared to significantly enhance recruitment of the scapular muscles of the shoulder complex. These exercises included shoulder elevation in the scapular plane, upright rowing, a press-up, and a push-up with a plus.[94] Neuromuscular control exercises and drills for the scapulothoracic musculature are also initiated during this phase. These activities are performed on a regular basis to ensure improvement in the volitional motor control and coordinated movement of the scapula. These exercises, originally described by Feldenkrais[47,112,140] and modified by Wilk et al.[148] are performed with the patient lying on the contralateral side. The involved shoulder is therefore free to move while the affected hand is placed on the table with the shoul-

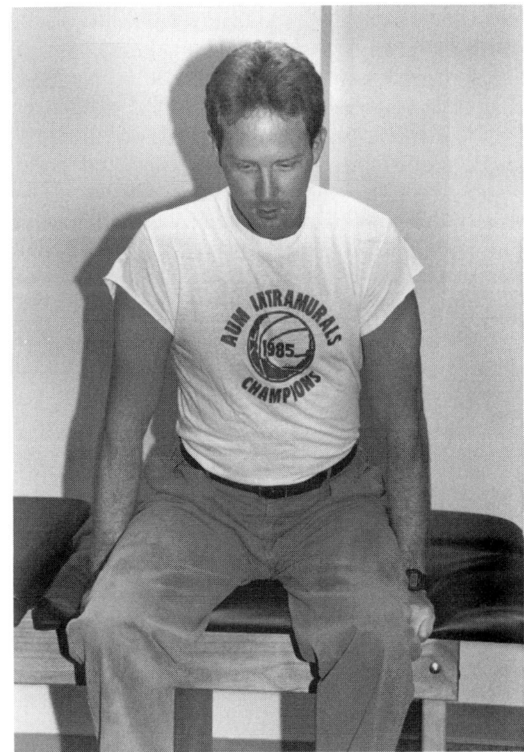


**Figure 8-11.** Isometric press-up movement in the sitting position.

der abducted to 90 degrees and internally rotated. The drill is for the patient to slowly elevate and depress the scapula and then to slowly retract and protract the scapula repeatedly. It is the quality of movement, not the quantity, that is important during the performance of these exercises. The goal is isolated, nonsubstituted movements of the scapula. Often, manual resistance is used initially to provide tactile stimulus in the desired direction of movement with these exercises (Fig. 8-12). The manual resistance serves to reinforce the appropriate direction of movement and enhance the quality of the exercise performed.

Additionally, biceps brachii function is emphasized during resisted elbow flexion exercises with exercise tubing. Because the long head of the biceps brachii has been shown to be a strong humeral head depressor and acts to steer the humeral head during active arm movements, these exercises are imperative.[82]

Submaximal isokinetics for the shoulder internal and external rotators are often initiated during this phase in either a standing, sitting, or supine position, with appropriate limitations imposed on the amount of rotation and the speed of exercise. Although a complete discussion of isokinetic exercise follows under the section on advanced strengthening, initiation of isokinetics during this phase allows for exercise at a comfortable velocity in a relatively safe and stable position. This type of exercise also serves to assist in the transition to unrestricted daily activities or to higher-level exercises and drills.

It is also extremely important to combine the single-plane submaximal, isotonic, and isokinetic strengthening exercises outlined above with multiplane, diagonal pattern activities using synergic movement such as with proprioceptive neuromuscular facilitation (PNF) exercises. This ensures an exercise progression philosophy that moves from basic concepts and exercises to more complex and difficult levels of physical activity. Table 8-4 highlights this exercise philosophy and provides the sequencing of activities from the most simple to the more complex exercises. A common diagonal pattern used in this progression is the D2 flexion/extension pattern with manual resistance incorporating rhythmic stabilization and slow reversal hold techniques[78, 126] (Figs. 8-13 and 8-14). During rhythmic stabilization, the static resistance angles commonly used are 30, 60, 90, and 140 degrees of shoulder elevation. This maneuver is used to accomplish a cocontraction within the rotator cuff musculature and enhance the dynamic stabilization of the humeral head. This D2 flexion pattern is employed because of the increased muscle activity of the posterior deltoid, infraspinatus, teres minor, trapezius, and rhomboids demonstrated during the performance of this movement pattern. This exercise maneuver is used to enhance

**Table 8-4**

**Philosophy of Exercise Progression**

| |
|---|
| Simple → complex |
| Proximal → distal |
| Single-plane → multiple-plane |
| Isometric stability → isometric movement |
| Stability → mobility |
| Controlled mobility → skill movements |
| Controlled environment → uncontrolled environment |
| Horizontal movements → vertical movements |
| Unidirectional movements → multi-directional movements |

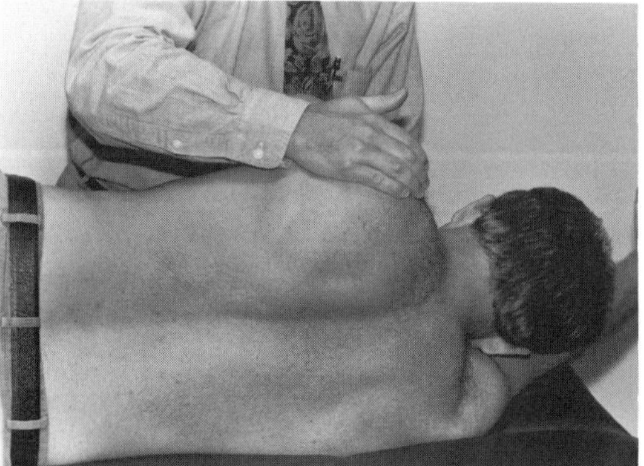

**Figure 8-12.** Neuromuscular control exercises for the scapulothoracic muscles against manual resistance; this movement is scapular retraction.

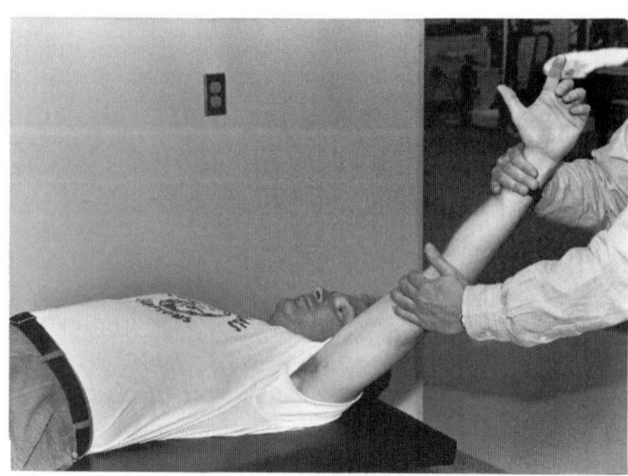

**Figure 8-13.** Proprioceptive neuromuscular facilitation exercise utilizing manual resistance during D2 extension.

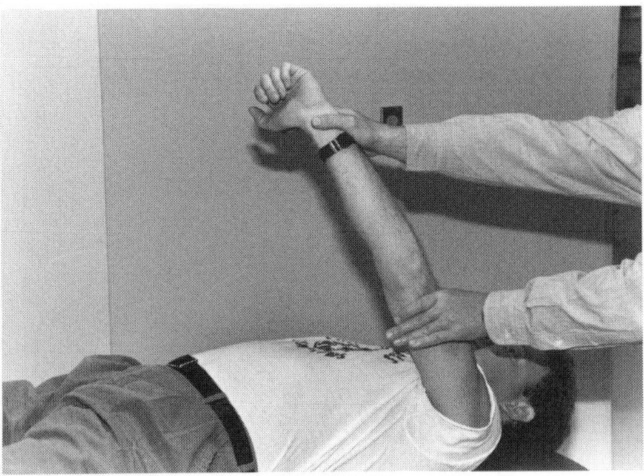

**Figure 8-14.** Proprioceptive neuromuscular facilitation exercise utilizing manual resistance during D2 flexion.

the efficiency of the glenohumeral joint force couples. The rehabilitation specialist should perform the D2 flexion pattern in various positions such as side lying, seated, and standing, as well as in the supine position.

During this phase of exercises, it is extremely important to continue glenohumeral joint complex stretching exercises to maintain and continually increase passive shoulder motion. Most often these exercises can be performed with a stick for shoulder flexion, external rotation, internal rotation, and continued self-stretching as described previously.

To progress from phase II to phase III exercises, the patient must exhibit (1) full nonpainful range of motion, (2) no pain or tenderness on clinical examination, and (3) strength that is 70 percent of the contralateral shoulder for the external and internal rotators and the abductors/adductors. The patient must exhibit these specific criteria before being deemed capable of performing the phase III exercise drills because of the stressful nature of the activities used in the next rehabilitative phase. Although most patients will progress to the end of phase II in this criteria-based rehabilitation program, progression to phase III activities is not appropriate for all patients. The general, nonathletic population and sedentary individuals may graduate from this phase with the ability to perform activities of daily living and function without the need for higher-level exercises and activities. Those industrial and athletic individuals who require greater strength, power, and endurance, as well as guidance in returning to strenuous activities, need to be progressed into the remaining two rehabilitative phases.

## Phase III: Advanced Strengthening Exercises

Phase three exercises are considered dynamic strengthening exercises and drills. The goals of this phase are increasing strength, power, and muscular endurance, improving neuromuscular control, and preparing the patient for functional activities. The emphasis of these exercises for the recreational or competitive athlete is on high-speed, high-energy strengthening drills, eccentric muscular contractions, and diagonal movements in functional positions.

The exercises performed in this phase include isotonic dumbbell movements, resistive exercise tubing movements with concentric/eccentric contractions, isokinetics, plyometrics, and the continuation of scapulothoracic neuromuscular control exercises. Resistive isotonic dumbbell exercises are continued, progressing up to 8 to 10 lb, five sets of 10 repetitions, emphasizing the rotator cuff and deltoid musculature.

The exercises performed with exercise tubing or Theraband during this phase include internal/external rotation in the 90/90 degree position (Fig. 8-15), which may be appropriate for the

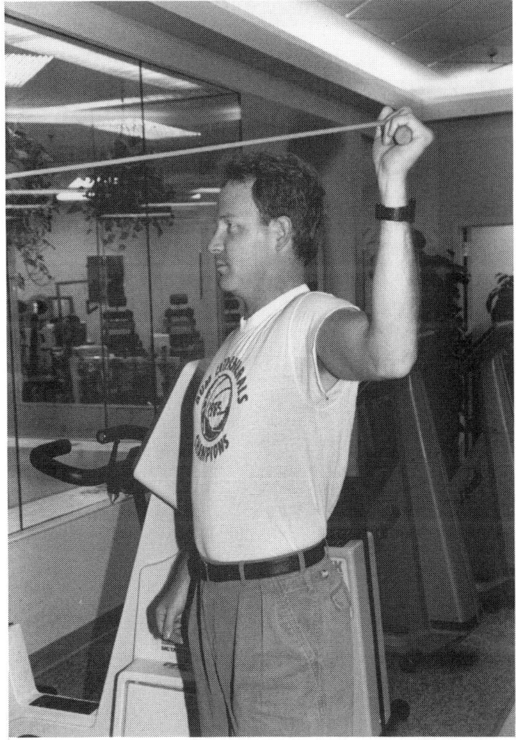

**Figure 8-15.** Shoulder external rotation in the 90-degree shoulder abduction and 90-degree elbow flexion (90°/90° position) position with exercise tubing.

overhead movements associated with an industrial worker or athlete. This exercise activity is progressed from the 0-degree abducted position, up to the modified neutral position, into the plane of the scapula, and when appropriate, on to the 90/90 degree abducted position. If the patient experiences discomfort in this 90/90 degree overhead position, the exercise activity is moved back to the scapular plane and down to 45 degrees of shoulder elevation, and glenohumeral stabilization activities are emphasized. In addition, tubing exercises are performed for the biceps (Fig. 8-16), latissimus dorsi, and teres major musculature (Fig. 8-17). Diagonal patterns are used with exercise tubing for D2 flexion, emphasizing both concentric and eccentric muscle activities (Figs. 8-18 and 8-19). Two to five sets of 10 to 15 repetitions for each of these exercises are usually performed as tolerated. The sets alternate between slow, deliberate concentric/eccentric muscular contractions and fast, high-speed, high-energy repetitions.

Often, these diagonal movements are performed with isometric holds at various points in the range of motion to strengthen the humeral head stabilizers and are described with manual proprioceptive neuromuscular facilitation techniques. Manual resistance is applied to the arm

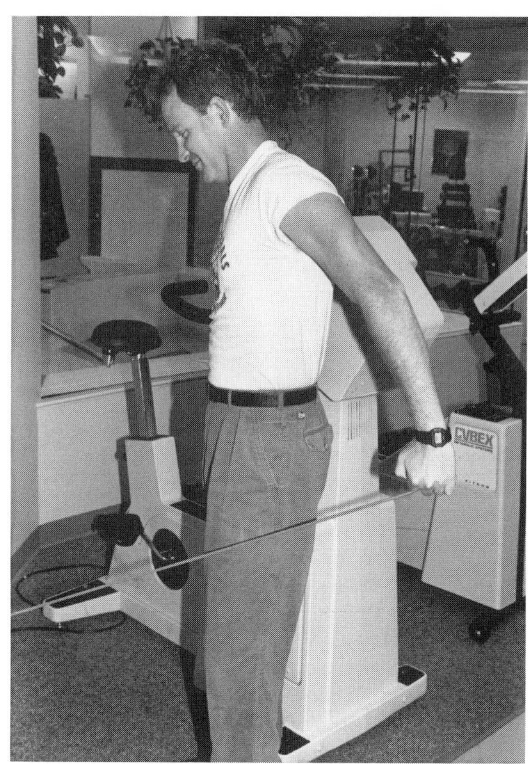


**Figure 8-17.** Resisted shoulder extension tubing movement for the latissimus dorsi and teres major.

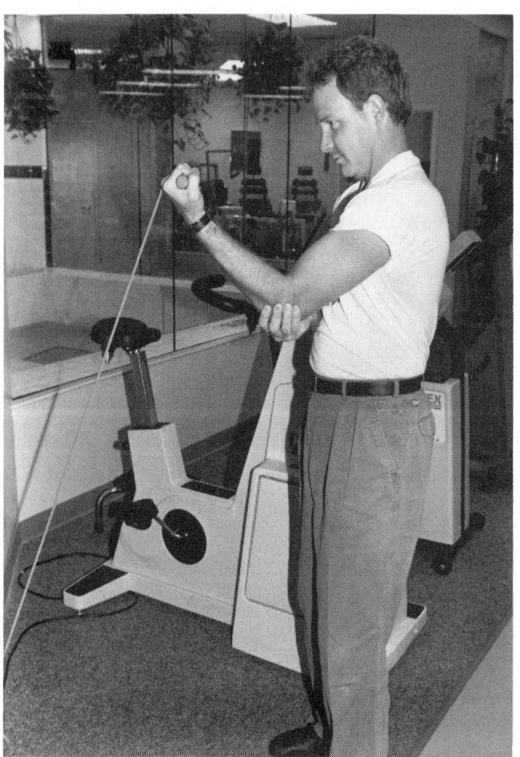

**Figure 8-16.** Biceps brachii strengthening with exercise tubing.

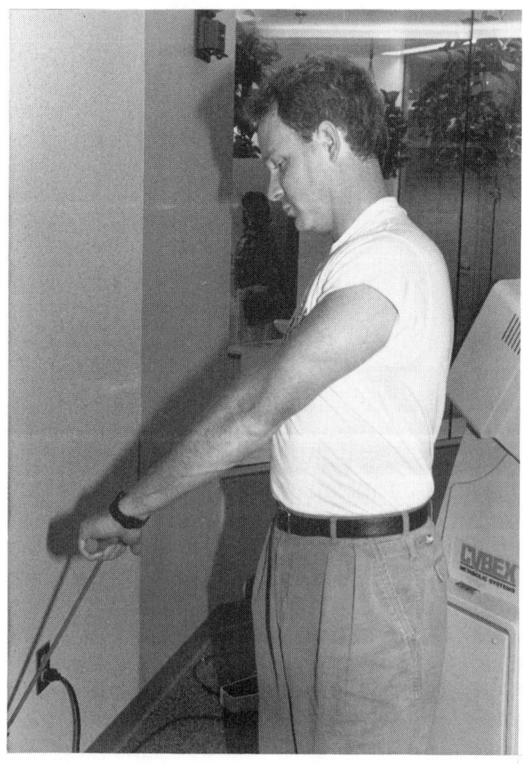


**Figure 8-18.** A D2 flexion PNF movement pattern with exercise tubing start position.

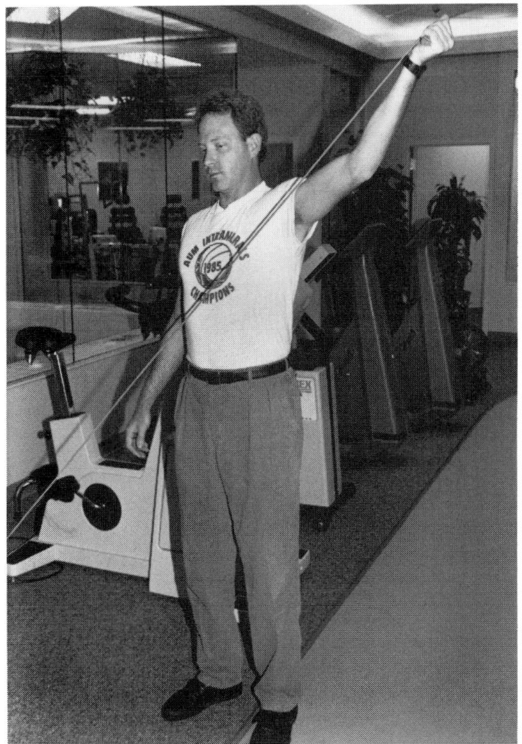

**Figure 8-19.** A D2 flexion PNF movement pattern with exercise tubing end position.

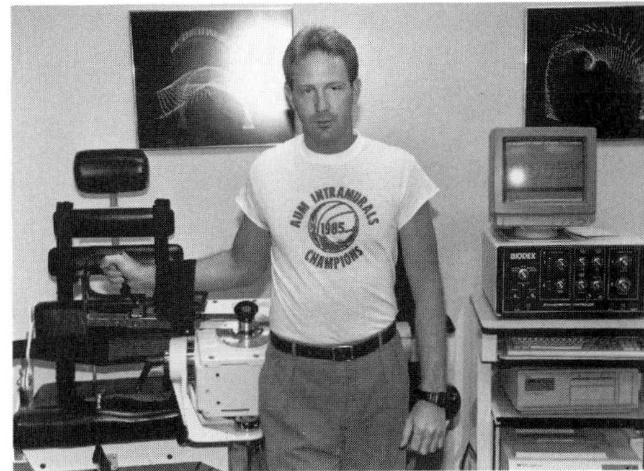

**Figure 8-20.** Isokinetic exercise for shoulder internal/external rotation in the modified neutral position.

while the patient performs tubing D2 flexion/extension patterns to augment the concentric or eccentric contraction as desired. Additionally, rhythmic stabilization can be employed at various points in the range with exercise tubing activities and manual resistance techniques.

## ISOKINETIC REHABILITATION

Isokinetic exercise has been shown to be extremely beneficial for improving muscle strength, power, and endurance through selective-speed training.[2,147,149,150] Additionally, the transition from the phase II intermediate exercises to the more demanding, advanced strengthening exercises used during phase III can be enhanced with the proper use of isokinetic exercise techniques. As outlined previously, submaximal isokinetics for the shoulder rotators in the modified neutral position (Fig. 8-20), progressing to the scapular plane (Fig. 8-21) and, when appropriate, to the 90-degree abducted position (Fig. 8-22), are initiated during the second rehabilitative phase once good dynamic glenohumeral function is attained. Utilizing isokinetics in this manner aids preparation of the upper extremity for the high-speed, high-energy strengthening activities used during this third phase of shoulder rehabilitation.

Isokinetic shoulder rehabilitation incorporates intermediate to functional contractile velocities (120 to 450 degrees/s) for five specific reasons[147]:

1. A majority of functional activities occur at or above these velocities.
2. Joint compressive forces are decreased as the speed of movement increases.
3. Neurophysiologic activity patterning occurs with the morphology of the muscle.
4. These speeds facilitate joint lubrication and decrease synovial fluid viscosity.
5. They can provide a physiologic overflow to slower isokinetic velocities where demands on the musculotendinous unit are greater.

The speed of exercise used initially is the maximal speed at which the patient can engage the machine to produce force without pain. It is from this point that a specific exercise program will be created using a velocity-spectrum reha-

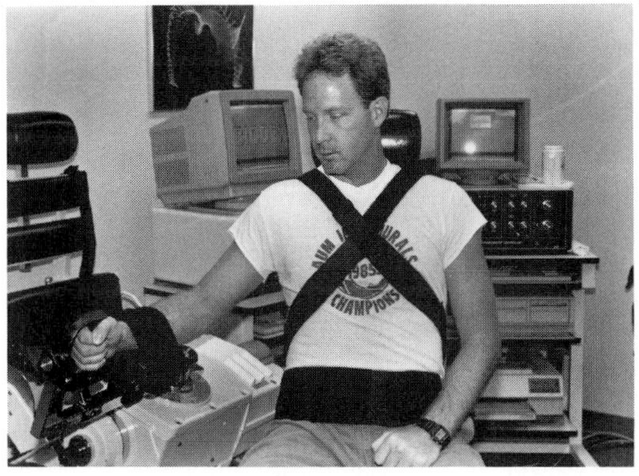

**Figure 8-21.** Isokinetic exercise for shoulder internal/external rotation in the scapular plane/midposition.

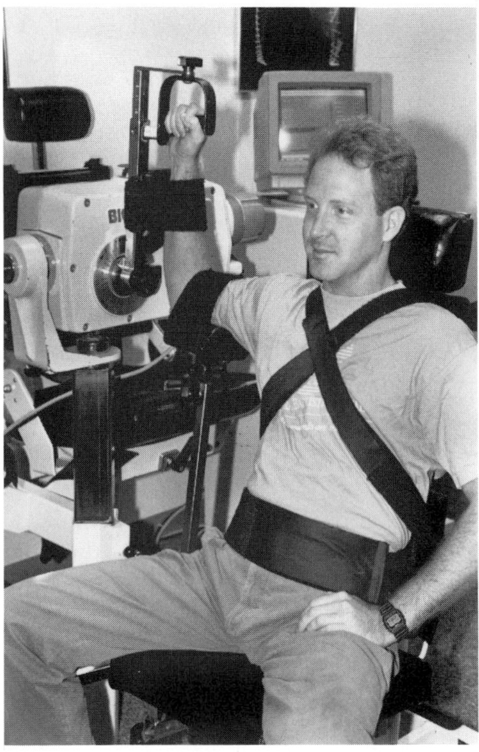

**Figure 8-22.** Isokinetic exercise for the shoulder internal/external rotators in the 90°/90° position.

**Table 8-5**

**Velocity Spectrum Approach to Isokinetic Rehabilitation**

| Intermediate Velocity Spectrum | | | | | | | | | | | |
|---|---|---|---|---|---|---|---|---|---|---|---|
| 120 | 150 | 180 | 210 | 240 | 240 | 210 | 180 | 150 | 120 | | |
| **Fast Velocity Spectrum** | | | | | | | | | | | |
| 180 | 210 | 240 | 270 | 300 | 300 | 270 | 240 | 210 | 180 | | |
| **Functional Velocity Spectrum** | | | | | | | | | | | |
| 300 | 330 | 360 | 390 | 420 | 450 | 450 | 420 | 390 | 360 | 330 | 300 |

*Note:* 10 repetitions are performed at each velocity.

bilitation approach for each activity. It has been suggested that isokinetic exercise training be performed 3 days a week with a day of active rest in between to produce optimal strengthening results.

This velocity-spectrum approach to rehabilitation incorporates the performance of 10 repetitions at each training speed through a spectrum of three to five isokinetic velocities. Table 8-5 outlines the three most commonly used isokinetic velocity spectrums by the authors. The intensity of this exercise activity progresses from submaximal to maximal contractions as allowed by the healing process, patient tolerance, and muscular performance.

Initially, isokinetic exercise programs should be performed concentrically until symptom-free maximal contractions can be elicited. At this time, some therapists use submaximal eccentric isokinetics for the external rotator and biceps musculature in an attempt to replicate the functional demands placed on the glenohumeral complex during repetitive overhead athletic/work activities.[147] Additional safety measures and closer monitoring of mechanical eccentrics are warranted because the forces applied are considerable and associated with strain to tendon tissue. Furthermore, forces are being generated by the isokinetic device and thus are not under the control of the patient, as they are in a concentric mode.

Shoulder internal/external rotation is probably the most commonly performed isokinetic exercise movement. Numerous authors have documented significant torque-value variations by altering the subject's test positions.[54, 57, 62, 122, 133] Soderberg and Blaschek[122] evaluated six test positions and concluded that the internal rotators (IR) exhibited increased torque production in a neutral position (0 to 20 degrees of abduction) and that the external-rotator (ER) torques were increased in both the 90/90 degree and neutral positions. Several investigators[62, 66, 133] have confirmed Soderberg's conclusions regarding IR torque production. Greenfield et al.[54] reported that the ER torque values were higher in the scapular plane versus the frontal plane. Therefore, clinicians must be aware of these significant variations in torque production when the arm position is altered.

In the search for an optimal position in which to test and exercise the shoulder Clark[31] evaluated the inter- and intrarater reliability of the isokinetic measurement of shoulder rotation with the shoulder placed in 45 degrees of abduction and 30 degrees of forward flexion. Justification for selecting this position was based on a review of the literature regarding isokinetics, shoulder anatomy, biomechanics, and pathophysiology. Utilizing this test and exercise position is strongly advocated for many shoulder patients for the following reasons:

This position can be used for isokinetic testing and exercise in patients unable to progress to higher levels of elevation. Scapular plane positioning at 45 degrees reduces tension on the capsuloligamentous complex and rotator cuff in addition to optimizing vascularity of the rotator cuff and avoiding the impingement arc.

The authors advocate using a continuum of IR/ER exercise and testing positions progressing from 0 degrees of shoulder abduction through the scapular plane and finally to the 90/90 degree position (Table 8-6). By using this continuum of exercise, the stability of the glenohumeral joint progresses from a level of maximal stability requiring minimal rotator cuff demands for dynamic stability to one of minimal stability necessitating maximal dynamic muscular stability. Clinicians need to be aware of the potential compromise of the rotator cuff and capsuloligamentous complex that is inherent in the 90/90 degree position. As with any form of exercise, a built-in feedback loop ensures that if symptoms develop at any stage, the activity is regressed to an asymptomatic level and readvanced only when adequate dynamic humeral head stability is achieved.

Additional isokinetic movements that may be beneficial to patient progression include the D2 flexion/extension pattern, shoulder abduction/adduction, shoulder flexion/extension, and elbow flexion/extension.

**Table 8-6**

**IR/ER Rehabilitation Position Continuum**

| Modified neutral |
|---|
| 0° |
| ↓ |
| Scapular plane |
| 45° |
| ↓ |
| 90°/90° |
| Functional position |

## ISOKINETIC SHOULDER TESTING

Isokinetic testing allows the clinician the ability to objectively assess muscular performance in a way that is both safe and reliable using either isolated or combined movement patterns. This objectivity ensures appropriate patient progression or regression, as well as assisting in the determination of functional questions such as, "When can I hit a golf ball?" "begin throwing?" "begin hitting a tennis ball?" or "return to overhead work activities?"

Consequently, isokinetics provide the clinician with objective and reproducible data to monitor patient improvement and plan patient progression. Although objective data are generated, it is critical for clinicians to understand that an isokinetic test is not a functional measure. Its sole purpose is to measure forces produced by the patient while performing specific movements.

To assess the muscular performance characteristics of the shoulder joint, clinicians must consider the positions that most frequently produce the type of injury involved and the demands placed on the shoulder during routine activities. Most commonly, the shoulder is placed at risk of sustaining an injury when elevation, abduction, and rotation are required while performing a wide variety of activities. Examples of these superimposed activities include throwing, tennis, swimming, volleyball, tackling, and a variety of work-related activities, such as painting and maintenance work. In these types of patients, it is recommended that testing and exercising be initiated in the midposition using the scapular plane and then, when appropriate and pain-free, progressing these patients to the 90/90 degree position.

In contrast for the patient who has sustained a shoulder injury involving either the capsule or rotator cuff and who performs only daily activities that do not necessitate repetitive overhead motions, testing is recommended in the plane of scapula only.

Wilk, Arrigo, and Andrews,[149] in identifying inconsistencies in the testing methodology of various published articles, have suggested a standardized isokinetic testing protocol for the shoulder. This standardized isokinetic testing protocol is referred to as the *Thrower's series*. The goal of this type of standardized testing protocol is to improve test-retest reproducibility,[21] as well as allowing clinicians the ability to share test data.[143,149] Clinicians need to be aware of the reliability of any and all protocols they may choose to use for testing the shoulder. There are 14 "variables" that must be standardized and controlled to ensure an objective, reliable, and reproducible isokinetic evaluation of the shoulder[149] (Table 8-7).

The first variable to evaluate is the planes of motion necessary test. In the overhead athlete/industrial worker, it has been reported that the shoulder's internal and external rotators, adductors/abductors, and horizontal abductors/adductors are the most critical motions to assess.[40,41,68,69,101,149] Therefore, isokinetic testing in the thrower's series recommends the evaluation of the shoulder's internal and external rotators, as well as the abductors and adductors.[149] Because isokinetic testing of the horizontal abductors and adductors is performed in either the supine and/or prone positions, these nonfunctional positions are not recommended in the normal testing sequence. In the low-demand shoulder patient, routine tests recommended include modified neutral or scapular plane internal/external rotation and shoulder flexion/extension because of the frequency of these motions during routine daily activities. The testing sequence is specifically standardized with the internal and external rotators always evaluated first, followed by either shoulder abduction/adduction or flexion/extension.

**Table 8-7**

**Standardized Isokinetic Testing Protocol**

1. Planes of motion to evaluate
2. Testing position/stabilization
3. Axis of joint motion
4. Client education
5. Active warmup
6. Gravity compensation
7. Rest intervals
8. Test collateral extremity first
9. Testing environment
   a. Standardized verbal commands
   b. Standardized visual feedback
   c. Free from distractions
   d. Tester skill
10. Testing velocities utilized
11. Test repetitions performed
12. System calibration
13. System level/stabilized
14. Use of windowed data/semihard end stop

It is necessary to test the shoulder in a position that closely resembles its position of function during routine activity while isolating the specific muscle groups involved. To both approximate functional positioning and ensure muscular isolation, most testing is performed in the seated position. This position allows for normal gravitational forces acting on the trunk and upper extremities and enhances glenohumeral joint stabilization. Some isokinetic systems are limited in their design and only allow for certain positions. When it is possible to modify positions, clinicians are encouraged to do so, keeping in mind the need for adequate stabilization and safety. Appropriate stabilization of the trunk, hip, lower extremities, and scapulothoracic joint during isokinetic testing of the shoulder is highly recommended.

The third critical parameter that needs to be addressed is to ensure that the axis of joint motion is aligned with the axis of rotation of the shaft of the dynamometer. Proper alignment is required for accuracy in torque measurement.[143] Although not yet documented for the shoulder, it has been demonstrated that changes in lever arm length of 2.5 in or greater during knee extension/flexion significantly alter torque production.[72,119,127] In testing shoulder abduction/adduction, the axis of the dynamometer should be aligned 1 to 2 cm distal to the acromioclavicular joint. The axis of rotation should be aligned 1 to 2 cm distal to the lateral aspect of the acromion during shoulder flexion/extension testing. In testing the IR/ER, the axis of rotation is aligned through the center of the olecranon and the shaft of the humerus.

The next parameter is to ensure that the subject is informed regarding the purpose and intent of isokinetic testing. The subject should be familiarized with the testing device, how it functions, and what results will be provided. An informed client will be less apprehensive and produce more consistent, reproducible results. Two investigators have demonstrated that subjects with previous isokinetic exposure elicit significantly improved responses during isokinetic testing. Mawdsly and Knapik,[89] in a series of seven test trials, reported significant differences between the torque values of the first testing session and those of the remaining six test trials. Wilk[142] has shown that subjects allowed one practice session prior to testing produced more consistent torque values in 83 to 88 percent of all test trials. Therefore, it is recommended that, whenever possible, clients undergo at least one isokinetic exposure prior to testing.

The fifth testing guideline is the use of an

active warmup prior to isokinetic testing. Although several studies have demonstrated no direct relationship between a warmup and increased isokinetic torque production,[34,139] there is definite basic science research that documents the need for an active warmup from a physiologic basis.[13,15,53,86] Based solely on basic exercise physiology principles, a standardized upper extremity warmup is recommended prior to isokinetic testing of the shoulder. An example of a graded active warmup activity includes a 5-minute upper body ergometer (UBE) session at 90 repetitions per minute at a 60 kg/m work load, as well as 5 submaximal isokinetic repetitions and 1 maximal repetition at each angular test velocity.[89]

The effects of gravity also must be addressed during isokinetic testing, and therefore, gravity compensation of the limb prior to testing is recommended. Significant differences have been shown during isokinetic testing of muscle groups that were gravity compensated when compared with those which were not.[26,51] Although no specific investigations have demonstrated this fact during shoulder testing, it is generally accepted that when gravity compensation is not used, the muscles assisted by gravity will show higher torque values, while the muscles working against gravity will demonstrate significantly smaller torque values. Also, as isokinetic angular velocities increase, so does the relative effect of gravity on torque values.[11,99]

The seventh parameter pertains to controlling the rest interval during testing. This must be addressed to ensure test reproducibility. Ariki et al.[11] have demonstrated that the optimal period of rest between each isokinetic test speed is 90 seconds, and therefore, this amount of rest should be employed during testing.

Testing the uninvolved side first is the next parameter that requires standardization. This serves three important functions:

1. It establishes a baseline of data for the involved side.
2. It evaluates the patient's willingness to be tested.
3. It serves to decrease patient apprehension by allowing exposure to an isokinetic movement on the contralateral extremity first.[33,143]

The testing environment should afford concentration and eliminate distractions. This is the eighth parameter to standardize. A designated room for testing is recommended to isolate the subject and tester from interruptions, distractions, or additional activities that may impede a consistent test trial. When this is not practical, clinicians need to ensure that the testing environment encourages consistent data collection by eliminating any obstacles that might influence test results.

The verbal commands provided each patient should be standardized to enhance test reproducibility. Johansson et al.[70] demonstrated that loud verbal commands resulted in greater isometric torque values when compared with softer verbal commands. This also has been stated empirically during manual resistance techniques.[78] Therefore, it is recommended that verbal commands during isokinetic testing be consistent, encouraging, and moderate in intensity. Perhaps the only practical way to ensure that this variable does not adversely affect reliability is for the clinician conducting the test to be silent during data collection.

The subject's knowledge of torque production results during testing is the third component of the testing environment that needs to be controlled. Several investigators have reported that knowledge of results during strength testing may enhance some parameters of performance.[49,50,58,85,107,131] Therefore, visual feedback in the form of knowledge of results can significantly influence testing performance and must be used consistently or not used at all during isokinetic testing. Since visual feedback has been shown to enhance torque values and promote earlier fatigue, its use is not recommended.[49,143]

The final component of the testing environment is the skill and experience of the examiner. An experienced tester can greatly allay subject apprehension, improve test reproducibility, and maximize the efficiency and efficacy of isokinetic shoulder assessment.

The tenth guideline is the selection of the angular velocities to be used during shoulder testing. Because of the extremely high angular velocities the shoulder obtains during throwing, golf, or tennis,[22,40,41,104] testing at slow isokinetic speeds may be inappropriate and, in fact, may impart undue forces on the glenohumeral joint.[44] Two primary factors need to be considered in choosing the speed at which one tests and exercises the shoulder. First, one must consider the fact that as the speed of contraction decreases, the compressive forces on the joint being tested increase. If the compressive forces are in excess of what the joint can tolerate, the potential for injury is greater. The second important factor to consider is the ability of the person being tested to perform the isokinetic test pain free, thereby ensuring valid assessment of muscle performance. The slower the speed of contraction, the greater the amount of torque produced as a result of an increase in fiber recruitment and neuromuscular response. These two factors are at times directly opposed to each other. However, in nearly all situations, striking a compromise allows one to select a speed that takes into consideration both these factors. Trials on the isokinetic device prior to data collection assist in determining which speeds are most appropriate. First and foremost, the speed selected should be comfortable in that it does not produce pain within the joint or joint-related structures. This will assist in determining if the speed selected causes potential harm to the shoulder. In light of these facts, it is recommended that testing be performed at angular velocities ranging from 90 to 450 degrees/s.

The number of repetitions performed during isokinetic shoulder testing also requires standardization. Davies[34] has noted previously that 10 isokinetic repetitions elicit an optimal training effect for both peak torque and average power parameters. Based on this observation, isokinetic evaluation of the shoulder is performed by us using 10 repetitions at 180 degrees/s, 15 repetitions at 300 degrees/s, and 10 repetitions at 450 degrees/s. We have demonstrated that peak torque for both internal and external rotation, as well as abduction and adduction, of the shoulder is produced during the second or third test repetition in 96 percent of all cases. However, 10 to 15 test repetitions are used during isokinetic shoulder testing to ensure the optimal assessment of total work and average power parameters.

The twelfth parameter to consider is the importance of isokinetic system calibration. Although most manufacturers recommend calibration every 30 days to ensure validity in testing measures, it is recommended that calibration of the testing system be conducted every 2 weeks.

The next guideline is to ensure that the isokinetic system is level and stabilized to the floor. A level and stable system will minimize the interference of artifact, overshoot, and oscillation during testing. Each of these abnormal recordings may lead to misinterpretation of test data, especially during shoulder abduction/adduction and flexion/extension testing.[146, 149, 150]

The fourteenth and final parameter concerns data collection during isokinetic testing of the shoulder. During shoulder abduction/adduction and flexion/extension testing, there exists the potential for a tremendous amount of end-stop oscillation and torque-curve spiking.[146, 150] These undesired torque spikes are produced by combining the long lever arm, high test speeds, and large torque values demonstrated during testing with an abrupt terminal endpoint. Any abrupt endpoint results in the spiking of the torque-curve graph far beyond the actual values produced.

Clinicians can control this troublesome factor by using a semihard (firm) end stop and windowing the isokinetic data collection during shoulder abduction/adduction testing. An end stop is used to cushion the end range and decelerate the lever arm during testing. A "firm" or semihard end stop results when the end-stop control is turned one-quarter turn from the hard end point. This type of end stop minimizes the excessive deceleration produced by a soft end stop, as well as the abrupt endpoint oscillation that occurs during testing with a hard end stop.[150] End-stop oscillation is also smoothed by windowing the test results, ensuring that any test data not obtained at the preset isokinetic test speed or at 95 percent of that speed will not be recorded.

The 14 components outlined in this testing protocol are presented so that clinicians are aware of all the variables that need to be controlled to ensure reliability in isokinetic testing. The thrower's series[31] assists in providing a framework on which to design a clinically functional, activity-specific, and consistent means of evaluating the shoulder isokinetically. The test protocol advocated by Clark[31] has yielded high levels of inter- and intrarater reliability (ICC = 0.88–0.99) and may be used as an alternative position for testing or exercising in patients who are symptomatic in higher degrees of elevation. Clinicians often must develop their own testing protocol given the specific isokinetic device they may have and the limitations their individual clinic presents. Their development of a specific protocol needs to be in recognition of the aforementioned principles, and they must maintain a consistent format for testing and exercising.

## INTERPRETATION OF TEST DATA

A copious amount of data are generated from an isokinetic evaluation of the shoulder. These data can be divided into three broad subtopics, including torque parameters, acceleration and deceleration characteristics, and muscular performance parameters. Each of these will be discussed and their relevance to test interpretation considered.

*Torque* can be defined as force times the perpendicular distance from the axis of rotation.

The term *peak torque*, therefore, expresses a single repetition event that is the highest point on the graph regardless of where it occurs in the range of motion.[33] The average torque of all the test repetitions performed during one set is referred to as the *mean peak torque*. Mean peak torque values ultimately may prove to be more valuable information regarding muscular performance than any single repetition peak torque value.

The test parameter referred to as *time rate to torque development* (TRTD) is an example of an acceleration parameter. This test parameter represents how quickly the subject can generate torque. The TRTD can be expressed as a factor of time, such as TRTD at 0.2 s, or as a factor of joint position, such as at any specific joint angle or predetermined torque value. This test parameter is beneficial in determining the acceleration capability of the shoulder's internal rotators when testing overhead athletes.

The next test parameter to consider is the *force decay rate* of the torque curve or the *deceleration capability* of the muscle group. On torque curve observation it should appear straight or slightly convex. A torque curve whose force decay rate is concave indicates an inability or difficulty in producing force near the end range of motion.

The next area of data interpretation is classified as *muscular performance parameters*, including total work, average power, and muscular endurance characteristics.[142] *Total work* is defined as torque times an arc of movement. It represents the volume of area contained under the entire torque curve. The term *maximum work repetition* is simply the one repetition during which the maximum amount of work occurred. *Average power* is torque times an arc of movement divided by time, or work divided by time. This parameter is represented in watts. Both work and power also can be expressed in relation to body weight, such as with work-to-body-weight ratios. Additionally, work can be expressed as the amount of work performed in the first third and the last third of a testing set. *Work fatigue percentage*, then, is the ratio of change between the amount of work performed during the first third and the last third of any test.

This vast amount of data creates a paradoxical situation for the clinician—how to effectively and accurately interpret the information available. There are three commonly used parameters for data interpretation of the shoulder. These are (1) bilateral data comparison, (2) unilateral data comparison, and (3) torque-to-body ratios. The current published literature has produced a significant amount of controversy in data comparison. This confusion can be attributed to the inconsistencies in the test positions used and the significant differences demonstrated between results gathered on various testing devices.[52,55,128,143,149] It is important for the clinician to remember that results of isokinetic testing cannot be compared directly from one device or system to another device or system.

Regarding the bilateral comparison of dominant versus nondominant shoulder peak torque, we have reported the results of isokinetic testing in 150 professional baseball pitchers.[145,146,150] Table 8-8 highlights the results regarding the bilateral mean peak torque comparisons of shoulder ER/IR and abductor/adductor testing.[145,146] During ER/IR testing, the throwing shoulder was shown to be equal to the nonthrowing shoulder. Although no significant peak torque differences were exhibited during shoulder abductor testing, the throwing shoulder's adductors were found to be significantly stronger at both test speeds, 180 and 300 degrees/s.[146]

Unilateral muscle ratios demonstrate the balance between the agonist and antagonist muscle groups. Several investigators have published data regarding ER/IR ratios for the shoulder.[2,33,66,145] Ivey et al.[66] reported a ratio of 66 percent at 60, 180, and 300 degrees/s. Cook[2] demonstrated an ER/IR ratio of 70 percent at 180 and 300 degrees/s on the throwing shoulder and a ratio of 83 and 87 percent at the respective test speeds for the nonthrowing shoulder. Similarly, Wilk et al.[145] described a throwing shoulder ER/IR ratio of 65 percent at 180 degrees/s, 61 percent at 300 degrees/s, and 64 and 70 percent, respectively, for the nonthrowing shoulder. Davies[33] reported a ratio of 66.6 percent at 60 and 300 degrees/s. The unilateral muscle ratio for the shoulder abductors/adductors has been reported at 2:1 by two authors.[2,66] Wilk et al.[146] found the abduction/adduction ratio for the dominant shoulder (throwing shoulder) to be 83 and 94 percent at 180 and 300 degrees/s, respectively. The nondominant shoulder abduction/adduction muscular ratios were 66 and 70 percent at the reported test speeds.[146]

The last torque parameter expressed in the literature is the ratio of torque to body weight. This parameter may actually prove more valuable in data interpretation because of the constant comparison to body weight as an nonfluctuating standard within the side being evaluated. Alderink and Kuck[2] demonstrated no significant difference in the peak torque-to-body-weight

**Table 8-8**

**Comparison of Mean Peak Torque ± SD (ft-lb) Between Dominant (D) and Nondominant (ND) Throwing Arms**

| | $n = 150$ | | | |
|---|---|---|---|---|
| | External Rotation | | Internal Rotation | |
| Test Speed | D, ft-lb | ND, ft-lb | D, ft-lb | ND, ft-lb |
| 180°/s | 34.5 ± 6.2 | 36.5 ± 6.8* | 53.9 ± 8.8 | 52.4 ± 9.5 |
| 300°/s | 29.3 ± 5.1 | 30.1 ± 6.3 | 49.0 ± 8.5 | 48.0 ± 10.4 |
| | $n = 59$ | | | |
| | Abduction | | Adduction | |
| Test Speed | D, ft-lb | ND, ft-lb | D, ft-lb | ND, ft-lb |
| 180°/s | 56.1 ± 12.5 | 58.6 ± 9.7 | 68.1 ± 12.6 | 62.5 ± 10.5* |
| 300°/s | 40.3 ± 15.7 | 38.4 ± 14.7 | 61.0 ± 12.5 | 54.6 ± 13.2* |

*Statistically significant difference ($p < 0.05$) between respective pairs.

ratios for the shoulder ER/IR and abductors/adductors. Davies[33] reported torque-to-body-weight ratios for the abductors/adductors in males and females at 60 degrees/s. These ratios were shown to be 25 percent for the abductors and 39 percent for the adductors in males, with female ratios being approximately 10 percent less than these values. We have been involved in two studies that assessed the peak torque-to-body-weight ratios of the shoulder's ER/IR and abductors/adductors.[145,146] The results of these investigations are highlighted in Table 8-9.

Because the isokinetic muscular performance parameters among various sports, age and skill levels, and pathologic conditions differ, descriptive data from several authors regarding tennis players[30,42,43,76,100] and swimmers are included in Tables 8-10, 8-11, and 8-12. These data are intended to assist the reader in interpreting isokinetic shoulder test data in various overhead athletic populations.

**Table 8-9**

**Comparison of Mean Peak Torque-to-Body-Weight Ratios Between Dominant (D) and Nondominant (ND) Throwing Arms**

| | $n = 150$ | | | |
|---|---|---|---|---|
| | External Rotation | | Internal Rotation | |
| Test Speed | D, % | ND, % | D, % | ND, % |
| 180°/s | 17.5 ± 2.9 | 18.7 ± 3.3* | 26.9 ± 4.3 | 26.5 ± 4.3 |
| 300°/s | 14.9 ± 2.4 | 15.1 ± 2.6 | 25.3 ± 7.3 | 24.4 ± 4.7 |
| | $n = 59$ | | | |
| | Abduction | | Adduction | |
| Test Speed | D, % | ND, % | D, % | ND, % |
| 180°/s | 28.0 ± 4.7 | 29.0 ± 4.9 | 34.0 ± 6.4 | 31.0 ± 5.8 |
| 300°/s | 20.0 ± 7.8 | 19.0 ± 7.2 | 30.0 ± 6.4 | 27.0 ± 6.6 |

*Statistically significant difference ($p < 0.05$) between respective pairs.

**Table 8-10**

### Isokinetic Muscular Performance Data of Collegiate Tennis Players

| | 60°/s | 180°/s | 210°/s |
|---|---|---|---|
| Males | | | |
| Eccentric PT/BW ratio ER | 80 | 80 | 77 |
| Eccentric PT/BW ratio IR | 99 | 91 | 96 |
| Concentric PT/BW ratio ER | 43 | 41 | 40 |
| Concentric PT/BW ratio IR | 59 | 49 | 50 |
| ER/IR ratio concentric | 59 | 49 | 50 |
| ER/IR ration eccentric | 84 | 92 | 81 |
| Ecc/conc ratio ER | 202 | 206 | 202 |
| Ecc/conc ratio IR | 183 | 202 | 201 |
| Females | | | |
| Eccentric PT/BW ER | 46 | 47 | 46 |
| Eccentric PT/BW IR | 56 | 56 | 57 |
| Concentric PT/BW ER | 25 | 22 | 22 |
| Concentric PT/BW IR | 34 | 27 | 25 |
| ER/IR eccentric | 87 | 93 | 89 |
| ER/IR concentric | 80 | 82 | 89 |
| Ecc/conc ratio ER | 103 | 107 | 119 |
| Ecc/conc ratio IR | 123 | 143 | 173 |

From Ellenbecker TS. Eccentric and concentric isokinetic strength characteristics of the rotator cuff. Annual American Physical Therapy Assoc. Meeting, Boston, Mass., 1991.

We have identified 11 key parameters for routine evaluation during the interpretation of an isokinetic shoulder evaluation. These parameters include

1. External rotator torque-body-weight ratios
2. Internal rotator torque-body-weight ratios
3. Bilateral external rotator comparisons
4. Bilateral internal rotator comparisons
5. External rotator/internal rotator ratios
6. Internal rotator acceleration (TRTD)

**Table 8-11**

### Isokinetic Muscular Performance Data of Collegiate Tennis Players

| | Dominant | | Nondominant | |
|---|---|---|---|---|
| | 60°/s | 300°/s | 60°/s | 300°/s |
| Internal rotation (PT) | 30 | 21 | 24 | 16 |
| External rotation (PT) | 18 | 13 | 17 | 11 |
| IR torque/body weight | 20 | 13 | 15 | 10 |
| ER torque/body weight | 12 | 8 | 11 | 7 |
| ER/IR | 61 | 65 | 70 | 69 |

From Chandler TJ, Kibler WB, Straccner EC, et al. Shoulder strength, power, and endurance in college tennis players. Am J Sports Med 1992;20(4):455.

**Table 8-12**

### Isokinetic Muscular Performance Data of Scholastic Swimmers

| | 120°/s | | | 180°/s | | |
|---|---|---|---|---|---|---|
| | IR | ER | ER/IR | IR | ER | ER/IR |
| Pretraining | 36 | 20 | 57% | 32 | 19 | 58% |
| Post 3-week training program | 42 | 32 | 75% | 41 | 30 | 73% |

*Note:* All values expressed represent peak torque in footpounds.
From Murphy TS, unpublished data, 1993.

7. Abductor torque-body-weight ratios
8. Adductor torque-body-weight ratios
9. Bilateral abductor comparisons
10. Bilateral adductor comparisons
11. Abductor/adductor ratios

Table 8-13 illustrates the acceptable percentile ranges for torque-to-body-weight ratios of the shoulder's external rotators (ER), internal rotators (IR), abductors (Abd), and adductors (Add). The ranges used to interpret bilateral shoulder comparisons are provided in Table 8-14. The unilateral muscle ratio test interpretation parameters for the ER/IR and Abd/Add ratios are outlined in Table 8-15. Additionally, the parameter of internal rotator acceleration is assessed by measuring the percentage of peak torque occurring at 0.2 s. Optimally, this time rate to torque development measure should be 90 percent of the total peak torque for internal rotation.

There exist several pitfalls that should be avoided when performing an isokinetic shoulder test. First, all testing should be performed in the identical position, at the same speeds, and using the same testing protocol, because when the test position or protocol is altered, the test results will be significantly affected.[21,31,143,149] The second pitfall is basing the data interpretation solely on bilateral peak torque comparisons to determine a patient's progress.[142,143] The review of the

**Table 8-13**

### Isokinetic Test Interpretation for Torque-to-Body-Weight Ratios

| | 180°/s | 300°/s |
|---|---|---|
| ER | 18–23% | 15–20% |
| IR | 27–33% | 25–30% |
| Abd | 26–32% | 20–26% |
| Add | 32–36% | 28–33% |

**Table 8-14**

**Isokinetic Test Interpretation for Bilateral Comparison Parameters**

| | 180°/s | 300°/s | 450°/s |
|---|---|---|---|
| ER | 98–105% | 85–95% | 90–100% |
| IR | 105–120% | 100–115% | 100–110% |
| Abd | 100–110% | 100–110% | — |
| Add | 120–135% | 115–130% | — |

literature presented in this chapter illustrates that bilateral comparisons are inconsistent and specifically altered by the test position used. The next pitfall is relying on torque-curve shapes to determine various pathologies. In our experience, after several hundred preoperative tests, specific torque-curve variations are not consistently generated by any specific shoulder pathology. Fourth, one cannot rely solely on peak torque measurements to determine a patient's status. Power, work, and time parameters must be considered to effectively determine muscular performance. The next potential pitfall occurs when clinicians fail to realize that this is not the only test. Clinicians must rely on their clinical examinations, functional tests, and ancillary special tests to assist in determining the overall condition of the shoulder. Lastly, the tester should window all test data to prevent misinterpretation from test artifact, oscillation, and overshoots.

This section on isokinetics has outlined the important variables and considerations that clinicians need to keep foremost in their minds when utilizing isokinetics with shoulder patients.

## PLYOMETRICS

Plyometric drills are also initiated during the advanced phase. *Plyometric drills* refer to quick, powerful movements involving a prestretch of the muscle, thereby activating the muscular stretch-shortening cycle.[14,23,151,152] Thus plyometrics are designed to increase the excitability of the neurologic receptors for improved reactivity of the neuromuscular system.[152] Adaptations of these plyometric principles can be used to enhance the specificity of training in any sport or activity that requires a maximum amount of muscular force in a minimal amount of time. These stretch-shortening drills also can be employed to enhance the amount of neuromuscular coordination in the unstable shoulder joint. All movements in competitive athletics involve a repeated series of stretch-shortening muscular contraction cycles.[71] This is especially true for the upper extremity athlete, such as the thrower, who relies on the prestretch of the internal rotators and adductors during the cocking phase prior to a concentric contraction of these muscles during the acceleration phase of throwing. This also applies to other overhead athletes, such as the tennis player, swimmer, and golfer, all of whom rely on the stretch-shortening cycle for arm speed and powerful, forceful movements.

The neurophysiologic basis of plyometric exercise incorporates the elastic and reactive properties of the muscle to generate maximal force during exercise performance.[14,23,151,152] This is accomplished in three phases: the eccentric or setting phase, the amortization phase, and the concentric response phase. The eccentric phase increases the muscle spindle activity, causing a prestretch of the muscle group being exercised. The second phase of the plyometric response is the amortization phase, which is the amount of time between the initiation of the yielding eccentric contraction and the beginning of the concentric contraction. The final phase of any plyometric exercise is the concentric response phase. This is the resulting contraction from the eccentric preloading of the muscle(s). An entire plyometric program for the upper extremity can be found in Table 8-16. A complete description of these exercises can be found in a paper by Wilk et al.[151] These plyometric exercises can be performed using a Plyoball and exercise tubing.

An example a plyometric drill for the shoulder's external rotators using exercise tubing is outlined. The subject starts with the arm in maximal external rotation and then slowly releases the isometric hold, allowing the arm to move into internal rotation (eccentric preloading phase). When the arm reaches horizontal (or 0 degrees of rotation), a quick concentric movement is performed, reversing the arm position into external rotation. This type of plyometric movement also can be performed for the internal rotators, biceps brachii, and D2 diagonal movement pattern.

Additional plyometric movements and drills can be performed with a Plyoball and Plyoback (Functionally Integrated Technology, Dublan,

**Table 8-15**

**Isokinetic Test Interpretation for Unilateral Muscle Ratios**

| | 180°/s | 300°/s | 450°/s |
|---|---|---|---|
| ER/IR | 63–70% | 65–72% | 62–70% |
| Abd/add | 82–87% | 92–97% | — |

**Table 8-16**

**Plyometric Drills for the Upper Extremity**

I. Warmup exercises
  - Med ball rotation
  - Med ball side bends
  - Med ball wood chops
  - Tubing ER/IR
  - Tubing diagonal pattern ($D_2$)
  - Tubing biceps
  - Push-ups

II. Throwing movements
  - Med ball soccer throw
  - Med ball chest pass
  - Med ball step and pass
  - Med ball side throw
  - Tubing plyos IR/ER
  - Tubing plyos diagonals
  - Tubing plyos biceps
  - Plyos push-ups (boxes)
  - Plyos (clappers)

III. Medicine ball wall exercises
  - Soccer throw
  - Chest pass
  - Side-to-side throw
  - Backward side-to-side throw
  - Forward two-hand through legs
  - One-hand baseball throw

Calif.). These movements include a two-handed overhead soccer throw (Fig. 8-23a), chest pass (Fig. 8-23b), baseball throw (Fig. 8-23c), and side-to-side throw[151] (Fig. 8-23d).

These plyometric drills and exercises provide the athlete with a functional progression toward unrestricted, sport-specific movements, such as throwing, tennis, and/or golf. These dynamic, high-energy exercises prepare the shoulder musculature for the microtraumatic stresses applied during most sporting and functional activities.

The specific criteria a patient must exhibit to progress from phase III to phase IV in the rehabilitation process are

1. Full, nonpainful ROM
2. No pain or tenderness on clinical examination
3. Satisfactory muscular strength, power, and endurance based on functional demands
4. A satisfactory clinical examination

## Phase IV: Return-to-Activity Exercises

The last phase of the rehabilitation program is the return-to-activity phase. The patient is encouraged to continue specific exercises to address any remaining strength deficits and to improve the muscular strength related to functional demands. In addition, the patient will initiate a progressive, gradual return to unrestricted functional activities using a controlled program specific to his or her individual needs.

For the athletic population, an interval sporting program must be initiated (Tables 8-17 and 8-18). The purpose of this type of interval program is to progressively and systematically increase the demands placed on the shoulder while performing the patient's intended sporting activity. For the throwing athlete, the number and types of throws, distance, and intensity, are monitored and progressed to facilitate a successful return to competition. This type of progressive activity can be adapted and outlined for any functional athletic rehabilitation program. For the overhead industrial patient, a gradual progression to strenuous work activities also would be extremely beneficial and may facilitate a successful return to symptom-free work endeavors.

# Postoperative Rehabilitative Considerations

This section is designed to apply the four-phased, criteria-based rehabilitation program previously outlined to specific rotator cuff surgical procedures. The aim is not to provide a "cook book" rehabilitative method but to apply the specific indications, precautions, and contraindications associated with the postoperative management of shoulder pathology. Individualized adaptations and alterations in the generalized rehabilitation guidelines will be specifically addressed for the procedures described.

## Mini-Open Rotator Cuff Repair

This type of surgical procedure uses a small deltoid-splitting incision that permits repair of the rotator cuff defect while minimizing trauma to the shoulder joint and deltoid in particular. The total length of the rehabilitation program will vary based on the severity of the tear, acute versus chronic condition, tissue status, strength and range of motion prior to surgery, age and general health of the patient, and the performance and activity demands to which the patient wishes to return. The most significant factors

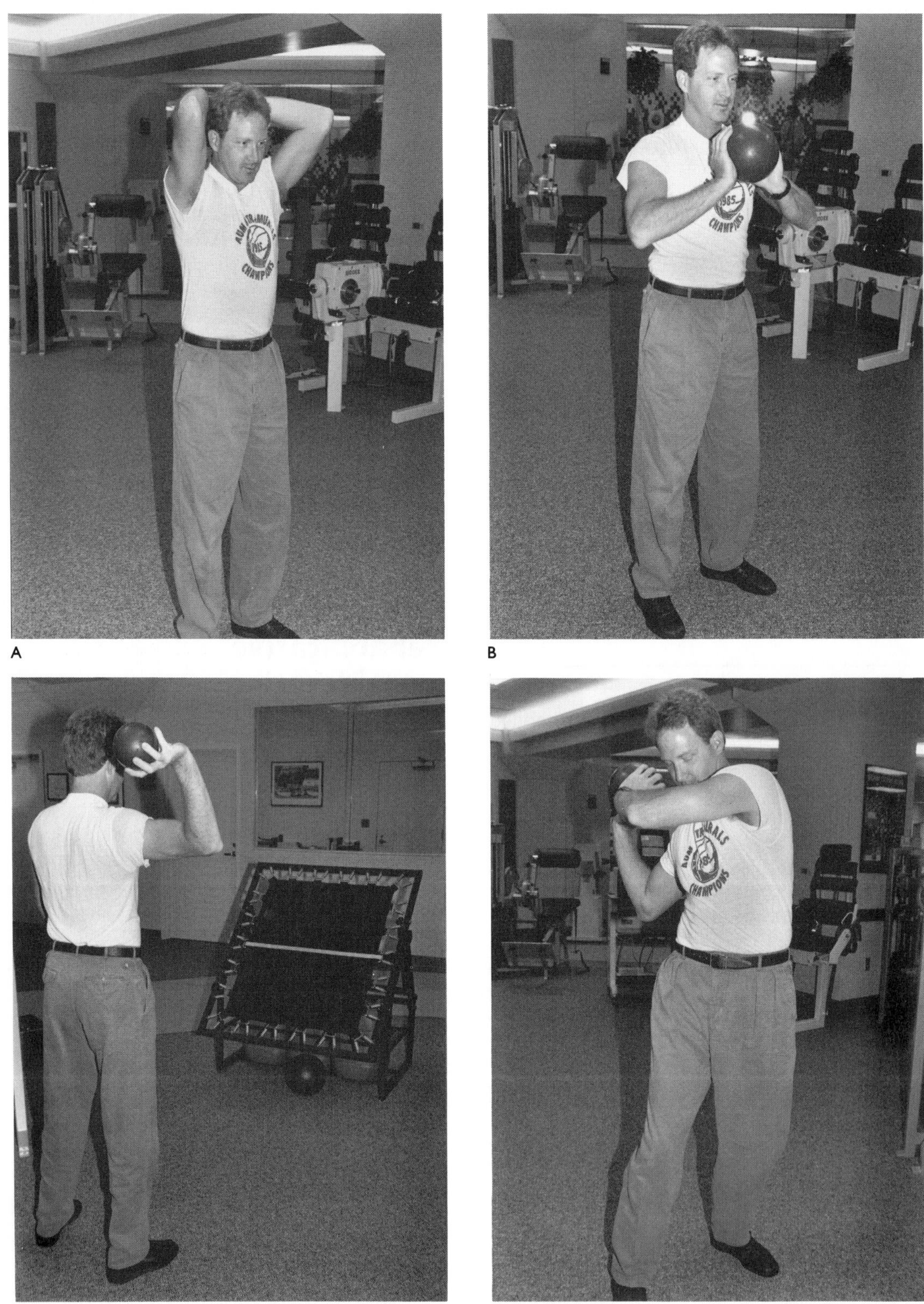


**Figure 8-23.** (a) Plyometric drill: two-hand overhead soccer throw in standing using a Plyoball and Plyoback. (b) Plyometric drill: two-hand chest pass. (c) Plyometric drill: one-hand baseball throw. (d) Plyometric drills: a side-to-side throw with trunk rotation.

**Table 8-17**

**Interval Throwing Program, Phase I**

| 45-ft Phase | 90-ft Phase | 150-ft Phase | 180-ft Phase |
|---|---|---|---|
| Step 1:<br>a. Warmup throwing<br>b. 45 ft (25 throws)<br>c. Rest 15 minutes<br>d. Warmup throwing<br>e. 45 ft (25 throws) | Step 5:<br>a. Warmup throwing<br>b. 90 ft (25 throws)<br>c. Rest 15 minutes<br>d. Warmup throwing<br>e. 90 ft (25 throws) | Step 9:<br>a. Warmup throwing<br>b. 150 ft (25 throws)<br>c. Rest 15 minutes<br>d. Warmup throwing<br>f. 150 ft (25 throws) | Step 11:<br>a. Warmup throwing<br>b. 180 ft (25 throws)<br>c. Rest 15 minutes<br>d. Warmup throwing<br>e. 180 ft (25 throws) |
| Step 2:<br>a. Warmup throwing<br>b. 45 ft (25 throws)<br>c. Rest 10 minutes<br>d. Warmup throwing<br>e. 45 ft (25 throws)<br>f. Rest 10 minutes<br>g. Warmup throwing<br>h. 45 ft (25 throws) | Step 6:<br>a. Warmup throwing<br>b. 90 ft (25 throws)<br>c. Rest 10 minutes<br>d. Warmup throwing<br>e. 90 ft (25 throws)<br>f. Rest 10 minutes<br>g. Warmup throwing<br>h. 90 ft (25 throws) | Step 10:<br>a. Warmup throwing<br>b. 150 ft (25 throws)<br>c. Rest 10 minutes<br>d. Warmup throwing<br>e. 150 ft (25 throws)<br>f. Rest 10 minutes<br>g. Warmup throwing<br>h. 150 ft (25 throws) | Step 12:<br>a. Warmup throwing<br>b. 180 ft (25 throws)<br>c. Rest 10 minutes<br>d. Warmup throwing<br>e. 180 ft (25 throws)<br>f. Rest 10 minutes<br>g. Warmup throwing<br>h. 180 ft (25 throws) |
| **60-ft Phase** | **120-ft Phase** | | Step 13:<br>a. Warmup throwing<br>b. 180 ft (25 throws)<br>c. Rest 10 minutes<br>d. Warmup throwing<br>e. 180 ft (25 throws)<br>f. Rest 10 minutes<br>g. Warmup throwing<br>h. 180 ft (25 throws) |
| Step 3:<br>a. Warmup throwing<br>b. 60 ft (25 throws)<br>c. Rest 15 minutes<br>d. Warmup throwing<br>e. 60 ft (25 throws) | Step 7:<br>a. Warmup throwing<br>b. 120 ft (25 throws)<br>c. Rest 15 minutes<br>d. Warmup throwing<br>e. 120 ft (25 throws) | | Step 14:<br>Begin throwing off the mound or return to respective position |
| Step 4:<br>a. Warmup throwing<br>b. 60 ft (25 throws)<br>c. Rest 10 minutes<br>d. Warmup throwing<br>e. 60 ft (25 throws)<br>f. Rest 10 minutes<br>g. Warmup throwing<br>h. 60 ft (25 throws) | Step 8:<br>a. Warmup throwing<br>b. 120 ft (25 throws)<br>c. Rest 10 minutes<br>d. Warmup throwing<br>e. 120 ft (25 throws)<br>f. Rest 10 minutes<br>g. Warmup throwing<br>h. 120 ft (25 throws) | | |

that guide the rehabilitation restrictions initially is the tissue status and the size of the rotator cuff tear. These tears can be classified into four groups: small (<1 cm), medium (1 to 3 cm), large (3 to 5 cm), and massive (>5 cm). The rehabilitation program following rotator cuff repair surgery is subdivided into three types of guidelines depending on the size of the tear repaired. A type I rehabilitative format is used when small tears are repaired, a type II program is used for medium tears, and large to massive tears are treated under type III guidelines (Tables 8-19, 8-20, and 8-21). Because the mini-open procedure provides limited exposure of the rotator cuff, only small to large tears may be repaired in this manner, and the massive tear treated under the type III guidelines requires full open exposure for adequate repair and therefore slower rehabilitation progression.

## TYPE I

Rehabilitation following type I mini-open rotator cuff repairs includes an immediate postoperative phase of 0 to 3 weeks. Initially, a sling is used for comfort during the first 1 to 2 weeks. Pendulum and active assisted range-of-motion exercises for the shoulder flexors and external/internal rotators in 0 degrees of abduction are performed initially to tolerance. Additionally, submaximal pain-free shoulder isometrics are also incorporated for strengthening, and local modalities are used as necessary. The 3- to 6-week time frame following this type of surgical repair advances active assisted range-of-motion exercises for the external/internal rotators to 45 degrees of abduction. Also, surgical tubing exercises are used for these same motions, and humeral head stabilization activities are emphasized. Scapula strengthening exercises are also initiated during this time

**Table 8-18**

**Interval Throwing Program, Phase II**

**Stage one: Fastball only**

Step 1:
- Interval throwing
- 15 Throws off mound 50%

Step 2:
- Interval throwing
- 30 Throws off mound 50%

Step 3:
- Interval throwing
- 45 Throws off mound 50%

Step 4:
- Interval throwing
- 60 Throws off mound 50%

Step 5:
- Interval throwing
- 30 Throws off mound 75%

Step 6:
- 30 Throws off mound 75%
- 45 Throws off mound 50%

Step 7:
- 45 Throws off mound 75%
- 15 Throws off mound 50%

Step 8:
- 60 Throws off mound 75%

(Use interval throwing to 120-ft phase as warmup.)

(All throwing off the mount should be done in the presence of your pitching coach to stress proper throwing mechanics.)

(Use speed gun to aid in effort control.)

**Stage two: Fastball Only**

Step 9:
- 45 Throws off mound 75%
- 15 Throws in batting practice

Step 10:
- 45 Throws off mound 75%
- 30 Throws in batting practice

Step 11:
- 45 Throws off mound 75%
- 45 Throws in batting practice

**Stage three**

Step 12:
- 30 Throws off mound 75% warmup
- 15 Throws off mound 50% breaking balls
- 45–60 Throws in batting practice (fastball only)

Step 13:
- 30 Throws off mound 75%
- 30 Breaking balls 75%
- 30 Throws in batting practice

Step 14:
- 30 Throws off mound 75%
- 60–90 Throws in batting practice 25% breaking balls

Step 15:
- Simulated game: progressing by 15 throws per workout

frame. Intermediate-phase exercises are incorporated from 7 to 12 weeks following this type I surgical repair. Active assisted external/internal rotation range of motion is advanced to 90 degrees of abduction 6 weeks following surgery. Full range of motion is desired between 8 and 10 weeks postoperatively. During this timetable, neuromuscular strengthening, shoulder isotonics, and upper body endurance activities are also initiated. The advanced strengthening phase normally ranges from 13 to 21 weeks after surgery. It is characterized by exercises to maintain full, nonpainful range of motion, improve shoulder complex strength and power, and allow a progressive gradual return to activities.

## TYPE II

Type II rotator cuff repairs are immobilized following surgery for the first 3 weeks in either a sling or an abduction brace according to the physician's direction. If an abduction brace is used, it is normally placed in 45 degrees of abduction and 0 degrees of rotation. Exercises incorporated initially following this type of repair include elbow/hand range-of-motion and strengthening exercises. Also included are active assisted shoulder activities, including flexion to tolerance and internal/external rotation in 30 to 45 degrees of abduction. Pain-free submaximal shoulder and elbow isometrics are also initiated immediately following this type of surgery for all major planes of motion. Seven to 14 weeks following these type II repairs, patients are advancing from the immediate motion to the intermediate phase. Exercise activities during this time frame are characterized by the initiation of internal/external rotation range-of-motion exercises in 90 degrees of abduction 6 weeks following surgery. Also, scapular strengthening, humeral head stabilization exercises, and shoulder isotonics are initiated as appropriate. Full range of motion is desired following these type II rotator cuff repairs between 10 and 12 weeks postoperatively. The rehabilitation guidelines for weeks 15 to 26 following this type of procedure include the continuation of all active assisted range-of-mo-

**Table 8-19**

**Type I Rotator Cuff Repair (Deltoid Splitting), Small Tear (less than 1 cm)**

I. **Phase I: Protective phase** (weeks 0–6)
  Goals: 1. Gradual return to full ROM
    2. Increase shoulder strength
    3. Decrease pain
  A. Weeks 0–3
    1. Sling for comfort (1–2 weeks)
    2. Pendulum exercises
    3. Active assisted ROM exercises (L-bar exercises)
    4. Rope and pulley for flexion (only)
    5. Elbow ROM, hand gripping
    6. Isometrics (submaximal, subpainful isometrics)
      a. Abductors
      b. External rotators
      c. Internal rotators
      d. Elbow flexors
      e. Shoulder flexors
    7. Pain control modalities (ice, high-voltage galvanic stimulation)
    Range of motion exercises are employed in a nonpainful range, gentle and gradual increase motion to tolerance.
  B. Weeks 3–6
    1. Progress all exercises (continue all above exercises)
    2. AAROM L-bar exercises
      ER/IR (shoulder at 45° abduction)
    3. Surgical tubing ER/IR (arm at side)
    4. Initiate humeral head stabilizing exercises

II. **Phase II: Intermediate Phase** (weeks 7–12)
  Goals: 1. Full, nonpainful ROM
    2. Improvement of strength and power
    3. Increasing functional activities; decreasing residual pain
  A. Weeks 7–10
    1. Active assisted ROM exercises (L-bar)
      a. Flexion to 170–180°
      b. ER/IR performed at 90° abduction of shoulder
        ER to 75–90°
        IR to 75–85°
      c. ER exercises performed with 0° abduction
        ER to 30–40°
    2. Strengthening exercises for shoulder
      a. Exercise tubing ER/IR arm at side
      b. Isotonics dumbbell exercises for
        Deltoid
        Supraspinatus
        Elbow flexors
        Scapula muscles
    3. Upper body ergometer
    Full range of motion is goal of weeks 8 to 10.
  B. Weeks 10–12
    1. Continue all above exercises
    2. Initiate isokinetic strengthening (scapulae plane)
    3. Initiate sidelying ER/IR exercises (dumbbell)
    4. Initiate neuromuscular scapulae control exercises

III. **Phase III: Advanced Strengthening Phase** (weeks 13–21)
  Goals: 1. Maintain full, nonpainful ROM
    2. Improve shoulder complex strength
    3. Improve neuromuscular control
    4. Gradual return to functional activities
  A. Weeks 13–18
    1. Active stretching program for the shoulder
      AAROM L-bar flexion, ER, IR
    2. Capsular stretches
    3. Aggressive strengthening program (isotonic program)
      a. Shoulder flexion
      b. Shoulder abduction
      c. Supraspinatus
      d. ER/IR
      e. Elbow flexors/extensors
      f. Scapulae muscles
    4. Isokinetic test (modified neutral position) (week 14)
      ER/IR at 180 and 300°/s
    5. General conditioning program
  B. Weeks 18–21
    1. Continue all exercises listed above
    2. Initiate interval sport program

IV. **Phase IV: Return to Activity Phase** (weeks 21–26)
  Goals: 1. Gradual return to recreational sport activities
  A. Weeks 21–26
    1. Isokinetic test (modified neutral position)
    2. Continue to comply to interval sport program
    3. Continue basic ten program for strengthening and flexibility

tion exercises, as well as progressive strengthening and upper body endurance activities. If required, interval sport programs usually can be incorporated between weeks 21 and 26 following surgery. The progression to a return to activity ranges from 26 to 30 weeks following surgery. Both strengthening and flexibility exercises should be continued as patients are progressed to unrestricted work and sporting activities.

## TYPE III

Often type III open rotator cuff repairs are initially immobilized in a brace at between 30 and 45 degrees of abduction. The brace is gradually progressed to a sling as directed by the physician, with some type of immobilization normally used during the first 4 to 6 weeks following surgery.

Exercises used during this first 8 weeks include passive range of motion and to active as-

**Table 8-20**

**Type II Rotator Cuff Repair (Deltoid Splitting), Medium to Large Tear (greater than 1 cm and less than 5 cm)**

I. **Phase I: Protection Phase** (weeks 0–6)
   Goals: 1. Gradual increase in ROM
   2. Increase shoulder strength
   3. Decrease pain and inflammation
   A. Weeks 0–3
      1. Brace or sling (physician determines)
      2. Pendulum exercises
      3. Active assisted ROM exercises (L-bar exercises)
         a. Flexion to 125°
         b. ER/IR (shoulder at 40° abduction) to 30°
      4. Passive ROM to tolerance
      5. Rope and pulley flexion
      6. Elbow ROM and hand gripping exercises
      7. Submaximal isometrics
         a. Flexors
         b. Abductors
         c. ER/IR
         d. Elbow flexors
      8. Ice and pain modalities
   B. Weeks 3–6
      1. Discontinue brace or sling
      2. Continue all exercises listed above
      3. AAROM exercises
         a. Flexion to 145°
         b. ER/IR (performed at 65° abduction) range to tolerance

II. **Phase II: Intermediate Phase** (weeks 7–14)
   Goals: 1. Full, nonpainful ROM (Week 10)
   2. Gradual increase in strength
   3. Decrease pain
   A. Weeks 7–10
      1. AAROM L-bar exercises
         a. Flexion to 160°
         b. ER/IR (performed at 90° shoulder abduction) to tolerance (>45°)
      2. Strengthening exercises
         a. Exercises tubing ER/IR (arm at side)
         b. Initiate humeral head stabilizing exercise
         c. Initiate dumbbell strengthening exercises
            Deltoid
            Supraspinatus
            Elbow flexion/extension
            Scapulae muscles
   B. Weeks 10–14 (full range of motion desired by weeks 10–12)
      1. Continue all exercises listed above
      2. Initiate isokinetic strengthening (scapulae plane)
      3. Initiate sidelying ER/IR strengthening exercises
      4. Initiate neuromuscular control exercises for scapular
   Patient must be able to elevate arm without shoulder and scapular hiking before initiating isotonics; if unable, maintain on humeral head stabilizing exercises.

III. **Phase III: Advanced Strengthening Phase** (weeks 15–26)
   Goals: 1. Maintain full, nonpainful ROM
   2. Improve strength of shoulder
   3. Improve neuromuscular control
   4. Gradual return to functional activities
   A. Weeks 15–20
      1. Continue AAROM exercises with L-bar Flexion, ER, IR
      2. Self capsular stretches
      3. Aggressive strengthening program
         a. Shoulder flexion
         b. Shoulder abduction (to 90°)
         c. Supraspinatus
         d. ER/IR
         e. Elbow flexors/extensors
         f. Scapula strengthening
      4. Conditioning program
   B. Weeks 21–26
      1. Continue all exercises listed above
      2. Isokinetic test (modified neutral position) for ER/IR at 180 and 300°/s
      3. Initiate interval sport program

IV. **Phase IV: Return-to-Activity Phase** (weeks 24–28)
   Goals: 1. Gradual return to recreational sport activities
   A. Weeks 24–28
      1. Continue all strengthening exercises
      2. Continue all flexibility exercises
      3. Continue progression on interval programs

sisted motion for shoulder internal/external rotation to tolerance in 45 degrees of abduction. As previously noted, elbow/hand range of motion and gripping are performed along with pain-free submaximal shoulder isometrics. Active assisted motion is initiated when tolerated. From 8 to 14 weeks following these type III repairs, rehabilitative emphasis is placed on humeral head control. Active assisted range-of-motion exercises are advanced to include shoulder flexion to tolerance and internal/external rotation in 90 degrees of abduction. Isotonic and scapular strengthening exercises are also incorporated as appropriate. Rehabilitative efforts during the 15 to 26 postoperative weeks are directed at obtaining full range of motion. This is desired between weeks 12 and 24 and varies according to physician direction based on the repair and the patient variables previously described. Also during this time frame, active assisted range-of-motion and

**Table 8-21**

**Type III Rotator Cuff Repair (Deltoid Splitting), Large to Massive Tear greater than 5 cm)**

I. **Phase I: Protection Phase** (weeks 0–8)
- A. Weeks 0–4
  1. Brace or sling (determined by physician)
  2. Pendulum exercises
  3. Passive ROM to tolerance
     - a. Flexion
     - b. ER/IR (shoulder at 45° abduction)
  4. Elbow ROM
  5. Hand gripping exercises
  6. Continuous passive motion (CPM)
  7. Submaximal isometrics
     - a. Abductors
     - b. ER/IR
     - c. Elbow flexors
  8. Ice and pain modalities
  9. Gentle AAROM with L-bar at week 2
- B. Weeks 4–8
  1. Discontinue brace or sling
  2. AAROM with L-bar
     - a. Flexion to 100°
     - b. ER/IR (shoulder 45° abduction) 40°
  3. Continue pain modalities

II. **Phase II: Intermediate Phase** (weeks 8–14)

Goals: 1. Establish full ROM (week 12)
2. Gradual increase strength
3. Decrease pain

- A. Weeks 8–10
  1. AAROM L-bar exercises
     - a. Flexion to tolerance
     - b. ER/IR (shoulder 90° abduction) to tolerance
  2. Initiate isotonic strengthening
     - a. Deltoid to 90°
     - b. ER/IR sidelying
     - c. Supraspinatus
     - d. Biceps/triceps
     - e. Scapula muscles
- B. Weeks 10–14
  1. Full ROM desired by weeks 12–14
  2. Continue all exercises listed above
  3. Initiate neuromuscular control exercises

  If patient is unable to elevate arm without shoulder hiking (scapulothoracic substitution), then maintain on humeral head stabilizing exercises.

III. **Phase III: Advanced Strengthening Phase** (weeks 15–26)

Goals: 1. Maintain full, nonpainful ROM
2. Improve strength of shoulder
3. Improve neuromuscular control
4. Gradual return to functional activities

- A. Weeks 15–20
  1. Continue AAROM exercises with L-bar Flexion, ER, IR
  2. Self capsular stretches
  3. Aggressive strengthening program
     - a. Shoulder flexion
     - b. Shoulder abduction (to 90°)
     - c. Supraspinatus
     - d. ER/IR
     - e. Elbow flexors/extensors
     - f. Scapula strengthening
  4. Conditioning program
- B. Weeks 21–26
  1. Continue all exercises listed above
  2. Isokinetic test (modified neutral position) for ER/IR at 180 and 300°/s
  3. Initiate interval sport program

IV. **Phase IV: Return-to-Activity Phase** (weeks 24–28)

Goals: 1. Gradual return to recreational sport activities

- A. Weeks 24–28
  1. Continue all strengthening exercises
  2. Continue all flexibility exercises
  3. Continue progression on interval programs

capsular stretching activities are continued along with the appropriate advancement of shoulder strengthening activities. Twenty-four to 30 weeks following the repair of these large to massive rotator cuff tears, all strengthening and stretching activities are continued, along with a gradual progression of all functional activities. As with all shoulder clients, the efficiency of the glenohumeral force couples is essential for a successful outcome—this is especially true with large surgically repaired rotator cuff tears or massive unrepaired tears.

# Summary

This chapter represents a program for strengthening the shoulder complex musculature and restoring of normal, symptom-free, functional activities. The program progresses from simple to complex in both exercise activities and the demands placed on the shoulder complex. In addition, the program is designed to maximize static stability of the glenohumeral joint before progressing to dynamic activities during complex movement patterns. The philosophy for this program of exercise progression can be found in Table 8-4. The primary function of the rotator cuff is one of humeral head stability during arm motion; this must be accomplished and mastered before any complex movements can be initiated and performed successfully. Additionally, one must not underestimate the importance of strengthening the scapulothoracic musculature to guarantee appropriate shoulder function. The reader is encouraged when rehabilitating a patient with shoulder dysfunction to incorporate an integrated treatment approach utilizing the principles described in this chapter for a successful outcome.

## References

1. Akeson WH, Woo SLY, Amiel D. The connective tissue response to immobility: biomechanical changes in periarticular connective tissue of the immobilized rabbit knee. Clin Orthop 1973; 93:356.
2. Alderink GJ, Kuck DJ. Isokinetic shoulder strength of high school and college aged pitchers. J Orthop Sports Phys Ther 1986;7(4): 163.
3. Altcheck DW, Skyhar MJ, Warren RF. Shoulder arthroscopy for shoulder instability. In: Barr JS, ed. American Academy of Orthopaedic Surgeons, Instructional course lecture. Vol. 27. St. Louis: CV Mosby, 1989:187.
4. Altcheck DW, Warren RF, Skylar MJ. T-plasty modification of the Bankart procedure for multidirectional instability of the anterior and inferior types. J Bone Joint Surg 1991;73A:105.
5. Andrews JR: Personal communication, December 1992.
6. Andrews JR, Broussard TS, Carson WG. Arthroscopy of the shoulder in the management of partial tears of the rotator cuff: a preliminary report. Arthroscopy 1985;1:117.
7. Andrews JR, Carson WG. The arthroscopic treatment of glenoid labrum tears in the throwing athlete. Orthop Trans 1984;8:44.
8. Andrews JR, Carson WG, McLeod WD. Glenoid labrum tears related to the long head of the biceps. Am J Sports Med 1985; 13(5):337.
9. Andrews JR, Gidamal RH. Shoulder arthroscopy in the throwing athlete, perspectives and prognosis. Arthroscopy 1987;6:656.
10. Andrews JR, Kupferman SP, Dillman CJ. Labral tears in throwing and racquet sports. Clin Sports Med 1991;10(4):901.
11. Arild PK, Davies GJ, Siewert MW, et al. Optimum rest interval between isokinetic and velocity spectrum rehabilitation speeds (abstract). Phys Ther 1985;65(5):735.
12. Aronen JG, Regan K. Decreasing the incidence of recurrence of first time anterior shoulder dislocations with rehabilitation. Am J Sports Med 1984;12(4):283.
13. Assmussen E, Boje O. Body temperature and capacity for work. Acta Physiol Scand 1945;10:1.
14. Assmussen E, Bonde-Peterson F. Storage of elastic energy in skeletal muscle in man. Acta Physiol Scand 1974;91:385.
15. Astrand PO, Rodal K. Textbook of work physiology: physiologic basis of exercise. 2nd Ed. New York: McGraw-Hill, 1977.
16. Baklim G, Paila M. Surgical treatment of rupture of the rotator cuff tendon. Acta Orthop Scand 1975;46:751.
17. Barrack RL, Skinner HB, Brunet DW. Joint kinesthesia in the highly trained knee. J Sports Med Phys Fitness 1984;24(1):18.
18. Bateman JE. The diagnosis and treatment of ruptures of the rotator cuff. Surg Clin North Am 1963;43(6):1523.
19. Bigliani LV, Kimmel J, McCann PD, Wolfe I. Repair of rotator cuff tears in tennis players. Am J Sports Med 1992;20(2):112.
20. Blackburn TA, McLeod WD, White B. EMG analysis of posterior rotator cuff exercises. Athl Train 1990;25:40.
21. Bly NN, Wells L, Grady D, et al. Consistency of repeated isokinetic testing: effect of different examiners, sites, and protocols. Isokinet Exerc Sci 1991;1(3):122.
22. Bradley J, Tibone JE. Electromyographic analysis of muscle action about the shoulder. In: Hawkins RJ, ed. Basic science and clinical application in the athlete's shoulder. Clin Sports Med 1991;10(4):789.
23. Bosco C, Komi P. Potential of the mechanical behavior of the human skeletal muscle through pre-stretching. Acta Physiol Scand 1979;106:467.
24. Bost FC, Inman VTG. The pathological changes in recurrent dislocation of the shoulder. J Bone Joint Surg 1942;24:595.
25. Bowen MK, Warren RF. Ligamentous control of shoulder stability based on selected cutting and static translation experiments. Clin Sports Med 1991;10(4):757.
26. Caizzo VJ. Alterations in the vivo force velocity curve. Med Sci Sports Exerc 1980;12(2):134.
27. Cash JD. Recent advances and perspectives on arthroscopic stabilization of the shoulder. Clin Sports Med 1991;10(4):871.
28. Caspari RB. Arthroscopic reconstruction for anterior shoulder instability. In: Paulos LE, Tibone JE, eds. Operative techniques in shoulder surgery. Baltimore: Aspen Publishers, 1991:57.
29. Cave EF, Burke JR, Boyd RJ. Trauma management. Chicago: Year Book Medical Publishers, 1974:437.
30. Chandler TJ, Kibler WB, Stracener EC, et al. Shoulder strength, power, and endurance in college tennis players. Am J Sports Med 1992;20(4):455.
31. Clark WA. Reliability of an alternative method for the measurement shoulder rotation strength. MGH Institute of Health Professions, M.S., 1985 University Microfilms International, Ann Arbor, Mich., 1987.
32. Codman EA. The shoulder. Boston: Thomas Todd, 1934.
33. Davies GJ. A compendium of isokinetics in clinical usage. 3rd Ed. Onolaska, Wisc.: S&S Publishers, 1987.
34. Davies GJ. Cybex II isokinetic dynamometer measurements on the acute effects of direct active warm-ups and direct passive warm-ups on knee extension/flexion and power. Presented at annual conference of American Physical Therapy Association, June 1978.
35. Debeyre J, Patt D, Emelik E. Repair of ruptures of the rotator cuff with a note on advancement of the supraspinatus muscle. J Bone Joint Surg 1965;47B:36.
36. Dehne E, Tory R. Treatment of joint injuries by immediate mobilization, based upon the spinal adaption concept. Clin Orthop 1971;77:218.
37. Dempster WT. Mechanisms of shoulder movement. Arch Phys Med Rehabil 1965;46:49.
38. DePalma AF, Callery G, Bennett CA. Variational anatomy and degenerative lesions of the shoulder bone. AAOS 1949;16:255.
39. DePalma AF, Cooke AJ, Prabhakar M. The role of the subscapularis in recurrent anterior dislocations of the shoulder. Clin Orthop 1967;54:35.
40. Dillman CJ. Biomechanics of pitching. Presented at the 1991 Injuries in Baseball Conference, Birmingham, Alabama, American Sports Medicine Institute, January 25, 1991.
41. Dillman CJ, Fleisig GS, Werner SL, Andrews JR. Biomechanics of the shoulder in sports: throwing activities. Pennington, N.J.: Postgraduate Studies in Physical Therapy, Forum Medicom, Inc., 1990.
42. Ellenbecker TS. Eccentric and concentric isokinetic strength characteristics of the rotator cuff. Presented at 1991 Annual Conference American Physical Therapy Association, Boston, Mass., June 1991.
43. Ellenbecker TS. A total aim strength profile of highly skilled tennis players. Isokinet Exerc Sci 1991;1:9.
44. Elsner RC, Pedegana LR, Lang J. Protocol for strength testing and rehabilitation of the upper extremity. J Orthop Sports Phys Ther 1985;4(4):229.
45. Eriksson E. Rehabilitation of muscle function after sport injury: a major problem in sports medicine. Int J Sports Med 1981;2:1.
46. Eriksson E, Haggmark T. Comparison of isometric muscle training and electrical stimulation supplementing isometric muscle training in the recovery after major knee ligament surgery. Am J Sports Med 1979;7:169.
47. Feldenkrais M. Awareness through movement. New York: Harper & Row, 1972.
48. Ferrari DA. Capsular ligaments of the shoulder. Am J Sports Med 1990;18:20.
49. Figoni SF, Christ CB, Massey BH. Effects of speed, hip and knee

angle, and gravity on hamstring to quadriceps torque ratios. J Orthop Sports Phys Ther 1988;9(8):287.

50. Figoni SF, Morris AF. Effects of knowledge of results on reciprocal isokinetic strength and fatigue. J Orthop Sports Phys Ther 1984;6:104.
51. Fillyaw M, Bevins T, Fernandez L. Importance of correcting isokinetic peak torque for the effect of gravity when calculating knee flexor to extensor muscle ratios. Phys Ther 1986;66:23.
52. Francis K, Hoobler T. Comparison of peak torque of the knee flexor and extensor muscle groups using the Cybex II and Lido 2.0 isokinetic dynamometers. J Orthop Sports Phys Ther 1987; 8(10):480.
53. Franks DB. Physical warm-up. In: Morgan WP, ed. Ergogenic aids and muscular performance. Orlando, Fla.: Academic Press, 1972.
54. Greenfield BH, Donatelli R, Wooden MJ, Wilken J. Isokinetic evaluation of shoulder rotational strength between plane of the scapula and frontal plane. Am J Sports Med 1990;18(22):124.
55. Gross MT, Huffman GM, Phillips CN, Wray JA. Intramachine and intermachine reliability of the Biodex, Cybex for knee flexion and extension peak torque and angular work. J Orthop Sports Phys Ther 1991;13(6):329.
56. Gross RM. Arthroscopic shoulder capsulorrhaphy; does it work? Am J Sports Med 1989;17:495.
57. Hageman PA, Mason DK, Rydlund KW, et al. Effects of position and speed on eccentric and concentric isokinetic testing of the shoulder rotators. J Orthop Sports Phys Ther 1989;11(2):64.
58. Hald RD, Battken EJ. Effects of visual feedback on maximal and submaximal isokinetic test measurements of normal quadriceps and hamstrings. J Orthop Sports Phys Ther 1987;9(2):86.
59. Hawkins RJ, Misamore GW, Hobeika PE. Surgery of full thickness rotator cuff tears. J Bone Joint Surg 1985;67A(9):1349.
60. Hawkins RJ, Schutte JP, Huckell GJ. The assessment of glenohumeral translation using manual and fluoroscopic techniques. Orthop Trans 1988;12:727.
61. Heikel HVA. Rupture of the rotator cuff of the shoulder; experiences of surgical treatment. Acta Orthop Scand 1968;39:477.
62. Hinton RY. Isokinetic evaluation of shoulder rotational strength in high school baseball pitchers. Am J sports Med 1988;16(3): 274.
63. Hovelius L. Recurrences after initial dislocation of the shoulder. J Bone Joint Surgery 1983;65A:343.
64. Howell SM, Galinat BJ, Renze AJ, Marone PJ. Normal and abnormal mechanics of the glenohumeral joint in the horizontal plane. J Bone Joint Surg 1988;70A(2):227.
65. Inman VT, Saunders JR, Abbott JC. Observations on the function of the shoulder joint. J Bone Joint Surg 1944;26:1.
66. Ivey FM, Calhoun JH, Rusche K, et al. Normal values for isokinetic testing of shoulder strength (abstract). Med Sci Sports Exerc 1988;16(2):274.
67. Jobe FW, Moynes DR. Delineation of diagnostic criteria and a rehabilitation program for rotator cuff injuries. Am J Sports Med 1982;10:336.
68. Jobe FW, Moynes DR, Tibone JE, et al. An EMG analysis of the shoulder in pitching: a second report. Am J Sports Med 1984; 12(3):218.
69. Jobe FW, Tibone JE, Perry J, et al. An EMG analysis of the shoulder in throwing and pitching: a preliminary report. Am J Sports Med 1983;11(1):3.
70. Johansson CA, Kent BE, Shepard KF. Relationship between verbal command volume and magnitude of muscle contraction. Phys Ther 1983;63(8):1260.
71. Johnson L. Instrument maker's education film. Okemus, Mich.: Instrument Maker Company, 1991.
72. Johnson RJ, Wilk KE. The effect of lever arm pad placement upon the isokinetic torque during knee extension and flexion. Phys Ther 1988;68(5):779.
73. Kaltenborn F. Manual therapy of the extremity joints. Oslo: Olaf Norlis Borkhandel, 1973.
74. Kapandji I. The physiology of joints. Vol. 1. Baltimore: Williams & Wilkins, 1970.
75. Kazas B, Relousky E. Prognosis of primary dislocation of the shoulder. Acta Orthop Scand 1969;40:216.
76. Kibler WB, McQueen C, Uhl T. Fitness evaluations and fitness findings in competitive junior tennis players. Clin Sports Med 1988;7(2):403.
77. Kisner C, Colby LA. Therapeutic exercise: foundations and techniques. Philadelphia: FA Davis, 1985.
78. Knott M, Voss D. Proprioceptive neuromuscular facilitation. New York: Hoeber Medical Division, Harper & Row, 1968:84.
79. Kumar VP, Balasubramaniam P. The role of atmospheric pressure in stabilizing the shoulder; an experimental study. J Bone Joint Surg 1985;67B:719.
80. Lindblom K. On pathogenesis of ruptures of the tendon aponeurosis of the shoulder joint. Acta Radiol 1939;20:563.
81. Lindblom K. Arthrography and roentgenography in ruptures of the tendons of the shoulder joint. Acta Radiol 1939;20:548.
82. Lucas DB. Biomechanics of the shoulder joint. Arch Surg 1973; 107(3):425.
83. Maitland G: Peripheral manipulation. 2nd Ed. Boston: Butterworth, 1977.
84. Make WJ. Bankart repair: an arthroscopic technique. Presented at the American Academy of Orthopaedic Surgeons, New Orleans, 1990.
85. Manzer CW. The effect of knowledge of output on muscle work. J Exp Psychol 1935;18:80.
86. Martin BV, Robinson S, Wiogoma DC, et al. Effect of warm-up metabolic responses to strenuous exercise. Med Sci Sports 1925;7:146.
87. Matsen FA, Thomas SC, Rockwood CA. Anterior glenohumeral instability. In: Rockwood CA, Matsen FA, eds. The shoulder. Philadelphia: WB Saunders, 1990:540.
88. Matsen FA. Subacromial Impingement. In Rockwood CA, Matsen FA, eds. The shoulder. Philadelphia: WB Saunders, 1990.
89. Mawdsley RH, Knapik JJ. Comparison of isokinetic measurements with test repetitions. Phys Ther 1982;62:169.
90. MacConaill MA, Basmajian JV. Muscles and movements: a basis for human kinesiology. Baltimore: Williams & Wilkins, 1969.
91. McArdle A, Katch FI, Katch VL. Exercise physiology: energy, nutrition, and human performance. 2nd Ed. Philadelphia: Lea & Febiger, 1985.
92. Morgan CD, Bordenstab AB. Arthroscopic Bankart suture repair: technique and early results. Arthroscopy 1987;3(2):111.
93. Moseley HF, Goldie I. The arterial pattern of the rotator cuff of the shoulder. J Bone Joint Surg 1963;45B:780.
94. Moseley VB, Jobe FW, Pink M, et al. EMG analysis of the scapular muscles during a shoulder rehabilitation program. Am J Sports Med 1992;20(3)128.
95. Neer CS II. Impingement lesions. Clin Orthop 1983;173:70.
96. Neer CS, Foster CR. Inferior capsular shift for involuntary inferior and multidirectional instability of the shoulder: a preliminary report. J Bone Joint Surgery 1980;62A:897.
97. Neer CS, McCann PD, MacFarlane EA. Earlier passive motion following shoulder arthroplasty and rotator cuff repair: a prospective study. Orthop Trans 1987;11:231.
98. Neer CS, Welsh RP. The shoulder in sports. Orthop Clin North Am 1977;8:583.
99. Nelson SG, Duncan PW. Correction of isokinetic and isometric torque recordings for the effects of gravity. Phys Ther 1983; 63:674.
100. Ng LR, Kramer JS. Shoulder rotator torques in female tennis and nontennis players. J Orthop Sports Phys Ther 1991;13:40.
101. Noyes FR, Mangine RE, Barber S. Early knee motion after open and arthroscopic ACL reconstruction. Am J Sports Med 1981; 15:149.
102. O'Brien SJ, Neyes MC, Arnocsky SP, et al. The anatomy and histology of the inferior glenohumeral ligament complex of the shoulder. Am J Sports Med 1990;18(5):449.
103. Ovesen J, Nielsen S. Anterior and posterior shoulder instability. Acta Orthop Scand 1986;57:324.
104. Pappas AM, Zawacki RM, Sullivan TJ. Biomechanics of baseball pitching: a preliminary report. Am J Sports Med 1985;13(4):216.
105. Partridge MJ. Joints: the limitation of their range of movement, and an explanation of certain surgical conditions. J Anat 1923; 108:346.
106. Perkins G. Rest and motion. J Bone Joint Surg 1954;45B:521.
107. Pierson WR, Rasch PJ. Effect of knowledge of results on isometric strength scores. Res Q 1964;35:313.
108. Poppen NK, Walker PS. Normal and abnormal motion of the shoulder. J Bone Joint Surg 1976;58A:195.
109. Rathbun JB, Macnab I. The microvascular pattern of the rotator cuff. J Bone Joint Surg 1970;52B:540.
110. Reeves B. Experiments on the tensile strength of the anterior capsular structures of the shoulder region. J Bone Joint Surg 1968;50B:858.

111. Rothman RH, Parke WW. The vascular anatomy of the rotator cuff. Clin Orthop 1965;41:176.
112. Rywerant Y. Improving the ability to perform: an instance of the Feldenkrais method of functional integration. Somatics 1977;37.
113. Saha AK. Dynamic stability of the glenohumeral joint. Acta Orthop Scand 1971;42:491.
114. Saha AK. Theory of shoulder mechanism. Springfield, Ill.: Charles C Thomas, 1961:54.
115. Saha AK. Mechanics of elevation of glenohumeral joint: its application in rehabilitation of flail shoulder in upper brachial plexus injuries and poliomyelitic and in replacement of the upper humerus by prosthesis. Acta Scand Orthop 1973;44:668.
116. Salter RB, Simmonds DF, Malcolm BW. The biological effects on continuous passive motion on the healing of full thickness articular cartilage defects. J Bone Joint Surg 1980;62A:1231.
117. Salter RB, Bell RS, Kealey F. The protective effect of continuous passive motion on living articular cartilage in acute septic arthritis: an experimental investigation in the rabbit. Clin Orthop 1981;159:223.
118. Schwartz RE, O'Brien SJ, Warren RF, et al. Capsular restraints to anterior-posterior motion of the abducted shoulder: a biomechanical study. Orthop Trans 1988;12(3):727.
119. Siewert MW, Arik PK, Davies GJ, et al. Isokinetic torque changes based on lever arm placement. Phys Ther 1985;65:715.
120. Sigholm G, Herberts P, Almstrom C, Kadifors R. Electromyographic analysis of shoulder muscle load. J Orthop Res 1984; 1:379.
121. Smith RH, Brunolti J. Shoulder kinesthesia after anterior glenohumeral joint dislocation. Phys Ther 1989;69:106.
122. Soderberg GJ, Blaschek MJ. Shoulder internal and external rotation peak torque production through a velocity spectrum in differing positions. J Orthop Sports Phys Ther 1987;8(11):518.
123. Spiegelman JJ, Woo SL-Y. A rigid body method for finding centers of rotation and angular displacements of planar joint motion. J Biomech 1987;20(7):715.
124. Steindler A. Kinesiology of human body under normal and pathological conditions. Springfield, Ill.: Charles C Thomas, 1955.
125. Symeonides PP. The significance of the subscapularis muscle in the pathogenesis of recurrent anterior-dislocation of the shoulder. J Bone Joint Surg 1982;54B:476.
126. Sullivan PE, Markos PA, Minor MD. An integrated approach to therapeutic exercise, theory and clinical application. Reston, Va.: Reston Publishing Company, 1982.
127. Taylor RC, Casey JJ. Quadriceps torque production on the Cybex II dynamometer as related to changes in lever arm length. J Orthop Sports Phys Ther 1986;8:147.
128. Thompson MC, Shingleton LG, Kegerreis ST. Comparison of values generated during testing of the knee using the Cybex II + and Biodex mode B-2000 isokinetic dynamometers. J Orthop Sports Phys Ther 1989;11(3):100.
129. Townsend H, Jobe FW, Pink M, Perry J. Electromyographic analysis of the glenohumeral muscles during a baseball rehabilitation program. Am J Sports Med 1991;19(3)264.
130. Uhthoff H, Piscopo M. Anterior capsular redundancy of the shoulder: congenital or traumatic? J Bone Joint Surg 1985;67B: 363.
131. Ulrich C, Burke RK. Effect of motivational stress on physical performance. Res Q 1957;28:403.
132. Van Linge B, Mulder JD. Function of the supraspinatus muscle and its relationship to the supraspinatus syndrome. J Bone Joint Surg 1963;45B:750.
133. Walmsley RP, Szybbo C. A comparative study of the torque generated by the shoulder internal and external rotators in different positions and at varying speeds. J Orthop Sports Phys Ther 1987;9:217.
134. Warren JP, Deng XH, Warren RF, Torzilli PA. Static capsuloligamentous restraints to superior-inferior translation of the glenohumeral joint. Am J Sports Med 1992;20(6):675.
135. Warren RF. Subluxation of the shoulder in athletes: symposium on injuries to the shoulder in the athlete. Clin Sports Med 1983; 2(2):339.
136. Warren RF, Kornblatt IB, Marchand R. Static forces affecting posterior shoulder stability. Orthop Trans 1984;8:89.
137. Warwick R, Williams PL, eds. Gray's anatomy. 35th Ed. Philadelphia: WB Saunders, 1973.
138. Watson-Jones, Sir R. Fractures and joint injuries. Edinburgh: E & S Livingstone, 1955:452.
139. Wiktursson-Moller M, Oberg B, Edstrand V, et al. Effect of warming up, massage and strengthening on range of motion and muscle strength in the lower extremity. Am J Sports Med 1983; 11:249.
140. Wildman G. Awareness in movement. Milwaukee: March 1989.
141. Wiley AM. Arthroscopy for shoulder instability and a technique for arthroscopic repair. Arthroscopy 1988;1:25.
142. Wilk KE. Isokinetic testing and exercise for the shoulder complex. Presented at Annual Conference Biodex Corporation, Ft. Lauderdale, Fla., October 3, 1991.
143. Wilk KE. Dynamic muscle strength testing. In: Amunsen LR, ed. Muscle strength testing: instrumental and noninstrument systems. New York: Churchill Livingstone, 1990:123.
144. Wilk KE, Andrews JR. Rehabilitation following arthroscopic subacromial decompression. Orthopaedics 1993;16(3):349–358.
145. Wilk KE, Andrews JR, Arrigo CA, et al. The internal and external rotator strength characteristics of professional baseball pitchers. Am J Sports Med 1993;21(1):61–66.
146. Wilk KE, Andrews JR, Arrigo CA, et al. The isokinetic abductor and adductor strength characteristics of professional baseball pitchers. Am J Sports Med. Accepted for publication 1994.
147. Wilk KE, Arrigo CA. Isokinetic testing and rehabilitation of microtraumatic shoulder injuries. In: Davies GD, ed. Compendium of isokinetics. 4th Ed. Onalaska, Wisc.: S&S Publishing, 1992.
148. Wilk KE, Arrigo CA. Current concepts in the rehabilitation of the athletic shoulder. J. Orthrop Sports Phys Ther 1993;(18):365–378.
149. Wilk KE, Arrigo CA, Andrews JR. Standardized isokinetic testing protocol for the throwing shoulder: the thrower's series. Isokinet Exerc Sci 1991;1(2):63.
150. Wilk KE, Arrigo CA, Kierns MA. Shoulder abduction/adduction isokinetic test results: window vs. unwindow data collection. J Orthop Sports Phys Ther 1992;15(2):107.
151. Wilk KE, Voight ML, Keirns MA, et al. Stretch shortening drills for the upper extremities; theory and clinical application. J Orthop Sports Phys Therapy (in press).
152. Wilt F. Plyometrics, what it is and how it works. Ath J 1975;55(5): 76.
153. Woo SL-Y, Matthews SU, Akeson WH. Connective tissue response to immobility. Arthritis Rheum 1975;18:257.
154. Yoneda B, Welsh RP, MacIntosh DL. Conservative treatment of shoulder dislocation in young males. J Bone Joint Surg 1982; 643:254.

Chapter 9

*James E. Zachazewski*
*Linda A. Steiner*
*Alex J. Petruska*

# Overhead Throwing and Other Related Motions



## Overhead Throwing Motion

Often the upper extremity is asked to provide a propulsive force to an object during athletic activity. The object propelled, most often a ball, may leave the hand directly or may be "launched" from some external device attached to the hand, as is the case with tennis or lacrosse. During any overhead propulsive activity, shoulder mobility

Martin J. Kelley and William A. Clark: ORTHOPEDIC THERAPY OF THE SHOULDER.

and ligamentous restraints, as well as the strength, endurance, and motor control of muscles specifically associated with the scapula and glenohumeral joint, are challenged.

The basic mechanics and phases of the throwing or pitching act have been studied and described by many authors[4,9,21,37,41,42,55,56,86,88] (Fig. 9-1). Others have completed electromyographic (EMG) studies[17,25,26,34,35] or have studied the dynamic[11,30] or passive[20,53,54,84] restraints of the shoulder during throwing or in relation to the types of injuries most commonly seen with throwing. Equal but opposite reaction forces and torques must be generated by muscle, tendon, and ligament about the joint to maintain stability and prevent injury.[21] If either the dynamic or passive restraints to these forces are compromised, injury may result. Working in concert, the integrity of these structures protects them from glenohumeral instability and the impingement syndrome. Changes in technique, poor flexibility, or fatigue (muscular and cardiovascular) may be sufficient to tip the critical balance necessary to avoid injury in the high-velocity, repetitive act of throwing.

The primary purpose of this section of the chapter will be to describe the various phases of overhead throwing in relation to biomechanics of the shoulder, the ligaments stressed, and muscle activity patterns. Associated activities, such as the tennis serve, waterpolo, and football, will be compared and contrasted as appropriate in the second section.

# Phases

Description of the throwing phases varies among authors. For purposes of this chapter, the phases of throwing will be divided up into windup, arm cocking (early and late), arm acceleration, and deceleration and follow-through as they relate to pitching a baseball (see Fig. 9-1) Common points

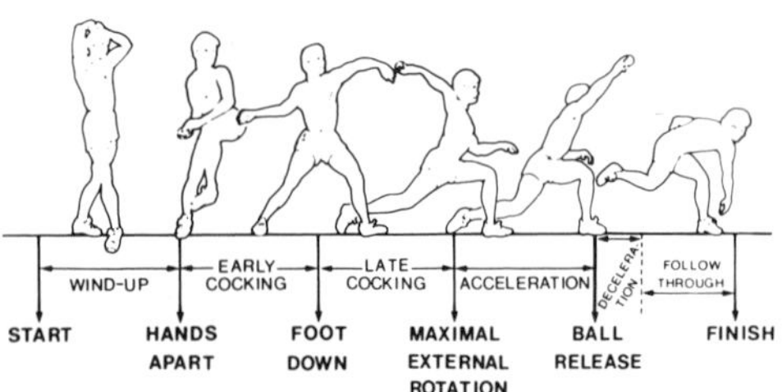


**Figure 9-1.** Phases of pitching. (Reprinted with permission from DiGiovine NM, Jobe FW, Pink M, et al. An electromyographic analysis of the upper extremity in pitching. J Shoulder Elbow Surg 1992;1:15.)

within each phase will be summarized from literature reviewed.[4,9,21,37,41,42,55,56,86,88] Specific points of interest will be credited to the originating author.

## WINDUP

The purpose of the windup phase is to place the body in an optimal position from which to start the throw. Attaining this optimal balanced position will allow the pitcher to achieve maximum efficiency, power, and speed. The windup is the time between the initiation of motion and when the ball is removed from the glove. It may be initiated from either the stance or stretch positions. As the hands move as a unit, the contralateral lower extremity comes off the ground. The ipsilateral leg and trunk then rotate approximately 90 degrees so that the pitcher is perpendicular to the batter. The contralateral hip and knee are fully flexed, and the pitcher is now in a balanced position from which to begin the next phase of the throw. The windup phase ends when the hands separate and the ball is brought out of the glove. Pappas et al.[55] have stated that this phase takes 0.5 to 1.0 seconds, while Nicholas et al.[49] have reported 1.3 seconds. Minimal muscle activity has been documented during this phase.[17,25,26,34,35]

## COCKING

The cocking phase may be divided into two distinct parts: early cocking and late cocking. This is a highly dynamic phase. The purpose of this phase is to place the arm into a position of 90 degrees of abduction and maximal external rotation and horizontal abduction. This position winds the fibrous tissues of the glenohumeral joint to create an elastic force and position the driving muscles at their full length.[56] It is from this position that energy generated from the different segments of the body is quickly and systematically passed to the ball from the lower extremities and trunk.[9,21] During all types of overhead throwing motions, the shoulder is abducted approximately 90 degrees. The apparently different points of release for the overhand, three-quarters arm, sidearm, and submarine throws are accounted for by lateral trunk flexion.[4,9,21,42]

Early arm cocking is characterized by abduction and external rotation of the shoulder as the ball is released from the glove. While this is happening, the contralateral lower extremity begins to stride out. Simultaneously, the hips, pelvis, and shoulders begin to rotate toward the target at which the pitcher is throwing.

Late arm cocking commences when the foot

of the contralateral leg (stride leg) contacts the ground. At foot contact, the hips, pelvis, and shoulders continue to rotate toward the target. The shoulder is in a position of approximately 90 degrees of abduction, 30 degrees of horizontal abduction, and 90 to 120 degrees of external rotation.[21,55] The hips and shoulders continue to rotate forward at their highest angular velocity as the arm continues into external rotation.[55] The entire arm remains behind the frontal plane, in line with the shoulders. As trunk rotation ends, the arm begins to accelerate. Late cocking ends and acceleration begins as the arm reaches a position of maximum external rotation, 160 to 175 degrees.[21,55] It is at this time that the greatest amount of energy is available to accelerate the arm. In this position, the internal rotators are maximally stretched and eccentrically loaded.[21] Static stabilizing structures are twisted into a dense fibrous band.[56] According to Pappas et al.,[55] the early and late cocking phases each require 0.5 to 1.0 seconds. The entire windup and cocking phases require approximately 1.5 seconds.[55]

The musculotendinous unit and capsuloligamentous complex (CLC) must generate opposing reaction forces about the joint to maintain stability and prevent injury.[21] Joint kinetic forces have been well summarized by Fleisig et al.[21] for late cocking, acceleration, and follow-through (Fig. 9-2a–f). A careful review of these figures provides the reader with a sound understanding of the torques (see Fig. 9-2a–c), forces (see Fig. 9-2d–f), and ranges of motion (see Fig. 9-2g–i) required at the shoulder during throwing. For example, the horizontal adduction torque generated by muscles such as the subscapularis and pectoralis major must dynamically resist the dis-

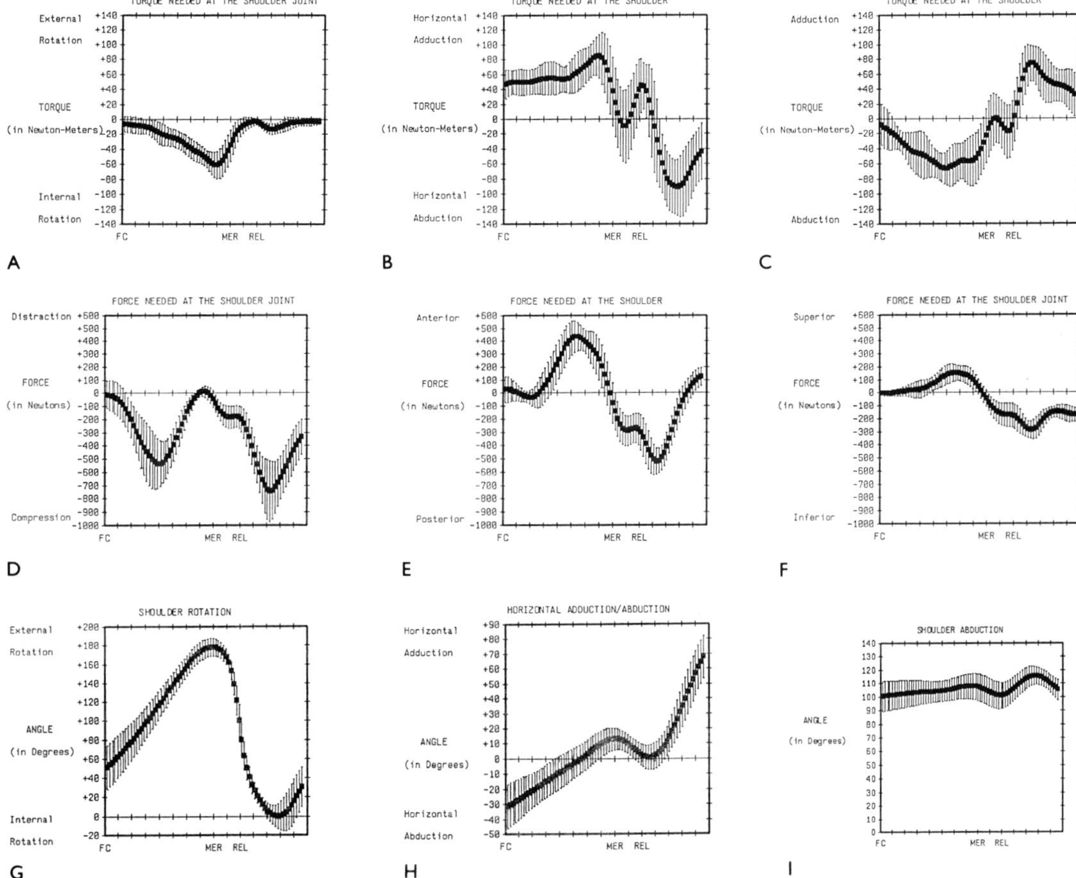


**Figure 9-2.** Summary of joint kinetics and kinematics at the shoulder while pitching. (Reprinted with permission of Fleisig GS, Dillman CJ, Andrews JR, et al. A biomechanical description of the shoulder joint during pitching. Sports Medicine Update 1991;Fall:10.) *Legend: FC*, foot contact; *MER*, maximal external rotation; *REL*, ball release. (a) External and internal rotation torque. (b) Horizontal abduction and adduction torque. (c) Abduction and adduction torque. (d) Compressive and distractive forces. (e) Anterior and posterior forces. (f) Superior and inferior forces. (g) External and internal rotation range. (h) Horizontal abduction and adduction range. (i) Shoulder abduction range.

traction force and while the infraspinatus and teres minor resist the anterior shear placed on the glenohumeral joint by trunk. At the same time the passive restraint provided by the glenohumeral ligaments and capsule must attempt to passively resist the same forces. If either the dynamic or passive restraints to these forces are compromised, abnormal humeral head translation could result in subluxation or possibly dislocation.

There is a dramatic increase in muscle activity during the entire arm cocking phase. Initial details regarding activity of the rotator cuff, completed by Jobe et al.[34,35] (Fig. 9-3), have been further detailed by other authors.[17,25,26] Details on specific muscle activity and the sequence of activation are presented in Table 9-1 and Figure 9-4a–d.

Sequential activation of muscles details their importance. During early cocking, arm elevation is accomplished by the deltoid, with little contribution from the rotator cuff other than the supraspinatus. As early cocking continues, there is an increase in activity of the supraspinatus, infraspinatus, and teres minor to begin to position the arm in external rotation. As late cocking begins and external rotation increases, the subscapularis and pectoralis major become active eccentrically to control external rotation and horizontal abduction. Activity continues in the supraspinatus, infraspinatus, and teres minor to control anterior strain against the glenoid rim and glenohumeral ligaments.[56] Because of their orientation and direction of action, activity of the infraspinatus and teres minor is perhaps most

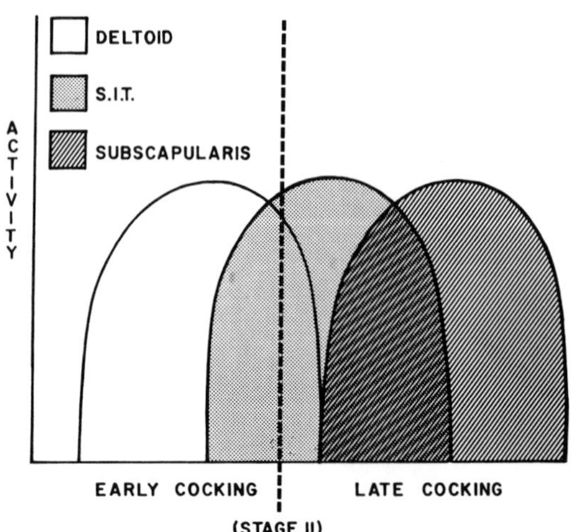


**Figure 9-3.** The sequential muscle activation pattern of cocking. (Reprinted with permission of Jobe FW, Tibone JE, Perry J, et al. An EMG analysis of the shoulder in throwing and pitching. Am J Sports Med 1983;11:3.)

important in controlling excessive shear and overload of the glenohumeral ligaments in this phase[11] (Fig. 9-5).

During the arm cocking phase, and especially in late cocking, the glenohumeral ligaments, in particular the inferior glenohumeral ligament (IGHL), undergo significant stress in limiting anterior shear and external rotation. The IGHL is a complex structure consisting of an anterior band, a posterior band, and an interposed axillary pouch (Fig. 9-6). When the arm is in 90 degrees of abduction and external rotation, as in the cocking phase, the IGHL, specifically its anterior band, is the primary restraint to anterior translation of the humeral head[20,53,54,84] (Fig. 9-7). If the inferior glenohumeral ligament or its labral attachment is compromised, subluxation or dislocation can occur because the barrier and compression effect created by an intact capsuloligamentous-labral complex is disrupted.

Terry et al.[84] have attempted to determine the function of the ligamentous restraints of the shoulder during simulated throwing activity. Their preliminary results appear to confirm the stabilizing requirements placed on the IGHL during the cocking phase[84] (Fig. 9-8). Although information and studies such as this are critical, the reader must utilize this information with caution at this time because of the wide variability of the data (mean versus standard deviation).

The kinetic study completed by Fleisig et al.[21] details the torque and forces applied by the trunk to the arm during late cocking (see Fig. 9-2a–f). Abduction torque generated is small (see Fig. 9-2c), the only requirement being to resist gravity and keep the arm abducted during throwing. Horizontal adduction and internal rotation torques (generated by eccentric contraction of the subscapularis, pectoralis major, latissimus dorsi, and teres major) are applied to the arm to balance and control the amount of horizontal abduction and external rotation being imposed on the arm as the athlete rotates the trunk toward the target in preparation for throwing (see Fig. 9-2a, b). As the trunk rotates, a distractive force is applied to the glenohumeral joint that must be resisted by a compressive force at the glenohumeral joint (see Fig. 9-2d). During cocking, an anterior shear force is imposed on the arm so that it maintains an appropriate relationship with the glenohumeral joint during trunk rotation. This shear force is resisted by restraint of the IGHL passively and contraction of the posterior muscles of the rotator cuff, most notably the infraspinatus and teres minor (see Table 9-1). Muscles that control scapular position and rotation (serratus anterior, trapezius, and levator scapulae) are also very active at this time, main-

**Table 9-1**

## EMG of Muscle Groups in the Upper Extremity during Pitching*

| | No. of Pitchers | Windup | Early Cocking | Late Cocking | Acceleration | Deceleration | Follow-Through |
|---|---|---|---|---|---|---|---|
| Scapular muscles | | | | | | | |
| Upper trapezius | 11 | 18 ± 16 | 64 ± 53 | 37 ± 29 | 69 ± 31 | 53 ± 22 | 14 ± 12 |
| Middle trapezius | 11 | 7 ± 5 | 43 ± 22 | 51 ± 24 | 71 ± 32 | 35 ± 17 | 15 ± 14 |
| Lower trapezius | 13 | 13 ± 12 | 39 ± 30 | 38 ± 29 | 76 ± 55 | 78 ± 33 | 25 ± 15 |
| Serratus anterior (sixth rib) | 11 | 14 ± 13 | 44 ± 35 | 69 ± 32 | 60 ± 53 | 51 ± 30 | 32 ± 18 |
| Serratus anterior (fourth rib) | 10 | 20 ± 20 | 40 ± 22 | 106 ± 56 | 50 ± 46 | 34 ± 7 | 41 ± 24 |
| Rhomboids | 11 | 7 ± 8 | 35 ± 24 | 41 ± 26 | 71 ± 35 | 45 ± 28 | 14 ± 20 |
| Levator scapula | 11 | 6 ± 5 | 35 ± 14 | 72 ± 54 | 77 ± 28 | 33 ± 16 | 14 ± 13 |
| Glenohumeral muscles | | | | | | | |
| Anterior deltoid | 16 | 15 ± 12 | 40 ± 20 | 28 ± 30 | 27 ± 19 | 47 ± 34 | 21 ± 16 |
| Middle deltoid | 14 | 9 ± 8 | 44 ± 19 | 12 ± 17 | 36 ± 22 | 59 ± 19 | 16 ± 13 |
| Posterior deltoid | 18 | 6 ± 5 | 42 ± 26 | 28 ± 27 | 68 ± 66 | 60 ± 28 | 13 ± 11 |
| Supraspinatus | 16 | 13 ± 12 | 60 ± 31 | 49 ± 29 | 51 ± 46 | 39 ± 43 | 10 ± 9 |
| Infraspinatus | 16 | 11 ± 9 | 30 ± 18 | 74 ± 34 | 31 ± 28 | 37 ± 20 | 20 ± 16 |
| Teres minor | 12 | 5 ± 6 | 23 ± 15 | 71 ± 42 | 54 ± 50 | 84 ± 52 | 25 ± 21 |
| Subscapularis (lower third) | 11 | 7 ± 9 | 26 ± 22 | 62 ± 19 | 56 ± 31 | 41 ± 23 | 25 ± 18 |
| Subscapularis (upper third) | 11 | 7 ± 8 | 37 ± 26 | 99 ± 55 | 115 ± 82 | 60 ± 36 | 16 ± 15 |
| Pectoralis major | 14 | 6 ± 6 | 11 ± 13 | 56 ± 27 | 54 ± 24 | 29 ± 18 | 31 ± 21 |
| Latissimus dorsi | 13 | 12 ± 10 | 33 ± 33 | 50 ± 37 | 88 ± 53 | 59 ± 35 | 24 ± 18 |
| Elbow and forearm muscles | | | | | | | |
| Triceps | 13 | 4 ± 6 | 17 ± 17 | 37 ± 32 | 89 ± 40 | 54 ± 23 | 22 ± 18 |
| Biceps | 18 | 8 ± 9 | 22 ± 14 | 26 ± 20 | 20 ± 16 | 44 ± 32 | 16 ± 14 |
| Brachialis | 13 | 8 ± 5 | 17 ± 13 | 18 ± 26 | 20 ± 22 | 49 ± 29 | 13 ± 17 |
| Brachioradialis | 13 | 5 ± 5 | 35 ± 20 | 31 ± 24 | 16 ± 12 | 46 ± 24 | 22 ± 29 |
| Pronator teres | 14 | 14 ± 16 | 18 ± 15 | 39 ± 28 | 85 ± 39 | 51 ± 21 | 21 ± 21 |
| Supinator | 13 | 9 ± 7 | 38 ± 20 | 54 ± 38 | 55 ± 31 | 59 ± 31 | 22 ± 19 |
| Wrist and finger muscles | | | | | | | |
| Extensor carpi radialis longus | 13 | 11 ± 8 | 53 ± 24 | 72 ± 37 | 30 ± 20 | 43 ± 24 | 22 ± 14 |
| Extensor carpi radialis brevis | 15 | 17 ± 17 | 47 ± 26 | 75 ± 41 | 55 ± 35 | 43 ± 28 | 24 ± 19 |
| Extensor digitorum communis | 14 | 21 ± 17 | 37 ± 25 | 59 ± 27 | 35 ± 35 | 47 ± 25 | 24 ± 18 |
| Flexor carpi radialis | 12 | 13 ± 9 | 24 ± 35 | 47 ± 33 | 120 ± 66 | 79 ± 36 | 35 ± 16 |
| Flexor digitorum superficialis | 11 | 16 ± 6 | 20 ± 23 | 47 ± 52 | 80 ± 66 | 71 ± 32 | 21 ± 11 |
| Flexor carpi ulnaris | 10 | 8 ± 5 | 27 ± 18 | 41 ± 25 | 112 ± 60 | 77 ± 42 | 24 ± 18 |

*Means and standard deviations, expressed as a percentage of the maximal manual muscle test.

Reprinted with permission of DiGiovine NM, Jobe FW, Pink M, et al. An electromyographic analysis of the upper extremity in pitching. J Shoulder Elbow Surg 1992;1:15.

taining appropriate scapular position and providing a stable base of support for the glenohumeral joint.

It is during this critical phase, which requires eccentric internal rotator muscle control, concentric external rotator activity, and integrity of the passive restraints to control position of the humeral head in the glenoid fossa, that injuries such as anterior instability and "impingement" syndrome may begin to develop.

## ACCELERATION

Acceleration begins when the arm has reached maximum external rotation and terminates with release of the ball. At the instant when external rotation and horizontal abduction end and internal rotation and horizontal adduction begin, the torque has been estimated to be up to 17,000 kg/cm.[56] Angular velocity has been demonstrated to be between 6000 degrees/s[55] and 7500 degrees/s.[21] This phase accounts for less than 2 percent of the actual time involved in the act of throwing.[55]

Ball release occurs with the shoulder between 40 and 60 degrees of external rotation. The shoulder is in a position of 90 to 110 degrees of abduction during the acceleration phase.[4,9,21,42,55,88] Maximum external rotation has been measured to be between 160 degrees[55] and 175 degrees[21] *relative to the trunk*. This measurement is a summation of many motions, including spine extension.[21] According to Perry,[56] the majority of acceleration may be due to a release of tension on a stretched anterior capsule. Muscle activity was reported originally to be significantly less during acceleration than during cocking.[34] Subsequent reports, however, detail substantial activity of scapular muscles and the subscapularis during this phase, demonstrating that muscle activity plays a pivotal role[17] (see Table 9-1 and Fig. 9-4a–d). Acceleration would appear to be initiated by muscles that were initially activated and functioning eccentrically to control external rotation during late cocking, specifically the subscapularis, latissimus dorsi, and sternal pectoralis major.[17,25,26,56] Scapular muscles are again very active in optimally positioning the glenoid and maintaining a stable platform from which the glenohumeral muscles can accelerate the humerus.

Following the initiation of acceleration, the strain applied to the anterior portion of the IGHL decreases as the capsuloligamentous complex untwists and the humerus rapidly moves into horizontal adduction and internal rotation. The strain is transferred to a number of different ligamentous structures, especially the posterior capsule (see Fig. 9-8). The anterior relaxation of the IGHL during acceleration theoretically places the anterosuperior labrum in greater jeopardy, a point that has been confirmed by an injury mechanism–pitching correlation.[84]

## DECELERATION AND FOLLOW-THROUGH

These phases begin the moment the ball is released and continue until the athlete has completed his or her throwing motion. These phases take approximately 350 ms, or 18 percent of the throwing cycle.[55]

It has been reported that during deceleration, internal rotation, horizontal adduction, and glenohumeral distraction occur at the shoulder.[21,42,55,56] Internal rotation at the shoulder makes it appear as if forearm pronation occurs after release.[21,42] After ball release, the arm is in front of the body, at which time the rotator cuff, posterior deltoid, and scapular muscles are positioned to decelerate the arm by resisting distraction (see Table 9-1, Fig. 9-2d, and Fig. 9-4a–d). A horizontal abduction torque is required to prevent excessive horizontal adduction (see Fig. 9-2b). Surprisingly, minimal rotational torque is applied to the arm by the trunk at the shoulder. This appears to be due to the fact that following release, the elbow is almost fully extended.

The remaining portion of follow-through, body follow-through, is more passive in nature. During this period, the body moves forward with the arm by moving into flexion and rotation. By allowing the body to follow the arm, the amount of horizontal abduction torque and compressive force required by the ligaments and musculature to resist horizontal adduction and distraction is reduced. Lack of body follow-through may increase the possibility of injury to the posterior rotator cuff, anterior labrum via a grinding effect, and posterior capsular complex.

Throughout this phase, passive resistance to

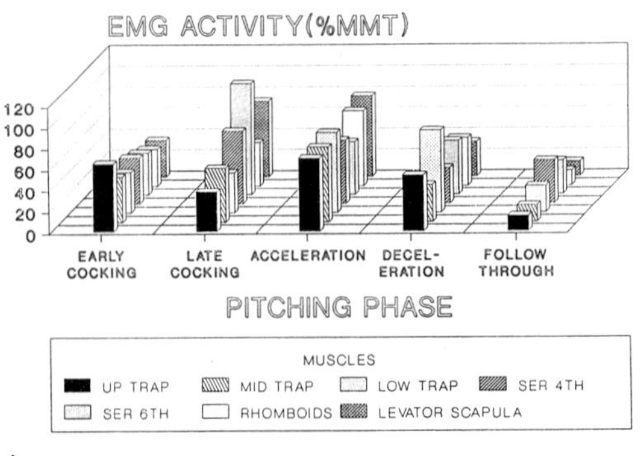


A

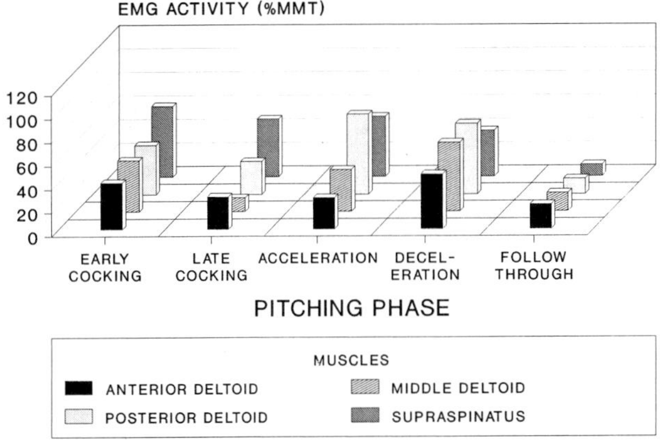


B

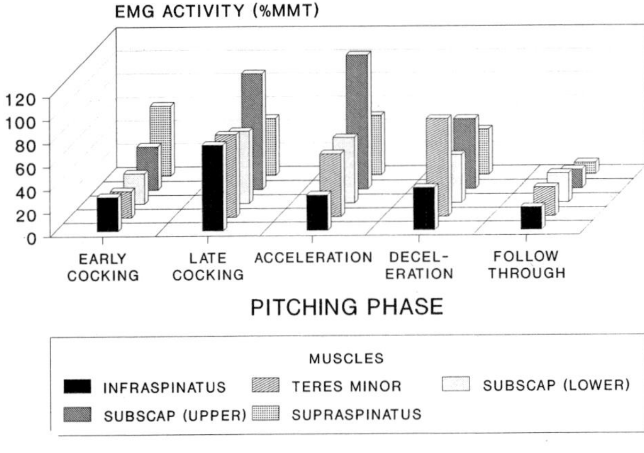


C

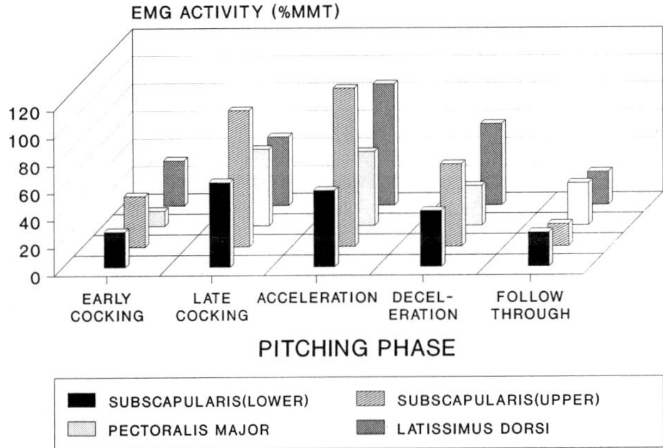


D

**Figure 9-4.** (a) EMG activity of scapular rotator muscles. (b) EMG activity of deltoids and supraspinatus. (c) EMG activity of rotator cuff. (d) EMG activity of internal humeral rotators. (Reprinted with permission of DiGiovine NM, Jobe FW, Pink M, et al. An electromyographic analysis of the upper extremity in pitching. J Shoulder Elbow Surg 1992;1:15.)

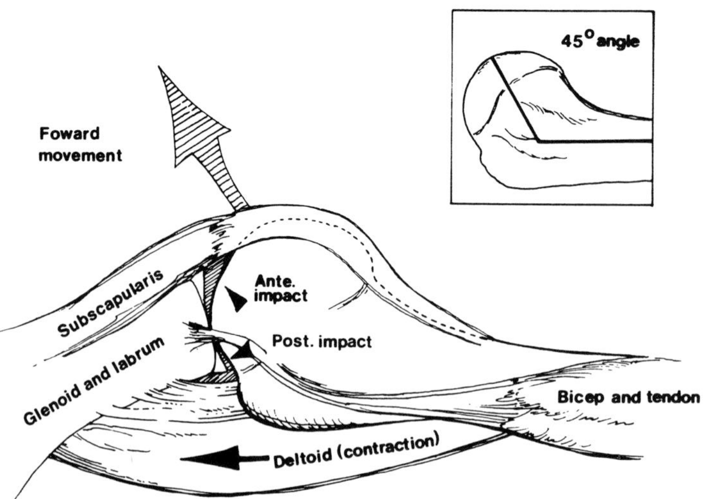


**Figure 9-5.** The mechanism of glenohumeral joint injury during the cocking action with abduction, horizontal abduction, and external rotation is shown. An anterior shear force is produced against the glenoid labrum and capsuloligamentous complex. (Reprinted with permission of Perry J. Anatomy and biomechanics of the shoulder in throwing, swimming, gymnastics and tennis. Clin Sports Med 1983;2:247.)

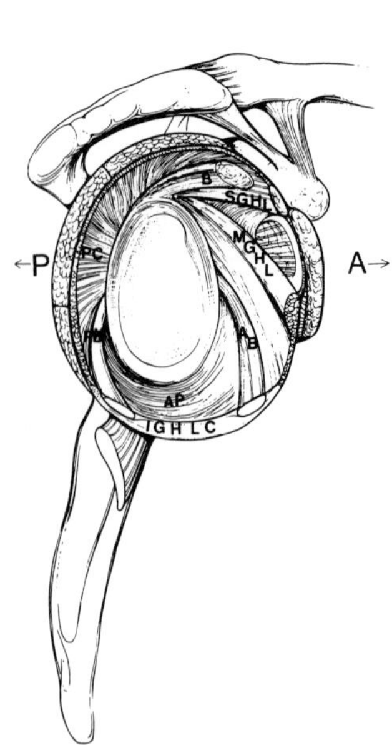


**Figure 9-6.** The shoulder capsule illustrating the location and extent of the IGHLC, inferior glenohumeral ligament complex. *A*, anterior; *P*, posterior; *B*, biceps tendon; *SGHL*, superior glenohumeral ligament; *MGHL*, middle glenohumeral ligament; *AB*, anterior band; *AP*, axillary pouch; *PB*, posterior band; and *PC*, posterior capsule. (Reprinted with permission of O'Brian SJ, Veves MC, Arnoczky SP, et al. The anatomy and histology of the inferior glenohumeral ligament complex of the shoulder. Am J Sports Med 1990;18:579.)

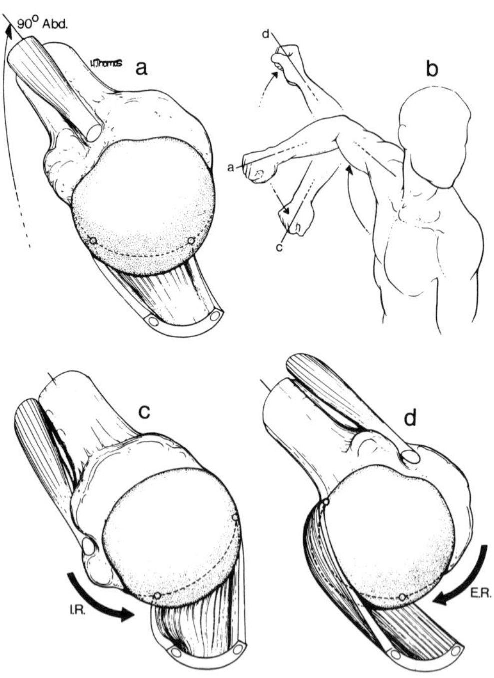


**Figure 9-7.** How the IGHLC functions to support the humeral head both anteriorly and posteriorly with the arm in abduction. (a) The arm is abducted 90 degrees and is in neutral rotation. (b,c) As the arm is internally rotated, the posterior band of the IGHLC fans out to support the humeral head posteriorly. (b,d) When the arm is externally rotated, the anterior band of the IGHLC fans out to support the humeral head anteriorly. (Reprinted with permission of O'Brian SJ, Veves MC, Arnoczky SP, et al. The anatomy and histology of the inferior glenohumeral ligament complex of the shoulder. Am J Sports Med 1990;18:579.)

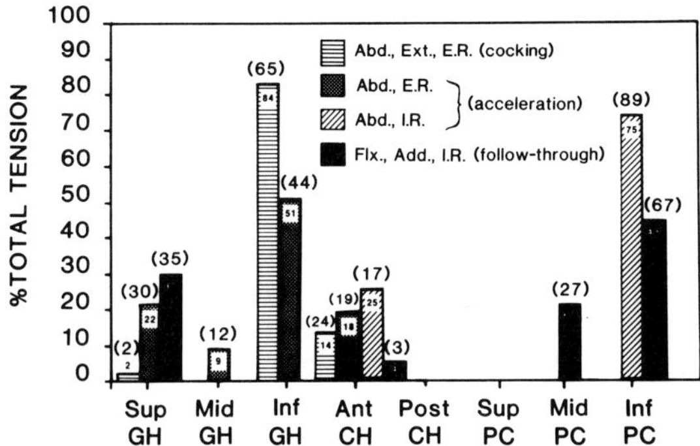


**Figure 9-8.** Strain gauge measurements during the complex motions of pitching: cocking, acceleration, and follow-through phases. Glenohumeral ligaments (*GH*), curacohumeral ligaments (*CH*), posterior capsule (*PC*). (Reprinted with permission from Terry GC, Hammon D, France P, et al. The stabilizing function of passive shoulder restraints. Am J Sports Med 1991;19:62.)

horizontal adduction, internal rotation, and distraction is transferred primarily to the posterior capsule as well as to some of the anterior capsule[84] (see Fig. 9-8). Dynamic restraint to forces imposed on the glenohumeral joint during follow-through is provided by the rotator cuff, biceps, pectoralis major, latissimus dorsi, and serratus anterior.[17,25,26,34,35,40,56]

# Muscle Activity: Selected Populations

The exact contribution that specific shoulder muscles make to the throwing sequence has been well summarized for normal individuals,[17,34,35] professional pitchers versus amateur pitchers,[26] and the normal stable shoulder versus the anteriorly unstable shoulder.[25] The contribution and timing of the activity of each of these muscles must be considered. Efficient and effective utilization of the muscles associated with the glenohumeral and scapulothoracic joints is required for optimal performance and injury prevention. Late cocking, acceleration, and follow-through are the most critical phases in which injury occurs or becomes apparent.

## LATE COCKING

Gowan et al.[26] compared EMG activity during pitching for the professional and the amateur athlete (Fig. 9-9a–d). Large differences are apparent for specific muscles. Activity is greater in the subscapularis muscle for the professional, while supraspinatus, biceps, serratus anterior, and pectoralis activity is less. Unfortunately, no

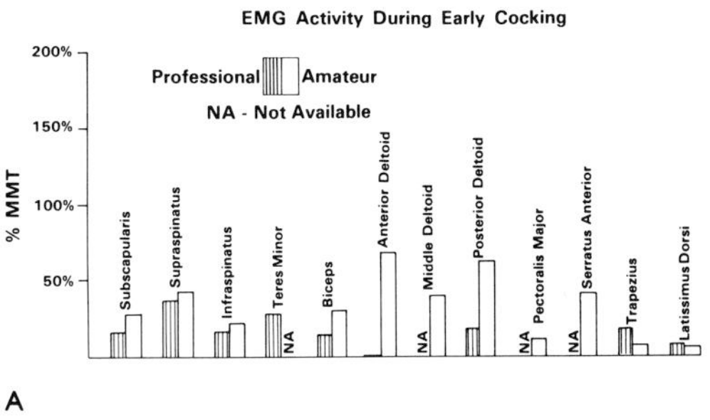


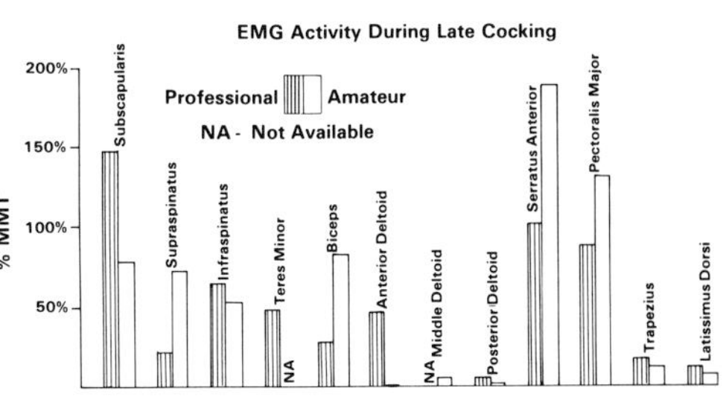


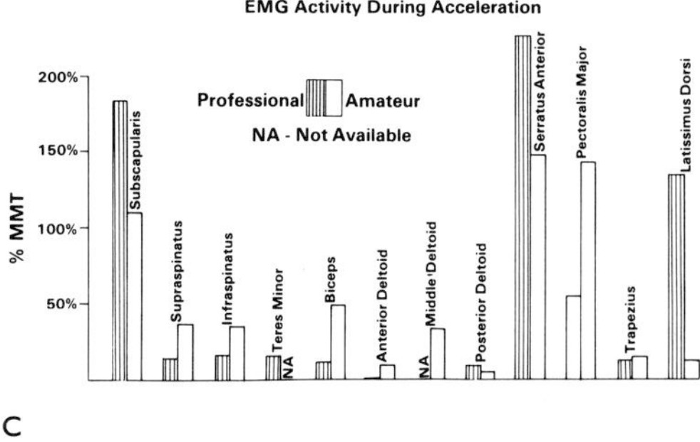


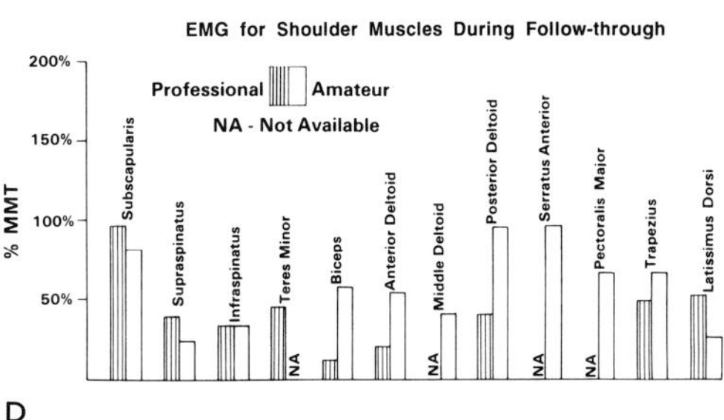


**Figure 9-9.** Average shoulder muscle EMG, professional versus amateur baseball pitchers. (a) Average EMG from shoulder muscles during early cocking. (b) Average EMG from shoulder muscles during late cocking. (c) Average EMG from shoulder muscles during acceleration. (d) Average EMG from shoulder muscles during follow-through. (Reprinted with permission from Gowan JD, Jobe FW, Tibone J, et al. A comparative electromyographic analysis of the shoulder during pitching: professional versus amateur pitchers. Am J Sports Med 1987;15:586.)

statistical analysis was applied in this study. Glousman et al.[25] completed a similar analysis comparing pitching in the normal athlete with a stable shoulder with that in individuals with documented anterior instability (Table 9-2). Individuals with anterior instability demonstrated significantly greater ($p < 0.05$) activity of the supraspinatus and significantly less activity of the pectoralis major, subscapularis, and serratus anterior muscles. Some scrutiny is required when interpreting this data, since all individuals who were unstable had positive apprehensive signs. Therefore, they would be reluctant to place their arms into the late cocking position, resulting in less activity of the internal rotators and serratus anterior. Increased activity of the supraspinatus might have been an attempt to provide greater dynamic stability.

The integrity and contraction of the subscapularis, latissimus dorsi, and pectoralis major may limit the load placed on passive ligamentous stabilizers. Poor neuromuscular control, altered timing, and insufficient strength and/or endurance of these dynamic stabilizers may be factors in the development or subsequent control of anterior instability. The therapist also must remember the impact that stretch weakness may have on the ability to contract these muscles to the extent required. In the individual with anterior instability, the significant increase in supraspinatus activity may be in an effort to stabilize the glenohumeral joint via compressive force.[10] The serratus anterior and scapular retractors are critical in controlling the position of the scapula. Decreased activity diminishes the protraction and upward rotation of the scapula that normally

**Table 9-2**

**Average EMG Values of Shoulder Muscles during Throwing in Individuals with Normal and Unstable Glenohumeral Joints**

| Phase Muscle Group | Windup | Early Cocking | Late Cocking | Acceleration | Follow-Through |
|---|---|---|---|---|---|
| **Biceps** | | | | | |
| Unstable | 8 | 21 | 35 | 32* | 18 |
| Normal | 8 | 17 | 26 | 12 | 13 |
| **Deltoid** | | | | | |
| Unstable | 7 | 35 | 10 | 26 | 37 |
| Normal | 7 | 39 | 6 | 32 | 41 |
| **Supraspinatus** | | | | | |
| Unstable | 12 | 45 | 51* | 37 | 43 |
| Normal | 12 | 36 | 21 | 13 | 40 |
| **Infraspinatus** | | | | | |
| Unstable | 9 | 30 | 52 | 37 | 39 |
| Normal | 9 | 15 | 65 | 16 | 35 |
| **Pectoralis major** | | | | | |
| Unstable | 3 | 7 | 58* | 61 | 27* |
| Normal | 3 | 11 | 85 | 55 | 67 |
| **Subscapularis** | | | | | |
| Unstable | 6 | 12 | 47* | 91* | 47* |
| Normal | 6 | 16 | 147 | 185 | 97 |
| **Latissimus dorsi** | | | | | |
| Unstable | 1 | 9 | 38* | 54* | 36 |
| Normal | 1 | 7 | 13 | 133 | 54 |
| **Serratus anterior** | | | | | |
| Unstable | 3 | 22 | 75* | 42* | 25* |
| Normal | 3 | 41 | 102 | 226 | 97 |

*Note:* All values expressed as a percent of maximal manual muscle test.
*$p < 0.05$; a statistically significant difference between groups exists.

Adapted from Glousman R, Jobe F, Tibone J, et al. Dynamic electromyographic analysis of the throwing shoulder with glenohumeral instability. J Bone Joint Surg 1988;70A:220.

begin during late cocking. In the late cocking phase, horizontal abduction begins while the humerus continues to rotate externally. Deficient rotation of the scapula places additional stress on both dynamic and passive anterior restraints. In addition, the subacromial space also can be compromised, potentially accentuating impingement.[34]

### ACCELERATION

Dynamically, acceleration is initiated by the subscapularis, pectoralis major, and latissimus dorsi muscles. Individuals with anterior instability demonstrated a significant decrease in activity of the subscapularis and latissimus dorsi. Activity of the serratus anterior was also found to be significantly less.[34] This alteration of muscle activity is most likely related to the subject's "apprehension" during late cocking. The serratus anterior fires during acceleration to provide a rigid platform from which to initiate glenohumeral internal rotation. Similar activity patterns are also demonstrated when comparing the professional pitcher with the amateur. One must question if the normal individual with a stable shoulder and the professional pitcher are able to make more efficient and effective use of their shoulder musculature to control external rotation and then accelerate the arm, rather than relying on recoil of the passive restraints. By doing this, do they protect the passive restraints?

### DECELERATION AND FOLLOW-THROUGH

During these phases, the pectoralis major, subscapularis, latissimus dorsi, and serratus anterior muscles all demonstrate significantly less activity in the individual with anterior instability. The lower trapezius, which is very active in the normal population,[17] was not assessed in those with anterior instability. Inability to optimally control these dynamic stabilizers during this phase may allow excessive distraction at the glenohumeral joint, resulting in overload to the posterior rotator cuff and posterior capsule.

The proper balance of strength, endurance, and timing of contraction between all muscles associated with the glenohumeral joint during throwing is critical. This balance appears to differ between the professional and amateur pitcher, as well as between individuals with and without anterior instability. The therapist must utilize knowledge of specific muscle activity patterns in the design of a comprehensive rehabilitation program.

# Other Overhead Sports

## Waterpolo

Shoulder injuries in waterpolo are similar to those in other overhead sports. The waterpolo competitor is at high risk because he or she must swim and throw. Data from the United States National Waterpolo Team have revealed a 36 percent incidence of rotator cuff tendinitis.

The upper extremity throwing motion is similar to baseball regarding phases of activity. There are critical differences in waterpolo, however. The ball is initially held out of the water with the opposite arm positioned in front of the ball for balance. Since the player is not touching the bottom of the pool, he or she is using an eggbeater kick in an attempt to maintain position and provide a somewhat stable platform from which to throw.

Rollins et al.[67] have completed a thorough cinemagraphic evaluation of waterpolo. These results will be presented in summary. During the windup phase, the arm is cocked. This cocking motion may happen repeatedly as the player goes through a series of faking motions/throws. During this motion, the humerus is typically abducted 90 degrees. Greater external rotation has been related to ball velocity.

Because no stable platform exists for the player to push off of during acceleration, all momentum must be generated by the eggbeater kick, body momentum, and arm acceleration. EMG studies have not been carried out to define any differences in muscle activity compared with pitching. The great requirement of acceleration through muscular effort may place a greater load on the myotendinous structures about the shoulder in comparison with passive restraints.

## Football

Wick et al.[88] have documented some of the kinematic differences between baseball pitching and football passing, demonstrating both similarities and differences (Table 9-3). This comparison requires further study in relation to the types of injuries suffered from passing a football compared with throwing a baseball.

## Tennis

The racquet is an additional link in the kinetic chain when comparing the tennis serve with the

Table 9-3

**Comparison of Kinematic Parameters of Baseball Pitching versus Football Passing**

| | Baseball ($n$ = 23) | Football ($n$ = 14) |
|---|---|---|
| **Foot contact parameters (deg)** | | |
| Shoulder external rotation* | 65 ± 29 | 88 ± 36 |
| Shoulder abduction | 103 ± 13 | 105 ± 17 |
| Shoulder horizontal adduction | −11 ± 24 | −2 ± 17 |
| **Delivery parameters** | | |
| **Angular variables (deg)** | | |
| Max external rotation | 175 ± 12 | 168 ± 12 |
| **Angular velocity parameters (deg/s)** | | |
| Max internal rotation* | 7365 ± 1503 | 4586 ± 843 |
| Max shoulder horizontal adduction | 657 ± 266 | 519 ± 165 |
| Max shoulder* | 1180 ± 294 | 1017 ± 177 |
| **Release parameters (deg)** | | |
| Shoulder external rotation* | 124 ± 22 | 145 ± 25 |
| Shoulder abduction* | 99 ± 8 | 114 ± 15 |
| Shoulder horizontal adduction* | 10 ± 8 | 21 ± 10 |
| Ball velocity (m/s)* | 74 ± 5 | 46 ± 4 |
| Duration of throw (s)* | .15 ± .03 | .20 ± .03 |

*$p$ = 0.05, significant difference.

Adapted from Wick H, Dillman C, Werner S, et al. A kinematic comparison between baseball pitching and football passing. Sports Med Update 1991;Spring:13.

overhand throw. The addition of this lever arm would appear to increase the stress placed at the shoulder. According to Leach,[39] however, much of the impact force is dissipated by the strings of the racquetball interface, the racquet frame, and the wrist and forearm so that less force is transmitted to the shoulder. This seems plausible, since a tennis player serves more often than a baseball pitcher pitches during each competition and is able to compete more often. The tennis player is able to compete on repetitive days, while pitchers often require a rest of 3 to 5 days between each start.

## PHASES

The serve may be divided into stages similar to the pitch.[37, 69] These stages are the windup, cocking-backscratch, acceleration-impact, and deceleration–follow-through[69] (Fig. 9-10).

### WINDUP

This is the preparatory phase of the stroke, and it lasts until the ball is tossed. During this phase, the shoulder is brought into abduction, extension, and external rotation. The trunk extends and the lower extremities rotate appropriately.

### COCKING-BACKSCRATCH

This phase begins as the ball leaves the hand and ends with maximal external rotation of the shoulder. The racquet appears to "scratch the back" due to a combination of its length and associated wrist and trunk motion. Scapular rotation increases during this phase.[69] Placement of the ball toss is important on the next phase, acceleration. If the ball is tossed too far backward, excessive abduction of the shoulder may result, increasing stress on the capsuloligamentous complex and rotator cuff.

### ACCELERATION-IMPACT

This phase is initiated as internal rotation begins and ends with ball impact. The upper extremity may be more vertically oriented at ball impact in the tennis serve during this phase compared with the acceleration–ball-release phase of pitching. Elliott[18] has stated that the upper extremity is elevated approximately 180 degrees in this phase. Elliot does not detail whether this position is relative to the ground or the position of the trunk. Elliott's conclusion is in direct contrast to that of Atwater,[4] who attributes much of the perception of upper extremity elevation to lateral trunk bending. Exact quantification of the position of shoulder abduction has not adequately been detailed.

Inappropriate trunk rotation or lateral flexion can again force excessive positioning of the shoulder. This is seen in the inflexible athlete, particularly the older participant.

### FOLLOW-THROUGH–DECELERATION

Follow-through and deceleration begin immediately following impact. Like throwing a baseball, follow-through should be complete to dissipate forces across the shoulder.

## MUSCLE ACTIVITY

Ryu et al.[69] have documented muscle activity during all phases or stages of serving (Table 9-4). The importance of muscle activation during each phase of the serve can be appreciated. The patterns demonstrated are similar to those of pitching. The contribution of the scapular muscles cannot be overemphasized in the ability of the participant to repetitively serve without injury.

From these results and the similarity to the phases of pitching, one might hypothesize that

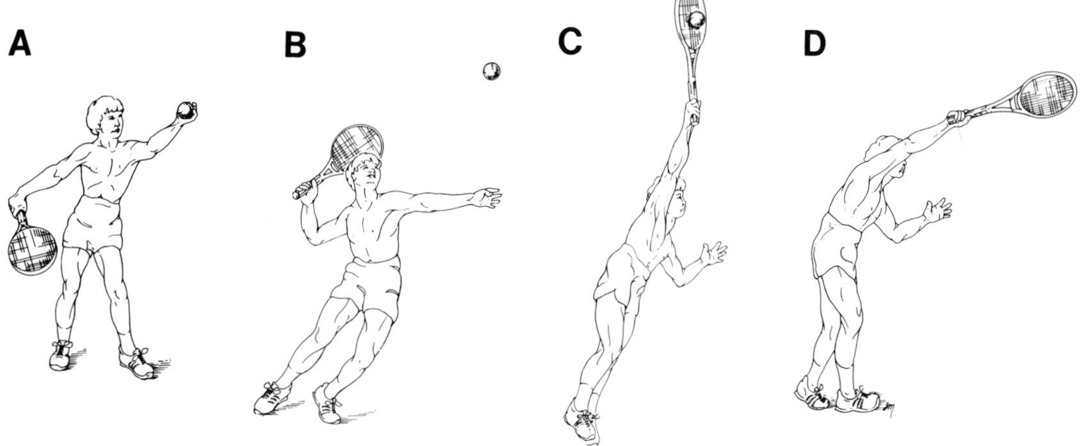


**Figure 9-10.** The four stages of the tennis serve. (a) Windup. (b) Cocking. (c) Acceleration. (d) Follow-through. (Reprinted with permission of Ryu RK, McCormick J, Jobe FW, et al. An electromyographic analysis of shoulder function in tennis players. Am J Sports Med 1988;16:481.)

other similarities exist regarding kinematic forces and stress placed on ligamentous restraints.

## Rehabilitative Considerations

When considering the biomechanics of any sport activity, internal and external forces must be balanced in an effort to avoid injury. The known factors involved in the activity must be compared with the unknown factors. The same balance must be considered in the rehabilitative process.

**Table 9-4**

**Average EMG Values of Shoulder Muscles during Tennis Serve: Stages Illustrated As I–IV**

| | Stages—%MMT | | | |
|---|---|---|---|---|
| **Muscles** | I | II | III | IV |
| Biceps brachii | 6 | 39 | 10 | 34 |
| Middle deltoid | 18 | 23 | 14 | 36 |
| Supraspinatus | 15 | 53 | 26 | 35 |
| Infraspinatus | 7 | 41 | 31 | 30 |
| Subscapularis | 5 | 25 | 113 | 63 |
| Pectoralis major | 5 | 21 | 115 | 39 |
| Serratus anterior | 24 | 70 | 74 | 53 |
| Latissimus dorsi | 16 | 32 | 57 | 48 |

Reprinted with permission from Ryu RK, McCormick J, Jobe FW, et al. An electromyographic analysis of shoulder function in tennis players. Am J Sports Med 1988;16:481.

The therapist cannot restore the integrity of the static restraints if pathologic ligamentous laxity exists, whether subtle or extreme. Therapeutic exercise programs for the throwing or overhand-specific athlete must be designed to facilitate proper muscle balance, strength, endurance, and timing of contraction *in an attempt* to prevent injury of ligamentous restraints and labrum or to control abnormal motion if laxity exists. The therapeutic exercise program must be designed around what is known about muscle function and the kinematic factors associated with the sport-specific overhead demands. Muscles of the rotator cuff and scapula must serve as dynamic stabilizers. Programs must appropriately address the position in which these muscles function as well as the force, velocity, acceleration, or deceleration associated with the activity.

Program design will vary depending on the individual philosophies of each clinician but should adhere to what is known from research regarding specific muscle groups and stress on the glenohumeral and scapulothoracic joints during throwing and serving. Scapular stability must first be gained prior to attempting to isolate muscles of the glenohumeral complex. Rhythmic stabilization utilizing body weight or free weights in an isometric manner is appropriate during the early phases of the rehabilitative course. Scapula proprioceptive neuromuscular facilitation patterns are useful at this stage. The program should progress from stress-free positions to more stressful positions as the athlete tolerates. Emphasis should be placed on proper mechanics in a controlled range of motion initially. Velocity of activity and range are progressed depending on the athlete's tolerance, provided the mechanics are correct and the activity is pain-free. As the program progresses, activity simulation is encouraged within the program utilizing rubber tubing, exercise equipment, and upper extremity plyometrics. Use of activity-simulation exercises such as these provides the important eccentric loading stresses, first at controlled velocities and then at changing velocities.

## Core Program

Based on EMG analyses, all muscles of the upper quarter require attention; however, critical muscles appear to be the supraspinatus, infraspinatus, teres minor, subscapularis, latissimus dorsi, pectoralis major, trapezius, and serratus anterior. A core group of critical exercises is required to effectively strengthen these muscles[8,10,46,85] (Table 9-5). Resistance, when appropriate, is provided by the use of hand weights, rubber tubing, or body weight.

In utilizing core rehabilitative exercises, initial program emphasis should be placed on building a base of strength and endurance of critical muscles with isolated activity. Endurance and correct motor control/function should be stressed early and throughout the program. Care must be taken to attempt to promote an appropriate scapulohumeral rhythm.

The ability to stabilize and control the glenohumeral joint in multiple positions, especially overhead positions, is critical. Rhythmic stabilization and alternating isometrics may be used to teach the athlete to control this position. Little resistance is required. Emphasis is placed on control. The Bodyblade also may be used to teach positional control and develop proprioceptive sense as well as strength and endurance. It has the advantage of being used in multiple positions (Fig. 9-11).

**Table 9-5**

**Core Exercises for a Rehabilitation Program**

| Exercise | Muscles Activated |
|---|---|
| "Scaption" | Anterior/middle deltoid |
| Internal Rotation | Supraspinatus<br>Subscapularis<br>Serratus anterior |
| External rotation | Anterior/middle deltoid<br>Supraspinatus<br>Infraspinatus<br>Serratus anterior<br>Rhomboids<br>Trapezius |
| Horizontal abduction in external rotation | Infraspinatus<br>Teres minor<br>Posterior deltoid<br>Upper/middle/lower trapezius |
| Rowing | Upper/middle/lower trapezius<br>Levator scapulae<br>Rhomboids<br>Posterior deltoid |
| Press-ups | Pectoralis major<br>Latissimus dorsi<br>Pectoralis minor |
| Push-ups with a plus | Pectoralis major<br>Pectoralis minor<br>Serratus anterior |

Developed from information presented in references 8, 10, 66, and 85.

## Endurance and General Conditioning

When the athlete has appropriate isolated muscle strength and good scapulohumeral mechanics, general upper extremity endurance and conditioning may begin. An upper body ergometer and general weight equipment may be used. Emphasis is again placed on activities that require use of the muscle groups involved in throwing. Flexibility of the upper extremity should be addressed with appropriate exercises.

Trunk and lower extremity strength and flexibility are also essential for the athlete who uses the arm to throw or serve. Since the legs and trunk are involved in the transference of energy during throwing and serving, ensuring optimal conditioning of these areas has ultimate performance enhancing and prophylactic effects on the shoulder.

## Summary

Appropriate biomechanics of the shoulder during throwing and serving are critical in maintaining integrity of the associated shoulder structures. The therapist must have a sound working knowledge of muscle activity and kinematics to evaluate, treat, and design an appropriate rehabili-

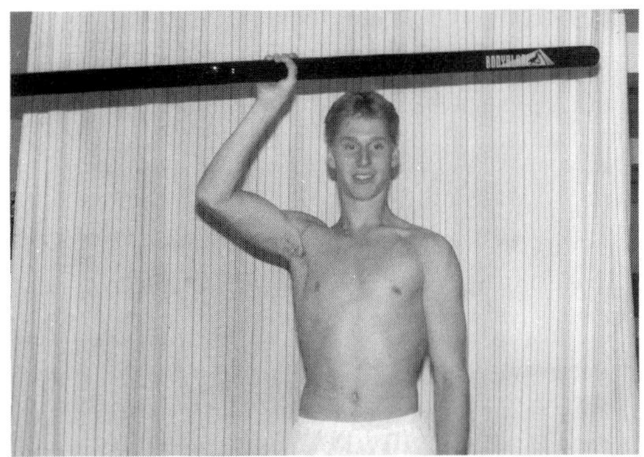

**Figure 9-11.** The Bodyblade is used to simulate a throwing motion. Oscillations by the blade during this simulation require the athlete to work on motor control, timing, and proprioceptive skills, as well as strength and endurance.

tative or conditioning program for the throwing athlete. The therapist should seek to be innovative in program design within the bounds of research detailing overhand specific characteristics.

# The Shoulder in Swimming

Swimming, like throwing, is essentially a propulsive activity involving overhead use of the upper extremity. As such, the shoulder is subjected to considerable forces. In addition, the swimmer must overcome the resistance, or drag, of the water on the body. While there is some disagreement on the exact contribution of the kick to forward motion, it is generally agreed that the arm stroke is the main source of propulsion in all swimming styles except the breaststroke. In the freestyle and butterfly, the arm motion has been estimated to account for as much as 85 percent of the propulsive power.[45] Thus shoulder girdle joints and soft tissues must be capable of meeting the repetitive demands of swimming. Failure to do so can result in dysfunction and pathology.

Of the four major swimming techniques, freestyle or crawl is the most common and has been studied the most extensively. The butterfly has been described as a bilateral freestyle with respect to arm action. The backstroke shares many of the same forces. Consequently, this section will focus primarily on freestyle mechanics with specific reference to the other strokes for comparison where relevant.

The phases and kinetics of the freestyle stroke have been described by many authors.[13,45,47,56,66,68,71] Muscle action has been studied by EMG[15,32,47,51,61,68] and by assessment of isokinetic torque changes in the swimming athlete.[44]

## Phases

Each swimming stroke has a characteristic arm pattern, but all four techniques exhibit two main phases: (1) the pull-through and (2) the recovery. A commonly adopted model[66] further breaks down the two phases into three stages each. Pull-through is composed of hand entry, middle pull-through, and late pull-through. Recovery consists of elbow lift, middle recovery and late recovery (Fig. 9-12). Richardson et al.[66] summarized the mechanics associated with each phase (Table 9-6). Upper extremity propulsive power in freestyle, butterfly, and backstroke is accomplished during the pull-through phase primarily through shoulder adduction, internal rotation, and extension. Recovery is characterized by abduction, external rotation, and flexion.[56]

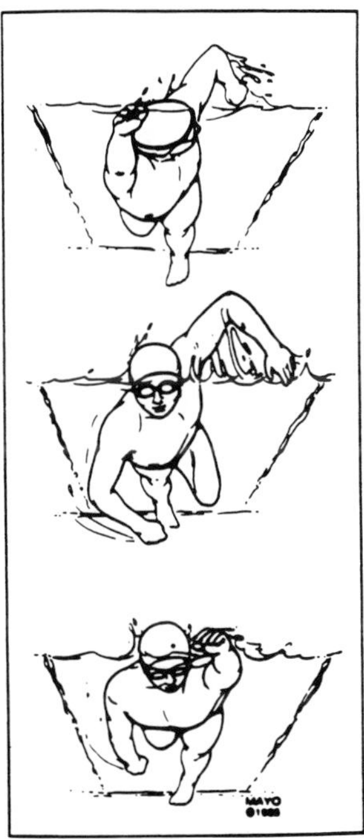


**Figure 9-12.** Stroke mechanics for freestyle swimming. For the right arm, three phases of pull-through are identified: hand entry (top), middle pull-through (middle), and late pull-through (bottom). For the left arm, the three stages of recovery are depicted: elbow lift (top), midrecovery (middle), and late recovery (bottom). (Reprinted with permission from Johnson E, Sim FH, Scott SG. Musculoskeletal injuries in competitive swimmers. Mayo Clin Proc 1987;62:289.)

**Table 9-6**

**Shoulder Mechanics in Swimming**

| Stroke and Phases | Description |
|---|---|
| Freestyle | |
| Pull-through phase | |
| Hand entry | Shoulder external rotation and abduction. Body roll begins |
| Middle pull-through | Shoulder at 90° abduction and neutral internal-external rotation. Body roll is at maximum of 40–60° from horizontal |
| End of pull-through | Shoulder internally rotated and fully adducted. Body has returned to horizontal |
| Recovery phase | |
| Elbow lift | Shoulder begins abduction and external rotation. Body roll begins in opposite direction from pull-through |
| Midrecovery | Shoulder abducted to 90° and externally rotated beyond neutral. Body roll reaches maximum of 40–60°. Breathing occurs by turning head to side |
| Hand entry | Shoulder externally rotated and maximally abducted. Body has returned to neutral roll |
| Backstroke | |
| Pull-through phase | |
| Hand entry | Shoulder external rotation and abduction. Body roll begins |
| Middle pull-through | Shoulder at 90° abduction and neutral internal-external rotation. Body roll maximum |
| End of pull-through | Shoulder internally rotated and abducted. Body roll horizontal |
| Recovery phase | |
| Hand lift | Shoulder begins abduction and external rotation. Body roll allows arm to clear water |
| Midrecovery | Shoulder at 90° abduction. Body roll maximum |
| Hand entry | Shoulder at maximum abduction. Body roll neutral |
| Butterfly | |
| Pull-through phase | Same as freestyle with the absence of body roll in all stages. To avoid shoulder flexion or extension, the hands are spread apart at the mid pull-through stage |
| Recovery phase | Again, similar to freestyle with the absence of body roll. Body lift allows both arms to clear the water. Shoulder flexion-extension does not occur. |

Reprinted with permission from Richardson AB, Jobe F, Collins HR. The shoulder in competitive swimming. Am J Sports Med 1980;8:159.

## PULL-THROUGH

This is the propulsive phase of the arm stroke and has been likened to the acceleration phase of throwing.[56] The arm follows an S-shaped curve through the water in 0.6 s in the experienced swimmer[32] to 1 s in the average swimmer.[51] Since the entire freestyle stroke is completed in 1.65 s (1.15 s for the butterfly), the pull-through phase accounts for 65 to 70 percent of the stroke time.[68]

### HAND ENTRY

Correct hand placement at hand entry is critical. The hand enters the water with the index finger first and the elbow high in a line between the head and shoulder.[71] Body roll begins. The shoulder is still externally rotated and abducted but moving toward internal rotation. At hand entry, the arm reaches forward and glides as the elbow extends. No propulsion occurs during this stage. It functions primarily to place the arm in preparation for the pull. Primary movers at hand entry have been studied by Pink et al.[61] and are illustrated in Figure 9-13. Phasic activity of these five muscles varies from 40 to 64 percent of their maximal isometric activity level. The serratus anterior, although not depicted, peaks from its constant low level of activity to upwardly rotate the scapula in a force couple with the upper trapezius and the rhomboids. The supraspinatus assists the middle and anterior deltoids to elevate the arm during the reach forward just after hand entry.

### MIDDLE PULL-THROUGH

The pull itself begins after the reach and ends as the palm nears the thigh in late pull-through.[71] Approximately 45 percent of the entire stroke is spent from hand entry to the position of a 90-degree arm/trunk angle at middle pull-through.[68] The body rolls to a maximum of 40 to 60 degrees from horizontal to the opposite side. The thumb points to the high part of the chest as the elbow flexes to move the hand and arm back, out, and down in the characteristic S curve. The elbow is ideally held above the level of the hand. This sweeping motion creates the powerful surge of propulsion and acceleration. EMG patterns of the primary movers have been detailed and are illustrated in Figures 9-14 through 9-17.[61] The pectoralis major peaks to provide the initial adduction, extension, and internal rotation. The teres minor assists extension and provides an external rotation counterbalance to the strong internal rotation force of the subscapularis and pectoralis major. At middle pull-through, the latissimus dorsi gains mechanical advantage for extension and increases its activity. Nuber et al.[51] report peak activity for the latissimus dorsi at middle

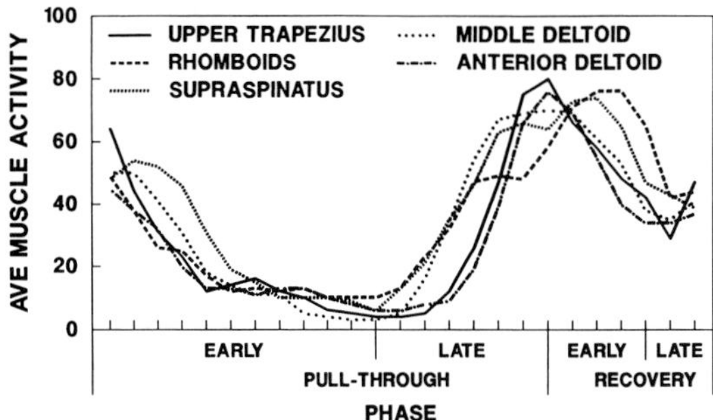


**Figure 9-13.** Primary movers at hand entry and exit. (Reprinted with permission from Pink M, Perry J, Browne A, et al. The normal shoulder during freestyle swimming: an electromyographic and cinematographic analysis of twelve muscles. Am J Sports Med 1991;19:569.)

pull-through, while Pink et al.[61] show peak activation later in this phase. The serratus anterior muscle is active throughout this phase to stabilize the scapula, thereby allowing the propulsive muscles to pull the humerus against a solid base (see Fig. 9-14). The activity of biceps brachii is reported inconsistently[51,68] in the literature. When the proper stroke technique of a flexed high elbow is maintained, peak activity for the biceps occurs from early to middle pull as the elbow flexes.[68] Biceps activity is much less in all other phases. The less efficient extended arm technique produced a constant, nonspecific high level of biceps activity throughout the entire stroke.[68] Nuber et al.[51] report inconsistent biceps activity throughout the stroke, with only a slight increase noted in the beginning of pull-through. The biceps appears to function in positioning the hand and assisting in depressing the humeral head as the shoulder muscles elevate the elbow.

## LATE PULL-THROUGH

This stage continues the propulsive part of the stroke. Body roll returns to horizontal. The hand is brought backward as the elbow and arm are maximally extended. The shoulder is maximally adducted and internally rotated. In this position, the supraspinatus and infraspinatus tendons are most prone to hypovascularity as the tendons are "wrung out" over the humeral head[36,62] (Fig. 9-18). The increased passive tension developed in the supraspinatus and infraspinatus tendon fibers can initiate or perpetuate inflammation. The latissimus dorsi is now at its best mechanical advantage and peaks at 75 percent of its maximum as it provides the final push of propulsion.[61] Pectoralis major activity declines but continues beyond resting level. The serratus anterior is significantly active throughout late pull as it eccentrically contracts to stabilize the scapula as the arm medially rotates. At the very end of pull-through, activity in the latissimus dorsi and pectoralis major muscles diminishes rapidly. Sequential firing of the deltoid fibers begins the change from the pull of shoulder extension to the lift of the humerus from the water in preparation for recovery. Ikai et al.[32] state that while less experienced swimmers use more muscular effort, more experienced swimmers have a more selective use of both the latissimus dorsi and teres minor during this phase.

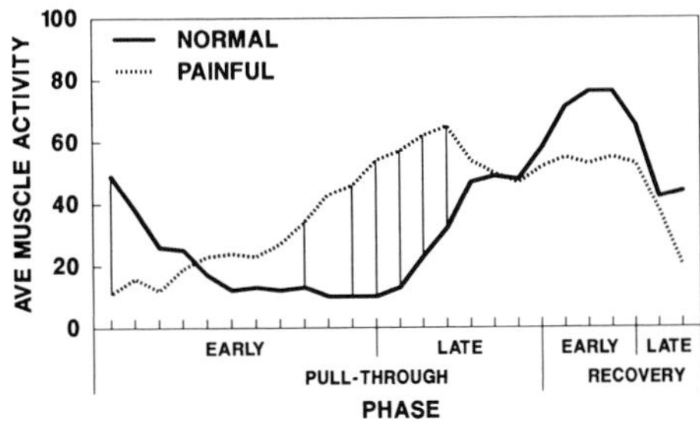


A

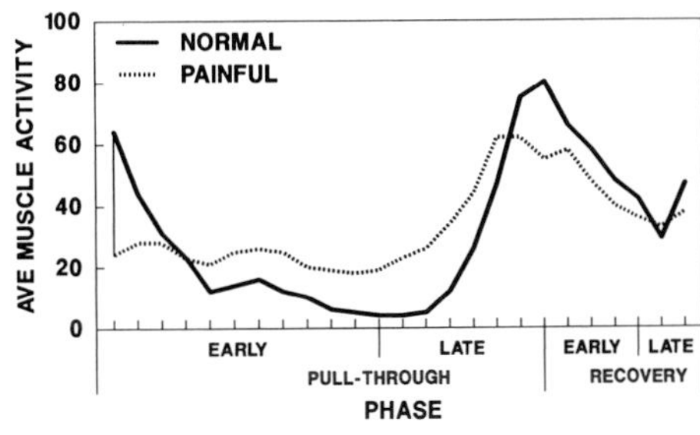


B

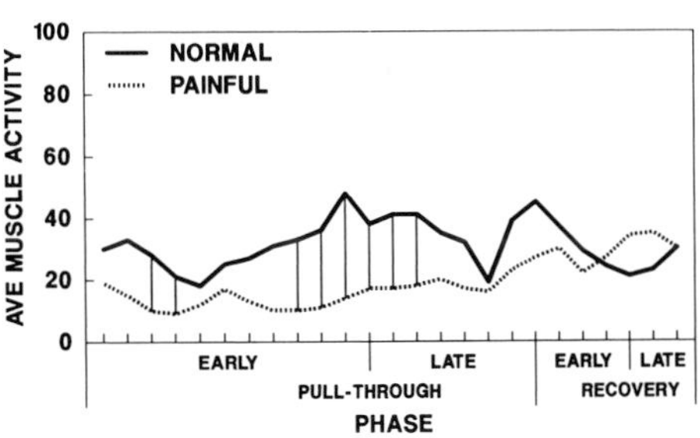


C

**Figure 9-14.** Muscle activity of the scapular muscles in the painful and the normal shoulders during the freestyle stroke. Vertical lines show periods of significant difference. (Reprinted with permission from Scovazzo ML, Browne A, Pink M, et al. The painful shoulder during freestyle swimming: an electromyographic and cinematographic analysis of twelve muscles. Am J Sports Med 1991;19:577.)

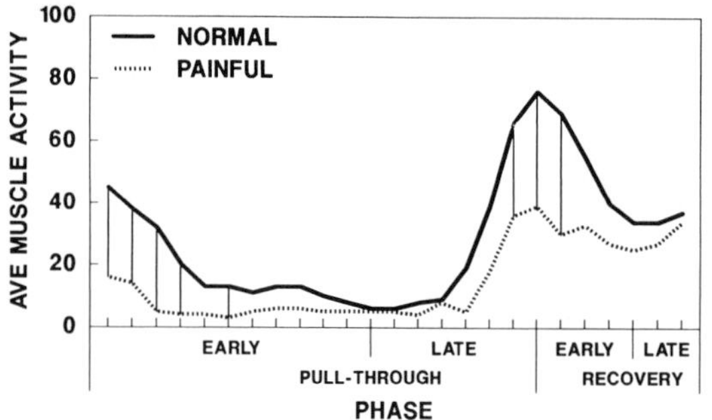


A

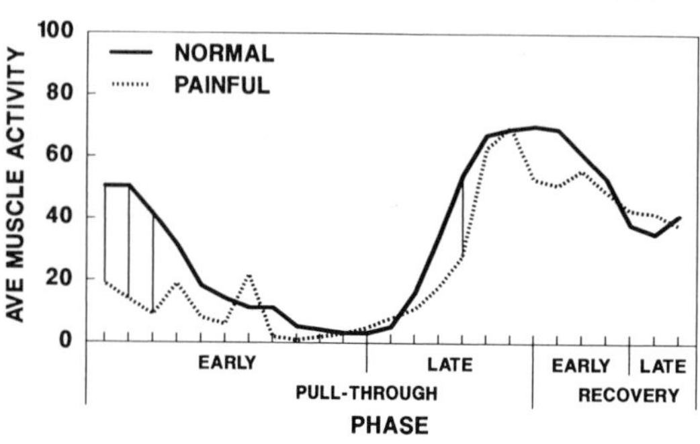


B

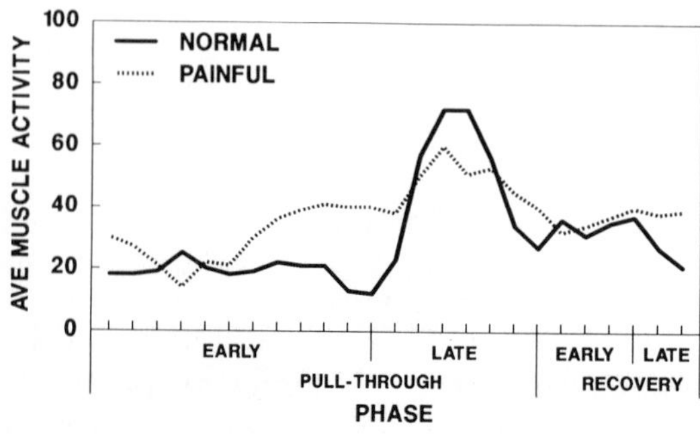


C

**Figure 9-15.** Muscle activity of the deltoids in the painful and the normal shoulders during the freestyle stroke. Vertical lines show periods of significant difference. (Reprinted with permission from Scovazzo ML, Browne A, Pink M, et al. The painful shoulder during freestyle swimming: an electromyographic and cinematographic analysis of twelve muscles. Am J Sports Med 1991; 19:577.)

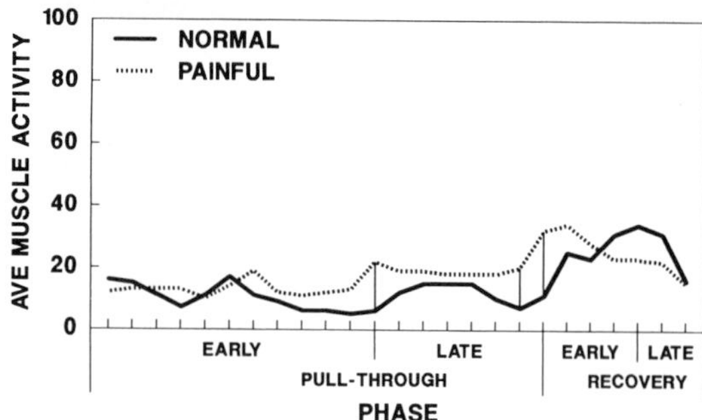


A

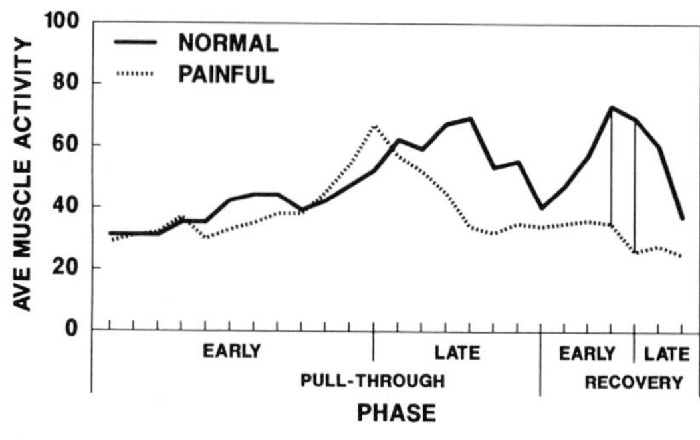


B

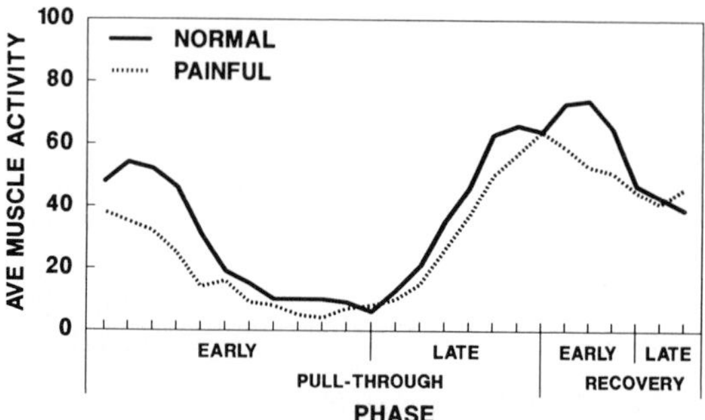


C

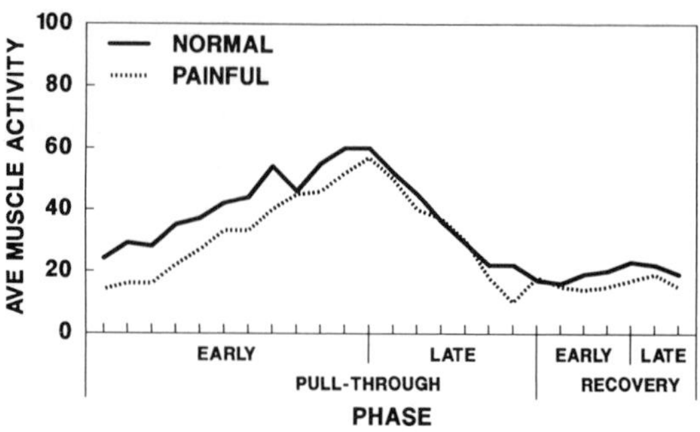


D

**Figure 9-16.** Muscle activity of the rotator cuff muscles in the painful and the normal shoulders during freestyle stroke. Vertical lines show periods of significant difference. (Reprinted with permission from Scovazzo ML, Browne A, Pink M, et al. The painful shoulder during freestyle swimming: an electromyographic and cinematographic analysis of twelve muscles. Am J Sports Med 1991;19:577.)

NORMAL AND PAINFUL - PECTORALIS MAJOR

AVE MUSCLE ACTIVITY
100
80
60
40
20
0
NORMAL
PAINFUL
EARLY
LATE
PULL-THROUGH
EARLY
LATE
RECOVERY
PHASE

A

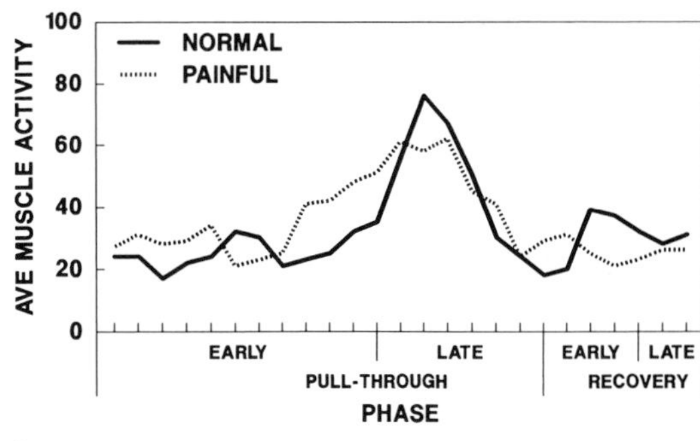


B

**Figure 9-17.** Muscle activity of the shoulder extensor muscles in the painful and the normal shoulders during the freestyle stroke. Vertical lines show periods of significant difference. (Reprinted with permission from Scovazzo ML, Browne A, Pink M, et al. The painful shoulder during freestyle swimming: an electromyographic and cinematographic analysis of twelve muscles. Am J Sports Med 1991;19:577.)

## RECOVERY

Recovery accounts for 30 to 35 percent of the total stroke.[51,68] It is a very rapid period of repositioning of the arm prior to the next stroke. It is comparable with the cocking phase of overhead throwing, except that the degree of external rotation is significantly less than in throwing.[56] Recovery is characterized by shoulder abduction and external rotation as the arm is elevated. This stage has been implicated as a major source of mechanical irritation in the glenohumeral joint of the swimmer, since the rotator cuff tendons can be impinged between the acromial arch and the humeral head.[13,19,22,38,65]

### ELBOW LIFT

Body roll begins in the direction of the arm that is beginning recovery. Adequate body roll is critical at this stage to minimize the amount of shoulder horizontal abduction required to initiate the elbow lift from the water (see Fig. 9-12). The glenohumeral joint begins to abduct and externally rotate from its previous position at maximal adduction/internal rotation. The same five prime movers are active at hand exit as at hand entry[61] (see Fig. 9-13). The posterior deltoid helps to initiate the elbow lift as the supraspinatus peaks in activity. The middle deltoid functions to elevate the arm. Both the rhomboids and the upper trapezius are active, retracting and elevating the scapula, respectively. Serratus anterior activity peaks as the arm is elevated.[72]

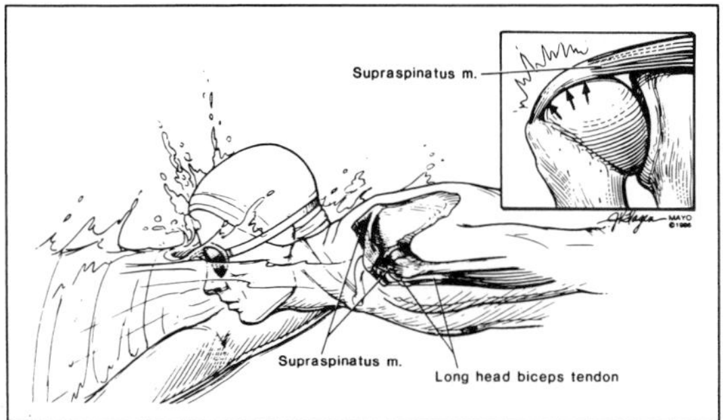


**Figure 9-18.** Adduction of the glenohumeral joint, as in late pull-through phase of freestyle swimming, is a mechanism that can cause "wringing out" of supraspinatus and biceps tendons. (Reprinted with permission from Johnson JE, Sim FH, Scott SG. Musculoskeletal injuries in competitive swimmers. Mayo Clin Proc 1987;62:289.)

### MIDDLE RECOVERY

Body roll reaches its maximum of 40 to 60 degrees for the second time as the head turns to breath in the direction of the arm in recovery phase. The scapula rotates upward and abducts as the humerus now externally rotates beyond neutral. Sufficient upward scapular rotation is critical to prevent mechanical subacromial space impingement until the humerus reaches maximal abduction as the arm is brought forward. Like the throwing athlete, but to a lesser degree, it is at this stage that the anterior capsuloligamentous complex is loaded and most susceptible to injury.[13] With arm abduction and external rotation, the inferior glenohumeral ligament occupies a more anterior position and serves as a primary restraint. The humeral head is positioned against the inferior glenohumeral ligament. While the forces in swimming do not equal the torques generated in the throwing motion, the swimmer repeats the activity thousands of time at each practice, which may predispose him or her to laxity. Some authors report that the supraspinatus and infraspinatus muscles are active throughout the recovery phase to externally rotate and abduct the arm.[47] More recent EMG analysis demonstrates that while both these muscles are active throughout recovery, supraspinatus activity peaks early at 66 to 74 percent of its peak 1-s EMG activity (during a manual muscle test [MMT]).[72] The supraspinatus functions primarily as an early abductor. The infraspinatus exhibits its highest activity at 34 percent of its peak 1-s EMG activity in middle recovery to externally rotate the humerus, as a humeral head depressor, and as an antagonist to the strong internal rotation moment of the subscapularis (see Fig. 9-16).

### LATE RECOVERY

Recovery ends with hand entry. The body is once more horizontal. The upper extremity is in the "catch" position previously described for the hand-entry phase. Just prior to hand entry, the glenohumeral joint is abducted and externally rotated. The serratus anterior activity increases (but does not peak) during late recovery as it assists scapular upward rotation. This activity allows for maximal arm elevation while minimizing impingement of the rotator cuff, bursa, and biceps tendon (Fig. 9-19).

## The Painful Shoulder in Swimming

The painful "swimmer's shoulder," so called originally by Kennedy et al.,[38] is traditionally ascribed to a tendinitis of the supraspinatus tendon and sometimes the long head of the biceps. This condition is created by one of two mechanisms: (1) mechanical impingement of the superior rotator cuff tendons and subacromial bursa[2,13,36,65,87] or (2) a "wringing out" of the vascularity of the rotator cuff tendon.[13,19,62] Extreme elevation and internal rotation of the flexed shoulder can result in impingement of the greater tuberosity against the anterior acromion and the coracoacromial arch.[48] Poor technique during recovery and early pull-through predispose a swimmer to this mechanical irritation. Extreme adduction and internal rotation create a temporary hypovascular area approximately 1 cm proximal to the insertion of the supraspinatus tendon as well as the biceps tendon.[62] Fatigue or faulty mechanics during middle to late pull-through may simulate these conditions.[13,19]

More recently, McMaster[43] described another dysfunction in the painful swimmer's shoulder. He demonstrated a functional instability in swimmers who do not exhibit true instability. It is characterized by damage to the anterior glenohumeral labrum in an arc between the superior and inferior glenohumeral ligaments. The swimmer notes pain at hand entry and catch, with maximal pain reported at middle pull-through in a position of adduction and internal rotation. McMaster hypothesizes that such swimming motions, when combined with anterior capsular laxity, may produce a subclinical anterior subluxation that damages the labrum. He differentiates this syndrome from the anterior subluxation associated with the flip turn of the backstroke (Fig. 9-20), in which the swimmer has a positive classic apprehension sign.[38,43] Complete shoulder dislocation is not a common finding in swimmers, but primary directional instability, either anterior or posterior, is common, as is multidirectional instability.[13]

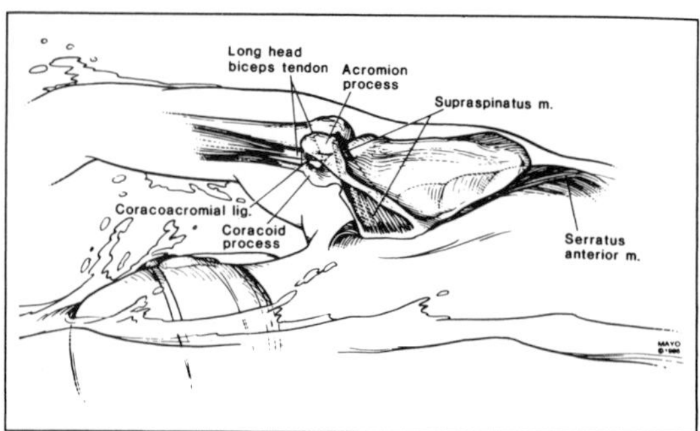


**Figure 9-19.** Impingement of supraspinatus and biceps tendons between humeral head and coracoacromial arch can occur the late recovery phase of the freestyle stroke. Serratus anterior activity allows greater shoulder range of motion and delays impingement of the greater tuberosity under the coracoacromial arch. (Reprinted with permission from Johnson JE, Sim FH, Scott SG. Musculoskeletal injuries in competitive swimmers. Mayo Clin Proc 1987;62:289.)

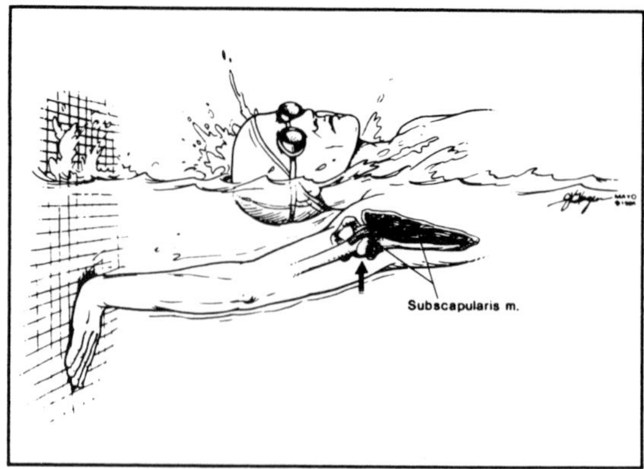


**Figure 9-20.** The backstroke flip turn is initiated by forceful shoulder internal rotation and forward flexion with the arm in extreme abduction and external rotation. The action places considerable stress on the anterior glenohumeral joint structures and can lead to anterior instability. (Reprinted with permission from Johnson JE, Sim FH, Scott SG. Musculoskeletal injuries in competitive swimmers. Mayo Clin Proc 1987;62:289.)

While numerous authors have correlated swimming injuries with possible faults in technique and fatigue, little work has been done to document biomechanical or EMG alterations in the swimmer with a painful shoulder. Scovazzo et al.[72] compared such data between pain-free and painful collegiate and masters-level competitive swimmers. Numerous changes were found in the painful swimmer in this study and are described below.

At hand entry, the painful swimmer's hand entered farther from midline with the humerus lower in the "dropped elbow" position often seen with Fatigue. This entry minimizes internal rotation and elevation. EMG studies (see Figs. 9-14 through 9-17) reflected significantly decreased activity in both the anterior and middle deltoids as well as the upper trapezius and rhomboids. The normal firing sequence and the EMG amplitude of the scapular muscles during propulsion were altered. During the pull-through phase, the painful swimmers exhibited decreased serratus anterior and increased rhomboid activity, resulting in a downward rotation of the scapula relative to that found in the nonpainful swimmer. Increased rhomboid activity also appeared to be in preparation for early hand exit and elbow lift. The painful swimmer thereby avoids the extreme range of internal rotation normally seen with full elbow extension at late pull-through. Infraspinatus activity occurs earlier and shows a greater amplitude as external rotation starts earlier and the infraspinatus works harder to counteract the internal rotation moment throughout pull-through. During recovery, anterior deltoid and subscapularis activity was diminished as the arm was allowed to drop and the swimmer avoided internal rotation.

No differences were found in the amplitude, sequence, or timing of firing in the posterior deltoid, supraspinatus, teres minor, pectoralis major, or latissimus dorsi. Since the pectoralis major and the latissimus dorsi are the muscles of propulsion, the painful swimmers appear to be maintaining their ability for propulsion by minimizing pain with a shortening of the arc of arm rotation.

# Preventative and Rehabilitative Considerations

As with all athletes, prevention of injury and dysfunction in the swimmer is preferable to rehabilitating a painful shoulder. Correct stroke technique,[14,19] a proper training schedule to prevent forced fatigue from overtraining,[19,36,71] adequate flexibility,[13,27,43,87] and sufficient, balanced muscle strength, activation, and endurance[13,19,87] have all been addressed as important in maintaining an injury-free glenohumeral joint.

## STROKE TECHNIQUE

The potential for mechanical impingement and tendinitis is accentuated with crossover of the hand beyond midline at hand entry and by moving across midline during early pull-through. Both positions increase glenohumeral internal rotation and adduction, placing increased stress on the shoulder soft tissues. Lack of body roll during recovery can create forced external rotation and horizontal abduction, increasing dynamic demands on the rotator cuff and challenging the static restraints. Excessive roll may increase crossover placement of the hand, causing increased internal rotation and horizontal adduction at hand entry and early pull-through. The kick significantly contributes to controlling and stabilizing body motion.[45] It should be examined along with the arm stroke in the painful swimmer. The effect of breathing pattern on the development of shoulder pain is inconclusive.[13,19,36,38] It has been suggested by one author that the combination of increased body roll away from the breathing side and decreased body roll away from the nonbreathing side may have an impact on the development of impingement factors on the nonbreathing side.[19]

## TRAINING INTENSITY

Typical competitive swim training distances have been reported to vary from 8000 to 20,000 yards for 5 to 7 days per week depending on the season.[36,38] Clearly, the swimmer's shoulder is subjected to pathology from overuse syndromes and from fatigue that can adversely affect stroke mechanics. High-quality workouts incorporating interval training and the use of kickboards, pull buoys, and stroke variations have been suggested to minimize shoulder and scapular muscle fatigue.[13,19] As with other athletes subject to overuse syndromes, swimmers should be counseled against progressing distance or speed too quickly. Falkel and Murphy[19] recommend midseason training reductions for in-season management of swimmer's shoulder.

## FLEXIBILITY

Three authors correlated glenohumeral joint inflexibility with an increased incidence of mechanical impingement in the swimmer.[7,27,87] Greipp[27] assessed anterior shoulder tightness in competitive swimmers. Beach et al.[7] reported hypomobility in internal rotation in most competitive swimmers in their study but a low, nonsignificant correlation to shoulder pain. They reported a higher incidence of impingement in those using the butterfly stroke than the freestyle. They attributed this finding to the inability of the swimmer to compensate for lack of flexibility with body roll during the butterfly. Warner et al.[87] implicate posterior capsule inflexibility in the development of impingement syndrome. Others have identified excessive flexibility in making the swimmer more susceptible to subclinical or outright glenohumeral subluxation.[13,43] Warner et al.[87] report a 68 percent incidence of impingement signs in addition to positive apprehension and capsular laxity in a group of swimmers with clinically unstable shoulders. The therapist needs to assess fully for the presence of inflexibility or laxity before designing a stretching program.

## MUSCLE BALANCE

As stated previously, the adductors and internal rotators are more active during propulsion than their antagonists. Normal ratios of isokinetic shoulder torque have been reported for external/internal rotation (2:3) and for adduction/abduction (2:1).[33] A study of nonswimming subjects and competitive collegiate swimmers revealed that swimmers have significantly increased overall torque production and shifts in these ratios.[44] In both men and women, torque ratios shifted to greater than 2:2 for adduction/abduction (Tables 9-7 and 9-8). External rotation/internal rotation ratios approached 1:2 for male swimmers (Table 9-9) and 3:5 for female swimmers (Table 9-10). In total torque production, the swimmers had greater torque in all muscle groups except external rotation. Beach et al.[7] demonstrated a significant correlation between swimmers' shoulder pain and decreased isokinetic endurance ratios of the external rotators and abductors. Relative weakness of the external rotators with respect to the internal rotators has been associated with shoulder pain from impingement.[87] In addition to strengthening the muscles of propulsion, "dry land" exercises are recommended for strengthening those muscles which are not used as forcefully in the stroke in an attempt to provide some muscle balance.

The role of the scapular muscles in providing a stable base for glenohumeral mobility in the freestyle and related strokes was discussed previously. The serratus anterior is active throughout the entire stroke cycle at amplitudes from 20 to 48 percent of its maximal isometric force.[61] Therefore, it is particularly susceptible to fatigue

**Table 9-8**

**Mean (SD) Values of Adduction/Abduction Ratios in Women**

| Testing Mode | Controls | Swimmers | $p$* |
|---|---|---|---|
| 30 Deg/s | | | |
| Right | 1.65 (0.21) | 2.13 (0.42) | 0.004 |
| Left | 1.57 (0.12) | 1.99 (0.24) | 0.000 |
| 180 Deg/s | | | |
| Right | 1.79 (0.3) | 2.06 (0.59) | 0.209 |
| Left | 1.83 (0.39) | 2.09 (0.47) | 0.187 |

*$p < 0.05$ is significant.

Reprinted with permission from McMaster WC, Long SC, Caiozzo VJ. Shoulder torque changes in the swimming athlete. Am J Sports Med 1992;20:323.

**Table 9-7**

**Mean (SD) Values of Adduction/Abduction Ratios in Men**

| Testing Mode | Controls | Swimmers | $p$* |
|---|---|---|---|
| 30 Deg/s | | | |
| Right | 1.53 (0.12) | 2.05 (0.43) | 0.0003 |
| Left | 1.44 (0.19) | 2.11 (0.04) | 0.0000 |
| 180 Deg/s | | | |
| Right | 1.70 (0.25) | 2.38 (0.82) | 0.0056 |
| Left | 1.58 (0.25) | 2.38 (0.72) | 0.0000 |

*$p < 0.05$ is significant.

Reprinted with permission from McMaster WC, Long SC, Caiozzo VJ. Shoulder torque changes in the swimming athlete. Am J Sports Med 1992;20:323.

**Table 9-9**

**Mean (SD) Values of External Rotation/Internal Rotation Ratios in Men**

| Testing Mode | Controls | Swimmers | $p$* |
|---|---|---|---|
| 30 Deg/s | | | |
| Right | 0.74 (0.11) | 0.53 (0.14) | 0.0003 |
| Left | 0.78 (0.11) | 0.57 (0.11) | 0.0001 |
| 180 Deg/s | | | |
| Right | 0.65 (0.14) | 0.45 (0.15) | 0.0017 |
| Left | 0.66 (0.13) | 0.55 (0.18) | 0.0543 |

*$p < 0.05$ is significant.

Reprinted with permission from McMaster WC, Long SC, Caiozzo VJ. Shoulder torque changes in the swimming athlete. Am J Sports Med 1992;20:323.

**Table 9-10**

**Mean (SD) Values of External Rotation/Internal Rotation Ratios in Women**

| Testing Mode | Controls | Swimmers | *p** |
|---|---|---|---|
| 30 Deg/s | | | |
| Right | 0.74 (0.10) | 0.63 (0.10) | 0.024 |
| Left | 0.74 (0.13) | 0.65 (0.13) | 0.144 |
| 180 Deg/s | | | |
| Right | 0.58 (0.11) | 0.57 (0.15) | 0.826 |
| Left | 0.65 (0.12) | 0.64 (0.19) | 0.926 |

*$p < 0.05$ is significant.

Reprinted with permission from McMaster WC, Long SC, Caiozzo VJ. Shoulder torque changes in the swimming athlete. Am J Sports Med 1992;20:323.

and should be trained with low resistance and multiple repetitions to enhance both strength and endurance. Both serratus and trapezius strengthening can be performed using resisted upper extremity proprioceptive neuromuscular facilitation patterns with tubing. Exercises previously described for the throwing athlete such as "scaption" and push-ups with a plus can be used for serratus strengthening.[46]

## Summary

To summarize, training and rehabilitation of the swimming athlete should emphasize instruction in correct stroke mechanics, specific stretching where appropriate, and selective strengthening of the rotator cuff and scapular muscles, particularly the serratus anterior, in addition to training of the primary muscles of propulsion. Furthermore, the recognition of overuse in the competitive and recreational swimmer is critical to preventing or at best reducing the likelihood of problems related to instability and rotator cuff damage. The notion of training needing to be painful must be dismissed. Athletes who complain of pain should be examined, and if it is determined that the shoulder is at risk for developing recurrent problems, modifications in training or technique should be instituted. The younger the athlete, the more important this is since these athletes are at risk due to the fact that their capasuloligamentous-labral complex is still maturing. The static and dynamic stabilizers of the glenohumeral joint need to be protected if the athlete desires longevity in this sport as well as in functional use of the arm.

# The Shoulder in Weight Lifting

High levels of athletic performance and the physical demands on the musculoskeletal structures of the shoulder necessitate effective sports conditioning programs. The goals of such programs are not only to maximize performance but also to reduce the risk and incidence of injury to the shoulder and a resulting loss of the athlete's ability to function in sports.

The use of resistance exercise with weights in the form of barbells, dumbbells, or weight machines has been popular for many years.[29] With the availability of modern sports medicine and exercise science, weight training as a sport and as a component of a comprehensive sports training program has become universally accepted.

According to Stone and Kroll,[80] "it has been clearly established in a number of studies that strength training has a beneficial effect on motor skills and sports performance." However, strength training exercises also can be a cause of injury to the athlete's shoulder, causing loss of sports participation time.

It is therefore essential that strength-building exercises be performed in a safe, controlled manner with proper supervision so that injury potential can be minimized and sports performance enhancement can be maximized.[57,58] People who participate in recreational weight lifting or strength training are generally unsupervised and uneducated about weight lifting technique and safety. This consideration increases their injury risk.

The object of this section on weight lifting will be to describe the various forms of weight lifting, the various exercises pertinent to the shoulder complex, and the benefits, injury risks, and modifications necessary when injury is present. Although the therapist may not be treating competing weight lifters or body builders, many of the exercises discussed are used in weight training for competing athletes, recreational athletes, and individuals involved in supervised or unsupervised rehabilitation.

## Weight Lifting Classifications

The exercises used in weight lifting can be classified under the following headings:

1. Body building
2. Power weight lifting

3. Olympic-style weight lifting[74]
4. Recreational, using resistance exercise machines[24]

These weight-lifting disciplines (except recreational weight lifting using resistive exercise machines) are competitive sports in and of themselves. The exercises and techniques used in these weight-lifting sports are employed by strength-training athletes to improve muscular strength and optimally develop motor skills. The synthesis of these weight-lifting disciplines for use in sports training might be termed *sports strength training*.[60] These weight-lifting exercises are also commonly used by the general public for fitness and recreational pursuits.

### BODY BUILDING

This weight-lifting discipline utilizes various exercises to maximally develop and sculpture the body's muscles in a symmetrical fashion so as to optimize the "ideal" total muscular development. In competition, participants pose in a choreographed routine to highlight their particular muscular development. Participants are judged on muscular development, symmetry, and balance of the body's muscle groups.

### POWER WEIGHT LIFTING

In the sport of power lifting, participants are required to perform three lifts, attempting one repetition maximum amounts for each lift. These three lifts are the bench press, the squat to parallel, and the dead lift. Each lifter is given three attempts at each lift, recording the heaviest lift for each exercise.

### OLYMPIC-STYLE WEIGHT LIFTING

In the sport of olympic lifting, participants are required to perform two lifts, again attempting one repetition of maximum amounts. These lifts are the snatch and the clean and jerk. Three attempts are made at each lift, recording the heaviest amount lifted.

### RECREATIONAL LIFTING

According to Garhammer,[24] "Machines used for weight training may not actually utilize weights of any kind. For example, air-compression cylinders, hydraulic mechanisms, springs, or elastic cables may provide resistance to movement. Of the vast variety of machines currently available for consumer use, however, those found most commonly in public exercise facilities are truly weight machines; that is, their use involves the lifting of weight plates as part of a weight "stack." When training with or lifting free weights, the resistance on the muscle is maximal only in the weakest part of the joint range of motion. The muscle is being stressed submaximally in joint positions of greater mechanical advantage and maximally in joint positions of lesser mechanical advantage. Variable-resistance weight machines were introduced in an attempt to provide resistance to the muscle maximally throughout the entire exercise range of motion. Through the use of cams or rolling pivots,[24] the lever arm length can be varied through the exercise motion, resulting in maximal muscle tension at any point in the range of exercise movement. The use of resistance exercise machines is advantageous because of ease of resistance adjustment, reduced injury potential, and joint and muscle group isolation.[24] This type of weight training is preferred by people interested in recreational fitness because each muscle group can be exercised on a separate machine. The lifter does not have to lift a free barbell or balance it. The lifter concentrates effort on moving the machine's lever system only, thereby focusing the exercise effort only on the target muscle group. If muscle failure occurs, the lifter is not obligated to hold the barbell or return it to the floor or a rack as in a free-weight exercise. The machine acts as a safety system for the lifter and reduces injury potential when compared with free-weight lifting.

In the next section, various lifts commonly used involving the shoulder will be described regarding osteokinematics, muscle activity, and soft-tissue effects.

## Specific Exercises

### BENCH PRESS

The bench press is perhaps one of the most widely used[24] and overused exercises in weight lifting (Fig. 9-21). In performance of the bench press, the lifter lies supine on a bench-press bench. The barbell is lifted off the support rack and stabilized at arm's length, above the base of the neck.[1] The shoulder is forward flexed to approximately 90 degrees and mildly internally rotated. At this point, the elbows are extended and locked, and the scapulae are stabilized by the bench. This might be called the *start/finish position* (see Fig. 9-21a).

In the *down phase*, the bar is slowly lowered in a controlled fashion until it lightly touches the chest area, just above the xiphoid process of the sternum.[1] In this bar-on-chest position, the shoulder is in a position of extreme extension,

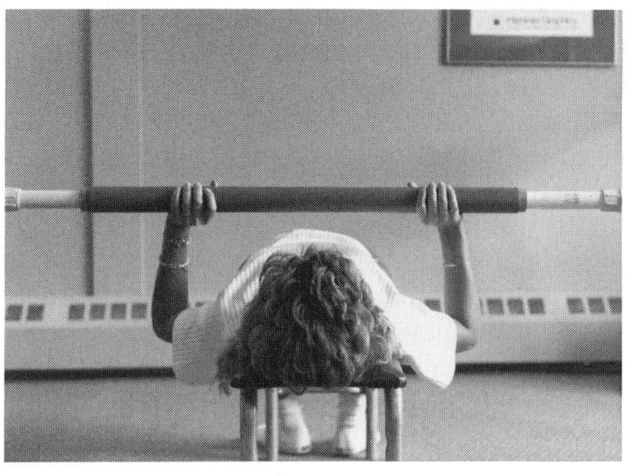

A

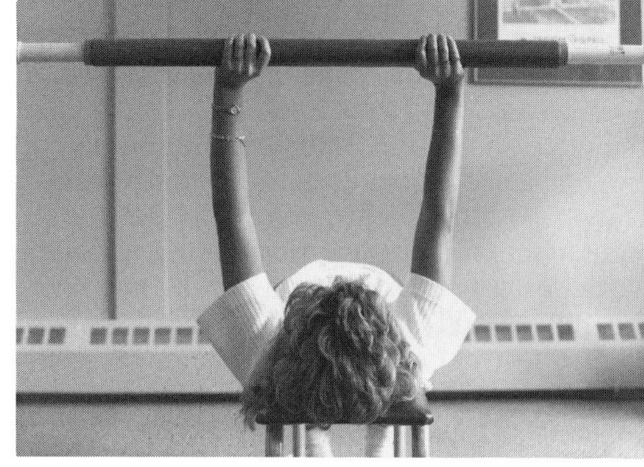

B

**Figure 9-21.** Bench press. (a) Start-finish position. (b) Bar-on-chest position.

horizontal abduction, and moderate external rotation (see Fig. 9-21b). Ideally, the forearm forms a right angle to the bar, and the elbows are flexed to 100 to 120 degrees. The wrists remain extended throughout the lift.

The *pressing phase* begins as the bar is pressed back to the starting position at arm's length. The primary muscles used and exercised in the bench press are the pectoralis major and minor, serratus anterior, triceps brachii, and anterior and middle deltoid. The trapezius, rhomboids, biceps, and latissimus dorsi muscles act as secondary stabilizers and synergists throughout the bench-press movement.[46]

The benefits of this exercise and the resulting muscular development would be most useful in contact sports where pushing is involved, such as football, wrestling, and hockey. Sports where reaching quickly or placing the hands in front of the body, such as basketball, volleyball, or boxing, would benefit from the bench press. Speed and power of the acceleration phase in throwing or racket sports might be enhanced by the development of the pectoralis major muscle.[35]

## POTENTIAL INJURIES AND PRECAUTIONS

Injury potential to the shoulder joint in the bench press is higher for heavier lifts, wider hand grip spacing, and faster rates of exercise speed. This is due to the higher shoulder joint torques developed under these conditions.[24] Muscle failure due to force overload, as in lifting a weight that is too heavy, or muscle fatigue occurring at the end of a high-repetition set, causes a shift of force and stress from the contractile components of the muscle to the musculotendinous junction, tendons, and capsuloligamentous structures. According to Ferrari,[20] "The middle glenohumeral ligament and anterior superior capsule can be stretched by heavy lifting that occurs in the position of external rotation, extension, and slight abduction that is used in the bench press" (this is the bar-on-chest" position) (see Fig. 9-21b). Also, the anterior attachment of the coracohumeral ligament that supports the long head of the biceps tendon is taught in this position. Ferrari states that this may produce recurrent subluxation of the long head of the biceps tendon.[20] Repetitive subluxation under heavy loading conditions can mechanically irritate and inflame the biceps tendon. Subluxation of the biceps tendon also could cause increasing stresses on the superior part of the glenoid labrum, as noted by Andrews et al.[2] This might ultimately lead to the so-called SLAP lesion. This acronym represents the clinical entity of a tear of the *s*uperior *l*abrum, *a*nterior and *p*osterior.

Howell et al.[31] state that in the maximally externally rotated and abducted position, the humeral head slides approximately 4 mm posteriorly from the center of the glenoid cavity. As the arm forward flexes and internally rotates, as in the pressing phase of the bench press, the humeral head normally glides anteriorly to the concentric center of the glenoid. If, over a period of time, the middle glenohumeral ligament and superior capsule have been attenuated due to the repeated stress of loading the shoulder in the bar-on-chest position, this might result in an eventual anterior shoulder subluxation and glenoid labrum erosion due to the loss of normal function of the anterior capsular restraints. In the athlete with anterior shoulder instability, the bench-press exercise may be contraindicated because as the individual lowers the bar approaching the bar-on-chest position, the humeral head will be translated and displaced anteriorly from the concentric center of the glenoid instead of the normal posterior displacement, as described alone.[31] This abnormal anterior translation could result at any point in the bench-press motion where the shoulder is loaded in the position of horizontal abduction, extension, and external rotation. Posterior subluxation or dislocation can occur in the start/finish position in the presence of the posterior capsular laxity of the shoulder. The rotator cuff and biceps tendon complex attempt to dynamically control humeral head translation. When attempting to control abnormal humeral head translations, as in the individual with instability, myotendinous overload can result, leading to fiber disruption and injury.

The acromioclavicular joint undergoes high levels of stress in the bench-press exercise. In the bar-on-chest position, forces are such that the acromioclavicular joint is being forced apart. As the pressing phase begins, the acromioclavicular joint surfaces become compressed together, reaching maximal at the start/finish position. According to Norris,[52] a higher incidence of acromioclavicular joint degeneration is present in weight lifters. Scavenius and Iverson[70] have recently documented osteolysis of the distal clavicle in a group of Danish weight lifters.

Ruptures of the pectoralis major and triceps brachii muscles at their musculotendinous junction are common among bench pressers.[73,89] This is due to the high levels of force production in these muscles during maximal or near-maximal lifts. These ruptures may be due to muscular fatigue caused by overuse or tension overload exceeding the capabilities of these tissues. An appropriate warmup period before lifting involving calisthenic exercises and submaximal lifting movements is essential for prevention of muscle- and tendon-related injuries. After the warmup period, individuals should practice flexibility exercises for all major muscle groups. A cooldown period after completion of strength training exercises should include additional flexibility exercises to prevent the tightening of muscles that can occur in the absence of a good stretching routine.

Muscle imbalance frequently occurs in athletes who overtrain the bench press while neglecting strengthening exercises for the posterior scapular stabilizers. This type of muscle imbalance can result in a forward shoulder girdle posture caused by developed tone and tightness in the pectoralis major and minor muscles. This forward posture of the shoulder girdle will cause lengthening and stretch weakness of the rhomboids, trapezius, and latissimus dorsi muscles. This type of muscle imbalance, in addition to the preceding postural deformity, can lead to dysfunctional scapulohumeral rhythm due to abnormal scapular resting position and the production of an inadequate force couple between the scapulothoracic and glenohumeral joints. Tendinitis also can occur due to a relative imbalance between the internal and external rotator muscles,[66] overuse, or a direct mechanical impingement on the coracoacromial arch due to inappropriate scapular rotation.

Variations of the bench press include the incline bench press, the decline bench press, and the chest fly exercise.

### INCLINE BENCH PRESS

The incline bench press is performed on a bench with an upward slant of about 60 degrees from the horizontal. This exercise is performed the same as the flat bench press except that the bar is pressed upward at a greater angle of forward flexion than the horizontal adduction of the bench press. This exercise is useful in body-building programs to develop the clavicular portion of the pectoralis major muscle and anterior deltoid.[76]

### DECLINE BENCH PRESS

The decline bench press is done on a bench with a downward slant of about 30 degrees. This downward slant of the bench forces the lifter to press the bar upward toward the waist area. This exercise is used in body-building programs to enhance the development of the lower costal fibers of the pectoralis major muscle.[78]

### CHEST FLY EXERCISE

The chest fly is an exercise using dumbbells to isolate the function and development of the pectoralis major muscles.[74] The lifter lies on a flat bench (incline and decline variations can be used), a dumbbell in each hand, in the start/finish position of the bench press. The weight is lowered into horizontal abduction and external rotation at the shoulder with elbow flexion. When the weight reaches the level of the shoulder (i.e., the frontal plane of the horizontal body), it is raised back to the start/finish position. Some lifters, however, like to lower the dumbbell well below the level of the shoulder into extreme horizontal abduction and external rotation. This practice of constant stress to the shoulder in horizontal abduction and external rotation can lead to, as described in the bench press section, pathologic stresses to the anterior capsuloligamentous structures with resulting anterior subluxation, dislocation, labral tearing, and biceps tendon or rotator cuff pathology.[2,3,20,31]

## OVERHEAD PRESSES

This category of lifts is comprised of the following lifts:

1. Military press
2. Behind-the-neck press
3. Push press
4. Jerk (press)

These lifts all have in common the fact that the barbell is pressed or pushed into an overhead position. The muscles used to accomplish this type of lift are common to all the exercise categories. The prime movers are the anterior and middle deltoid, supraspinatus, subscapularis, upper trapezius, serratus anterior, and triceps.[85] The rest of the shoulder muscles act as stabilizers to assist the prime mover muscles. Overhead pressing exercises in the standing position all require strong stabilization of the entire body utilizing trunk and hip musculature.

### MILITARY PRESS

In the military press (Fig. 9-22a), the lifter stands erect with the barbell held across the front of the shoulder, resting on the clavicles. The wrists are in extension, the forearms pronated, and the humerus slightly forward flexed. From this position, the bar is pressed directly upward, passing closely by the nose (in an attempt to keep the bar in line with the center of gravity of the body) and directly over the head. In this finish position, the shoulder is fully elevated, and the scapula is laterally rotated, abducted and elevated (see Fig.9-22b). The elbow is locked in extension, and the forearm and wrist remain pronated and extended, respectively. To complete the lift, the barbell is lowered to the starting position with the bar held across the clavicles.[80]

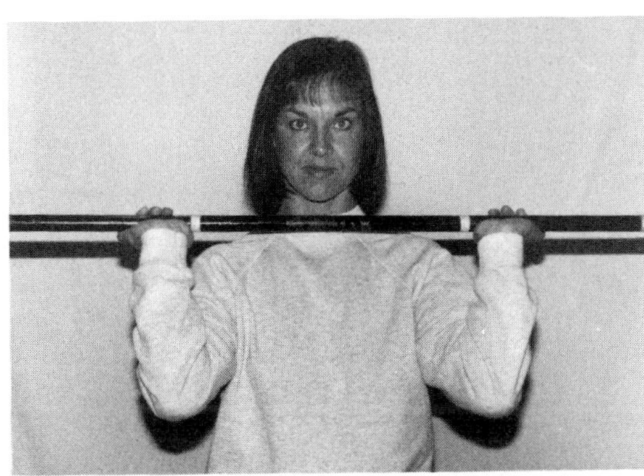

A

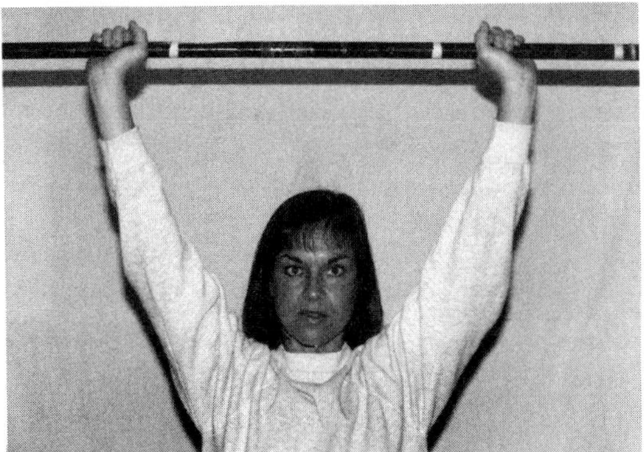

B

**Figure 9-22.** Military press. (a) Start-finish position. (b) Overhead position.

### BEHIND-THE-NECK PRESS

The behind-the-neck press is similar to the military press except that, in the starting position, the barbell is held in a position resting on the upper trapezius, "behind the neck." In this lift, the finish position is the same as in the military press, except that the humerus passes more in the frontal plane of abduction than in the military press, which passes between the frontal and sagittal planes. It is believed by some body builders that the behind-the-neck press better potentiates and isolates the middle deltoid muscle and that the military press better isolates the anterior deltoid muscle, although there are no conclusive data to support such an assertion. The behind-the-neck press does, however, require higher levels of shoulder flexibility in abduction and external rotation as the humerus passes to the over head position. It is important to remember, as noted by Hawkins and Kennedy,[28] that "activities involving repetitive use of the arms above the horizontal may produce the impingement syndrome." This is particularly true when heavy weights are used. This exercise clinically seems to produce higher rates of subacromial impingement and greater stress on the capsuloligamentous restraints than the military press. Primary instability can result with repetitive lifting and is many times clinically manifested as shoulder impingement and rotator cuff tendinitis in the weight-lifting athlete. When instability and/or impingement are present, the lifter is often unable to perform the behind-the-neck press, but is able to perform the military press. This is perhaps due to the greater degree of horizontal abduction and external rotation required in the behind-the-neck lift. The military press occurs closer to the scapular plane of movement, resulting in less twisting of the rotator cuff and capsuloligamentous complex. This concept is clinically useful when treating or advising the person with a previous history of glenohumeral dislocation/subluxation, rotator cuff pathology, or surgical intervention. If strengthening of the shoulder is desired in the overhead position, progression to the military press is advisable as opposed to behind-the-neck press.

### JERK (PRESS)

The jerk is a component of the olympic-style competitive lift: the clean and jerk.[6] The clean phase of this lift will be described in a later section.

For the jerk, the lifter stands in the same starting position as in the military press. The jerk lift begins with flexion at the knees and hips. This can be referred to as the dip phase. (Fig.9-23a) The lifter then forcefully accelerates the hips and knees into extension, imparting upward momentum to the barbell. At the peak of the hip and knee extension, the lifter raises up on the toes with the ankle joint in plantar flexion. This can be referred to as the leg drive phase. (Fig.9-23b) The lifter then jumps slightly, leaving the feet and dropping the body under the bar while at the same time maximally elevating the humerus and extending the elbows, resulting in the barbell being held overhead. This can be referred to as the split phase of the jerk (Fig. 9-23c). In this position with the barbell held overhead, the hip and knee of the forward leg are flexed, while the hip and knee of the backward leg are relatively extended. In the recovery phase, the forward limb is drawn backward by forcefully pushing off the forward foot. The backward limb is then drawn forward to meet the forward limb. In the finish position, the lifter stands erect, feet parallel, and the barbell overhead, as seen in the other overhead lifts. The barbell is then usually dropped to the floor to complete the clean-and-jerk sequence. The jerk lift described above is also referred to as the split jerk. The weights used in the jerk lifts are usually much higher than any of the other overhead lifts. The lifter must dip under the barbell to reach the overhead position because the weights are too heavy to press with upper body strength alone. They are considered full-body lifts that train speed and muscular power.[24] Of course, because the weights lifted are higher, the stresses placed on the shoulder, as outlined earlier, will be higher. These higher shoulder stresses will increase the injury risk in this weight-lifting population.

## WEIGHT-LIFTING PULLS

The term *pulls* in weight lifting refers to the action when the lifter raises a barbell from thigh level upward to the level of the chest.

### UPRIGHT ROW

In performing the upright row,[6] the lifter stands erect, holding the barbell with the arm by the side, with the elbows extended and the forearms pronated. The hands are held so that the thumbs are touching the outer thigh. A narrower grip also can be used if desired. To begin the lift, the shoulder is internally rotated and abducted, the elbows and wrists are flexed, and the forearms remain pronated. The bar is raised very close to or touching the front of the torso until it reaches its maximum height at approximately the nipple line.

This exercise requires strong action of the deltoid muscle and upper trapezius and elbow flexors as prime movers. Other scapular muscles and trunk stabilizers are also important as secondary muscles. Significant use of the shoulder external rotators is required to stabilize the humeral head and to overcome the internal rotation torque. The upright row is an excellent developer of the prime mover muscles, but certain injuries often occur. Because the humerus is abducted with internal rotation, shoulder impingement can occur if the greater tuberosity with the overlying rotator cuff tendons and bursa comes in contact with the undersurface of the acromion process.[28,39] Generally, in this position, it is recommended that the lifter not exceed 80 to 90 degrees of abduction to avoid injury to the rotator cuff. Strains of the deltoid, upper trapezius, and levator scapulae muscles can occur, as well as medial and lateral epicondylitis at the elbow due to the strong grip required while pulling the bar upward.

### THE CLEAN

The clean lift is an example of application of the upright rowing exercise as a means to transfer the barbell from the top of the thigh to the bar across the chest position, that is, the starting position of the military press and jerk lifts. In clean-and-jerk competition, the lifter must transfer the weight from the floor to the across the shoulder position and then perform the jerk portion of the lift. In sports training programs, the clean is used to train full body strength, developing speed and power for the explosive movements required for running and jumping.[6,58,60] There are two types of weight-lifting cleans. They are the clean and the power clean.

In performing the power clean, the lifter is positioned over the barbell (Fig. 9-24a). This begins the lift-off phase. The elbows are extended, and the shoulders are forward flexed and in neutral rotation. The forearms are pronated. The hips and knees are flexed, and the ankles are dorsiflexed. The back is held in extension, sometimes in lumbar lordosis. The barbell is raised off the floor by extending the hips and knees. In the pull-through-the-knees phase, the barbell is raised to the level of the knees, with the hips and

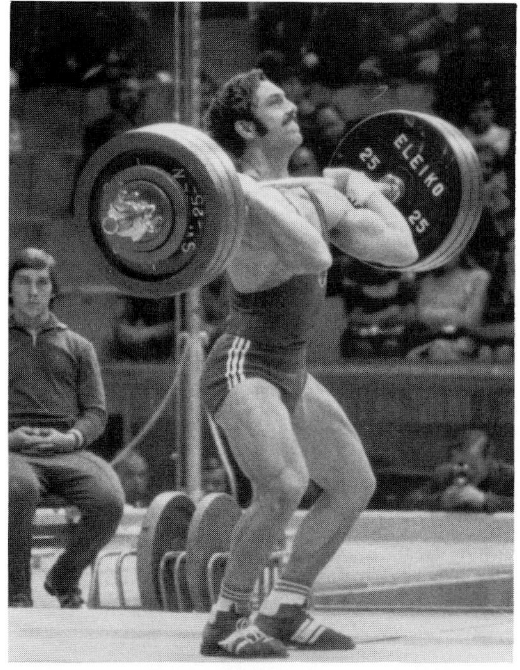


A

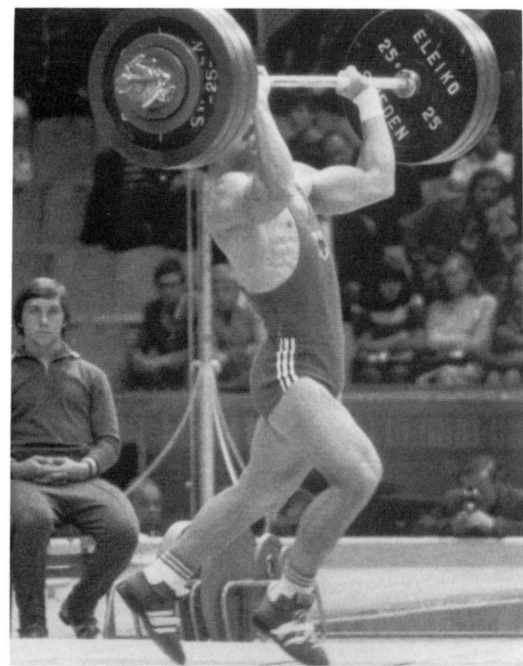


B

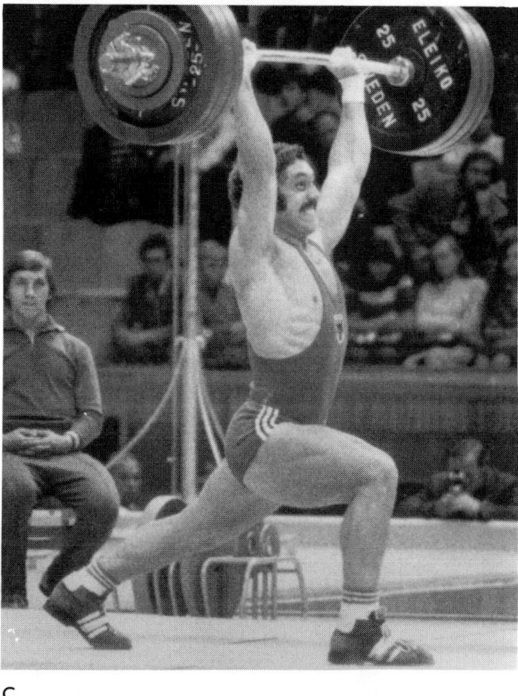


C

**Figure 9-23.** Jerk press. (a) Dip phase. (b) Leg drive. (c) Split phase. (Reprinted with permission from Bruce Klemens, Oak Ridge, N.J., 1988.)

knees still flexed, but less than in the lift-off phase. The shoulders remain flexed in neutral rotation. At this point in the lift, the barbell is allowed to simply hang from the shoulders with no direct muscle action at the shoulders or elbows.[6, 82–84] In the scoop phase, the pelvis is thrust forward, extending further the hips and knees (see Fig.9-24b). The barbell now rests across the midthigh with the arms by the sides. In the pull phase, the lifter performs the movement of the upright row as described earlier. At the same time, the lifter fully extends the hips and knees and raises up on the toes with the ankles in plantar flexion in an upward jumping movement

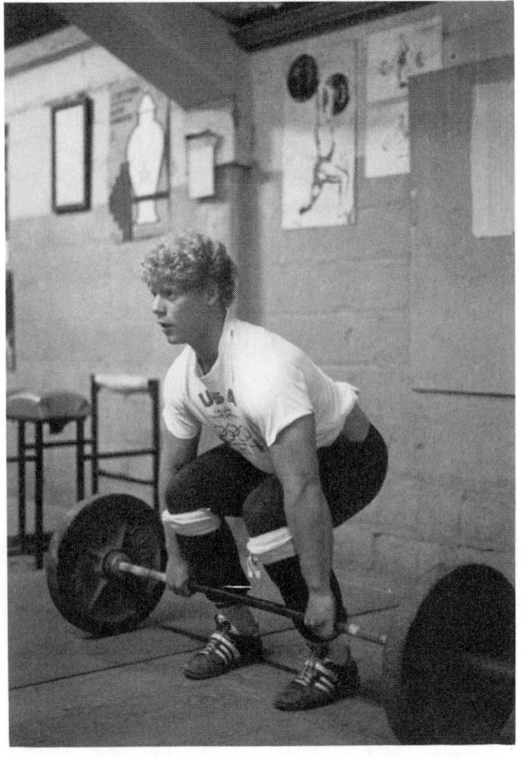
A

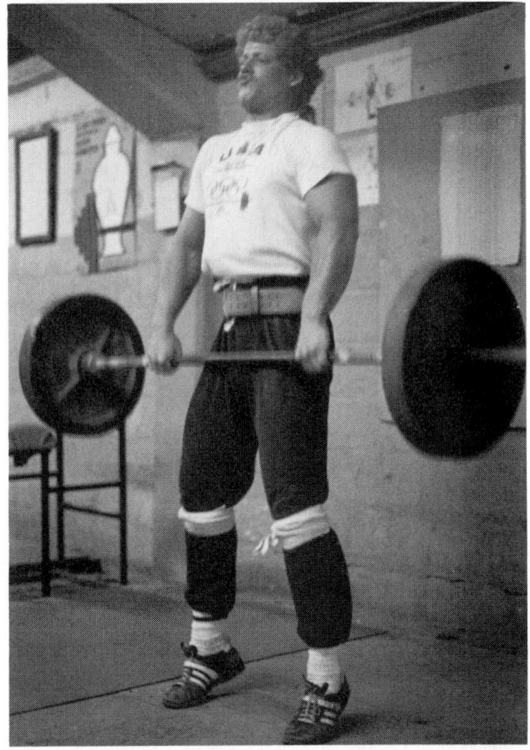
B

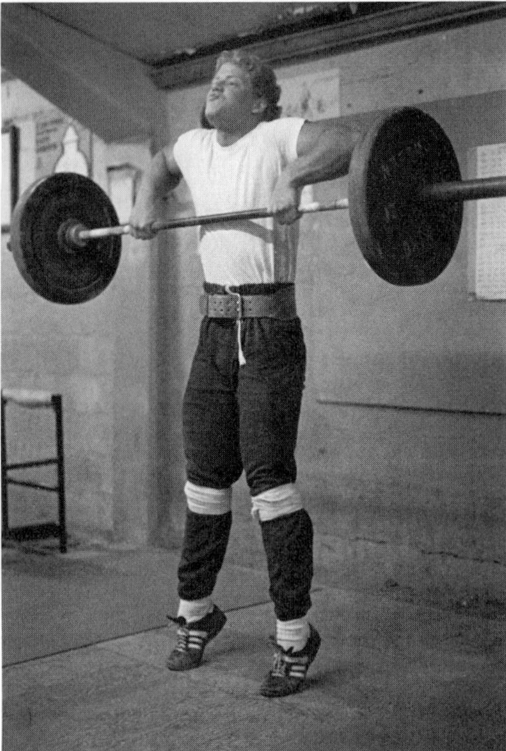
C

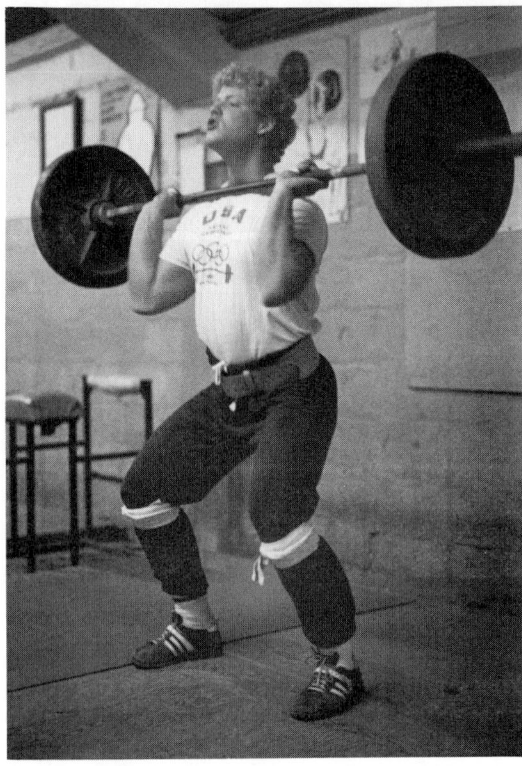
D

**Figure 9-24.** Power clean and jerk sequence. (a) Lift-off phase. (b) Scoop phase. (c) Pull phase. (d) Catch position in partial squat. (Reprinted with permission of Baker G, ed. The United States Weight Lifting Federation coaching manual, Vol. I: Technique. Colorado Springs, Colo.: USWLF, 1988.)

(see Fig. 9-24c). Because of this action, the lifter's feet are off the ground, allowing time for a shift of the base of support from a narrow base to a wider base as the lifter lowers the body under the rising bar. At this time, the catch phase begins (see Fig.9-24d). The lifter quickly reflexes the hips and knees and begins to squat underneath the elevated barbell. The shoulder goes from a position of abduction and internal rotation to a position of adduction and relative external rotation. At this point, the barbell has arrived at the position across the clavicles. The shoulder is then forward flexed slightly to stabilize the barbell against the clavicles. The elbows are fully flexed, forearms pronated, and wrists extended. The lifter then extends the hips and knees to the finish position, standing upright with the barbell. A press overhead may now be done, or the barbell may be lowered to the starting position for another repetition of the power clean.

In the clean lift, the lifter performs the same sequence as described for the power clean until the catch phase. Instead of catching the barbell in a partial squat position, the lifter progresses into a full squat position after the catch. This maneuver is done because the weight being lifted is much heavier than the weight used in a power clean; therefore, the lifter is unable to gain as much vertical barbell height in the pull phase. This necessitates that the lifter drop deeper under the lower rising barbell. The full squat position is used as a transition phase where the lifter becomes steady before rising to the finish position in a front squat recovery movement.

## THE SNATCH

The snatch is a competitive olympic lift that is used in many sports strength training programs.[6] As can be observed from Figure 9-25a, the handgrip spacing for the snatch is much wider than that used in the power clean or clean and jerk. In the starting position, the lifter bends over the bar. The hips and knees are flexed much further than for the cleans; there is also more forward lean of the torso. Both these conditions are required because of the wider hand-grip spacing. The shoulders are in a position of abduction and internal rotation, the elbows are fully extended, and the forearms are pronated. The lift-off, pull-through-the-knees, and scoop phases all progress similar to the clean lifts. The shoulder remains in its position of abduction and internal rotation throughout these phases. As noted earlier, through the scoop phase, the barbell essentially hangs from the upper limbs through the hand grips. In the pull phase (differentiated from the clean pulls as the snatch pull), the elbows are flexed, the shoulder girdle is elevated, and the humerus is further abducted and internally rotated, pulling the barbell upward toward the face (see Fig. 9-25b). The hips and knees extend fully, and the lifter raises up on the toes, jumps slightly upward off the ground, and lands back on the ground with a widened base of support. In the catch phase (see Fig. 9-25c), the lifter drops straight downward by quickly reflexing the hips and knees, in fact, heading toward the full squat position. Simultaneously, the shoulders pass from their position of abduction and internal rotation in the pull phase to a final position of full abduction with maximal external rotation. The elbows pass from flexion in the pull phase to full extension in the final catch position. The forearms are now supinated, and the wrists are maximally extended. The lifter rises out of the overhead squat position to finish the lift in the standing position with the barbell overhead.

A variation of the snatch, called the *power snatch*, is also commonly used in strength training programs. The difference between the two lifts is the same as the difference between the clean and the power clean. That is, in the catch phase, the lifter flexes the hips and knees into a *partial* squat position to catch the bar instead of the *full* squat position. The snatch lifts require a high degree of shoulder girdle muscle strength to be performed at the competitive level. In a sports training program, the snatch and its training variations can be used effectively to develop strength about the shoulder. However, due to the extreme position of abduction and external rotation required in the overhead position, this lift is not recommended where shoulder instability, laxity, or impingement is present. The overhead position of the snatch with a wide hand grip places the shoulder into a provocative position regarding stability. According to Gambardella and Jobe,[23] the highest stresses are placed on the anterior and inferior capsule and labrum in this position. An intact anterior band of the inferior glenohumeral ligament is necessary to keep the humeral head from sliding anteriorly from its position on the glenoid.[31,53] Impingement can occur if there is injury to these capsuloligamentous and labral structures due to excessive movement of the humeral head on the glenoid.[28,39a] Primary impingement can occur as the humerus moves from internal to external rotation in the position of abduction in the pull phase to catch phase sequence. In the starting position, lift-off, pull-through-the-knees phases, there are significant inferior forces on the glenohumeral joint, placing tension on the supraspinatus and superior capsule. In the person with inferior or multidirectional instability, these lifting actions can

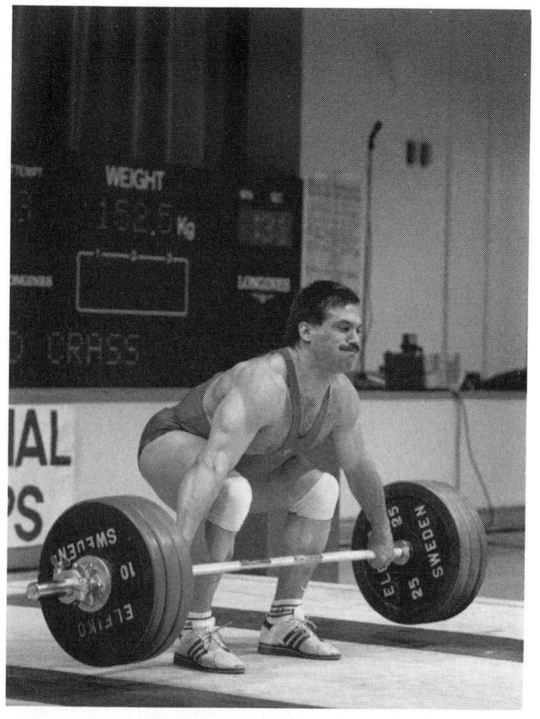


A

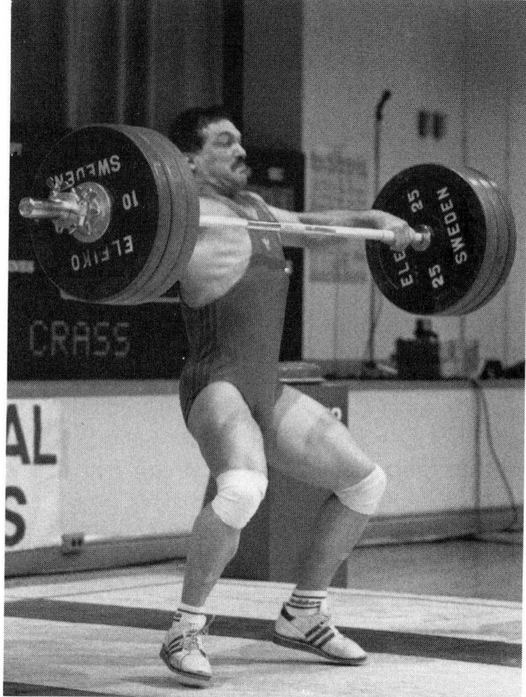


B

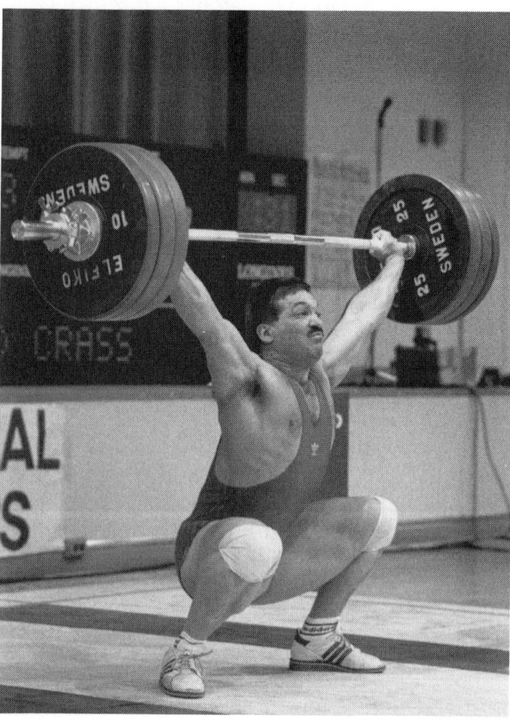


C

**Figure 9-25.** Snatch. (a) Start position ready for lift-off. (b) Pull phase. (c) Catch position in full overhead squat. (Reprinted with permission from Bruce Klemens, Oak Ridge, N.J., 1988.)

place the glenohumeral joint at risk for subluxation or dislocation.

When normal shoulder structure and function are present, the snatch can be used effectively as part of a comprehensive and varied shoulder strength-building program. Proper technical instruction and supervision are necessary to minimize injury potential when performing difficult technical lifts such as the snatch and the clean and jerk.[6,81–83]

## OTHER LIFTS

### FRONT RAISE

The front raise is an exercise used to develop the anterior deltoid and clavicular pectoralis major muscles.[74] To perform the front raise, the lifter stands with a dumbbell in each hand. The arms are adducted, the elbows extended, and the forearms in neutral rotation with the thumb facing forward. The lifter raises the weight forward with humeral flexion. The weight can be raised to 90 degrees or to full flexion (Fig. 9-26). Flexion to 90 degrees will isolate the anterior deltoid–clavicular pectoralis major component, while raising the weight to 180 degrees also will use the trapezius, serratus anterior, and interscapular muscles to a greater extent.

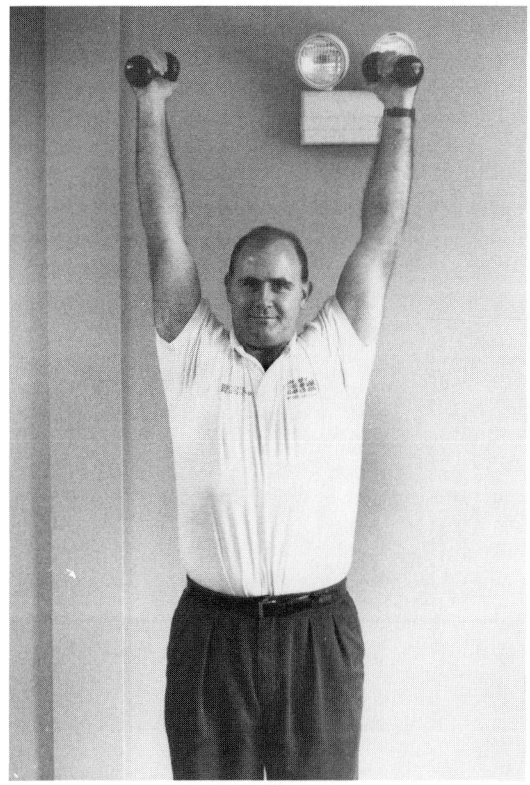

**Figure 9-26.** Front raise, overhead position.

Many body builders perform this exercise with the weight in the palm-down position. This position places the humerus into more internal rotation while forward flexion occurs. This position can cause coracoacromial impingement, especially in the range of shoulder flexion between 85 and 120 degrees.[39a] The use of the thumb-forward position enhances external rotation of the humerus and aides in the avoidance of rotator cuff impingement by allowing the greater tuberosity to clear the coracoacromial structures.

### SIDE RAISE

The side raise is an exercise used to develop the middle deltoid muscle of the shoulder.[74] To perform the side raise, the lifter stands in the same position as the starting position for the front raise with a dumbbell in each hand. With the elbows straight or slightly bent, the weight is raised sideways in the coronal plane. The weight should only be raised to 90 degrees of abduction and the hand held in a position where the thumb points straight upward (i.e., the arm would be supinated when by the side) (Fig. 9-27).

Body builders commonly experience shoulder impingement and rotator cuff tendinitis from improper technique. First, if the forearm is in a position of neutral rotation with the arm by the side, the humerus is in a position of relative internal rotation when compared with the anatomic position (forearm supinated) recommended above. Second, if this position is assumed and the lifter attempts to raise the arms past 90 degrees of abduction in the coronal plane, subacromial impingement will be more likely to occur than if the humerus were in neutral or external rotation.[31]

### LAT PULL-DOWNS

The lat pull-down is an exercise used to develop the latissimus dorsi muscles. Other muscles used for this exercise include the interscapular

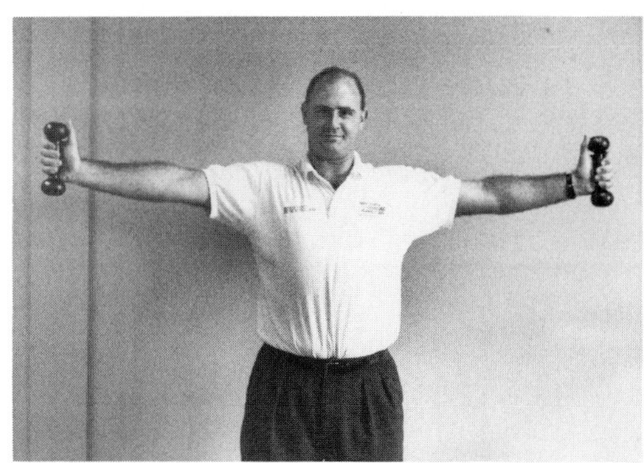

**Figure 9-27.** Side raise, abduction to 90 degrees.

muscles, elbow flexors, and the muscles of gripping. In this exercise, the lifter sits or kneels on the floor holding a bar connected to a weight pulley machine.

In the start-finish position, the lifter holds the bar connected to the weight machine cable with a wide grip with the palms facing forward. The shoulders are externally rotated and abducted to about 165 degrees. The elbows are extended, and the forearms are pronated. The exercise movement proceeds as the lifter pulls the bar downward toward a position behind the neck (Fig. 9-28a). The elbows are pulled downward and backward, causing shoulder extension, scapular adduction, and elbow flexion. The shoulder remains in a position of external rotation and abduction in this position. This exercise may, like exercises discussed earlier involving abduction and external rotation, cause difficulty or pain for the lifter with shoulder impingement or anterior capsuloligamentous-labral pathology. The start-finish position might cause subacromial impingement due to the extreme coronal plane abduction. An intact band of the inferior glenohumeral ligament complex[53] is necessary to prevent anterior subluxation in the position with the bar behind the neck. In these circumstances, the lifter should use a narrower grip and position himself or herself so that the bar is pulled further forward in front of the neck in the start-finish position (see Fig. 9-28b). This places the humerus toward the plane of the scapula, requiring less "twisting" on the rotator cuff and capsuloligamentous complex. This adaptation may lessen the chances of subacromial impingement. To further avoid the possible anterior subluxation, the lifter can instead pull the bar down in front of the neck to the clavicles. This would place the humerus in more relative internal rotation, lessening the stress on the capsular structures.

## CABLE ROW

In the cable row, the lifter sits facing a weight stack–cable machine. The feet are supported against a wood block placed against the machine. The lifter grasps a bar or handles; the forearms are pronated if using a bar or in neutral rotation if using handles.

In the start-finish position, the elbows extended, the shoulders are in forward flexion and internal rotation and the scapulae are protracted and abducted. The rowing motion begins as the lifter pulls toward the chest by forcefully adducting and retracting the scapulae, extending the shoulders and flexing the elbows. This exercise strongly exercises the rhomboids, middle and lower trapezius,[46] as well as the shoulder extensors: latissimus dorsi, teres major, and posterior deltoid. Strong action of the elbow flexors is required in the cable row exercise.

This exercise would be the exercise of choice to provide muscular balance with the muscles used in the bench press. The scapular adductors and retractors used in the cable row would balance the strong function of the serratus anterior and pectoralis minor used in the bench press.[46] The strong use of the shoulder extensors of the cable row would balance the action of the pectoralis major and minor and anterior deltoid action in the bench press. Elbow flexors and extensors also would find balance in these two opposing exercises. This balance between antagonistic muscle groups is an important principle to observe in all strength-building programs.[58–60]

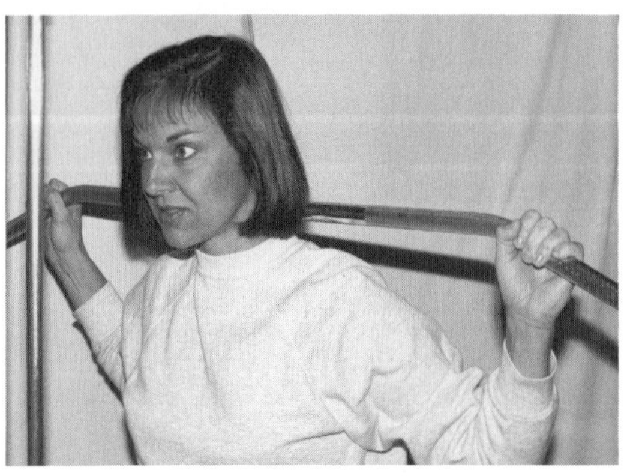

A

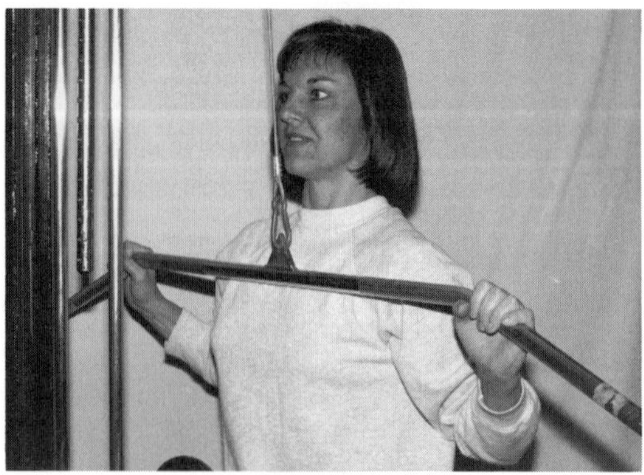

B

**Figure 9-28.** Lat pull-downs. (a) Behind-the-neck position. (b) Position in front of the neck.

# Summary

The use of weights as resistance for strength-building exercises is a popular and effective form of training for the enhancement of sports performance as well as for general fitness and recreation. The application of weights for strength training ranges from individual muscle group exercises such as those used in resistive weight machines and body-building exercises to the complex and high-risk lifts used in power lifting and olympic-style programs. Individuals with injury or preexisting pathologic conditions of the shoulder can utilize many of the exercises discussed in this chapter in their rehabilitation if proper precautions and adaptations are observed. Care must be taken during or following a strength program that exercises provide proper balance between antagonistic muscle groups.

# References


1. Algra B. An in-depth analysis of the bench press. J Nat Strength Cond Assoc 1982;4:6–11, 70–72.
2. Andrews JA, Carson WG, McLeod WD. Glenoid labrum tears related to the long head of the biceps. Am J Sports Med 1985; 13:337.
3. Andrews JA, Kuplerman SP, Dillman CJ. Labral tears in throwing and raquet sports. Clin Sports Med 1991;10:906.
4. Atwater AE. Biomechanics of overarm throwing movements and of throwing injuries. Exerc Sport Sci Rev 1979;7:43.
5. Bach BR, Warren RF, Wickiewicz TL. Triceps rupture: a case report and literature review. Am J Sports Med 1987;15:285.
6. Baker G, ed. The United States Weight Lifting Federation coaching manual, Vol. 1: Technique. Colorado Springs, Colo.: USWLF, 1988.
7. Beach ML, Whitney SL, Dickoff-Hoffman SA. Relationship of shoulder flexibility, strength and endurance to shoulder pain in competitive swimmers. J Orthop Sports Phys Ther 1992;16:262.
8. Blackburn TA, McLeod WD, White B, et al. EMG analysis of posterior rotator cuff exercise. Athl Train 1990;25:40.
9. Braatz JH, Gogia PP. The mechanics of pitching. J. Orthop Sports Phys Ther. 1987;9:56.
10. Bradley JP, Tibone JE. Electromyographic analysis of muscle action about the shoulder. Clin Sports Med 1991;10:789.
11. Cain PR, Mutschler TA, Fu FH, et al. Anterior stability of the glenohumeral joint: a dynamic model. Am J Sports Med 1987; 15:144.
12. Chang DE, Buschbaker LP, Edlich RF. Limited joint mobility in power lifters. Am J Sports Med 1988;16:280.
13. Ciullo JV, Stevens GC. The prevention and treatment of injuries to the shoulder in swimming. Sports Med 1989;7:182.
14. Counsilman JE. The science of swimming. Philadelphia: Prentice-Hall, 1968.
15. Dalla Pria Bankoff A, Vitti M. Simultaneous EMG of latissimus dorsi and the sternocostal part of pectoralis major muscles during the crawl stroke. Electromyogrgr Clin Neurophysiol 1978;18:289.
16. Derwin B. The snatch: technical description and periodization program. J Nat Strength Cond Assoc 1990;12:6.
17. DiGiovine NM, Jobe FW, Pink M, et al. An electromyographic analysis of the upper extremity in pitching. J Shoulder Elbow Surg 1992;1:15.
18. Elliott BC. Tennis strokes and equipment. In: Vaught CL, ed. Biomechanics of Sports. Boca Raton, Fla.: CRC Press, 1989:263.
19. Falkel JE, Murphy TC. Case principles: swimmer's shoulder. Sports Injury Management 1988;1:109.
20. Ferrari DA. Capsular ligaments of the shoulder: anatomical and functional study of the anterior superior capsule. Am J Sports Med 1990;18:20.
21. Fleisig GS, Dillman C, Andrews JR. A biomechanical description of the shoulder joint during pitching. Sports Med Update 1991; Fall:10.
22. Fowler PJ, Webster MS. Shoulder pain in highly competitive swimmers. Orthop Trans 1983;7:170.
23. Gamberdella RA, Jobe FA. Diagnosis and treatment of shoulder injuries in throwers. In: Nicholas JA, Hershman EB, eds. The upper extremity and spine in sports medicine. St Louis: CV Mosby, 1990:751.
24. Garhammer J. Weight lifting and training. In: Vaught CL, ed. Biomechanics of sports. Boca Raton, Fla.: CRC Press, 1989.
25. Glousman R, Jobe FW, Tibone J, et al. Dynamic EMG analysis of the throwing shoulder with glenohumeral instability. J Bone Joint Surg 1988;70(A):220.
26. Gowan ID, Jobe FW, Tibone J, et al. A comparative electromyographic analysis of the shoulder during pitching: professional versus amateur pitchers. Am J Sports Med 1987;15:586.
27. Greipp JF. Swimmer's shoulder: the influence of flexibility and weight training. Phys Sports Med 1985;13(8):92.
28. Hawkins RJ, Kennedy JC. Impingement syndromes in athletes. Am J Sports Med 1980;8:151.
29. Hoffman B. Better athletes through weight training. York, Pa.: Strength and Health Publishing Company, 1959.
30. Howell SM, Kraft TA. The role of the supraspinatus and infraspinatus muscles in glenohumeral kinematics of anterior shoulder instability. Clin Orthop 1991;263:128.
31. Howell SM, Galinat BJ, Renzi AJ, et al. Normal and abnormal mechanics of the glenohumeral joint in the horizontal plane. J Bone Joint Surg 1988;70A:27.
32. Ikai M, Ishii M, Miyashita M. An electromyographic study of swimming. Res J Phys Ed 1964;7:47.
33. Ivey FM, Calhoun JH, Rusche K, et al. Isokinetic testing of shoulder strength: normal values. Arch Phys Med Rehabil 1985;66:384.
34. Jobe FW, Tibone JE, Perry J, et al. An EMG analysis of the shoulder in throwing and pitching. Am J Sports Med 1983;11:3.
35. Jobe FW, Moynes DR, Tibone JE, et al. An EMG analysis of the shoulder in pitching: a second report. Am J Sports Med 1984; 12:218.
36. Johnson JE, Sim FH, Scott SG. Musculoskeletal injuries in competitive swimmers. Mayo Clin Proc 1987;62:289.
37. Keggerreis S, Jenkins WL, Maline TR. Throwing injuries. Sports Injury Management 1989;4:1.
38. Kennedy JC, Hawkins R, Krissoff WB. Orthopaedic manifestations of swimming. Am J Sports Med 1978;6:309.
39. Leach R. Tennis serve compared with baseball pitching. In: Zarins B, Andrews JR, Carson WG, eds. Injuries to the throwing arm. Philadelphia: WB Saunders, 1985:311.

39a. Leach R. The impingement syndrome. In: Zarins B, Andrews JR, Carson WG, eds. Injuries to the throwing arm. Philadelphia: WB Saunders, 1985:122.

40. Matzen FA, Harryman DT, Sidles JA. Mechanisms of glenohumeral instability. Clin Sports Med 1991;10:783.
41. McCue FC, Gieck JH, West JO. Throwing injuries of the shoulder. Athletic Training 1977;4:202.
42. McLeod WM. The pitching mechanism. In: Zarins B, Andrews JR, Carson WG, eds. Injuries to the throwing arm. Philadelphia: WB Saunders, 1985:22.
43. McMaster WC. Anterior glenoid labrum damage: a painful lesion in swimmers. Am J Sports Med 1986;14(5):383.
44. McMaster WC, Long SC, Caiozzo VJ. Shoulder torque changes in the swimming athlete. Am J Sports Med 1992;20:323.
45. Miyashita M. Arm action in the crawl stroke. In: Lewlllie L, Clarys JP, eds. Proceedings of the second international symposium on biomechanics of swimming. Baltimore: University Park Press, 1974.
46. Moseley JB, Jobe FW, Pink M, et al. EMG analysis of the scapular rotator muscles during a shoulder rehabilitation program. Am J Sports Med 1992;20:128.
47. Moynes DR, Perry J, Antonelli DJ, Jobe FW. Electromyography and motion analysis of the upper extremity in sports. Phys Ther 1986;66:1905.
48. Neer CS. Anterior acromioplasty for chronic impingement syndrome in the shoulder. J Bone Joint Surg 1972;54A:41.
49. Nicholas J, Grossman RB, Hershman EB. The importance of a simplified classification of motion in sports in relation to performance. Orthop Clin North Am 1977;8:499.
50. Nirschl RP: Shoulder tendinitis. In: Pettrone F, ed. Symposium on

upper extremity injuries in athletes. St. Louis: CV Mosby, 1986: 322.

51. Nuber GW, Jobe FW, Perry J, et al. Fine wire electromyography of the shoulder during swimming. Am J Sports Med 1986;14:7.
52. Norris T. History and physical examination of the shoulder. In: Nicholas JA, Hirschman EB, eds. The upper extremity and spine in sports medicine. St Louis: CV Mosby, 1990:41.
53. O'Brien SJ, Veves MC, Arnoczky SP, et al. The anatomy and histology of the inferior glenohumeral ligament complex of the shoulder. Am J Sports Med 1990;18:449.
54. O'Connell PW, Nuber GW, Mileski RA, et al. The contribution of the glenohumeral ligaments to anterior stability of the shoulder joint. Am J Sports Med 1990;18:579–584.
55. Pappas AM, Zwacki RM, Sullivan TS. Biomechanics of baseball pitching: A preliminary report. Am J Sports Med 1985;13:216–222.
56. Perry J. Anatomy and biomechanics of the shoulder in throwing, swimming, gymnastics and tennis. Clin Sports Med 1983;2: 247–270.
57. Petruska AJ. Rehabilitation of rotator cuff tendinitis. Sports Injury Forum, Sports Medicine Systems 1986;4(4):3.
58. Petruska AJ. Strength training for sport. Sports Injury Forum, Sports Medicine Systems. 1986;4(7).
59. Petruska AJ. Physical conditioning for sports participation: injury prevention through total fitness. Sports Injury Forum, Sports Medicine Systems 1987;4(10):3.
60. Petruska AJ. The strength and conditioning specialist is sports. Sports Performance Specialties, Westboro, Mass.: 1989.
61. Pink M, Perry J, Browne A, Scovazzo ML, Kerrigan J. The normal shoulder during freestyle swimming: an electromyographic and cinematographic analysis of twelve muscles. Am J Sports Med 1991;19:569.
62. Rathbun JB, McNab I. The microvascular pattern of the rotator cuff. J Bone Joint Surg 1970;52B:540.
63. Richardson AB. The mechanics of swimming: the shoulder and the knee. Clin Sports Med 1986;5:10.
64. Richardson AB. Overview of soft tissue injuries of the shoulder. In: The upper extremity and spine in sports medicine. Nicholas JA, Hirschman EB, Eds. C. V. Mosby Co., 1990:221.
65. Richardson AB. Overuse syndromes in baseball, tennis, gymnastics, and swimming. Clin Sports Med 1983;2:379.
66. Richardson AB, Jobe FW, Collins HR. The shoulder in competitive swimming. J Am Sports Med 1980;8:159.
67. Rollins J, Puffer JC, Whiting WC, et al. Waterpolo injuries to the upper extremity. In: Injuries to the throwing arm. Zarins B, Andrews JR, Carson WG, Eds. WB Saunders Co., 1985:311.
68. Rouard AH, Billat RP. Influences of sex and level of performance on the freestyle stroke: an electromyography and kinematic study. Int J Sports Med 1990;11:150.
69. Ryu RK, McCormick J, Jobe FW, et al. An electromyographic analysis of shoulder function in tennis players. Am J Sports Med 1988;16:481.
70. Scavenius M, Iverson BF. Non-traumatic clavicular osteolysis in weight lifters. Am J Sports Med 1992;16:481.
71. Schubert M. Competitive swimming techniques of champions. Sports Illustrated Winner's Circles Books. New York: TimeLife, 1990.
72. Scovazzo ML, Browne A, Pink M, et al. The painful shoulder during freestyle swimming: an electromyographic and cinematographic analysis of twelve muscles. Am J Sports Med 1991; 19:557.
73. Sherman OH, Snyder SJ, Fox JM. Tricep tendon avulsion in a professional body builder. Am J Sports Med 1984;12:328.
74. Smith T. Junior weight training. North Palm Beach, Fl.: The Athletic Institute, 1985.
75. Stiggins C, Allsen P. Exercise methods, notebook no. 9: lat pulldown. J Nat Strength Cond Assoc 1983;5:69.
76. Stiggins C, Allsen P. Exercise methods, notebook no. 42: dumbbell incline press. J Nat Strength Cond Assoc 1989;11:77.
77. Stiggins C, Allsen P. Exercise methods, notebook no. 43: seated rowing. J Nat Strength Cond Assoc 1989;11:82.
78. Stiggins C, Allsen P. Exercise methods, notebook no. 21: decline press. J Nat Strength Cond Assoc 1985;4:79.
79. Stiggins C, Allsen P. Exercise methods, notebook no. 7: seated overhead press. J Nat Strength Cond Assoc 1983;5:69.
80. Stone WJ, Kroll SW. Sports conditioning and weight training. 2nd ed. Des Moines, Iowa: Wm C Brown Company, 1988.
81. Takano B. Coaching optimal technique in the snatch and clean and jerk, part I. J Nat Strength Cond Assoc 1987;9(5):50.
82. Takano B. Coaching optimal technique in the snatch and clean and jerk, part II. J Nat Strength Cond Assoc 1987;9(6):57.
83. Takano B. Coaching optimal technique in the snatch and clean and jerk, part III. J Nat Strength Cond Assoc 1988;10(1):54.
84. Terry GC, Hammon D, France P, et al. The stabilizing function of passive shoulder restraints. Am J Sports Med 1991;19:26.
85. Towsend H, Jobe FW, Pink M, et al. EMG analysis of the glenohumeral muscles during a baseball rehabilitation program. Am J Sports Med 1991;19:264.
86. Tullos H, King JW. Throwing mechanism in sports. Orthop Clin North Am 1973;4:709.
87. Warner JP, Micheli LJ, Arselenian LE, et al. Patterns of flexibility, laxity, an strength in normal shoulders and shoulders with instability and impingement. Am J Sports Med 1990;18:336.
88. Wick H, Dillman C, Werner S, et al. A kinematic comparison between baseball pitching and football passing. Sports Med Update 1991;Spring:13.
89. Zeman SC. Tears of the pectoralis major muscle. Am J Sports Med 1979;7:343.

Chapter 10

*David W. Clifton, Jr.*

# Occupational Shoulder Injury Management



## Occupational Injuries

Rehabilitation of a shoulder injury can be a complicated endeavor. This task is made significantly more difficult when directed toward patients who have shoulder pathology and need to return to the occupational setting.

The interdependency of three key factors dictate whether a patient will experience a favorable outcome. These are

1. The congenital and structural makeup of the shoulder complex
2. Posttraumatic effects on structure
3. Postural and biomechanical effects on structure

For many clinicians, the primary focus of traditional treatment has been to address the trauma, with little attention paid to the ergonomic risk factors and their relationship to anatomic structure and physiologic processes. Traditional therapies have treated symptoms (i.e., muscle spasm, decreased range of motion, weakness, and inflammation) often through a host of "palliative" modalities while overlooking the proximate risk factors. Proximate risk factors include repetitive motion, vibration, external compression, exertional force, and nonphysiologic positions/postures. It is critical that these factors be considered in both the design and implementation of a treatment program. Berry-

Martin J. Kelley and William A. Clark: ORTHOPEDIC THERAPY OF THE SHOULDER.

hill[8] provides an excellent overview of the factors associated with return-to-work success rates. He describes the interdependency between clinical and work-site issues and cites four success indicators:

1. Demands of the workplace, i.e., risk factors
2. Disease category involvement, i.e., strains, fractures
3. Stage of recovery, i.e., acute, subacute, chronic
4. Functional abilities, i.e., job-related deficits

This chapter will review available literature and discuss an integrative approach incorporating ergonomic principles into shoulder rehabilitation programs. Since work-related injury is often cumulative in nature versus a single incident or trauma, the primary focus will be on cumulative trauma disorders, specifically, associated microtraumas.

# Cumulative Trauma Disorders

Cumulative trauma disorders (CTDs) are a class of musculoskeletal disorders involving damage to the tendons, tendon sheaths, synovial lubrication of the tendon sheaths, and the related bones, muscles, and nerves of the hands, wrists, elbows, shoulders, back, and neck. CTDs are the result of microtraumas leading to "a clinical syndrome where the effects of wear and tear are beyond the body's repair or healing processes."[32]

The shoulder complex, owing to its unique anatomic design and functional capability, is subject to a number of cumulative trauma disorders. The scope of this chapter will not enable a comprehensive review of all shoulder CTDs but will address several of the more common varieties. However, the ergonomic principles discussed will have applicability to virtually all categories of shoulder CTDs as well as noncumulative trauma conditions.

# Anatomic Considerations

The shoulder's primary function is to place the hand for functional tasks, yet a delicate balance exists between basic joint movement and control by the static and dynamic components. Since the glenohumeral joint is the shallowest of all major joints, its mobility capabilities constantly challenge the capsuloligamentous complex (CLC) and the rotator cuff. When compromise of these soft-tissue envelopes occurs, significant impairment results, particularly when considering the frequency and intensity demands placed on our shoulders during functional tasks (Fig. 10-1).

Rotator cuff tendonopathy and thoracic outlet syndrome are frequently applied diagnoses to the occupational patient and are of keen interest to the work therapist who must develop functionally based rehabilitation programs without exacerbating the patient's symptoms during the process. A brief review of shoulder anatomy related to these injury classifications demonstrates the incongruency between anatomy and workplace design, both of which directly affect successful work therapy outcomes.

The following anatomic review will be general, since a more detailed anatomic overview can be found in earlier chapters.

## ROTATOR CUFF TENDONOPATHY

Charles Neer[32] popularized the term *impingement syndrome* and classified it as three stages of rotator cuff and subacromial bursae degeneration related to age. He described impingement as a mechanical compression of the rotator cuff, subacromial bursae, and/or biceps tendon by the components of the coracoacromial arch. The bursae and the supraspinatus and biceps tendons are most frequently the victim of impingement because of their location. The supraspinatus insertion at the greater tuberosity and the bicipital tendon lie anterior to the coracoacromial arch when the shoulder is in neutral position. When forward flexion is executed, the soft tissues pass beneath the arch, making it vulnerable to impingement. This mechanical phenomenon exacerbates an already tenuous condition, since the rotator cuff is commonly

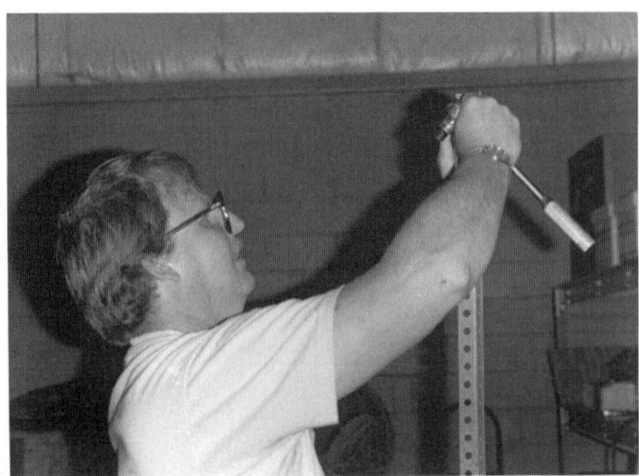

**Figure 10-1.** Position of functional task that stresses the shoulder structures.

believed to undergo degeneration due to attrition, questionable vascular supply, and decreased tensile strength. Neer[32] described three different stages of impingement, noted for the incessant changes of the cuff and associated structures over time with cumulative trauma. In stage I, there is reversible edema and hemorrhage, often seen in younger patients (i.e., under 25 years). If this condition persists, it enters stage II, resulting in fibrosis and thickening of the tendons and bursae; this is typically seen in the 25- to 40-year-old age groups. With continued cumulative trauma, one runs the risk of entering stage III. In this stage, bone spurs and tendon ruptures are common in the older worker (i.e., over 40 years age). At this stage, the degree of tissue involvement makes ergonomic modifications and rehabilitation less effective in resolving symptoms, and surgical intervention may be necessary. Traditional "palliative" modalities may be efficacious during stage I, but their effect becomes limited during the later stages.

The rotator cuff functions to move the humerus while dynamically stabilizing the glenohumeral joint. When rotator cuff function is compromised, the force-couple relationship with the deltoid is disrupted, resulting in superior humeral head migration against the coracoacromial arch and culminating in tissue trauma. Posterior capsule tightness common in these conditions adds further compression to the subacromial structures, particularly during overhead functional tasks. Adding insult to injury is the positive correlation between weight lifted to compressive forces and ischemia while in static postures.[20]

Anatomic and arthrokinematic flaws, tendon physiology, and workplace demands combine to predispose the shoulder to impingement syndromes. One of these risk factors alone may not lead to a problem, but in combination they often results in impingement syndromes best characterized as *cumulative trauma disorders*.

## THORACIC OUTLET SYNDROME

A second category of impingement syndrome afflicts the brachial plexus region of the shoulder. Thoracic outlet syndrome (TOS) has been linked to a host of structures. Jaeger et al.[25] assert that "all neurovascular structures that pass through the thoracic outlet are at risk of compression." These include the subclavian artery and vein, the brachial plexus itself, and the sympathetic efferent nerves. A great deal of confusion surrounds the use of semantics descriptive of TOS partly because of the anatomic variety. Many terms are used interchangeably to describe similar symptoms. Jaeger et al.[25] list the following: scalenus anticus syndrome, scalenus medius band syndrome, Sibson's fascia/scalenus minimus syndrome, costoclavicular compression syndrome, hyperabduction syndrome, acroparesthesis syndrome, Paget-Schroeder syndrome, and cervical rib syndrome. Despite the plethora of anatomic descriptors, from an ergonomics standpoint, all are treated similarly, most notably by eliminating or reducing the trauma associated with overhead repetitive and static activities.

As with rotator cuff syndrome, the earlier ergonomic/biomechanical stressors are addressed, the better is the outcome. In thoracic outlet syndrome, if compression persists and conservative treatment fails, there is a likelihood of irreversible neurovascular damage, as evidenced by the poor results frequently found with any number of surgical interventions. Although the debate rages on as to which anatomic structure is involved and the surgical procedures of choice, it is advisable for the work therapist to focus on the worksite risk factors.

## OCCUPATIONAL CERVICOBRACHIAL DISORDERS

Occupational cervicobrachial disorders (OCDs) are a third common category of CTDs. This is really a symptom complex and not a clinical diagnosis, since it encompasses characteristics of several disorders, such as myositis, arthritis, tendinitis, and TOS. This classification of CTDs is generally seen in the sedentary and light assembly-line worker, as opposed to rotator cuff pathology, which typically affects material handlers.[29] Video display terminal operators are one of the fastest growing occupational groups experiencing OCDs (Fig. 10-2).

Luck and Andersson[29] describe three grades of OCD based only on myofacial changes, commonly found among sedentary and light assembly workers (Table 10-1). Grade I involves a strain-type injury due to static loading that is symptomatic while working. Grade II is more involved, and symptoms persist for several days even when not working. Grade III is an advanced stage involving permanent myopathy and fibrosis. Sustained and/or repetitive forward flexion and elevation are biomechanical causation factors.

The work therapist not only should identify the involved tissues but also should evaluate and employ ergonomic principles when treating (Fig. 10-3). This is a dramatic shift away from the medical model, wherein the patient and his or her condition are the focus of attention, and to-

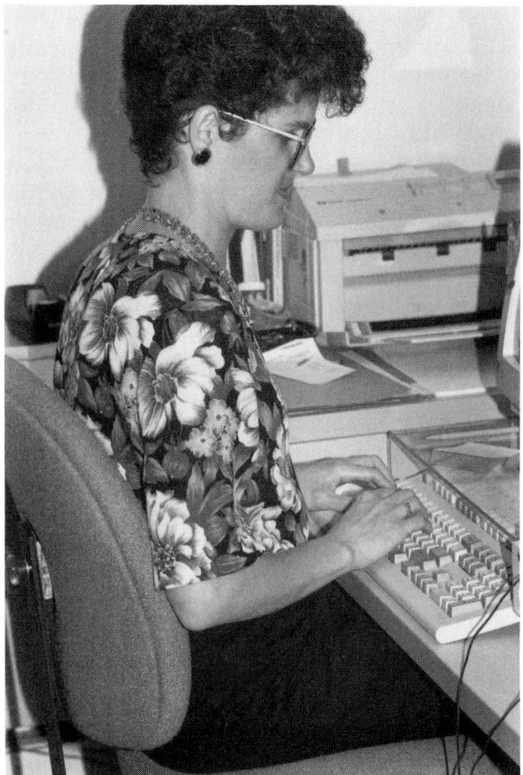

**Figure 10-2.** Typical position of video terminal user.

ward an ergomedical model, wherein ergonomics and rehabilitation are synergistic. Of course, during the acute or subacute stage of injury or disease, the choice of pain modality requires an assessment of involved structures, thereby following a traditional medical model.

**Table 10-1**

**Pathophysiologic Grading System of OCDs**

| | |
|---|---|
| **Grade I (mild)** | Shoulder girdle muscle pain that occurs during work or similar activities and resolves a few hours later. No finding on physical examination. |
| **Grade II (moderate)** | Shoulder girdle muscle pain that persists for several days after work. Muscle belly and insertional tenderness on examination. |
| **Grade III (severe)** | Shoulder girdle muscle pain that is constant for weeks or longer. Multiple tender areas. Palpable induration indicative of muscle fibrosis. Muscle belly contracture. Reduced range of motion of myogenic origin. |

Reproduced with permission from Luck JV, Andersson GBJ. Occupational shoulder disorders. In: Rockwood CA, Matsen FA, eds. The shoulder. Philadelphia: WB Saunders, 1990.

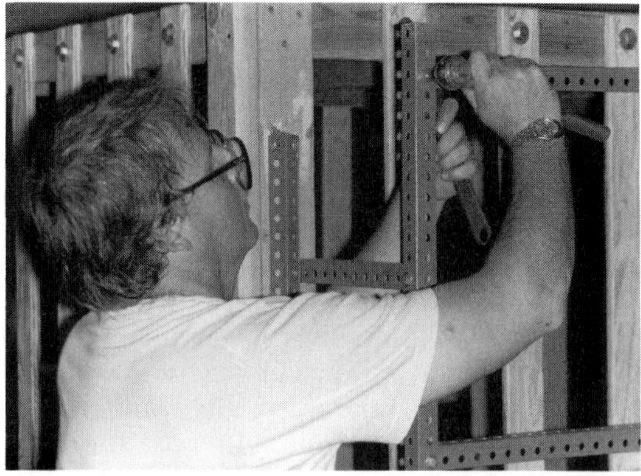

A

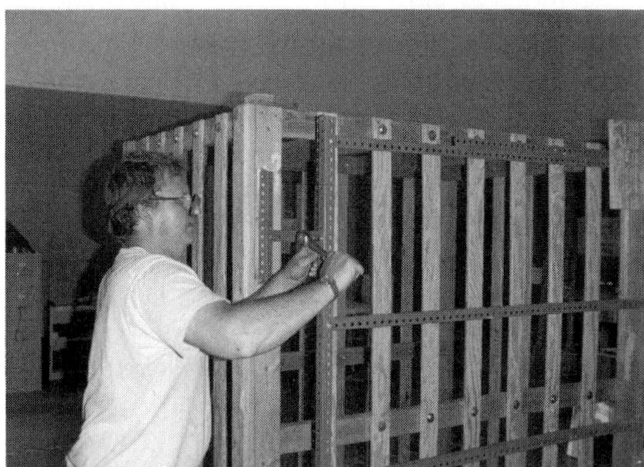

B

**Figure 10-3.** Inappropriate (a) and appropriate (b) positioning.

Through employee training, proper selection of workers (preplacement and return-to-work functional capacity evaluation) and ergonomic considerations, the therapist and injured worker can avoid some of the static postures and dynamic motions that are encouraged by poor ergonomics.

## Systems Approach

The ultimate goal of every work therapy program is a return of the worker to gainful employment. This is accomplished through the appropriate match of a worker to the work site and, reciprocally, the work site to the worker following rehabilitation. Functional capacity evaluation typifies the *worker approach* or human factors, while ergonomics addresses the *work-site approach. Job assessment* and *functional assess-*

*ment* are interdependent and will be jointly examined as a *systems approach* to disability management. The systems approach will address three key areas:

1. Analysis of occupational risk factors
2. Client functional assessment
3. Development of a return-to-work program

# Occupational Risk Factors

The literature is replete with studies of occupational risk factors relative to upper extremity injury or, in the case of CTDs, "disease." Because of their slow, insidious, and often unknown etiology, cumulative trauma disorders are considered to be "diseases" versus "injury" by the Occupational Safety and Health Administration (OSHA), and recordkeeping requirements must reflect this distinction.

Armstrong[6] has identified repetitiveness, force, mechanical stress, posture, temperature, and vibration as the most common risk factors associated with cumulative trauma disorders (Fig. 10-4). Van Wely[42] developed a table of posture-pain relationships from studies of symptoms. Additionally, the interactive nature of postures and work loads in various occupational categories has been studied extensively.[5,7,14,18,20,36]

Hayberg and Wegman[18] describe prevalence rates for shoulder-neck diseases by occupational groups. The study of vibration disorders has received attention and has been the focus of attempts to develop exposure standards with mixed results. Berger and Kleinert[7] assert that "the main reasons for the lack of progress in this disease [vibration induced] are the highly subjective nature of the symptoms, the lack of any reproducible technique of quantifying vibration exposure, and the difficulty in setting safe standards for vibration."

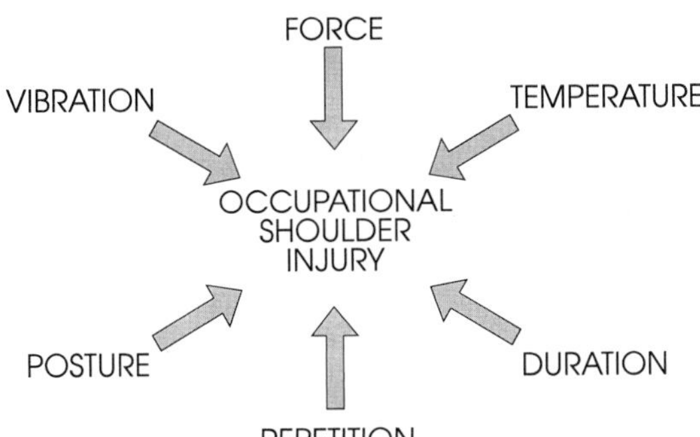


**Figure 10-4.** Ergonomic risk factors.

However, the effects of vibration have been highly correlated with vasomotor disturbances and osteoarticular lesions. Futatsaka et al.[14] found that lower frequencies (less than 40 Hz) led to osteoarticular lesions in some subjects, while higher frequencies (40 to 300 Hz) were correlative with vasomotor diseases. Pelmear et al.[36] conclude that there is minimal medical evidence linking vibration to specific disorders but have suggested it as a causative factor in vascular and neurologic damage. A number of authors have acknowledged the difficulty in identifying acceptable exposure levels with occupational risks.[5,24,37]

Past efforts to quantify/qualify occupational risk factors have included the National Institute for Occupational Safety and Health's (NIOSH) "Vibration Standards,"[33] NIOSH's "Maximum Permissible Limits for Lifting,"[34] OSHA's "Ergonomic Guidelines for the Red Meat Industry,"[35] and the American National Standards Institute's (ANSI's) "Standard for Human Factors Engineering of Visual Display Terminal Workstations."[3] Current efforts include the ANSI Z-365 Project[4] for the control of cumulative trauma disorders. This ANSI project involves three subcommittees: surveillance, medical management, and work analysis and design. These groups have been charged with the task of developing "standards to control cumulative trauma disorders arising from manual lifting, assembly, manipulation of tools, machinery and other devices and other stresses to muscles, nerves, and tendons."

The results of these and other efforts to establish exposure standards and abatement strategies will have a direct impact on work therapists and their efforts to return injured workers to gainful employment.

Occupational risk factors have received industry-specific study (Table 10-2). Herberts et al.[20] have conducted one of the more extensive epidemiologic studies of shoulder pain in welders. Welders make a good study group because their work often involves both repetitive and static overhead activities. Herberts' study compared welders with clerical workers and found shoulder pain to be significantly more prevalent in the welders (27 percent of welders had shoulder pain). This study produced some interesting findings that are relevant to rehabilitation programs:

1. Pain was localized to the supraspinatus, and there was no redistribution of the muscle load to other synergistically operating muscles.

**Table 10-2**

**Occupational Risk Factor Studies by Industry**

| Industry | Study |
|---|---|
| Automobile | Stetson (1986), Tennen (1986) |
| Carpenters | Astrand et al. (1968) |
| Castings plant | Silverstein (1987) |
| Garment workers | Marcotte (1989), Punnett (1985), Sokas (1989), Wick (1986) |
| Assembly | Konz (1967), Ortengren (1975), Radwin (1985) |
| Mechanical | Kudrinka et al. (1979) |
| Postal | Gomer et al. (1987) |
| Meatpacking | Dropf (1975), Finkel (1985), Hales (1989), National Safety Council (1978), UFCW (1980), Viikare-Juntura (1983) |
| Telecommunications | McKenzie (1975) |
| Video Display/ Keyboard Operators | Cakir (1980), Cushman (1984), Grandjean (1982), Helander (1985), Hunting (1982), Life (1984), Nakaseko (1985), Onishi (1985), Rowe (1987), Salvendy (1984), Smith (1984), Walsh (1981) |
| Poultry Processing | Armstrong (1987), Richardson (1988) |
| Welders | Petersen (1976) |
| Grocery | NIOSH Shoprite Study, Orgel (1990) |
| Glass Manufacturing | NIOSH HETA Study No. 89-137-2005 |

2. Experience of the welder serves to lower muscle fatigue through training and ergonomically improved work technique.
3. Neither the number of welding years or the rated level of shoulder muscle load were found to be important etiologic factors.

OSHA, in its "Ergonomics Guidelines for Meatpacking Plants,"[35] suggests that "finding solutions to the problems posed by ergonomic hazards may well be the most significant workplace safety and health issue of the 1990s." Therefore, the work therapist would be well advised to increase competencies within the ergonomic arena. A shift from clinically based thinking (i.e., treating symptoms) toward ergonomically based thinking should result in significant improvements in clinical outcomes, particularly decreased reinjury rates.

Perhaps, the greatest amount of attention has been paid to the effect of repetition. A number of authors have suggested a linkage between repetition and cumulative trauma syndromes.[5,13,19,30,40] The work therapist must exercise caution in the development and implementation of a work therapy program in order to avoid exacerbation or reinjury. A program that reproduces the proximate risk factors (i.e., repetition of overhead lifting) may likely compromise patient outcome.

# Client Assessment

## IMPAIRMENT VERSUS DISABILITY

Although one can "engineer out" many occupational risk factors, personal risk factors for shoulder CTDs cannot be engineered out. Therefore, the work therapist must determine if and when an injured employee can return to gainful employment. Work therapists have many disability assessment tools available to them but must choose the most reliable measures that accurately predict the injured worker's success in meeting or exceeding job requirements as a predicate to a return to work. A common source of controversy within the disability assessment system involves the interchangeable use of two distinct terms: *impairment* and *disability*. Medical providers are often called on to provide professional opinions regarding the disability status of clients. The work therapist offers this opinion based on data collected during a work-capacity or functional evaluation. However, these data often addresses the specific impairments which may or may not have bearing on disability status. Although these evaluations should include physical demand assessments they commonly fall short of adequately describing the client's actual job.

The therapist must begin by differentiating impairments from disabilities. The AMA[2] definition for impairment is:

> A purely medical condition. Permanent impairment is any anatomic or functional abnormality or loss after maximal medical rehabilitation has been achieved.

Therapists have traditionally measured impairment (i.e., ROM, strength deficits, edema) while leaving disability ratings to physicians. Times have changed and therapists are called upon with increasing frequency to render opinions regarding disability. Even the AMA[2] has acknowledged that disability ratings require a team approach and are not in the exclusive domain of the physician. According to the AMA "permanent disability is not a purely medical condition."[2] A patient is 'permanently disabled' or 'under permanent disability' when his actual or presumed ability to engage in gainful activity is reduced or absent because of 'impairment' which, in turn, may or may not be combined with other factors." Furthermore, disability is not a legal medical definition that requires an administrative decision process. "Disability" has been defined as, "an individual is disabled only if he or she meets the requirements of a specific disability benefits program or policy."

The AMA[2] acknowledges that disability is an administrative decision stating, "In general, it is not possible for a physician using medical information alone, to make reliable predictions about the ability of an individual to perform tasks or to meet functional demands." Of critical importance to the work therapist is the observation that a client with an impairment does not necessarily possess a disability. According to the American Medical Association (AMA),[2] "It is unrealistic to presume that all these impairments, especially those of a minor nature, will necessarily at some time result in disability."

Understanding these definitions is a prerequisite to the selection of any assessment methodology. Work therapists have a cadre of traditional assessment tools which, for the most part, measure impairment and rarely disability. For instance, range of motion measures joint integrity by examining the status of the capsuloligamentous complex (CLC) and osteokinematics, while muscle performance measures strength in terms of muscle fiber recruitment, chemical reactions, and innervation (Table 10-3).

In order to assess disability accurately, the work therapist must use the injured worker's functionally based job description, better known as a *job analysis*. This will require nontraditional assessment measures that may need to be customized to each worker's situation (Table 10-4). It is unrealistic to presume that one test battery will suffice for all injured workers. The *Dictionary of Occupational Titles*[11] has over 26,000 job descriptions, with minimal reference to functional tasks. Therefore, each client's physical job demands must be taken into consideration when developing a test. This is particularly critical given the implications of the Americans with Disabilities Act.

**Table 10-3**

**Traditional Assessment Measures**

- ROM measures
- Strength measures
- Endurance measures (subjective fatigue criterion)
- Perceived exertional measures
- Flexibility measures
- Subjective pain responses
- Activities of daily living assessments

**Table 10-4**

**Nontraditional Assessment Measures**

- Work-capacity evaluation
- Functionally based EMG/positional EMG
- Vibration measures
- Tremor metrics
- Precision movement measures
- Physiologic fatigue criterion (i.e., pulmonary function studies, stress tests)
- Computerized strength prediction models for manual materials handling

Nontraditional assessment measures more closely address the issue of disability by correlating impairment with functionality (disability). Work-capacity evaluation, which uses a functional job description as the "blueprint for recovery," exemplifies this assessment approach.

A constellation of variables interacts to create an enormous challenge to the therapist in the assessment of occupational shoulder girdle injuries. Peculiar to the shoulder are anatomic characteristics which, when combined with occupational risk factors, serve to heighten the chance of injury/reinjury. Anatomic idiosyncrasies of the shoulder girdle become aggravating factors when they occur in the presence of proximal causal factors (occupational risk factors). The relationship between occupational job demands and upper extremity performance has been studied by a number of researchers. The results of these studies provide a rationale for functional assessment and job analysis as a two-stage process. However, a number of current functional assessment schemes have not been validated and do not yield predictive data.

Some authors have discovered that although there is a significant correlation between isometric strength and dynamic strength, there is little correlation between dynamic strength capacity and precision motor performance.[27,38] Sigholm et al.[39] studied electromyographic (EMG) changes with shoulder muscle load (Fig. 10-5). The influence of hand tool weight and arm position on shoulder muscle load determined by EMG yielded the following results:

**Percentage increase of EMG level when hand load is increased by 1 Kg.**

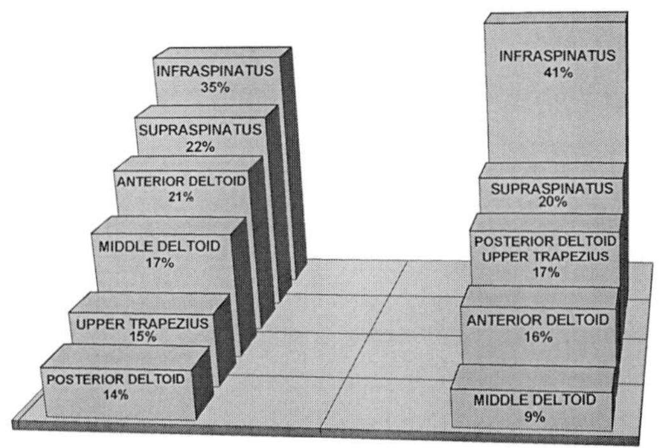


**FLEXION** **ABDUCTION**

**Figure 10-5.** Shoulder muscle activity. (Data from Sigholm G, Herberts P, Armstrong C, Kadefors R. Electromyographic analysis of shoulder muscle load. J Ortho Res. 1984;1(4):82.)

1. The short rotator muscles stabilizing the shoulder joint were found to be more hand-load-dependent than the deltoid muscle.
2. Experienced workers performing the same tasks were able to avoid fatigue in all studied muscles except for the supraspinatus.
3. Supraspinatus EMG activity was no different when positioned in abduction and flexion.
4. The degree of upper arm elevation was found to be the most important parameter determining muscle load.
5. Upper arm rotation and elbow flexion are of little importance for shoulder muscle loading.
6. The infraspinatus was heavily fatigued with overhead work in addition to supraspinatus.

In another study, Wiker et al.[44] postulated the correlation between arm posture and human movement capability. The low correlation between subject strength capability and posturally based decrements has tremendous impact on work therapists who frequently use strength as a predictor of functional capability. Work therapists frequently emphasize pounds lifted but neglect postural considerations. Regardless of one's strength capability, there were significant decrements in movement performance when hands were postured above shoulder level. Movement performance degraded immediately and was not linked to any plane of movement (i.e., sagittal versus coronal). The use of heavier equipment also was found to be highly correlative with performance decrements.

A second interesting finding of this study was that localized muscle fatigue was not associated with movement capabilities when the hands were positioned above the shoulders. Lastly, expressed subjective discomfort was not correlated with movement decrements. The implication of this study is that selecting stronger workers will not improve speed or accuracy of performance in above-shoulder assembly tasks. Yet rehabilitation programs frequently emphasize strength increases as a cornerstone of goal achievement.

This presents the clinician with an interesting paradox; on one hand, ergonomics is engineering heavy objects out of the workplace, while work therapies generally strive to increase weight lifted.

There have been a number of attempts to develop models for the prediction of muscle strength and performance. However, a significant number have addressed spinal conditions, while few have involved upper extremity models, especially the shoulder. Imran[23] studied predictive models of upper extremity rotary and linear pull strength, specifically elbow flexion and peak shoulder extension forces. Three primary variables were studied: velocity of movement, speed of contraction, and skeletal position of contracting segments. The shoulder was tested in nine different positions. It was generally found that shoulder forces decrease as elbow angle increases. The teres major and latissimus dorsi muscle groups developed greater tension capabilities when prestretched above the horizontal position (90 degrees of shoulder elevation). It also was noted that positions above the horizontal plane (130 to 170 degrees) produced greater forces than those below the horizontal plane (10 to 50 degrees). The author attributes this to a combination of mechanical leverage and length-tension relationship. This study concluded that "maximum strength of linear isokinetic pull and its components (elbow flexion/shoulder extension) can be predicted fairly accurately from pull velocity, skeletal configuration of the arm, and certain anthropometric variables."

Electromyography provides the work therapist with an assessment tool that allows job task-function interfacements. The literature relative to EMG activity forceful tasks is plentiful when compared with the study of less stressful or precision-based tasks. Gomer et al.[17] examined the effects of localized muscle fatigue in a machine-paced keyboard operation. This study supports the contention that EMG can provide physiologic data about occupational stress. Specifically, these data suggest that even small differences in microtrauma inducement can lead to earlier fatigue and CTD symptoms. Four assessment methodologies were used in reaching this conclusion: behavioral measures of localized fatigue, EMG study, self-reported physical discomfort, and work-related performance. The keyboard group that fatigued early

- Exhibited less accuracy in keyboard functions
- Rated visual and mental workload as higher
- Possessed greater tremor in postwork hand steadiness tests
- Reported greater discomfort in fingers, hands, wrists, and arms

It is universally understood that movements involve synergistic firing of multiple muscle groups, with some serving the role of stabilizers and others performing a joint movement function. Both the degree of contraction and the strength of a contraction in a muscle are dependent on the summation of the actions of the large number of motor units innervated.

Khalil[27] developed an assessment methodology that allowed for the simultaneous monitoring of integrated muscular activity. Total muscular effort expended in performing an industrial task was quantified via a computer circuit (total integrated muscular activity method, or TIMA). Although this technology is not available to most clinicians, this work clearly illustrates a physiologic flaw in traditional single-muscle-group testing through manual or electromechanical measures. Muscle performance testing apparatuses often attempt to measure output in a linear single-plane fashion. The reality of the workplace, however, is that job tasks are influenced by a plethora of variables and are rarely linear single-plane motions. Sapega[38] cautions that "in the orthopedic literature pertaining to testing of muscular performance, improper terminology often is used, testing methods that are inaccurate or misleading are described, and unproved assumptions are made regarding the functional importance of the parameters of various quantitative tests." Clinicians can gain insight into how to design a client assessment and rehabilitation methodology by examining the causative factors linked to shoulder pain. For instance, rates of muscle fatigue may allow the therapist to design a strengthening program that addresses the weak links of a synergist movement. EMG results have demonstrated the following arm position–fatigue relationships[21]:

- The anterior deltoid and trapezius fatigue increases as abduction increases.
- The supraspinatus fatigues significantly less at 45 degrees of abduction than at 0 or 90 degrees of abduction.
- The infraspinatus fatigues faster than other shoulder girdle muscles.

These data strongly reinforce the notion that ergonomic intervention is required to optimize upper extremity positioning at work in order to reduce injurious affects of muscle fatigue. Yet a work therapy program that focuses on selective strengthening along specific points of a motion arch may be unrealistic and thus inadequate in addressing the needs of the injured worker. Researchers acknowledge that sufficient epidemiologic evidence has not been produced to precisely identify risk factors, and practitioners of EMG recognize the potential for individuals demonstrating different muscle activity patterns. This lack of consensus serves to confound attempts at safely matching an injured worker to his or her job and further justifies a customized approach versus traditional treatment protocols.

A customized treatment program needs to consider the following questions:

1. What are the patient's symptoms, and how do specific postures and muscle loads influence these symptoms?
2. What are the specific functional tasks/subtasks that this patient must perform in the workplace?
3. Does a treatment program that avoids symptomatic postures and loads reflect the actual physical job demands?
4. Should the job(s) be redesigned to accommodate the patient?
5. Should specific restrictions be placed on the individual upon a return to work?

The purpose of this discourse has been twofold: (1) to caution the clinician against oversimplification in client assessment, and (2) to encourage clinicians to pursue ergonomic study of the work site and to conduct research to validate functional capacity assessment. Singleton[41] summarizes the first point well in stating, "force-velocity relationships are difficult to apply to living organisms whose muscles do not operate in isolation but rather in a system involving complex geometrical arrangements among skeletal attachments." Chaffin's[9] definition of *occupational biomechanics* describes the second process well: "the study of the physical interaction of workers with their tools, machines and materials, so as to enhance the worker's performance while minimizing the risk of future musculoskeletal disorders."

This section has not outlined a specific functional capacity evaluation because of the absence in the literature of validity studies and the belief that the functionally based evaluation must be individualized. Lechner et al.,[28] in a comparative analysis of commercially available functional capacity evaluations (FCEs), reached the following conclusions:

- "To date, none of the existing FCEs has a systematic objective method for quantifying causative data."
- "At this point, most FCEs do not have an objective method or formula for predicting who will benefit from the expense of such a program."
- "Neither static nor dynamic torque productions of muscles have been shown to be good predictors of functional capacity."
- "No intrarater reliability data for the FCEs we reviewed have been published in a peer-reviewed journal."
- "Many of the existing FCEs have the potential to offer distinct advantages over the informal assessments that they replaced."

The authors point out that in the absence of validity and reliability testing, even a well-designed FCE may offer little improvement over preexisting informal testing. However, the clinician who uses a functional job analysis as the "blueprint for rehabilitation" may be the beneficiary of greater content validity than the traditional therapist who relies on strength, range-of-motion, and pain measures to ascertain disability levels.

# Return to Work (RTW)

## THE WORKERS' COMPENSATION SYSTEM: DISINCENTIVES TO A RETURN TO WORK

Despite the best clinical and ergonomic efforts, many injured workers fail to return to gainful employment for a number of reasons. The workers' compensation system can present a variety of confounding obstacles that must first be understood if they are to be overcome. Given the same diagnosis, injury severity, and clinical treatment approach when compared with a non-workers' compensation case, a workers' compensation injury may not achieve expected outcomes.

Workers' compensation is a disability system best described as a *payer-based system* that focuses on treatment after the injury has occurred. Despite being treatment-driven, the workers' compensation system does not always ensure prompt, aggressive intervention.

Over 44 states include some reference to vocational rehabilitation within their workers' compensation laws, yet delayed rehabilitation remains one of the most powerful disincentives to expected clinical outcomes. In many cases, by the time a referral reaches the work therapist, the condition is advanced, and residual problems are present. Residual problems such as decreased strength, endurance, and functional capacities may have more to do with delayed rehabilitation than with the original trauma itself. Many authors have reported an inverse relationship between time spent on disability and likelihood of a successful return to work.[1,12,16,22,43]

Wadell[43] reports that following 6 months of unemployment, only 50 percent of injured workers will return to work, while after 2 years, the chances are negligible. A second common problem when dealing with workers' compensation is best described by Galvin[15]: "at the outset it is important to recognize that to delay rehabilitation is to jeopardize rehabilitation." In the disability system of workers' compensation, there are many, varied reasons for delayed rehabilitation. Eaton[12] describes a number of obstacles to rehabilitation stemming from workers' compensation systems:

- Development of an inactive lifestyle
- Dependence on monetary benefits
- Misconceptions about one's rights/benefits
- Negative self-esteem
- Threats to a person's vocational identity
- Adoption of the "sick role" for secondary gain
- Indifference of claims adjustors

One means of reducing disability severity is through early intervention and continued employment of the injured worker when feasible. Unfortunately, referral sources such as insurers, employers, physicians, and rehabilitation specialists frequently perceive work therapy programs as a last resort. Work-hardening centers subsequently receive referrals of clients who are well into the chronic stage of injury after other measures have been exhausted.

Experienced practitioners of work therapy appreciate that successful outcomes are to a large degree determined by the presence of incentives and disincentives to rehabilitation. For instance, a shoulder injury in an athlete may result in a dramatically different outcome for reasons other than diagnosis or clinical skill. Table 10-5 compares the injured athlete and the injured worker and generally describes the disincentives common to the occupationally injured worker.[10]

## RETURN-TO-WORK CONSIDERATIONS

Return-to-work (RTW) considerations can be thought of as a triad incorporating work therapy, job analysis, and work-site modifications (Fig.

**Table 10-5**

**A Comparison of an Injured Worker with an Injured Athlete**

| Injured Athlete | Injured Worker |
|---|---|
| Preconditioned for job (e.g., preseason camp) | Not conditioned for job |
| Had to make team (i.e., functional ability)? | Few have functional pre-employment (preplacement tests) |
| "Impairment" emphasis | Often possess a "disability" |
| Younger | Older |
| Cause of injury not questioned | "Causality" a key debate under workers' compensation |
| "Medical necessity" not questioned | "Medical necessity" often questioned |
| Money not an issue | Money often an issue (i.e., secondary gain) |
| May seek accelerated recovery | May seek delayed recovery |
| Trust of system, coach, trainer, medical team | Distrust of system, insurance company, employer, medical team |
| No attorney involvement | Attorney involvement |
| Few comorbidity problems | Comorbidity common (degenerative joint, diabetes, cardiac problems) |

10-6). Functional job analysis is the key to determining a proper fit between an injured worker and his or her job. Job analysis provides the necessary factual basis to enable an expedient but safe return to work. All too often, disability managers make the critical error of arbitrarily developing an RTW standard without performing an analysis of the job's critical task demands. Additionally, the medical community often fails to incorporate "functionally based" tests of the worker. Furthermore, a worker's medical standard in one job title or jurisdiction cannot be blindly applied to the same job classification in a different position. Often, the job must accommodate the needs of the injured worker. The basic elements of an ergonomics program are listed in Table 10-6.

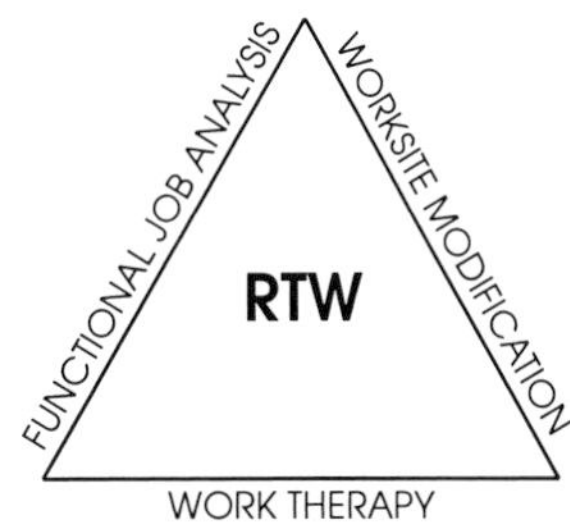


**Figure 10-6.** Return-to-work triad. (Adapted from Isernhagen Work Systems, Duluth, Minn.)

## JOB ACCOMMODATION

Job accommodation comes in many forms: work restriction, job restructuring, job or work-site modification, or support services. The clinician should routinely ask the following questions before returning an injured worker to a job requiring some form of accommodation:

1. Are accommodations actually required for the safe and efficient performance of the job? Or are they based on unproven assumptions?
2. Are accommodations physically possible for the required position?
3. Are accommodations financially feasible?
4. Are accommodations practical, cost-effective, and reasonable?
5. What medical, functional, and safety implicators are present in the proposed accommodations?
6. Has an occupational health professional reviewed and approved the accommodations?
7. Has management and supervisory staff been consulted with regard to the proposed accommodation?
8. Can additional suggestions, information, or other assistance be provided by a rehabilitation specialist?
9. Has a written record been established for each accommodation? And is it on file in the medical, engineering, personnel, and safety departments?
10. Are there employment concerns that preclude a specific accommodation (i.e., seniority, collective bargaining, incentive pay)?

Accommodations are accomplished via a number of methods.

### Work Restrictions

The employer may limit the worker from performing certain physical tasks or shield the worker from a host of environmental conditions. Lift restrictions and obstacle free lifting are examples of accommodation. Time restriction from performing stressful tasks may include job rotation and/or enlargement.

### Job Restructuring

Job restructuring involves the elimination of unsafe duties from the worker's essential tasks. A job analysis should preceed job restructuring and may include

- Use of questionnaires regarding job stresses

**Table 10-6**

**Basic Elements of an Ergonomics Program**

| |
|---|
| Management commitment |
| Written plan |
| Employee involvement |
| Complaint/suggestion mechanics |
| Prompt injury or symptom reporting |
| Safety and health committee |
| Ergonomic task force |
| Regular program review and follow-up |
| Analysis of injury trends |
| Use of employee surveys |
| Development of benefit-cost reports |
| Development of incentive programs for healthy behaviors |
| Work-site analysis |
| OSHA 200 log review |
| Ergonomic checklist/walk-through |
| Light-duty/modified-duty job identification |
| Annual work-site tour |
| Engineering controls |
| Workstation design |
| Work methods design |
| Tool design |
| Administrative controls |
| Work-practice modifications |
| New employee conditioning |
| Job enlargement |
| Job rotation |
| Job sharing |
| Frequent rest periods |
| Relief personnel |
| Facility/equipment maintenance |
| Written preventive maintenance plan |
| Regular performance tests |
| Specific performance mechanics |
| Effective housekeeping |
| Medical management |
| Injury/illness record keeping |
| Employee symptoms surveys |
| Systematic employee evaluation |
| Postoffer evaluation |
| Modified duty identification |
| Early work therapy |
| Functional job analysis |
| Training programs |
| All affected employees |
| All new hires or returning-to-work employees |
| Plant engineers |
| First-line supervisors |
| Health personnel |
| Management |

- Observation of different workers on the same task
- Employee interviews
- Task inventories/ergonomic checklists
- Time/motion studies
- Technical studies

Keeping all lift tasks below the NIOSH action limit (AL) is an example of job restructuring.

**Job or Work-Site Modification**

This accommodation method involves changing the methods and means of task accomplishment. Job-site modifications are often perceived as being overly expensive when in reality they are inexpensive. According to the National Rehabilitation Institute of America[31] (Chicago), the average work-site redesign costs less than $500, while the average tool redesign is less than $45. Examples of modifications include raising table heights, lift-assist devices, relocation of equipment controls, etc. (Fig. 10-7).

**Support Services**

A fourth form of accommodation is the provision of support services to the injured employee. An additional person(s) may be necessary in order for the worker to perform the actual task for the injured worker. An example would be the forklift operator who remains available to raise the height of a pallet stack while the worker depallitizes the load.

The clinician, following a disability assessment, should summarize in precise terms the client's functional limitations and work restrictions. Developing an "Employee Notice of Work Restriction" signoff form serves to foster greater adherence by the injured worker and management.

# Summary

In summary, the integration of ergonomics and biomechanical analysis into RTW decision making serves to match a worker's functional capacities to job demands/performance requirements. No two workers are alike, nor are their jobs; therefore, each program must consider congenital/structural makeup, posttraumatic effects on structure, and postural/biomechanical/ergonomic effects on structure. Work therapists demand a greater knowledge of ergonomics if successful clinical outcomes are to be achieved.

This chapter has proposed the integration of client assessment data with work-site analysis data in an effort to safely address the occupational shoulder injury. The work therapist is encouraged to combine nontraditional assessment methodologies with information gathered through

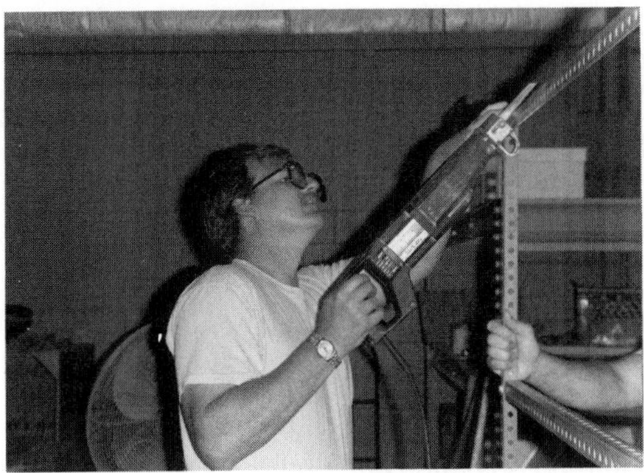

**Figure 10-7.** Although shoulder position is appropriate, the use of a ladder to modify the work site would reduce cervical strain.

job analysis. A conceptual model has been proposed that recognizes the importance of the physical demand characteristics of work.

## Case Studies

### Case 1

Joseph is a 27-year-old steel company laborer who complains of symptoms consistent with cumulative trauma disorder predominated by neural symptoms. He was only employed for a period of 30 days when he began to complain of multiple symptoms. He had worked previously as a car salesman, spending a great deal of time at a desk. Chief complaints included

- Numbness in both arms
- Losing strength in arms/hands
- Shoulder pain bilaterally
- Tingling in both arms/hands
- Occasional neck pain
- Numbness in right hand in digits 2 to 5

Significant clinical findings included

- Mottled skin on both hands
- Decreased sensation to light touch throughout hands
- Positive Tinel's sign at elbow and wrist bilaterally
- Good grip strength bilaterally
- No focal weakness in either upper extremity
- No focal neurologic deficits
- Forward head combined with kyphosis
- Obesity

Diagnostic tests were negative for carpal tunnel syndrome (sensory nerve conduction velocities), cervical spine osseous problems (x-ray), and rotator cuff tears (MRI). His physician diagnosed multiple crush injury mechanically induced by repetitive motion and sustained postures.

Joseph had undergone a preplacement screening, which included

- Standard medical tests, that is, spirometry, drug screening, vision tests, audiometric tests, chest x-ray, medical history, and vital signs
- Grip/pinch testing with a Jamar dynamometer
- Trunk muscle performance testing with an isokinetic protocol (not validated by clinical research in refereed journals)
- Clinical observations regarding materials handling, work style, biomechanics, posture assessments
- Hand dexterity/coordination testing, that is, Minnesota Rate of Manipulation Test

At the time of employment, the worker was judged to be comparably matched with the physical job demands as a steel fabricator. He was cleared by the examining physician for full unrestricted duty and scored within the 70 to 90 percentiie range on all tests. However, functional job analysis was not used as the blueprint for preplacement testing; therefore, fitness for duty was an extrapolation from the previously described test measures.

The worker originally suspected carpal tunnel syndrome and blamed his symptoms on one specific job task, eccentrically loading/unloading steel plates with the use of 24-in tongs. However, subsequent complaints involved the neck, shoulder, and arms. A time motion study determined that during his 30 days of employment, the time spent on the tong-related task totaled 1 hour.

A comprehensive ergonomic analysis was conducted of the multiple job tasks performed by the employee. There was a total of 19 subtasks involved in his steel fabrication department. Each subtask represented a complex of ergonomic stressors.

The ergonomic analysis classified the job tasks in the moderate to heavy range for cervicobrachial disorders and shoulder injury risk but in the minimal risk category for carpal tunnel syndrome. Also, the worker did not fit the profile for carpal tunnel risk (diabetes, history of previous injury, female). Repetitive forward reaching with the objects suspended a significant distance from the body (more than 16 in) was the primary ergonomic stressor and could account for the multiple crush-type symptoms. This worker also had to sustain postures that placed the arms above 90 degrees with a distal weight exceeding 10 lb.

This case underscores several important issues:

1. Individuals who may functionally qualify for a job position(s) are not insulated from injury if placed into poorly designed jobs.
2. Job positions perceived to be the cause of an injury may prove to be relatively free from risk factors.
3. Ergonomically induced injuries rarely settle into one joint but affect multiple points along the kinetic chain.
4. Medical providers must avoid looking at an injured worker from the context of one joint or diagnosis and must look beyond the human factors.
5. Preplacement evaluations should use the functional job analysis as a blueprint for testing to ensure content validity.

Joseph's work therapy program was designed as a "systems approach" to injury management. The systems approach used in this case involved the following:

*Biomechanical Problems*

- Repetitive forward reaching
- Sustained overhead lifting/holding
- Repetitive bending
- Repetitive carrying

*Cardiovascular Problems*

- Working around a hot furnace all day led to early fatigue.
- Rapid pacing of tasks led to early fatigue.
- Compensation on a "piece work" or incentive basis led to early fatigue in addition to poor work habits.
- Worker was a cigarette smoker.
- Worker was obese.

*Psychophysiologic Problems*

- Fear of specific job tasks and their alleged causation of symptoms
- Tendency to work despite pain rather than with it
- Difficulty with pacing skills
- Difficulty with quality of work leading to the need to repeat tasks

*Musculoskeletal Problems*

- Pain in bilateral wrists, hands, elbows, shoulders, and cervicothoracic spine
- Loss of sensation in multiple dermatomal patterns, which is especially critical because of glove use during the handing of hot steel
- Early localized muscle fatigue

This particular symptom complex is extremely common among moderate to heavy manufacturing industries.

### THERAPY PROGRAM

Joseph's plan of care involved a short course of pain-abatement procedures/modalities, which included thermal, mechanical, and physical agents. The bulk of his care involved job simulation to recondition his musculoskeletal system via functional tasks versus traditional uniplanar strengthening. "Industrial PNF" serves to describe the approach of combining tasks in functional combinations, including

- Rotary and linear tasks
- Static and dynamic motions
- Concentric and eccentric activities
- Continuous and interrupted movement patterns

Ergonomically stressful postures were avoided during work therapy (i.e., sustained overhead reaching). Specific ergonomic recommendations were given to the employer.

## Case 2

This injured worker was a 47-year-old baggage handler for a major airline diagnosed with a left rotator cuff strain with upper extremity crush injury. The mechanism of injury involved a pronated left forearm with internal rotation of the shoulder as his arm was pulled by a roller on a belt loader.

His chief complaint was of left shoulder pain and restricted motion, for which he was taking aspirin and ibuprofen. Shoulder ROM was as follows: abd 0–90 degrees, ER 0–90 degrees, IR 0–30 degrees, ext 0–60 degrees, and flx 0–130 degrees. Clinical findings included

- Positive left rotator cuff impingement
- Negative Tinel's sign at wrist, elbow, and shoulder
- Negative Adson's manuever and Elvey's test
- Good pulses
- Decreased left grip strength
- Crepitus, left elbow
- Paresthesis of the median nerve distribution below left elbow
- Left hand coldness
- Positive Yergason's left

Secondary problems included right C3–C4 herniated nucleus pulposus and central L3–L4 HNP. EMG tests were positive for multiroot damage in confirmation of suspected crush injury.

This case illustrates the complexity of many

industrial injuries wherein there are multiple diagnoses and comorbidities.

### THERAPY PROGRAM

An assortment of palliative modalities was designed to reduce pain while shoulder joint mobilization addressed both pain and restoration of accessory motions. A graded therapeutic exercise program was initiated to enhance overall joint motion and strength while avoiding excessive compression forces in the shoulder or muscle strain to the rotator cuff muscle. Pendulums, overhead pullies (AAROM, AROM), wand exercises for rotation improvement, and a full upper extremity reconditioning program were instituted.

When ROM and strength was restored to normal, a work therapy program was begun to provide instruction in various principles of motion economy. The following principles were reviewed and practiced using the functional job analysis as a guidepost:

- Begin and complete tasks with both hands.
- Motion of the arms should occur in symmetrical patterns.
- Sequence of motion should have the least amount of breaks or disruptions, that is, smooth, uninterrupted materials handling.
- Transfer tasks to larger muscle groups (i.e., when lifting a heavy piece of luggage, utilize the upper back and scapular muscles, not just the posterior deltoid and rotator cuff).
- Use controlled ballistic motions. Baggage handlers are notorious for using abrupt ballistic movements with the upper extremities in nonphysiologic positions.
- Arrange movements to avoid resistance to gravity (i.e., allow a bag to reach the end of a conveyor belt eccentrically lower versus hoisting up and then lowering to ground).
- Adjust work heights to accommodate many anthropometric types.

This client's reconditioning program emphasized the preceding motion economy principles through job task simulations. These tasks used comparable weights, object dimensions, spatial considerations, pacing elements, and other "real life" circumstances. Because this worker did not have true focal muscle weakness, a work-conditioning program substituted for a traditional weight program (i.e., isokinetics). Unlike, conventional strengthening programs, joints were not stabilized to facilitate isolated movement. In industry, it is rare to have a task that calls for the recruitment of just one muscle group, and stabilization is not feasible.

Instead, actual materials and equipment were used in a mock-up of the baggage handler's job. These included

- Materials handling with emphasis on lift heights commensurate with the industry-standard baggage cart
- Carrying suitcases, boxes, bags, etc.
- Complete simulation of the underbelly of an airplane with the client in an all-fours position
- Pushing and pulling of hand trucks and carts

There are some rare instances when ergonomic redesign is not feasible; this represents one such case, wherein the underbelly of a jet cannot be altered to accommodate the worker. In instances such as this, the work therapy program should emphasize more of the human factors, such as adherence to the aforementioned motion economy principles. And in some cases, transfer to a different job or vocation altogether is necessary. We can not engineer the perfect ergonomic environment, nor can we engineer out one's genetic background. Therefore, it is critical that each and every work injury patient receive a customized program. For this reason, we have chosen not to provide a recipe or protocol of care that could be applied to all steel manufacturers or baggage handlers.

## Case 3

This case study did not involve a patient but rather an intervention strategy addressing the problems of an incumbent worker. Its inclusion here is to encourage work therapists to offer their expertise before a person becomes a patient. The ergonomic principles outlined in this chapter can be applied at any point along the injury spectrum, from preemployment to a return-to work decision involving the injured worker (Table 10-7).

With the United States shifting away from a manufacturing power to a service-based economy, an increasing number of employees are reporting symptoms consistent with posturally and repetition-induced disorders. Many clients of work therapy centers can be classified as performing light to moderate tasks that are not necessarily associated with a one-time trauma or episode. Instead, these persons perform repetitive tasks often in a sedentary posture, creating a series of microtraumas that ultimately lead to symptomology and, in many cases, disability. This group is largely ignored by those who equate work therapy with materials handling only.

A joint ergonomic-medical (physical therapy) assessment of computer workstations was con-

**Table 10-7**

**Injury Intervention spectrum**

| Preloss | Injury Occurs | RTW |
|---|---|---|
| Preplacement or posthire evaluation | Entry WCE | WCE |
| Ergonomic design | Work therapy<br>Ergonomics<br>Rehabilitation | Ergonomics |
| Employee cumulative trauma education | | |
| Heightened management awareness | Cumulative trauma education | Disability evaluation |
| | Heightened management awareness | Modified duty |

ducted on behalf of a workers' compensation insurance company. The rehabilitation nurse and claims manager recognized the need to address the complaints of claims adjustors. In one unit alone, five claims adjustors had reported symptoms consistent with any number of cumulative trauma disorders. The Ergo-Med evaluation consisted of three components:

1. Physical therapy evaluations to determine the functional capacity of five employees. A symptom survey also was performed.
2. Ergonomics evaluations of the five computer workstations to analyze the ergonomic risk factors associated with the employee job activities.
3. A customized joint physical therapy–ergonomics awareness training session with the employees to review the recommendations and to provide education/training regarding postures, exercises, and proper ergonomic adjustments to minimize musculoskeletal strain and visual fatigue.

This program satisfied the requirements for disability management described by Jarvikoski and Lehelma[26]:

- It is directed toward the chronic or permanent functional limitation or disability.
- It is directed toward the individual with symptoms threatening chronic functional limitations or disability.
- It is intended to restore working or functional capacity.
- It is intended to prevent deterioration.
- It includes measures that maximize an individual's own resources.
- It serves to remove obstacles that were imposed by one's environment.

# References

1. Akabas SH, Gottleib A, Yasser R. Preventive rehabilitation: untapped horizon for vocational rehabilitation agencies. Am Rehabil 1979;5(2):20.
2. AMA guide to the evaluation of permanent impairment. Chicago: AMA, 1984.
3. American national standard for human factors engineering of visual display terminal workstations. ANSI/HFS 100-1988. Santa Monica, Calif.: Human Factors Society, Inc., 1988.
4. ANSI Z-365 Project. Secretariat, National Safety Council. 444 N. Michigan Ave., Chicago, Ill., 60611.
5. Armstrong TJ, Foulke J, Joseph B, Goldstein S. An investigation of cumulative trauma disorders in a poultry processing plant. Am Ind Hyg. Assoc J 1982;43:103.
6. Armstrong TJ. Ergonomics and cumulative trauma disorders. Hand Clin 1986;2(3):553.
7. Berger AC, Kleinert JM. Work-related vascular injuries and diseases. In: Occupational hand and upper extremity injuries and diseases. Philadelphia: Hanley and Belfus, 1991.
8. Berryhill BH. Returning the worker with an upper extremity injury to industry: a model for the physician and therapist. J Hand Ther 1990;3(2):56.
9. Chaffin DB, Andersson G. Occupational biomechanics. New York: John Wiley and Sons, 1984.
10. Clifton D. Critical issues for determining successful work hardening outcomes. Phys Ther Pract 1992;1(3):53.
11. Dictionary of occupational titles. 4th Ed. Washington: U.S. Department of Labor, Employment and Training Administration, 1977.
12. Eaton MW. Obstacles to the vocational rehabilitation of individuals receiving workers' compensation, J Rehabil 1979;4592:59.
13. Finkel ML. The effects of repeated mechanical trauma in the meat packing industry. Am J Ind Med 1985;8:375.
14. Futatsuka M, Sakurai T, Matsumoto, Comparative study of vibration disease among operators of vibrating tools by factor analysis. Br J Ind Med 1985;42:260.
15. Galvin DE. Employer-based disability management and rehabilitation initiative: a rehabilitation research review. Washington: NARC National Institute of Handicapped Research, U.S. Department of Education, 1986.
16. Gates LB, Yecheskel T, Akabas SH. Optimizing return to work among newly disabled workers: a new approach toward cost containment. Benefits Q 1989;5(2):19.
17. Gomer FE, Silverstein LD, Berg WK, Lassiter DL. Changes in electromyographic activity associated with occupational stress and poor performance in the workplace. Hum Factors 1987; 29(2):131.
18. Hagberg M, Wegman. Prevalence rates and odds ratios of shoulder-neck diseases in different occupational groups. Br J Ind Med 1987;448:602.
19. Hales T, et al. NIOSH HETA Report No. 88-180-1958. John Morrell and Co., 1989.
20. Heberts P, Kadefors R, Anderson G, Petersen I. Shoulder pain in industry: an epidemiological study on welders. Acta Orthop Scand 1981;52:299.
21. Herberts P, Kadefors R, Broman H. Arm positioning in manual tasks: an electromyographic study of localized muscle fatigue. Ergonomics 1980;23(7):655.
22. Hester EJ, Decelles PG. The worker who becomes disabled: a handbook of incidence and outcomes. Topeka, Kas.: The Menninger Foundation, 1985.
23. Imran SN. Predictive models of upper extremity rotary and linear pull strength. Hum Factors 1988;30(1):83.
24. Isernhagen SJ. Work injury prevention and management. Rockville, Md.: Aspen Publications, 1988.
25. Jaeger SH, Singer DI, Whiteneck SH. Nerve injury complications: management of neurogenic pain syndromes. Hand Clin 1986; 2(1):217.
26. Jarvikoski A, Lehelma E. Early rehabilitation and its implementation at the workplace. Int J Rehabil Res 1981;4:519.
27. Khalil TM. An electromyographic methodology for the evaluation of industrial design. Hum factors 1973;15(3):257.

28. Lechner D, Roth D, Straaton K. Functional capacity evaluation in work disability. Work 1991;1(3):37.
29. Luck JV, Andersson G. Occupational shoulder disorders. In: Rockwood C, Matsen F, eds. The shoulder. Vol. 2. Philadelphia: WB Saunders, 1990.
30. Luopajarvi T, Kvorinka I, Virolainen M, Holmberg M. Prevalence of tenosynovitis and other injuries of the upper extremities in repetitive work. Scand J Work Environ Health 1979;5(suppl 3):48.
31. National Rehabilitation Institute. Chicago, Illinois.
32. Neer CS. Impingement lesions. Clin Orthop 1983;173:70.
33. NIOSH criteria for a recommended standard: occupational exposure to hand-arm vibration. Cincinnati: U.S. Department of Health and Human Services, Centers for Disease Control, National Institute for Occupational Safety and Health, Division of Standards Development and Technology Transfer, pub. no. 89–106, 1989.
34. NIOSH work practices guide for manual lifting. Cincinnati: U.S. Department of Health and Human Services, Centers for Disease Control, National Institute for Occupational Safety and Health, Division of Biomedical and Behavioral Science, 1981.
35. OSHA ergonomic program management guidelines for meatpacking plants. OSHA 3123. Washington: USDOL/OSHA, 1990.
36. Pelmear PL, Leong D, Taylor W, et al. Measurement of vibration of hand-held tools: weighted or unweighted? J Occup Med 1989; 31:902.
37. Rodgers SH. Ergonomic design for people at work. New York: Van Rostrand Reinhold, 1986.
38. Sapega A. Muscle performance evaluation in orthopaedic practice. J Bone Joint Surg 1990;72A(10):1562.
39. Sigholm G, Herberts P, Armstrong C, Kadefors R. Electromyographic analysis of shoulder muscle load J Orthop Res 1984; 1(4):379.
40. Silverstein BA. The prevalence of upper extremity cumulative trauma disorders in industry. Ann Arbor: University of Michigan, Occupational Health and Safety Engineering Department, 1985.
41. Singleton WT. The body at work. Cambridge: Cambridge University Press, 1982.
42. Van Wely P. Design and disease. Appl Ergon 1969;1:262.
43. Waddell G. A new clinical model for the treatment of low back pain. Spine 1987;7:732.
44. Wiker SF, Langolf GD, Chaffin DB. Arm posture and human movement capability. Hum Factors 1989;31(4):421.


# Bibliography


Armstrong TJ, Radwin RG, Hansen DJ. Repetitive trauma disorders: job evaluation and design. Hum Factors 1986;28(3):325.

Astrand I, Guharay A, Wahren J. Circulatory response to arm exercise with different arm positions. J Appl Physiol 1968;25:528.

Chaffin DB. Localized muscle fatigue: definition and measurement. J Occup Med 1973;15:346.

Davis PR, Stubbs DA. A method of establishing safe handling forces in working situations. In: Safety in materials handling. Washington: U.S. Department of Health, Education and Welfare, 1978:34.

Eastman Kodak Company. Ergonomic design for people at work. Vol. 1. Belmont, Calif.: Lifelong Learning Publications, 1983.

Eastman Kodak Company. Ergonomic design for people at work. Vol. 2. New York: Van Nostrand Reinhold, 1986.

Hunting W, Grandjean E, Maeda K. Constrained postures in accounting machine operators. Appl Ergon 1980;11:145.

Jensen RC, Klein BP, Sanderson LM. Motion-related wrist Disorders traced to industries, occupational groups. Monthly Labor Review 1983;Sept:13.

Johnson SL. Ergonomic design of handheld tools to prevent trauma to the hand and upper extremity. St Louis: Mosby–Year Book, 1991:527.

Konz S. Design of workstations. J Ind Eng 1967;18:413.

Konz S. Work design. Columbus, Ohio: Grid Publications, 1979.

Onishi N, Sakai K, Kogi K. Arm and shoulder muscle load in various keyboard operating jobs of women. J Hum Ergol 1982;11:89.

Putz-Anderson V. Cumulative trauma disorders: a manual for musculoskeletal diseases of the upper limbs. NIOSH. New York: Taylor and Francis, 1988.

Rasch PJ. Relationship of arm strength, weight, and length to speed of arm movement. Res Q 1954;25:328.

Reynolds DD, Angevine EN. Hand-arm vibration: II. Vibration transmission characteristics of the hand and arm. J Sound Vibr 1977;51:237.

Sato H. Functional characteristics of human skeletal muscle revealed by spectral analysis of the surface electrogram. J Electromyogr Clin Neurophysiol 1982;22:459.

Schwartz RK. The medical return-to-work prescription: are the ignorant leading the blind? Work 1991;1(3):84.

Snook SH. The design of manual handling tasks. Ergonomics 1978A; 21:963.

Steinbrocker O, Argyrose TG. The shoulder-hand syndrome: present status as a diagnostic and therapeutic entity. Med Clin North Am 1958;42:1533.

Williams K. Functional capacity evaluation of the upper extremity. Work 1991;1(30):48.

# Chapter 11

*Martin J. Kelley*

# Case Studies



This chapter will demonstrate how the literature, concepts, and techniques presented in the preceding chapters are clinically applied to patients previously treated by the author. Four case studies, two nonoperative and two postoperative, have been chosen. The primary pathologies presented are rotator cuff tendonopathy and glenohumeral instability, yet the challenge of capsuloligamentous tightness is also revealed. Explanation for and rationale of evaluation findings and treatment approaches are discussed. Prior to the case studies, valued rehabilitation philosophies of the author will be reviewed.

## Rehabilitation Philosophies

Regardless of whether the patient is an athlete, laborer, or sedentary, regardless of age or if the patient is postinjury or postoperative, certain rehabilitation philosophies are closely followed. First, pain is always respected and rarely encouraged. The onset of pain following the introduction of a new exercise or a technique probably indicates the need for reevaluation of the recent intervention. Therefore, modalities, techniques, or exercises are introduced one or two at a time. In doing so, one can identify effective treatment interventions when the patient shows progress or problematic interventions when increased discomfort is reported. Second, performing a thorough evaluation to identify pathology, tissue reactivity, and functional deficits is critical to establishing an effective program. However, constantly reevaluating tissue reactivity is equally essential. Determining tissue reactivity qualifies the irritability of the involved structures and is based on both subjective and objective testing

Martin J. Kelley and William A. Clark: ORTHOPEDIC THERAPY OF THE SHOULDER.

(i.e., pain with resistance, impingement sign). The patient's reactivity therefore becomes the guide for program progression and efficacy of treatment. Intimate with assessing tissue reactivity is identifying if a patient reaches an *iatrogenic plateau*, which essentially means further recovery is hampered by the very same process that allowed some degree of recovery, the rehabilitation process. The plateau is characterized by stagnating mild tissue reactivity. By allowing the patient a short but full rest from exercise lasting 4 to 10 days, the tissue recovers, as does the patient's progress. Manual therapy, by resistive training or soft-tissue or joint mobilization, allows continuous reevaluation while treating. The real-time feedback gained by manual contact allows immediate modification of the therapist's techniques and exercise or the patient's movement patterns and is essential in discovering subtle and sometimes blatant problems that only arise with repetitive motion or those which manifest with fatigue.

Third, the progression of shoulder position or motion plane during exercise or with manual therapy is from the *nonprovocative* to *provocative*. Stress and safety zones are identified in Figure 11-1. The plane of the scapula lies within the safety zone. These nonprovocative and provocative positions vary based on pathology or surgery, but most commonly, the least provocative position is somewhere between 20 and 55 degrees of scapular plane abduction. Keeping the humerus below 55 degrees prevents subacromial impingement, and avoiding full adduction minimizes excessive tension across the

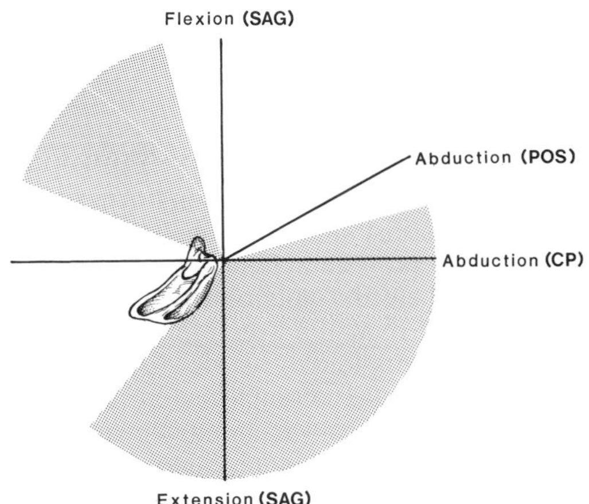


**Figure 11-1.** Stress zones (shaded areas) and safety zones (open areas).

**Table 11-1**

**Plane of the Scapula Rehabilitation Characteristics**

- Improved joint surface congruity
- Reduced rotational tension to the capsuloligamentous-labral complex and rotator cuff
- The supraspinatus and deltoid are optimally aligned for elevation
- Correlates with many functional activities

supraspinatus–coracohumeral ligament complex. The plane of the scapula is advantageous for use in manual therapy techniques and exercise performance for several reasons (Table 11-1). Utilization of the POS reduces tensile and torsional stresses to the rotator cuff and CLC and therefore is an inherently stable position for the glenohumeral joint if working with an individual with instability. Additionally, the natural optimal alignment for elevation of the supraspinatus and deltoid is utilized when strengthening in the scapular plane. Provocative positions are typically at end ranges, where the athlete or laborer must function, particularly 90 degrees of coronal plane abduction (or posterior) and full external rotation. This position not only stresses the CLC and twists the rotator cuff but also can cause supraspinatus impingement at the coracohumeral arch as well as against the posterior glenoid rim.[12]

Fourth, striving for balanced scapular muscle function is constantly emphasized in addition to integration of appropriate scapular muscle function into all dynamic exercises, from simple rotator cuff exercises to sport-specific manual resistance and isokinetics. We have found this principle to be most effective in returning the overhead athlete to competition, the laborer to work, and the sedentary individual to required activities.

Lastly, the patient's rehabilitation program is individualized based on reactivity, hyperelasticity/hypoelasticity, personality, goals, and surgical concerns/complications.

# Case 1

## 20-Year-Old College-Level Softball Catcher Right Hand Dominant

### HISTORY

Six months previous to the evaluation the patient began to notice pain in the right anterior shoulder during and following throwing. The patient complained of no previous history of pain or trauma in either shoulder. She saw an orthopedic surgeon 2 months previous to this evaluation. Plain x-rays were taken, but were negative and no injection was given. She was diagnosed as having multidirectional instability and impingement. She was told to rest, but after 3 weeks, she attempted to play, only to experience an increase in symptoms when throwing. She was referred to another physical therapy facility 3 weeks previous to this evaluation and reported minimal relief of symptoms. Therapy consisted of strengthening using elastic bands and free weights, followed by ice.

Her main complaints at the time of evaluation were pain with overhead activities and throwing, particularly during the late cocking phase. She complained of occasional "achiness" at rest. She could sleep on the right side but occasionally did wake. She was taking no medicine at the time. She did have a history of a T10 vertebral body compression fracture 3 years ago and was told flexion of the thoracic spine would be beneficial.

# EVALUATION

## OBSERVATION IN STANDING

No significant muscle contour changes noted.

### Posture Evaluation

Significant forward shoulders R > L, moderate forward head, and increased thoracic kyphosis.

## CERVICAL ROM

Within normal limits and painless.

## ACTIVE SHOULDER MOTION

Full and normal scapulohumeral rhythm. Pain during flexion started at 150 degrees and during abduction at 90 degrees. Pain increased toward end range over bicipital groove. Functional internal rotation to T3.

## RESISTED MOTIONS

Overall deltoid and rotator cuff strength was 4/5. Slight pain was present with abduction at 0, 45, and 90 degrees; slight pain with flexion at 0 and 45 degrees; moderate pain with external rotation at neutral and at external rotation end range; no pain with internal rotation. Elbow, wrist, and hand muscle strength was 5/5. Serratus anterior was graded as 5/5, but middle and lower trapezius were graded as 4−/5 on the right.

## SPECIAL TESTS

The following tests or signs were positive: Impingement sign (Neer) and multiangle impingement sign at 20 and 40 degrees from the sagittal plane. Resisted abduction/IR. (All these test produced anterolateral pain.) Speeds test produced bicipital tendon pain. Sulcus sign was positive for subluxation and was painful. Apprehension sign was painful but did not give rise to a sense of instability. Relocation test did relieve pain.

## STABILITY AND JOINT ASSESSMENT

| | Anterior/ER | | | | Posterior/IR | | | | Inferior | | | |
|---|---|---|---|---|---|---|---|---|---|---|---|---|
| | L | R | L | R | L | R | L | R | L | R | | |
| Load shift | I+ | I+ / | NA | | II | II / | | | I+ | I+ / | | |
| 45-degree position | II | II / | Tr | Tr+ | II | II / | Tr | Tr+ | I+ | I+ / | | |
| 90-degree coronal | II | II / | Tr | Tr+ | II | II / | Tr | Tr | I+ | I+ / | | |

Trace (Tr)—slight
I—1/2 distance
II—sublux
III—dislocate

Patient demonstrated both physiologic and pathologic laxity.

## PASSIVE SHOULDER MOTION

Patient demonstrated excessive external rotation of 120 degrees bilaterally. True 180 degrees of elevation was present. Slight pain was noted with passive end range of elevation and moderate pain at external rotation end range. Patient had hyperflexion at the wrist and excessive hyperextension of the elbows and knees.

## PALPATION

Trigger point was found in the infraspinatus muscle belly which reproduced anterior shoulder pain. Moderate tenderness and significant tenderness were found at the supraspinatus insertion and biceps tendon (groove and intraarticular), respectively.

## REFLEXES

Reactive and symmetrical

## SENSATION

Normal

# ASSESSMENT AND RATIONALE

Patient presented with classic multidirectional instability demonstrated by generalized hyperelastic tissue and nontraumatic onset of symptoms. Most likely the anteroinferior ligaments were elongated in March from repetitive throwing. Tendinitis symptoms arose due to attempted dynamic stabilization compensation. She did present with a positive impingement sign demonstrating painful compression of irritated tendinous/bursal tissue. The mechanism of impingement was probably abnormal humeral head excursion resulting in mechanical impingement, not because acromial hooking or spurring was present. Stability testing revealed a perceived increased translation in all directions with load shift and in 45 degrees and 90 degrees of joint glide assessment. When compared to the opposite side the transalotory motion appeared symmetrical, however, a painful click was experienced with anterior and inferior gliding. When external and internal rotations were combined with gliding, slight increased motion was noted on the right both anteriorly and posteriorly, respectively. Therefore, the symmetric increased translation demonstrates physiologic laxity while the increased unilateral translation found when combined with rotation demonstrates pathologic laxity. Possibly a SLAP lesion or irritated anterior labral attachments were the cause of this painful click. It was doubtful that a Bankart lesion existed, since there was no history of trauma. A positive relocation test is indicative of posterior glenoid rim impingement of the supraspinatus or possibly labral compression and/or CLC stretching. When positive, anterior subluxation may be suspected[5] although this test is not specific for instability since it can be positive in those with supraspinatus lesions.[9] Resisted motions were slightly uncomfortable in all directions except for external rotation, which was moderately painful, and internal rotation, which was painless. These findings, in conjunction with tenderness of the biceps and supraspinatus tendons, also demonstrated a low level of rotator cuff/biceps tendon irritation. It should be noted that in her previous rehabilitation she was allowed to externally rotate to the full range when performing resisted external rotation exercises with the arm adducted. We have found this to increase tendinous tension and mechanical irritation to the biceps and supraspinatus (based on extrapolation from Clark et al.[1] The patient also demonstrated weakness of the middle and lower trapezius. These muscles are essential for appropriate positioning of the glenoid to enhance osseous support and reduce stress on the static stabilizers during the cocking phase. Commonly the middle and lower trapezius are weak in the overhand athlete resulting in domination by the scapular elevators (upper trapezius, rhomboids, levator scapulae, and serratus anterior), the pectoralis minor (which causes anterior tilting), and the serratus anterior's strong abduction pull (causing over orientation of the glenoid toward the sagittal plane, increasing stress on the CLC). Trigger point of the infraspinatus was found, and diagnostic ischemic compression was performed. Following this, she had slightly less pain with active motion and upon resisted external rotation.

## TREATMENT AND RATIONALE

| Treatment | Rationale |
|---|---|
| **Session 1**<br>Patient was initially treated with phonophoresis using 10% hydrocortisone cream followed by ice massage in an alternating time sequence of 5, 2, 3, and 2 minutes. The arm was placed in approximately 20 degrees of hyperextension while slightly internally and externally rotating the humerus for better exposure of the involved tendons. A dermal patch was utilized for 5 days. The patient was taken off all strengthening exercises. Ischemic compression to the infraspinatus was performed. | Chronic inflammatory reaction present. Reduce inflammation by modalities, dermal patch, and terminating irritating exercise. The altering of ultrasound and ice is done for a contrast effect to aid in blood flow. |
| **Session 2**<br>Continued phonophoresis and ice, began scapular PNF, with emphasis on middle and lower trapezius. | Started strengthening scapular muscles due to weakness and requirement for throwing. These exercises should not provoke symptoms. |
| **Session 3**<br>Exam revealed full and painless elevation, and resisted motions were strong and painless except when an eccentric load was applied to the external rotators. Assessment revealed increased relative strength secondary to reduced pain upon resisted motion. Still slight tenderness of the infraspinatus belly but no referred pain was noted.<br><br>*Treatment*: Continued scapular PNF added quadruped and rhythmic stabilization to strengthen serratus anterior and | Infraspinatus trigger point deactivated. Inflammation significantly reduced, so began to progress strengthening to scapular muscles as well as cuff and deltoid. Emphasized trapezius and serratus because appropriate glenoid positioning reduces stress on the CLC. Began isolated strengthening to glenohumeral dynamic stabilizes and began resistance across elbow for direct strengthening, but also indirect strengthening and synergistic control of the scapular muscles. |

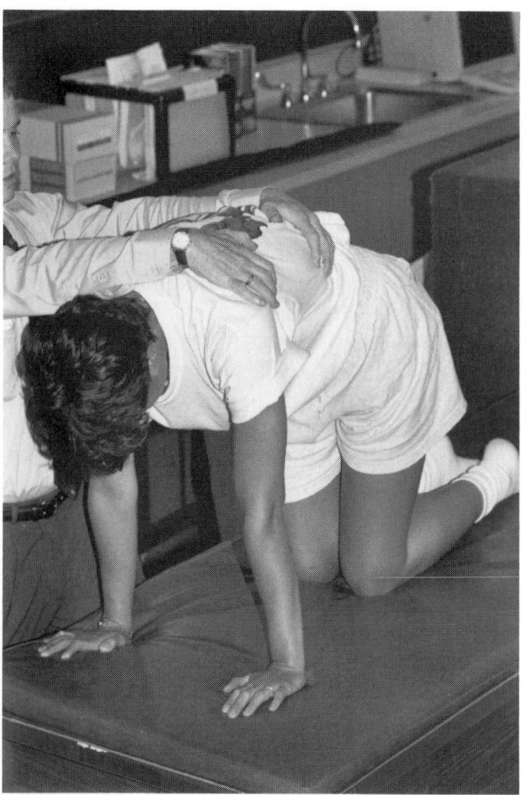

**Figure 11-2.** Quadruped positioning for strengthening the right serratus anterior by displacing trunk weight over the right upper extremity.

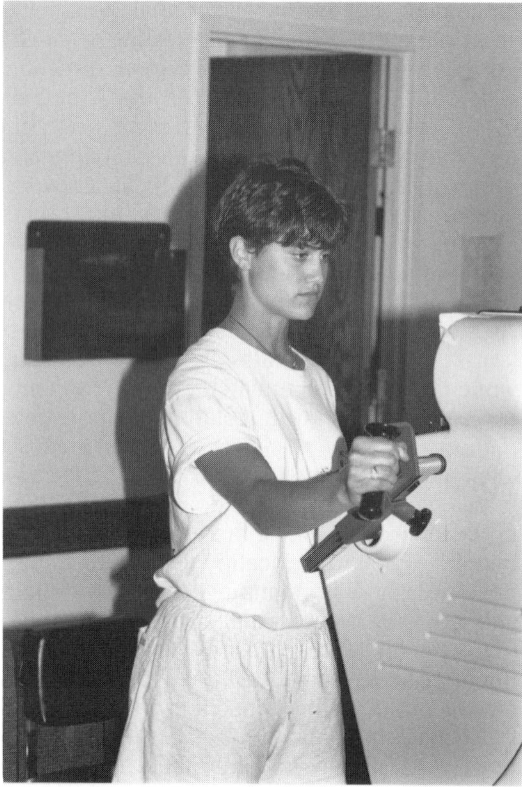

**Figure 11-3.** Standing while using the upper body ergometer to avoid the impingement arc.

glenohumeral muscles (Fig. 11-2). Added isolated manual resistance to the middle trapezius by pulling into scapular adduction. Began rhythmic stabilization manual resistance in 45 degree POS through 90 degrees with emphasis on scapular stabilization. Home program using elastic bands IR, ER to 30 degrees, extension, biceps and triceps. All these exercises were performed out of the impingement arcs, emphasizing scapular positioning.

**Sessions 4–6**

Began upper body ergometer for warmup (standing) (Fig. 11-3). Progressed to Bodyblade at side and elbow to 90 degrees. Began manual resistance for IR/ER at 45 degrees of abduction in the POS beginning submax → max. Quadruped to triped position. Upper extremity D1 and D2 to 90 degrees, submax → max. Began variable resistance exercises for biceps (preacher), front pull-downs from 90 degrees, and rows to the coronal plane. Continued with scapular muscle strengthening. D/C'd phonophoresis after session 3.

The rotator cuff could be directly challenged through the range in POS, progressing up to 90 degrees. Triped was in impingement arc but is a relatively static position regarding motion. All exercise improved dynamic stability in less provocative positions. The patient was constantly monitored regarding symptoms.

**Sessions 7–10**

Reevaluation revealed full and painless elevation, strong and painless resisted motions, and no pain with palpation. Continued to progress the above to maximal resistance and approached full range motion. Began wall ball. Progressed on UBE ending with a 6- to 10-minute session. Began isokinetic training at 90 degrees/s for IR/ER at 20-degrees in POS. Began submax and progressed to max output; also progressed speeds from 90 to 180 degrees/s.

Patient responded extremely well, so began further emphasis on endurance. Wall ball works the musculature at 90 degrees, emphasizing a "dynamic isometric" of the rotator cuff and deltoid while the elbow moves in space. Isokinetics were performed at 20 degrees to decrease tension on the supraspinatus tendon.

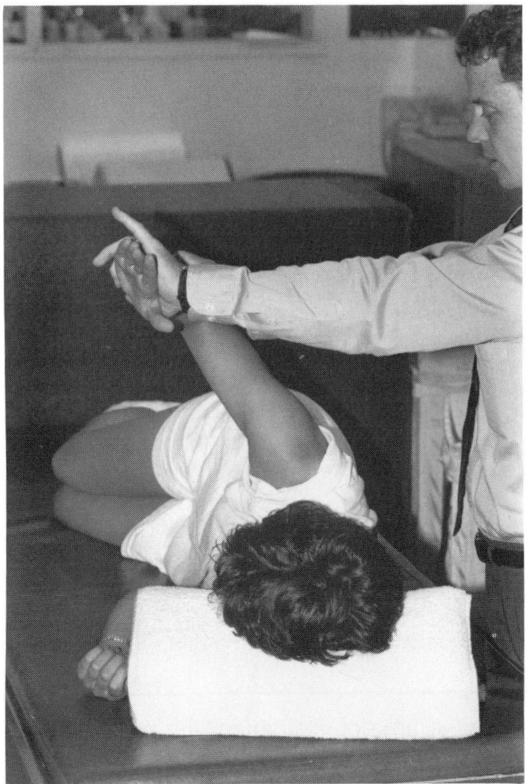

**Figure 11-4.** Manual resistance isometrics in 90 degrees of POS.

Side-lying; placed the arm in 90-degree POS; performed manual resistance simulating the throwing motion (Fig. 11-4). Started with multiangle isometrics at 20-degree intervals to the sagittal plane and back. Progressed to short arc concentric/eccentric and slow reversal holds. Submax → max and progressed to 90/90-degree position. Supine, began rhythmic stabilization at 120 degrees in POS and progressed to 160 degrees. Progressed positioning toward the coronal plane.

Dynamic stabilization in functional position moving from less provocative to more provocative.

**Sessions 11–13**

Progressed to throwing in kneeling with manual resistance and palpation for feedback particularly to the scapular muscles. Continued with home program with elastic bands; progressed to 90-degree POS → 90/90 simulating the throwing motion. Continue with aggressive strengthening and endurance activities. Progressed Bodyblade training to more provocative positions. Began plyometrics with chest pass (4 lb. ball) and progressed to patient catching at 90 degrees in the POS (2 lb. ball).

Still achieving strength and endurance requirements while working toward activity goal. Emphasis on middle and lower trapezius activity to achieve scapular muscle balance and prevent abnormal scapular elevation, anterior tilting, and abduction. Plyometric training performed to maximize functional stretch-shortening of the internal rotators.

**Session 14**

Throwing with tennis ball

| | **High Arc** | **3/4 Arc** |
|---|---|---|
| 20 ft | 10× | |
| 40ft | 10× | 10× |
| 60ft | 10× | 10× |

Evaluating throwing technique and response to activity goal when performed submaximally.

**Session 15**

Patient with increased symptoms did not tell me she had been throwing a soft ball the day before session 14. Returned to treatment at sessions 6 to 10.

Reduced irritative activities allowing tissues to recover. Progressed back to activity goal positions as long as she remained symptom-free.

**Sessions 16–21**

Symptoms reduced and progressed to intensive strengthening of shoulder musculature. Returned to resistance in the late cocking phase and elevated positions using manual resistance, elastic bands, and the Bodyblade. Continued with endurance training and home program.

**Sessions 22–30**

Returned to previous throwing program with tennis ball and progressed to a soft ball; experimented with sidearm throwing, which she tolerated well. Weaned off therapy and incorporated her coach into program. Progressed distance, reduced arc, and increased speed of throwing. Patient had less symptoms with sidearm throw at the expense of a quick release. Patient was followed up 3 months later during spring ball and was able to return to normal throwing technique, although she had to monitor number of throws to second base during practices. She was eventually able to return to her normal throwing technique yet still had to limit throws during practices to prevent symptom onset. She was painfree during and following competition throughout the next two seasons.

Return to activity goal. Initially required a change in throwing technique, which did reduce symptoms in throwing.

# Case 2

## 54-Year-Old Professor Right Hand Dominant

### HISTORY

Patient complained of left shoulder pain and decreased motion beginning approximately 4 months previously. He reported an incident in which he slipped and reached up to grab the railing, forcing his arm into elevation and internal rotation. The primary pain was achy in nature, located about the lateral deltoid. He reported occasional cervical and upper trapezius pain, but this did not radiate. Discomfort intensified with use of the arm, particularly during overhead activities. He reported significant night pain, particularly if sleeping on the left side. He had to give up racquetball 2 months ago. Aspirin provided temporary relief of symptoms. He was seen by an orthopedic surgeon 1 week previously; x-rays were negative, but he obtained 75 percent relief of overhead pain with an impingement test; a suspension of Lidocaine and Kenalog had been injected subacromially. The patient was told he had adhesive capsulitis and possibly a rotator cuff tear.

At the time of evaluation, the patient essentially had the same complaints as described above, but the pain intensity was 50 percent of the preinjection status. He also reported a noticeable improvement in motion since the injection.

## EVALUATION

### OBSERVATION IN STANDING

No significant muscle contour changes were noted.

**Posture**

Significant forward head, forward shoulder, and increased kyphosis.

### CERVICAL ROM

Full and painless; cervical provocative tests were negative.

### ACTIVE SHOULDER MOTION

Flexion was to 130 degrees; coronal plane abduction was 100 degrees; and POS abduction was to 125 degrees. Pain experienced at 80 degrees and increased to end range.

### RESISTED MOTIONS

Abduction and flexion were moderately weak and slightly painful in all positions. External rotation was moderately weak and slightly painful. Internal rotation was slightly weak but moderately painful. Abductors, flexors, and external rotators were graded as 4−/5. Internal rotators were graded as 4/5. All other musculature was graded as 5/5.

**SPECIAL TESTS**

Multiangle impingement sign painful throughout. Resisted abduction/internal rotation was painful and weak. Positive speed test but not for anterior (biceps) pain. Relocation test significantly reduced pain until overpressure was applied into external rotation. Less pain noted with reverse impingement sign. Horizontal adduction reproduced subacromial pain.

**STABILITY AND JOINT GLIDE ASSESSMENT**

No instability; joint glide decreased in all directions.

**PASSIVE SHOULDER MOTION**

Glenohumeral abduction: 0–80 degrees
Flexion scapulohumeral (S-H): 0–120 degrees
Abduction (coronal) (S-H): 0–100 degrees
Abduction (POS) (S-H): 0–130 degrees
External rotation at neutral: 0–35 degrees
External rotation at 80 degrees (coronal): 0–30 degrees
External rotation at 80 degrees (POS): 0–65 degrees
Internal rotation at 80 degrees: 0–30 degrees

Pain was experienced before end range was felt, demonstrated by fast and slow muscle guarding. With gentle stretching, a capsular end feel was appreciated.

**PALPATION**

Tenderness over the supraspinatus insertion and biceps tendon

**REFLEXES**

Reactive and symmetrical

**SENSATION**

Normal

## ASSESSMENT AND RATIONALE

Patient presented with significant limitations in all planes of motion yet had signs and symptoms consistent with rotator cuff pathology. The following discussion will relate clinical findings to the literature, clinician anecdotal experience, and differentiating between a rotator cuff tear and true adhesive capsulitis.

The patient had a somewhat unusual presentation for adhesive capsulitis, since his external rotation motion at 0 degrees was greater than at the elevated position of 80 degrees. Also, his external rotation motion at 80 degrees in the POS was 35 degrees greater compared with the coronal plane external rotation. A 30 degree difference can sometimes be appreciated between the two planes because of the decreased twisting of the CLC when in the POS, but the end feels and pain experienced between the two planes were significantly different in this individual. Pain along with fast and slow muscle guarding was present at all end ranges, although a capsular end feel was felt to be present 5 to 10 degrees further into the range; this demonstrated moderate reactivity. Pain and fast muscle guarding were significantly less in POS external rotation end range, even with overpressure.

Resisted motions revealed pain and weakness in abduction, flexion, external rotation and internal rotation. In stage I, adhesive capsulitis pain with resisted motions can be experienced because of the capsule's intimate relationship with the rotator cuff tendons (extrapolated from Clark[2]). When the CLC and synovium are inflamed, tension created by the cuff muscles during a contraction pull on the inflamed tissue causing pain. Certainly a rotator cuff (i.e., supraspinatus) lesion could cause pain during resisted motions, as seen in this patient, because of the force translation through the lesion and due to the supraspinatus tendon's fiber interlacing to the infraspinatus and subscapularis.[1] In the presence of rotator cuff tedonopathy, the degree of weakness and pain will depend on the extent of the lesion (i.e., tendinitis versus full-thickness tear), size of the tear, and reactivity. Typically, weakness is not associated with true adhesive capsulitis.

Although the patient presented with a positive impingement sign, it is of little value in differentiating between adhesive capsulitis and a rotator cuff lesion, since pain can be elicited in both cases due to the position. The CLC is stretched, and the subacromial tissue is compressed.[9] He did have a positive relocation test, which we have found positive in many patients with rotator cuff lesions without instability. The mechanism was probably due to the irritated portion of the rotator cuff–bursae complex being reoriented to the coracoacromial arch, relieving compression and reducing pain. Rotator cuff impingement against the posterior glenoid rim occurs at end-range external rotation when performed at 90 degrees of coronal plane abduction. Therefore, posterior humeral displacement during the relocation test relieves the impingement.[12] This mechanism also could explain the difference in pain and range of motion found between external rotation in the POS and coronal plane. External rotation in 90 degrees of POS abduction does not engage the supraspinatus against the posterior glenoid rim.

These findings were not consistent with true adhesive capsulitis for the following reasons: (1) Typically, a greater loss of motion is seen in external rotation at 0 degrees compared with external rotation in elevation in a patient with adhesive capsulitis; (2) the significant relief of pain obtained with the subacromial injection, although we do acknowledge pain relief can be gained with a subacromial injection in true adhesive capsulitis; (3) the degree of muscle weakness was not consistent with adhesive capsulitis; (4) an identified falling incident consistent with rotator cuff pathology; (5) a positive relocation test. For these reasons, the patient was felt to have a rotator cuff lesion, probably a partial- of small full-thickness cuff tear with secondary capsulitis.

## TREATMENT AND RATIONALE

| Treatment | Rationale |
|---|---|
| **Sessions 1–3** | |
| Patient was treated with hot pack to shoulder while supine, arm at 45 degrees of POS abduction. He was instructed to perform 30-s stretches into a *slightly* painful external rotation range for 10 minutes (Fig. 11-5). Treated with phonophoresis using 10% hydrocortisone alternating with ice massage in a 5, 2, 3, and 2 minute time sequence. Grade I and II glides were performed in all directions in the loose-pack position (LPP). Ice for 15 minutes while riding bike. | Heat and prolonged stretch have been shown to be more effective than either alone.[8] Stretching in 45 degrees in the POS reduces twisting on CLC and rotator cuff[6] yet still allows tissue elongation. Anti-inflammatory and vasodilitation achieved with phonophoresis and ice. Mobilization performed for neurophysiologic effect relieves pain.[7] |
| **Sessions 4–7** | |
| Patient continued to do well, he reported relief of pain and demonstrated increased motion. Resisted motions were only slightly weak, but resisted internal rotation was most painful when performed at neutral; resisted abduction/internal rotation was weak and painful at both 90 and 45 degrees, with 90 degrees more symptomatic. Continued with modalities, began transverse friction massage (TFM) over the supraspinatus. Patient continued to show favorable response with introduction of TFM, so began pain-free isometrics in all directions. Progressed joint mobilization to grade III and IV, moving from the LPP to end ranges. | Symptom from contractile lesion appeared to be resolving. Since reactivity was reduced, TFM was started to possibly assist in making scar more pliable.[3] Isometrics to strengthen. Mobilization intensified to stretch tight CLC. |
| **Sessions 8–10** | |
| ROM still improving; passive flexion was 0–150 degrees, abduction (POS) was 0–155 degrees, external rotation at 90 degrees was 0–55 degrees, external rotation at 0 degrees was 0–55 degrees, internal rotation was 0–45 degrees and functional internal rotation to L3. Resisted motions were strong and painless. Resisted abduction/internal rotation was slightly painful with eccentric load. Relocation test and impingement sign were positive.<br>Although patient was improving, he still had some fast muscle guarding at end ranges and was beginning to have more night pain. Therapist/physician discussion was in agreement that a second injection would be helpful. This was performed after session 8.<br>Following injection, patient demonstrated a significant reduction in pain at end range and at night. Began rhythmic stabilization at 45 degrees POS; then began elastic band exercises for the rotator cuff and deltoid. | Eccentric loading of muscle has greater sensitivity when assessing contractile lesions. Patient was improving, however was demonstrating increased reactivity at end range. We thought that a second injection would further quell residual inflammation. Progressed resistance exercise as tolerated with emphasis on scapular muscle integration into all exercise. |
| **Sessions 11–18** | |
| Discontinued phonophoresis after 10 sessions; continued grade IV mobilizations in all directions combined with prolonged stretching (Fig. 11-6). Used relocation test positioning (posterior glide while stretching into external rotation at 90 degrees) to regain motion. Began manual resistance for rotators and biceps/triceps. Progressed to PNF D1/D2 | Inflammation significantly reduced after second injection, so phonophoresis terminated. Emphasis on ROM using mobilization and stretch. Relocation position reduced rotator cuff and CLC irritation but allowed stretching of anterior/inferior CLC. Strengthening gradually progressed in range and resistance. |

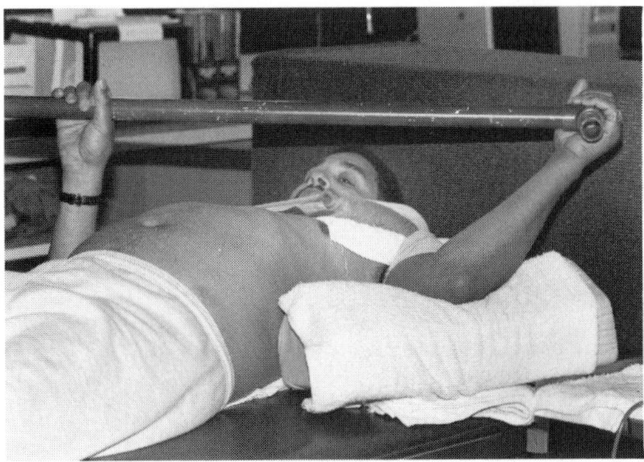

**Figure 11-5.** Passive stretching into external rotation.

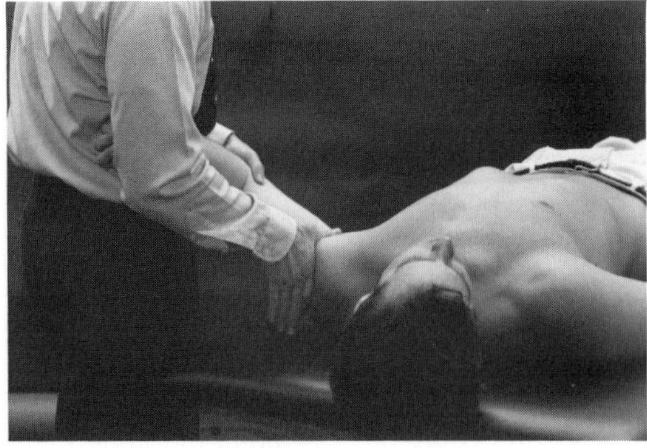

**Figure 11-6.** End-range mobilization performing inferior glide in 90 degrees of POS abduction and external rotation.

patterns up to 90 degrees → endrange and submax → max. Patient pain free in all resisted exercise.

**Session 19**

Assessment revealed functional elevation with slight scapular and trunk substitution to 170 degrees. Passively, flexion was 0–150 degrees, abduction (coronal) was 0–120 degrees, abduction (POS) was 0–150 degrees, external rotation at 90 degrees was 0–70 degrees, external rotation at 90 degrees in POS was 0–90 degrees, external rotation at 0 degrees was 0–75 degrees, internal rotation was 0–55 degrees, and functional internal rotation was to T10. External rotation end range was slightly painful, and all had capsular end feels. Resisted motions were strong and painless, although very slight weakness could be felt of the external rotators compared with the uninvolved side. Although full range was not achieved, the patient was released and asked to return in 4 weeks.

ROM significantly improved with capsular end feels at end range. Although range not full, he was motivated and independent in his home program. His rotator cuff was no longer reactive, so it was felt that time, remodeling of collagen, and continued stretching would result in the continued return of motion.

**Session 20**

Patient missed 4-week follow-up and returned 8 weeks from session 19. He presented with passive flexion of 0–165 degrees, abduction (coronal) was 0–145 degrees abduction (POS) was 0–165 degrees, external rotation at 90 degrees was 0–85 degrees. These ranges were within 5 degrees of the uninvolved side. All resisted motions were strong and painless, even external rotation. Resisted abduction/internal rotation at 90 degrees was painless but was slightly weaker than the other side. Impingement sign was negative.

Over the 8 weeks, the patient was "fairly" consistent with ROM exercises and showed a significant return of motion. We feel that in most individuals treated for a restricted CLC once (1) proper biomechanics have been initiated, (2) reactivity has significantly reduced, and (3) they are independent with their program, they can be released for several weeks and reevaluated. If significant progress has been made, they can be discharged with the belief they will continue to regain motion.

# Case 3

## 21-Year-Old Student Right Hand Dominant

### HISTORY

The patient was seen 4 weeks after right shoulder anterior capsular shift. The patient reported initially "popping his shoulder out" 5 years previously while reaching up for a pass when playing basketball. He rolled on the ground and reported that it "popped back in without much discomfort." He experienced several subluxation episodes over the subsequent 3 years but then had a traumatic event while playing recreational rugby 2 years ago. Apparently, while his arm was in a position of abduction and external rotation, someone landed on the posterior aspect of his shoulder. Following this, the shoulder had to be reduced in the emergency room, and the patient was told that he anteriorly dislocated the shoulder (subcoracoid). He did report one unstable episode on his other side. He received physical therapy consisting of strengthening exercises for 2 months following the traumatic event 2 years ago. Over the next 2 years, he experienced multiple (>15) subluxation episodes and had to significantly limit his recreational activities. His most recent event occurred while turning in bed. Although he reported feeling stronger, subluxations continued when the arm was placed in abduction and external rotation. He had seen several orthopedic surgeons over the years, and a Bristow procedure had been recommended. Recent x-rays revealed a small Hill-Sachs defect and slight erosion of the anterior glenoid. Because of continued instability and restricted activities, he decided to have surgery. The surgical notes described an extremely patulous capsule without a true Bankart lesion, although the anterior labrum was significantly frayed. He had remained in the sling since surgery but began pendulum exercises and external rotation stretching to neutral in 45 degrees of POS abduction 2 weeks prior to entering physical therapy.

## EVALUATION

### OBSERVATION IN STANDING

No significant postural faults noted, although slight atrophy to the shoulder girdle musculature was noted and significant atrophy of the anterior deltoid.

### CERVICAL ROM

Within normal limits and painless

### ACTIVE SHOULDER MOTION

Elevation was to 90 degrees with scapular substitution.

### RESISTED MOTIONS

1+/5 strength was noted of the anterior deltoid, but the middle and posterior heads were firing well. Grossly, strength was graded as 3+ to 4/5 for other shoulder muscles. Elbow, wrist, and hand muscle strength was 4+/5.

### SPECIAL TESTS

Most special tests were deferred at 4 weeks postoperatively. Patient had negative Tinel's sign at the thoracic outlet, medial arm, elbow, and wrist. Negative Adson maneuver.

### STABILITY AND JOINT GLIDE ASSESSMENT

Anterior and posterior glides assessed and found to be restricted, although assessment was difficult due to apprehension.

### PASSIVE ROM

Glenohumeral abduction: 0–80 degrees
Flexion (S-H): 0–95 degrees
Abduction (S-H): 0–85 degrees
External rotation at neutral: 0 degrees
External rotation at 85 degrees: 0–20 degrees
Internal rotation at 85 degrees: 0–25 degrees
Horizontal adduction: 0–80 degrees

### PALPATION

No significant findings

### REFLEXES

Reactive and symmetrical

### SENSATION

Normal

## ASSESSMENT AND RATIONALE

Patient provided a history consistent with underlying multidirectional instability and subsequent traumatic anterior dislocation. The traumatic episode resulted in further stretching of an already hyperelastic capsuloligamentous complex (CLC). The postoperative examination revealed significant atrophy and weakness (graded 1+/5) of the anterior deltoid. This finding was consistent with an iatrogenically induced neurapraxia of the axillary nerve branch supplying the anterior deltoid. This occasionally occurs following surgery due to prolonged retraction of the anterior deltoid in an attempt to gain exposure of the CLC. Range-of-motion restrictions were characteristic following this type of procedure. The end ranges were painful, and both fast and slow muscle guarding was noted. After gentle stretching at end range, a capsular end feel could be appreciated at all end ranges. Even though the surgeon "fixed" the shoulder in 30 degrees of external rotation, the patient presented with external rotation to neutral in adduction. A major reason for this type of limitation was positioning the arm into internal rotation (sling) following surgery. Although the suture lines need to be protected, we question whether this idiopathic contracture is necessary. Possibly it should be promoted in certain patients (i.e., revision capsular shift). A "gunslinger brace" or earlier and frequent positioning to neutral is more appropriate.

The clinician need only refer to previously recommended postoperative immobilization and positioning for ACL reconstructions, all in the name of protecting the fixation.

# TREATMENT AND RATIONALE

| Treatment | Rationale |
| --- | --- |
| **Session 1**<br>Began with moist heat for 10 minutes, performing 15-s intermittent stretching into external rotation at 45 degrees of POS abduction. Grade I and II joint mobilizations were performed in all directions Began submaximal (50–75 percent) isometrics for the shoulder external rotators, extensors, elbow flexors, and extensors. All resisted exercises were painless. Home program stretching continued but added supine AAROM flexion to 90 degrees and external rotation performed at 15 degrees of abduction. Patient seen two times a week for 2 weeks. | POS is the plane in which the least amount of tension is placed across the CLC[6] and the anterior shear force is reduced. Therefore, less tension is placed across the suture line, and there is less chance of promoting suture line disruption or subluxation. Heat and stretch are performed together to maximize effect. Began mobilizations to reduce pain and promote neurophysiologic relaxation. Isometrics for strength but not internal rotation, since the subscapularis was incised and sutured during surgery. |
| **Sessions 2–5**<br>Began scapular PNF with emphasis on the middle and lower trapezius. Continued as above; on session 4 began manual resistance for the glenohumeral rotators at 45 degrees POS. Performed rhythmic stabilization and progressed to a short arc (submaximally). Patient tolerated well, so began on Theraband in all directions. Began to see slight increased recruitment of anterior deltoid fibers. | Patient only seen two times a week, since much of work could be performed at home, and adequate time still needed to allow healing, particularly since he demonstrated significant hyperelasticity. Manual resistance was tolerated well; this hands-on approach provides constant feedback about pain and ability to resist. |
| **Sessions 6–11**<br>Began to see three times weekly. Continued with joint mobilization, progressing to grade III and IV. More attention placed on posterior CLC due to tightness (Fig. 11-7). Progressed range of manual resistance for rotators and POS abduction to 90 degrees and progressed to end range. Began D1/D2 patterns to 90 degrees submax → max with emphasis on D1 for anterior deltoid recruitment. Neurapraxia was resolving. Began Bodyblade. Began standing UBE at low resistance at session 9. | Began three times due to more aggressive mobilization and strengthening required. Although he was hyperelastic, he demonstrated significant tightness of all regions of the CLC. Posterior aspect tightness was impressive. Continued resistance work in the POS, since the supraspinatus is at a biomechanical advantage.[5,6] As tolerated, moved out of the POS for stretching and strengthening. Utilized position-dependent nature of the CLC.[10,11] Began endurance work on UBE. |
| **Sessions 12–20**<br>PROM at session 12: glenohumeral abduction was 0–85 degrees, flexion was 0–140 degrees, external rotation at 90 degrees (coronal) was 0–45 degrees, external rotation at 90 degrees (POS) was 0–65 degrees, external rotation at 0 degrees was 0–25 degrees, internal rotation at 90 degrees was 0–25 degrees, horizontal adduction (HA) was 0–95 degrees. More emphasis placed on stretching at home in all directions. Resisted motions were strong and painless, strength was graded as 4/5. Anterior deltoid continued to return. | ROM improving, although still fairly tight in external rotation and internal rotation. More aggressive stretching begun. We feel the therapist has an incredible effect on "dialing in" the limitations or lack of them in these patients. With constant monitoring of range and end feels individualization is achieved. At 3 months postoperatively, his end feel began to change, so stretching was reduced but continued with aggressive strengthening, which was well tolerated. Resistance and range were progressed slowly. |

A

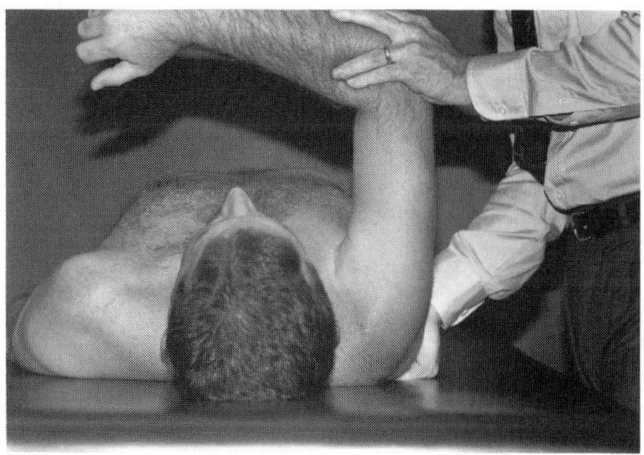

B

**Figure 11-7.** Assessing posterior capsule tightness. (a) Normal horizontal adduction. (b) Significant tightness.

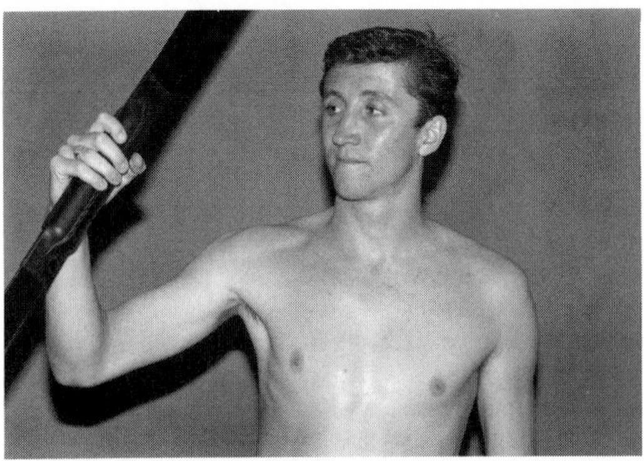

**Figure 11-8.** Bodyblade exercise performed at approximately 60 degrees of elevation in the plane of the scapula.

Grade IV mobilization continued in all directions. Manual resistance to full range and maximal force. Progressed to variable-resistance machines for biceps/triceps, rower, pull-downs (90 degrees → full). Continue to progress time and resistance on UBE, progressed Bodyblade to elevated positions (Fig. 11-8), wall ball, and rowing ergometer. Progressed to isokinetics at 20 degrees of abduction in the POS, 90 degrees/s, submaximally. By session 19, flexion range had improved to 150 degrees, external rotation at 90 degrees was 0–55 degrees and at 0 degrees was 0–40 degrees, internal rotation was 0–35 degrees, and horizontal adduction was 0–105 degrees. Patient made good gains in range and began to demonstrate a more pliable end range. Began to deemphasized stretching.

**Sessions 21–26**

Continued with aggressive strengthening. Progressed isokinetic speeds to 180 degrees/s, performing velocity spectrum training. External rotation range at 90 degrees was 0–65 degrees. Began to stretch more aggressively in all directions.

**Session 27**

Now 4 months postoperatively PROM at glenohumeral abduction was 0–100 degrees, flexion was 0–160 degrees, external rotation at 90 degrees was 0–70 degrees, external rotation at 0 degrees was 0–50 degrees, internal rotation was 40 degrees, and horizontal adduction was 110 degrees. Strength was 5/5. Anterior deltoid was almost symmetrical. Patient discharged with full program of exercise to continue.

Nine months from surgery, the patient was asked to return for reexamination.

| **PROM** | **R** | **L** |
|---|---|---|
| Glenohumeral abduction | 110 | 115 |
| Flexion | 165 | 180 |
| External rotation at 90 degrees | 85 | 110 |
| External rotation at 0 degrees | 65 | 85 |
| Internal rotation | 45 | 65 |
| Horizontal adduction | 120 | 135 |

Although end feels changed, his range was progressing too slowly, so returned to stretching. At 4 months his range was felt to be appropriate. Individuals who possess generalized hyperelasticity, such as this individual, will continue to increase range for at least a full year; thus we expected his ranges to improve. Our goal with this individual was to maintain some limitation of range of 10 to 20 degrees in all planes, compared with the other side, at the end of a year, not at the time of discharge. As seen with his 9-month measurement, he looked on target. He was extremely pleased with his function and was without limitation other than hard throwing.

Strength was 5/5 with complete recovery of the anterior deltoid.

We feel that these patients can and should be moved sooner in their rehabilitation. Caution is required in those patients who demonstrate "pathologic" hyperelastic tissue. We have had good success with this type of approach without instability recurring. The key is to individualize the treatment.

# Case 4

## 55-Year-Old Train Mechanic Right Hand Dominant

### HISTORY

This patient was seen for an evaluation 8 weeks after right shoulder open rotator cuff repair and acromioplasty. He reported injuring the shoulder at work 9 months previously when a lever he was trying to turn broke, causing his arm to forcefully jerk into flexion and horizontal adduction. He did have a history of several painful incidences over the preceding 3 years, precipitated by aggressive overhead work. He was seen in occupational health and was told that he had "separated his shoulder." He reported significant discomfort, which was treated with anti-inflammatories. He had been injected twice in 3 months following the injury and experienced good immediate relief with the first injection, but symptoms returned over the subsequent 3 weeks. The second injection was less effective. Approximately 1 month following the incident he was sent to physical therapy. He was placed on an AAROM program and resistive exercises using elastic bands. He was instructed in and told to continue with the "scaption" exercise, even though it was "really painful." He also was placed on the upper body ergometer in a sitting position but after three to four sessions had to stop because of pain and weakness. He continued with this type of therapy for 4 months, but because of continued symptoms, he was sent for a second orthopedic consultation. An MRI was performed that demonstrated a full-thickness supraspinatus tear. This finding, in conjunction with a remarkable physical examination, led to surgery. Preoperative physician notes discuss limited elevation to 130 degrees and external rotation to 20 degrees. The notes also mention significant atrophy of the spinati. Postoperative care consisted of using a sling for 4 weeks, but pendulums, passive flexion, and passive external rotation were performed at home since day 2. When he was seen by the surgeon at 8 weeks and was to start elastic band exercises, significant strength and range deficits were noted, as well as poor function of the arm. It was at this time the he was sent for formal physical therapy.

The patient's complaints at the time of the physical therapy evaluation were minimal pain at rest, although he still had difficulty sleeping at night due to pain. He felt extremely weak and could not use the arm easily for the activities of daily living secondary to pain and weakness. He was taking no medication at the time. The job he wished to return to required him to lift up to 70 lbs overhead and frequent use of the hand overhead with tools weighing several ounces to 15 lb.

### EVALUATION

#### OBSERVATION IN STANDING

Significant atrophy of the supraspinatus and infraspinatus. Apparent defect of the deltoid at the anterolateral acromion insertion (Fig. 11-9).

#### CERVICAL ROM

Within normal limits and painless

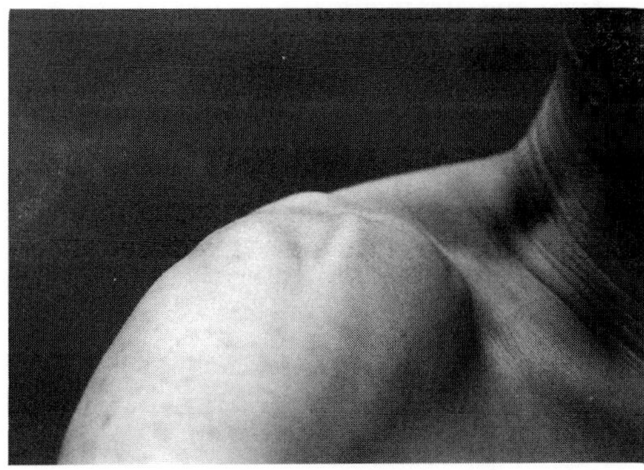

**Figure 11-9.** Defect of anterior deltoid.

## ACTIVE SHOULDER MOTION

Flexion was to 120 degrees, coronal plane abduction to 100 degrees, and POS abduction to 110 degrees. Functional internal rotation to the sacrum. All end ranges were painful, and scapular substitution was noted with elevation.

## RESISTED MOTIONS

Abduction and flexion tests were weak and significantly painful in all positions. External rotation was significantly weak and painful. Internal rotation was slightly painful and strong. All other resisted motions were strong and painless. Strength of the abductors and external rotators was graded as 2+/5 and the internal rotators 4/5. All other musculature of the upper extremity was graded as 4+ to 5/5.

## SPECIAL TESTS

The patient had a positive Neer impingement sign and pain through the full multiangle impingement sign. Resisted abduction/internal rotation was weak and painful at 90 and 45 degrees. Subacromial pain was present with passive horizontal adduction.

## STABILITY AND JOINT GLIDE ASSESSMENT

Joint glide was moderately reduced in all directions.

## PASSIVE SHOULDER MOTION

Glenohumeral abduction: 0–90 degrees
Flexion (S-H): 0–125 degrees
Abduction (S-H): 0–110 degrees
External rotation at neutral: 0–35 degrees
External rotation at 90°: 0–60 degrees
Internal rotation at 90°: 0–40 degrees

All end ranges were painful, and a "hard" capsular end feel was felt.

## PALPATION

Tenderness of the supraspinatus insertion

## REFLEXES

Reactive and symmetrical

## SENSATION

Normal

# ASSESSMENT AND RATIONALE

The patient presented with significant range-of-motion restrictions in all planes, reduced glides, and established firm capsular end feels. Pain was present at all end ranges. He had significant atrophy of the infraspinatus and supraspinatus in conjunction with significant weakness. There appeared to be a defect in the deltoid as it inserted into the anterolateral acromion. This defect was at the septum of the anterior and middle deltoid. An open procedure had been performed taking down the anterior deltoid and splitting the deltoid at the septum. It was difficult to say how badly the deltoid attachment had been compromised, since normal scar tissue sometimes gives this altered appearance following this approach. Also, the patient had a very defined deltoid bilaterally and demonstrated a deep septum on the uninvolved side.

The clinician needs to consider the preoperative history when assessing these postoperative findings. It was clear that the correct diagnosis and care were delayed, as well as inappropriate therapy provided preoperatively. Preoperatively he had obvious motion restrictions, yet no mobilizations or even focused stretching was done; he had obvious signs of cuff irritation yet was instructed to continue with the internal rotation "scaption" exercises, which excessively challenged his cuff as well as caused repetitive mechanical irritation. Lastly, therapy was blindly continued without reassessing progress.

The pain and restricted motion did not appear to be active capsulitis in nature but seemed to be related to poor subacromial gliding and established contracture of the rotator cuff and CLC. Although a noticeable strength deficit is expected in an uncomplicated rotator cuff repair at 8 weeks, this individual's weakness was excessive. The limited motion and weakness in this individual correlated directly with preoperative motion and strength deficits. A general rule of thumb is that the ROM expected postoperatively is equal to that seen preoperatively.[4] This is why it is prudent to maximize ROM and strength before surgery. A delay in entering this patient into therapy postoperatively, especially in light of his previous ROM restrictions, also perpetuated and/or produced the ROM and strength problems. The patient was seen three times weekly.

# TREATMENT AND RATIONALE

| Treatment | Rationale |
|---|---|
| **Sessions 1–9**<br>Began with moist heat for 10 minutes, performing 15-s intermittent stretching into external rotation at 45 degrees of POS abduction. Grade II and III mobilizations were performed in all directions. As pain decreased, mobilizations were increased to grade IV, and more aggressive prolonged stretching in all directions was performed. Home program emphasized prolonged stretching of 60 to 90 seconds. Also, had patient begin using pulley to assist with elevation stretches. He was taken off of all strengthening exercises except for the biceps and triceps until the fourth session. Evaluation at session 4 revealed a significant reduction of pain with resisted motions, although weakness persisted. Scapular PNF was performed after first session. Began rhythmic stabilization in 45 degrees of POS abduction. Progressed to free weights for external rotation (using bolster), flexors, abductors (in POS), and extensors. Patient was having slight discomfort, particularly with external rotation. Continued to use elastic bands for internal rotation. Progressed to manual resistance for the rotators and abductors in the POS. | Heat and stretching performed together in POS. Mobilizations done for pain relief and then progressed for stretching effect.[7] All rotator cuff strengthening exercises discontinued until pain and reactivity reduced and then progressed to free weights (1 to 3lb) and Theraband for strengthening. Scapular PNF was performed without pain and progressed to pain-free rotator cuff and deltoid strengthening using the advantageous properties of the scapular plane. Bolster was used during isotonic program to reduce tension of the rotator cuff. |
| **Sessions 10–20**<br>Patient was making steady gains in ROM. Active elevation was to 150 degrees but with scapular substitution. PROM at session 10: glenohumeral abduction was 0–95 degrees, flexion was 0–140 degrees, external rotation at 90 degrees was 0–65 degrees, external rotation at neutral was 0–40 degrees, internal rotation at 90 degrees was 0–30 degrees, and horizontal adduction was 0–95 degrees. Strength was abductors 3+/5, external rotation 3/5, internal rotation 4/5, and flexors 3+/5. Functional lifting revealed he could lift 20 lb into elevation to 90 degrees on the left compared with 3lb on the right. This roughly computes to 40 and 6ft · lb (moment arm distance from humeral head to weight was about 2 ft) left and right, respectively. This equals an 85 percent deficit. Patient's deltoid demonstrated significant hypertrophy with only slight gains in supraspinatus and infraspinatus mass. The deltoid was contracting almost exclusively without assistance from the pectoralis major. Began strengthening clavicular head of pectoralis major and encouraged recruitment during elevation. Continued with aggressive stretching and strengthening.<br>At session 18 isometric testing of external rotation and internal rotation strength revealed 21 and 8 ft · lb for the external rotation, left and right, respectively. Internal rotation was 32 and 22ft · lb for the left and right, respectively. This computed to a 62 percent external rotation deficit and a 32 percent internal rotation deficit. Abductor strength was 38 and 12ft · lb, left and right, respectively, which was a 69 percent deficit. Amazingly, the patient was reporting no pain and no difficulty with the activities of daily living other than significant fatigue when maintaining the arm above shoulder level. | Continued to emphasize ROM and restoration of CLC pliability by joint mobilization and stretching. Position dependency idea of the CLC was utilized to maximize stretching effect. Although strength was improving, significant strength deficits remained despite deltoid hypertrophy. The poor return of the spinati was probably due to the extent of atrophy preoperatively. Fatigue was a major complaint, so recruitment was encouraged from the clavicular head of pectoral to assist in elevation. It has been found that secondary muscles will change function or increase activity when deficits exist. Isometric testing during session 18 was performed on LIDO Active. |
| **Sessions 21–30**<br>ROM continued to improve with prolonged stretching and position-dependent mobilization. Continued with manual resistance in POS and progressed to D1 upper extremity | Had attempted PNF patterns previously, but they caused increased symptoms. Modifications were made during this stage, which he tolerated, resulting in continued gains. |

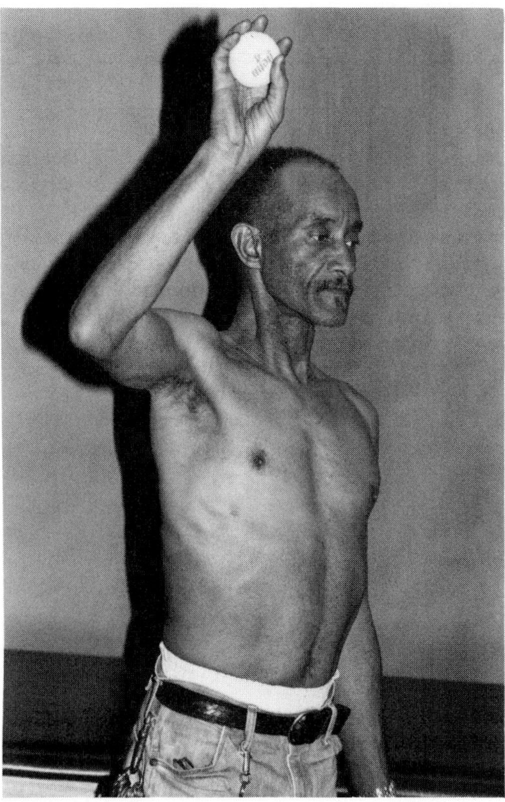

**Figure 11-10.** Wall ball exercise.

pattern to 90 degrees submaximally. Patient demonstrated biceps irritation, so modified resistance. Began use of Bodyblade in slight abduction (15 degrees) and progressed to 45 degrees. Began work-simulated activities up to 90 degrees.

Bodyblade allows excellent "stabilization" strengthening for the rotator cuff.

**Sessions 31–40**

Emphasized strengthening at elevation end range since fatigue was still a problem. Began wall ball (Fig. 11-10), upper body ergometer in standing, Bodyblade to 90 degrees, and manual resistance isolating end-range elevation. Work-simulated activities were performed above shoulder level, although ergonomic modification was still encouraged. Surprisingly, the patient eventually made excellent endurance gains above 90 degrees despite significant visible atrophy of the spinati. Patient was able to return to work as train mechanic without need for further treatment.

End-range strength and endurance were encouraged, since this was necessary for occupational demands. This patient had an unexpectedly excellent result in part because of his high motivation level and diligence with the home program.

# References


1. Clark JC and Harryman DT. Tendons, ligaments, and capsule of the rotator cuff. J Bone Joint Surg 1992;74A:713–733.
2. Clark JC, Sidles JR, and Matzen FA, III. The relationship of the glenohumeral joint capsule to the rotator cuff. Clin Orthop 1990; 254:29.
3. Cyriax J. Diagnosis of soft tissue lesions. In: Textbook of orthopaedic medicine. 8th Ed. Vol. 1. Baltimore MD: Williams & Wilkins, 1970.
4. Ellman H, Hanker G, and Bayer M. Repair of the rotator cuff: end-result study of factors influencing reconstruction. J Bone Joint Surg 1986;68A(8):1136.
5. Jobe FW, Moynes DR. Delineation of diagnostic criteria and a rehabilitation program for rotator cuff injures. Am J Sports Med 1982;10(6):336–339.
6. Johnston TB. The movements of the shoulder joint. A plea for the use of the "plane of the scapula" as the plane of reference in movements occurring at the humero-scapular joint. Br J Surg 1937;25:252.
7. Maitland GD. Peripheral manipulation. 3rd ed. London, England: Butterworth & Co., 1991.

8. Sapega AA, Quedenfeld TC, Moyer RA, et al. Biophysical factors in range-of-motion exercises. Phys Sports Med 1981;9:57.
9. Speer KP, Hannafin JA, Altchek DW, et al. An evaluation of the shoulder relocation test. J Should and Elbow Surg 1994;22:177.
10. Terry GC, Hammon D, France P, Norwood LA. The stabilizing function of the passive shoulder restraints. Am J Sports Med 1991;19:26–34.
11. Turkel SJ, Panio MW, Marshal JL. Stabilizing mechanism preventing anterior dislocation of the glenohumeral joint. J Bone Joint Surg 1981;63A:1208.
12. Walch G, Boileau P, Noel E, Donell T. Impingement of the deep surface of the supraspinatus tendon on the posterior glenoid rim: an arthroscopic study. J Should and Elbow Surg 1992;1:239.

# Index